OXFORD MEDICAL PUBLICATIONS

Clinical Paediatric Nephrology

Clinical Paediatric Nephrology
3rd Edition

Edited by

NICHOLAS J.A. WEBB DM FRCP FRCPCH
Consultant Paediatric Nephrologist,
Department of Paediatric Nephrology,
Royal Manchester Children's Hospital,
Pendlebury, Manchester M27 4HA, UK

and

ROBERT J. POSTLETHWAITE FRCP FRCPCH
Consultant Paediatric Nephrologist,
Department of Paediatric Nephrology,
Royal Manchester Children's Hospital,
Pendlebury, Manchester M27 4HA, UK

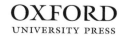

OXFORD
UNIVERSITY PRESS

OXFORD

UNIVERSITY PRESS

Great Clarendon Street, Oxford OX2 6DP
Oxford University Press is a department of the University of Oxford.
It furthers the University's objective of excellence in research, scholarship,
and education by publishing worldwide in

Oxford New York

Auckland Cape Town Dar es Salaam Hong Kong Karachi
Kuala Lumpur Madrid Melbourne Mexico City Nairobi
New Delhi Shanghai Taipei Toronto

With offices in

Argentina Austria Brazil Chile Czech Republic France Greece
Guatemala Hungary Italy Japan Poland Portugal Singapore
South Korea Switzerland Thailand Turkey Ukraine Vietnam

Oxford is a registered trade mark of Oxford University Press
in the UK and in certain other countries

Published in the United States
by Oxford University Press Inc., New York

© Oxford University Press 2003

The moral rights of the authors have been asserted

Database right Oxford University Press (maker)

First edition published 1986 by Wright
Second edition published 1994 by Butterworth - Heinemann

This edition first published 2003
Reprinted 2003 (twice, once with corrections), 2005, 2006

A catalogue record for this title is available from the British Library

Library of Congress Cataloging-in-Publication Data
(Data available)

ISBN-13: 978-0-19-263287-6
ISBN-10: 0-19-263287-6

10 9 8 7 6 5

Typeset by Newgen Imaging Systems (P) Ltd., Chennai, India
Printed in Great Britain
on acid-free paper by
Antony Rowe Ltd.,
Chippenham, Wiltshire

Contents

List of contributors

G Michael Addison PhD FRCPath; Consultant Chemical Pathologist, Department of Biochemistry, Royal Manchester Children's Hospital Pendlebury, Manchester M27 4HA, UK

Ellis D. Avner MD; Professor and Chairman of Paediatrics, Department of Pediatrics, Rainbow Babies and Children's Hospital, Case Western Reserve University, Cleveland, Ohio 44106-6003, USA

Eileen M. Baildam FRCP FRCPCH MRCGP; Consultant Paediatric Rheumatologist, Department of Paediatric Rheumatology, Booth Hall Children's Hospital, Manchester M9 7AA, UK

T James Beattie FRCP (Glas) FRCPCH; Consultant Paediatric Nephrologist, Department of Paediatric Nephrology, Royal Hospital for Sick Children, Yorkhill Glasgow G3 8SJ, UK

The late Malgorzata Borzyskowski* FRCP FRCPCH; Consultant Neurodevelopmental Paediatrician, Newcomen Centre, Guys Hospital, London SE1 9RT, UK

Mark G. Bradbury MRCP MRCPCH; Consultant Paediatric Nephrologist, Department of Paediatric Nephrology, Royal Manchester Children's Hospital, Pendlebury, Manchester M27 4HA, UK

Paul A. Brogan BSc(Hon) MRCP MSc; Clinical Research Fellow and Specialist Registrar in Paediatric Nephrology, Great Ormond St Hospital for Children and Institute of Child Health, London WC1N 1EH, UK

Helen Carty FRCR FRCPI FRCP FRCPCH FFRRCSI; Professor of Paediatric Radiology, Department of Radiology, Alder Hey Children's Hospital, Liverpool L12 2AP, UK

Imti Choonara MD MRCP FRCPCH; Professor of Child Health, Academic Division of Child Health, University of Nottingham, Derbyshire Children's Hospital, Derby DE22 3NE, UK

Jane E. Connell BMedSci MRCP MRCPCH; Specialist Registrar in Paediatric Medicine, Royal Manchester Children's Hospital, Pendlebury, Manchester M27 4HA, UK

Malcolm Coulthard PhD FRCP FRCPCH; Consultant Paediatric Nephrologist, Department of Paediatric Nephrology, Royal Victoria Infirmary Newcastle upon Tyne, NE1 4LP, UK

Katherine MacRae Dell MD; Assistant Professor of Paediatrics, Department of Pediatrics, Rainbow Babies and Children's Hospital, Case Western Reserve University, Cleveland, Ohio 44106-6003, USA

Alan Dickson BSc FRCS; Consultant Paediatric Urologist, Department of Paediatric Urology, Royal Manchester Children's Hospital Pendlebury, Manchester M27 4HA, UK

Michael J. Dillon FRCP FRCPCH; Professor of Paediatric Nephrology, Department of Paediatric Nephrology, Great Ormond Street Hospital for Children, London WC1N 3JH, UK

Alfred Drukker MD PhD; Past Head of the Division of Paediatric Nephrology, Shaare Zedek Medical Centre, Emeritus Professor of Paediatrics, Hebrew University- Hadassah Medical School, PO Box 8504, Jerusalem 91084, Israel

Allison A. Eddy MD; Professor of Paediatrics, University of Washington, Head, Division of Paediatric Nephrology, Children's Hospital and Regional Medical Center, Seattle 98105, USA

* Dr Borzyskowski sadly died after a long illness during the final stages of production of this book.

D. Mary Eminson FRCPsych FRCPCH; Consultant Child and Adolescent Psychiatrist, Child and Adolescent Mental Health Service, Royal Bolton Hospital, Bolton BL4 0JR, UK

Jonathan H.C. Evans FRCP FRCPCH; Consultant Paediatric Nephrologist, Children and Young Peoples Kidney Unit, Nottingham City Hospital, Nottingham NG5 1PB, UK

M. Khurram Faizan MB BS.; Paediatric Nephrology Fellow, Children's Hospital and Regional Medical Center, University of Washington, Seattle 98105, USA

Margaret M Fitzpatrick MD FRCP FRCPCH; Consultant Paediatric Nephrologist, Department of Paediatric Nephrology, St James's University Hospital Leeds LS9 7TF, UK

David Frank FRCS; Consultant Paediatric Urologist, Department of Paediatric Urology, Bristol Royal Hospital for Sick Children, Bristol BS2 8BJ, UK

Rasheed Gbadegesin MD FMCPaed (Nig); Lecturer and Consultant Paediatrician, College of Medicine University of Ibadan, University College Hospital, Ibadan, Nigeria

Chulananda D.A. Goonasekera MD MRCP DCH PhD MPhil MRCPCH FCARCS (Ire) Consultant Anaesthesiologist and Intensivist, Senior Lecturer and Head, Department of Anaesthesiology, Faculty of Medicine, University of Peradeniya, Sri Lanka

Jean-Pierre Guignard MD; Professor of Paediatric Nephrology, Département médico-chirurgical de Pédiatrie, Centre Hospitalier Universitaire Vaudois, CH-1011 Lausanne, Switzerland

George B Haycock FRCP FRCPCH; Rothschild Professor of Paediatrics, Department of Paediatrics, Guys Hospital, London SE1 9RT, UK

Richard C.L. Holt BSc MRCP MRCPCH; Clinical Research Fellow in Paediatric Nephrology, Manchester Institute of Nephrology and Transplantation, Manchester Royal Infirmary, Manchester M13 9WL, UK

Carol Inward MD MRCP MRCPCH; Clinical Research Fellow, Children's Kidney Centre, University Hospital of Wales, Cardiff CF14 4XW, UK

Caroline Jones MD MRCP MRCPCH; Consultant Paediatric Nephrologist, Department of Paediatric Nephrology, Alder Hey Children's Hospital Liverpool L12 2AP, UK

Bronwyn Kerr FRACP FRCPCH; Consultant Clinical Geneticist, Department of Clinical Genetics, Royal Manchester Children's Hospital, Pendlebury, Manchester M27 4HA, UK

Stephen J. Kerr FRACP FRCPCH; Consultant in Paediatric Intensive Care, Department of Intensive Care Medicine, Alder Hey Children's Hospital, Liverpool L12 2AP, UK

Nine V.A.M. Knoers MD PhD; Consultant in Clinical Genetics, Department of Human Genetics, University Medical Centre Nijmegen, 6500 HB Nijmegen, The Netherlands

Heather Lambert PhD FRCP FRCPCH; Consultant Paediatric Nephrologist, Department of Paediatric Nephrology, Royal Victoria Infirmary, Newcastle upon Tyne NE1 4LP, UK

Malcolm A. Lewis FRCP MRCPCH; Consultant Paediatric Nephrologist, Department of Paediatric Nephrology, Royal Manchester Children's Hospital, Pendlebury, Manchester M27 4HA, UK

Hilary Lloyd FRCPsych; Consultant Child and Adolescent Psychiatrist, Department of Child and Adolescent Psychiatry, Royal Manchester Children's Hospital, Pendlebury, Manchester M27 4HA, UK

David V. Milford DM FRCP FRCPCH; Consultant Paediatric Nephrologist, Department of Nephrology, Birmingham Children's Hospital, Birmingham B4 6NH, UK

Leo A.H. Monnens MD PhD; Professor of Paediatric Nephrology, Departments of Human Genetics, University Medical Centre Nijmegen, 6500 HB Nijmegen, The Netherlands

M Zulf Mughal FRCP FRCPCH; Consultant Paediatrician and Honorary Senior Lecturer in Child Health, Department of Paediatrics and Child Health, St Mary's Hospital, Manchester M13 0JH, UK

Robert J. Postlethwaite FRCP FRCPCH; Consultant Paediatric Nephrologist, Department of Paediatric Nephrology, Royal Manchester Children's Hospital, Pendlebury, Manchester M27 4HA, UK

Susan P A Rigden FRCP MRCPCH; Consultant Paediatric Nephrologist, Department of Paediatrics, Guys Hospital, London SE1 9RT, UK

Alan M. Robson MD FRCP FRCPCH FAAP; Professor of Pediatrics, Louisiana State University Health Sciences Center, Tulane University School of Medicine, Medical Director Children's Hospital, New Orleans, LA 70118, USA

Manoj Shenoy MS DNB MCh-Paed Surg FRCS FRCS-Paed Surg.; Clinical Fellow in Paediatric Urology, Children and Young Peoples Kidney Unit, Nottingham City Hospital, Nottingham NG5 1PB, UK

Jodi M. Smith MD; Acting Assistant Professor of Paediatrics, University of Washington, Division of Paediatric Nephrology, Children's Hospital and Regional Medical Center, Seattle WA 98105, USA

Graham C. Smith MA MRCP FRCPCH; Consultant Paediatric Nephrologist, Children's Kidney Centre, University Hospital of Wales, Cardiff CF14 4XW, UK

Rajendra N Srivastava FRCP; Consultant Paediatric Nephrologist, Indraprastha Apollo Hospitals, Sarita Vikar, New Dehli 110 044, India

Richard S. Trompeter FRCP FRCPCH; Consultant Paediatric Nephrologist, Department of Paediatric Nephrology, Great Ormond Street Hospital for Children, London WC1 3JH, UK

William van't Hoff BSc MD MRCP FRCPCH; Consultant Paediatric Nephrologist, Department of Paediatric Nephrology, Great Ormond Street Hospital for Children, London WC1 3JH, UK

Alan R. Watson FRCP FRCPCH; Consultant Paediatric Nephrologist and Special Senior Lecturer, Children and Young Peoples Kidney Unit Nottingham City Hospital, Nottingham NG5 1PB, UK

Nicholas J.A. Webb DM FRCP FRCPCH; Consultant Paediatric Nephrologist, Department of Paediatric Nephrology, Royal Manchester Children's Hospital, Pendlebury, Manchester M27 4HA, UK

Mark Woodward MD FRCS (Eng); Specialist Registrar in Paediatric Urology, Department of Paediatric Urology, Bristol Royal Hospital for Sick Children, Bristol BS2 8BJ, UK

Neville Wright DMRD FRCR; Consultant Paediatric Radiologist, Department of Paediatric Radiology, Alder Hey Children's Hospital, Liverpool L12 2AP, UK

Abbreviations

AAMI	American Association for the Advancement of Medical Instrumentation
aBMD	areal bone mineral density
ABPM	ambulatory blood pressure monitoring
ACE	angiotensin converting enzyme OR antegrade colonic enema
ACKD	acquired cystic kidney disease
ACR	American College of Rheumatology
ACT	activated clotting time
ACTH	adrenocorticotrophic hormone
ADH	antidiuretic hormone
ADPKD	autosomal dominant polycystic kidney disease
AFP	α-fetoprotein
AGN	acute glomerulonephritis
AGT	alanine-glyoxylate aminotransferase
AME	apparent mineralocorticoid excess
ANA	antinuclear antibody
ANCA	antineutrophil cytoplasmic antibody
ANH	antenatal hydronephrosis
AP	antero-posterior
APSGN	acute post-streptococcal glomerulonephritis
APTT	activated partial thromboplastin time
AQ-2	aquaporin-2
ARB	angiotensin receptor antagonists
ARF	acute renal failure
ARPKD	autosomal recessive polycystic kidney disease
ASOT	antistreptolysin-O titre
ATII	angiotensin II
AT_1	angiotensin-1 receptor
AT_2	angiotensin-2 receptor
ATM	acute transverse myelitis
ATN	acute tubular necrosis
AUS	artificial urinary sphincter
AV	arterio–venous
AVP	arginine vasopressin
BHS	British Hypertension Society
BILAG	British Isles Lupus Assessment Group
BMC	bone mineral content
BOR	branchio–oto–renal (syndrome)
BP	blood pressure
BSA	body surface area
BXO	balanitis xerotica obliterans
CAH	congenital adrenal hyperplasia
CAPD	continuous ambulatory peritoneal dialysis

CaSR	calcium-sensing receptor
CAVH	continuous arterio-venous haemofiltration
CAVHD	continuous arterio-venous haemodialysis
CCF	congestive cardiac failure
CCPD	continuous cycling peritoneal dialysis
CCU	clean-catch urine
CDI	central diabetes insipidus
CES	cat-eye syndrome
CF	cystic fibrosis
cfu	colony forming units
CI	confidence interval
CIC	clean intermittent catheterization
CMV	cytomegalovirus
CNS	central nervous system OR congenital nephrotic syndrome
CRF	chronic renal failure
CsA	ciclosporin A
CSF	cerebrospinal fluid
CSW	cerebral salt wasting
CT	computed tomography
CVVH	continuous veno-venous haemofiltration
CVVHD	continuous veno-venous haemofiltration and dialysis
DDAVP	1-deamino-8-D-arginine vasopressin
DGC	dorsal grey commissure
DI	diabetes insipidus
DIDMOAD	diabetes insipidus and mellitus, optic atrophy and deafness
DKA	diabetic ketoacidosis
DMS	diffuse mesangial sclerosis
DMSA	dimercaptosuccinic acid
DRC	direct radionuclide cystography
DRTA	distal renal tubular acidosis
DSD	detrusor sphincter dyssynergia
DTPA	diethylenetriaminepentaacetic acid
DVSS	dysfunctional voiding symptom score
DXA	dual-energy X-ray absorptiometry
EAR	estimated average requirement
EBV	Epstein–Barr virus
ECF	extracellular fluid
ECG	electrocardiogram
ECMO	extracorporeal membrane oxygenation
EEG	electroencephalogram
EF	ejection fraction
EM	electron microscopy
EMU	early morning urine
ENaC	epithelial sodium channel
ERPF	effective renal plasma flow
ESR	erythrocyte sedimentation rate
ESRD	end stage renal disease
ESRF	end stage renal failure
ESWL	extracorporeal shock-wave lithotripsy
FAH	fumaryl acetoacetase
FBC	full blood count

FE_{Na}	fractional excretion of sodium
FGF-2	fibroblast growth factor-2
FHH	familial hypocalciuric hypercalcaemia
FISH	fluorescence *in situ* hybridization
FRNS	frequently relapsing nephrotic syndrome
FSGS	focal segmental glomerulosclerosis
GAS	group A beta-haemolytic streptococcus
GBM	glomerular basement membrane
GCKD	glomerulocystic kidney disease
GFR	glomerular filtration rate
GH	growth hormone
GI	gastrointestinal
G-6PD	glucose-6-phosphate dehydrogenase
GRA	glucocorticoid remediable hyperaldosteronism
GR/HGD	glyoxalate reductase/D-glycerate dehydrogenase
HBV	hepatitis B virus
HD	haemodialysis
HIV	human immunodeficiency virus
HIVN	human immunodecifiency virus nephropathy
HLA	human leucocyte antigen
11β-HSD	11β-hydroxysteroid dehydrogenase
HSP	Henoch–Schönlein purpura
HSV	herpes simplex virus
HUS	haemolytic uraemic syndrome
HVDRR	hereditary vitamin D-resistant rickets
ICCS	International Children's Continence Society
ICF	intracellular fluid
ICP	intracranial pressure
ICU	intensive care unit
IDDM	insulin-dependent diabetes mellitus
IF	immunofluorescence
INS	infantile nephrotic syndrome
ISF	interstitial fluid
ISKDC	International Study of Kidney Disease in Children
i.u.	international units
i.v.	intravenous(ly)
IVC	inferior vena cava
IVF	*in vitro* fertilization
IVP	intravenous pyelogram
IVU	intravenous urogram
JCA	juvenile chronic arthritis
JN	juvenile nephronophthisis
LM	light microscopy
$β_2M$	$β_2$-microglobulin
MAG3	mercaptoacetyltriglycine
MCD	minimal change disease
MCDK	multicystic dysplastic kidney
MCNS	minimal change nephrotic syndrome
MCU	micturating cystourethrogram
MCUG	micturating cystourethrography
MIBG	metaiodobenzylguanidine

MIDAC	Microalbuminuria In Diabetic Adolescents and Children
MIF	Müllerian inhibitory factor
MN	membranous nephropathy
MPA	microscopic polyangiitis
MPGN	membranoproliferative (mesangiocapillary) glomerulonephritis
MRA	magnetic resonance angiography
MRI	magnetic resonance imaging
MSU	mid-stream urine
NDI	nephrogenic diabetes insipidus
NE	nocturnal enuresis
NIH	National Institutes of Health
NSAIDs	non-steroidal anti-inflammatory drugs
NSHP	neonatal severe hyperparathyroidism
NTBC	2-(2-nitro-4-trifluoromethylbenzoyl)-1,3-cyclohexanedione
$1,25(OH)_2D_3$	1,25-dihydroxyvitamin D_3
25(OH)D	25-hydroxyvitamin D
OI	Osteogenesis imperfecta
ORT	oral rehydration therapy
PA	postero–anterior
PAN	polyarteritis nodosa
PBS	prune belly syndrome
P_{Cr}	plasma creatinine
PCR	polymerase chain reaction
PD	peritoneal dialysis
PDA	patent ductus arteriosus
PDDR	pseudovitamin D-deficiency rickets
PG	prostaglandin
PGD	pre-implantation genetic diagnosis
PH1	primary hyperoxaluria type 1
PHA	pseudohypoaldosteronism
PHP	pseudohypoparathyroidism
P_i	inorganic phosphate
PICU	paediatric intensive care unit
PKD	polycystic kidney disease
PM	primary megaureter
PMC	pontine micturition centre
PMN	polymorphonuclear (leucocytes)
P_{Na}	plasma sodium
PNET	primitive neuro-ectodermal tumour
P_{osm}	plasma osmolality
pQCT	peripheral quantitative computed tomography
PRTA	proximal renal tubular acidosis
PSAGN	post-streptococcal acute glomerulonephritis
PSC	pontine storage centre
PT	proximal tubule
PTH	parathyroid hormone
PTSD	post-traumatic stress disorder
PTT	partial thromboplastin time
PUJ	pelvi-ureteric junction
PUV	posterior urethral valves
QCT	quantitative computed tomography

RBCs	red blood cells
RDA	recommended daily allowance
RFLP	restriction fragment length polymorphism
rhGH	recombinant human growth hormone
rHuEPO	recombinant human erythropoietin
RI	resistive index
RPD	renal pelvic diameter
RPGN	rapidly progressive glomerulonephritis
RRT	renal replacement therapy
RTA	renal tubular acidosis
r-TPA	recombinant tissue-type plasminogen activator
SA	surface area
SAG	serum anion gap
SCBU	special care baby unit
SCIC	self clean intermittent catheterization
SDNS	steroid-dependent nephrotic syndrome
SDS	standard deviation score
SG	specific gravity
SIADH	syndrome of inappropriate ADH secretion
SLE	systemic lupus erythematosus
SLEDAI	Systemic Lupus Erythematosus Disease Activity Index
SPA	suprapubic aspiration
SPECT	single-photon emission computed tomography
SRI	somatostatin receptor imaging
SSCA	single-strand conformational analysis
SSCP	single-strand conformation polymorphism
SSNS	steroid-sensitive nephrotic syndrome
SVD	standard vertex delivery
TBW	total body water
TDM	therapeutic drug monitoring
THAM	trometamol
TIMP-2	tissue inhibitor of matrix metalloproteinase-2
TPN	total parenteral nutrition
TRF	terminal renal failure
TRP	tubular reabsorption of phosphate
TS	tuberous sclerosis
TTKG	transtubular potassium gradient
UAG	urine anion gap
U_{Ca}	urinary calcium
U_{Cl}	urinary chloride
U_{Cr}	urinary creatinine
U_K	urinary potassium
U_{Na}	urinary sodium
U_{osm}	urine osmolality
U_{pH}	urine pH
URA	unilateral renal agenesis
US	ultrasound
USS	ultrasound scan
UTI	urinary tract infection
UTO	urinary tract obstruction
UVB	ultraviolet B

V2	vasopressin type 2
VDDR	vitamin D-dependent rickets type 1
VDR	intranuclear vitamin D receptor
VF	ventricular fibrillation
VMA	vanillylmandelic acid
V2R	vasopressin type 2 receptor
VT	verocytotoxin
VTEC	VT-producing *Escherichia coli*
VUD	video-urodynamic study
VUJ	vesico-ureteric junction
VUR	vesico-ureteric reflux
WBC	white blood cell
XLH	X–linked familial hypophosphataemic rickets

1 | The child with abnormal urinalysis, haematuria and/or proteinuria

David V. Milford and Alan M. Robson

Examination of urine

Urinary abnormalities may be obvious or covert, and may or may not be associated with renal or urological disorders of significant consequence to the child. Although the routine screening of all children for urinary abnormalities has not been demonstrated to be useful, it has been undertaken in Japan [1], and it is increasingly common for urine to be tested in general practice, outpatient and accident and emergency departments even if the presenting illness is not clearly related to the urinary tract. Consequently, increasing numbers of children are referred for investigation of microscopic haematuria or proteinuria, and some of these will be found to have renal disease. Urine testing may be undertaken by visual inspection, dip-testing using impregnated sticks, microscopy of unstained or Gram-stained urine, culture and laboratory analysis for protein and other urinary components.

Visual examination

Visibly bloodstained urine (macroscopic haematuria) may contain only very small amounts of blood, while apparently clear urine may contain significant numbers of red blood cells (microscopic haematuria). Bright-red bloodstaining, with or without clots, is indicative of heavy bleeding and is often associated with renal or urinary tract trauma, although it can occasionally be caused by glomerular disease. Commonly, there is a change to a brown colour as haemoglobin is converted to acid haematin as a result of chemical reaction with urinary acids. It is important to confirm that the visual finding of red urine is as a consequence of haematuria by dipstick analysis, and to distinguish haematuria from haemoglobinuria and myoglobinuria by demonstrating red cells on microscopy. Some drugs (e.g. rifampicin), foods (e.g. beetroot and some food colourings) and inborn errors of metabolism

(e.g. porphyria and alkaptonuria) may also give a red or brown discoloration to the urine, mimicking haematuria. Urate crystals in the urine of infants may cause a pink discoloration to nappies and cause alarm to parents who mistake the appearances for haematuria. Finally, the possibility that the haematuria may be factitious should be considered (Table 1.1).

Blood may be noted at the commencement of micturition, suggesting a urethral cause for the bleeding and requiring cystoscopy to make the diagnosis. Haematuria tends to be noted throughout voiding when there is a renal diagnosis, while terminal haematuria suggests a bladder cause, such as a bladder calculus or, rarely, schistosomiasis. Some paediatric urologists recognize a group of boys who present with terminal haematuria, with or without dysuria, who may have a ragged appearance to the posterior urethra on cystoscopy; these are diagnosed as having non-specific urethritis but the diagnosis does not have the same connotations as in adults and is not associated with a recognized pathogen.

Inspection of the urine may reveal it to be cloudy because of pyuria associated with a urine infection, because of calcium phosphate crystals in cooled urine or, more rarely, gravel composed of calcium salts, uric acid, cystine or struvite.

Table 1.1 Causes of red urine where no haematuria is present

Haemoglobinuria
Myoglobinuria
Drugs, e.g. rifampicin
Foods, e.g. beetroot and food colourings
Inborn errors of metabolism, e.g. porphyria and alkaptonuria
Urate crystals
Factitious haematuria/Münchausen syndrome by proxy

Key points: Examination of urine

- It is important to confirm that red urine is due to haematuria by the demonstration of red blood cells on urine microscopy (Table 1.1).

- Urate crystals in the urine of infants may cause a pink discoloration to nappies.

- Factitious haematuria should be considered in the differential diagnosis.

Dipstick testing of the urine

Urine testing sticks have entered widespread use because of their convenience and their increasing reliability, and it is now common practice to use dipsticks which can test many different urinary components. However, it is important to ensure they are stored in a dry environment in a moisture-proof container to maintain their efficacy, and to adhere to the manufacturer's instructions for their use. The use of an automated reading device ensures the stick is read at the correct time and avoids inter-observer variation while providing a print-out of the results for the medical records.

Blood is detected by the peroxidase-like action of haemoglobin, causing tetramethylbenzidine in the reagent strip to change to a green-blue colour. As little as $150\,\mu g/l$ of free haemoglobin can cause this reaction; consequently, a negative result excludes significant haematuria. Because the degree of haemolysis is variable, it is not possible to correlate reagent pad colour changes with the number of red cells in the urine. Reducing agents such as ascorbic acid reduce the sensitivity of the test and may give a false-negative result, while oxidizing agents give a false-positive result (Table 1.2).

Urinary protein is detected by causing a colour change following binding to tetrabromophenol in the reagent pads. Albumin demonstrates better binding characteristics to the dye than do other proteins, so that dipstick results correlate better with the level of albuminuria than with total proteinuria. Indeed, a negative dipstick test for protein does not exclude the presence in the urine of low concentrations of globulins, haemoglobin, Bence Jones protein, mucoproteins or low molecular weight 'tubular' proteins such as retinol-binding protein. Although a quantitative measure of protein excretion is ascribed to the varying degrees of colour change, these are very approximate and quantification should be undertaken using a laboratory method. The test may be falsely negative if the urine is very dilute: misinterpretation of such a false-negative result can be avoided if any negative dipstick result for protein is viewed with caution in urines with a specific gravity below 1.002, while a concentrated urine may produce a false-positive result, as may very alkaline urine. False-positive tests for protein may also occur in the presence of gross haematuria, pyuria and bacteriuria; as a result of contamination of the urine with antiseptics such as chlorhexidine or benzalkonium, which are the agents most frequently used for skin cleansing when obtaining a clean-catch urine sample; any quaternary ammonium compound, such as a detergent, especially if present in high concentration; and a limited number of drugs, such as phenazopyridine. Oversoaking of the reagent strip or excessive delay in reading the colour change both give false-positive results, highlighting the importance of adhering to the correct technique for dip-testing (Table 1.2). Finally, the concentration of urinary salts modifies the quantitative accuracy of the dipstick.

A confident assessment of urinary protein excretion can only be made by testing urine produced

---

Table 1.2　Causes of misleading dipstick tests for haematuria and proteinuria

False-positive results	False-negative results
Haematuria	
Oxidizing agents	Reducing agents
Proteinuria	
Highly concentrated urine	Very dilute urine
Alkaline urine (pH > 8)	Acid urine (pH 4.5)
Gross haematuria, pyuria, bacteriuria	Non-albumin proteinuria
Dipstick left in urine too long	
Delay in reading dipstick	
Contamination and drugs:	
quaternary ammonium compounds such as	
antiseptics, chlorhexidine or benzalkonium	

while recumbent (e.g. first morning sample) as some individuals excrete protein in the urine while in the upright posture (postural or orthostatic proteinuria). Vigorous exercise and fever may increase urinary protein excretion for non-pathological reasons.

The use of urine dipsticks as a screening test for urinary tract infection is discussed in Chapter 11.

Glucose is detected in urine by a glucose oxidase–peroxidase-linked reaction with a graded colour change. This provides a lower limit of detection of approximately 0.5 mmol/l but may be inhibited by some substances in the urine.

Reagent pads sensitive to pH, ketones, osmolality, bilirubin and urobilinogen are usually included on Multistix® (Ames Company) but are of limited use and provide qualitative rather than quantitative information.

Microscopy

Urine microscopy is easy to do [2] and provides a rapid answer, but is less frequently undertaken because microscopes are not widely available in clinical areas and there is unfamiliarity with the technique. This is compounded by the provision of a microscopy service by microbiology departments and a perception by junior doctors that a laboratory opinion is necessary if the results will determine the therapeutic approach. Fresh, uncentrifuged urine should be examined in a counting chamber (e.g. Fuchs–Rosenthal), although a formal count is not necessary for most clinical situations.

Occasional red cells may be seen in the urine of healthy children, but should not exceed 5 cells/μl [3]. The morphology of the red cells may help identify the origin of bleeding, as dysmorphic cells indicate glomerular bleeding and may be identified by ordinary light microscopy [4], although phase-contrast microscopy is the definitive technique [5,6]. However, few practitioners would allow this examination to determine subsequent management.

Normal children have fewer than 10 white blood cells/μl in a midstream specimen of urine, although neonates can have up to 50 cells/μl. Unstained white blood cells have a granular cytoplasm, which easily distinguishes them from circular red blood cells, which have a bland cytoplasm. Although neutrophils usually predominate, increased numbers of eosinophils may be found in cases of allergic interstitial nephritis.

Epithelial cells may have their origins from tubules, the collecting system, bladder or perineum.

The squamous epithelial cells reported by experienced urine microscopists are large polygonal cells and their presence indicates that the sample may have been contaminated by contact with the perineum or foreskin. Under these circumstances, urine culture often results in a mixed bacterial growth.

Casts are easily broken by centrifugation and so are best seen in unspun urine. They have a cylindrical structure and consist of cellular debris bound by Tamm–Horsfall protein and are classified by the predominant cellular constituent. Erythrocyte casts are pathognomonic of glomerular bleeding and either appear as a clump of red cells with abundant haemoglobin, easily seen on microscopy, or as components of granular casts with disintegrating red cells. White-cell casts have a dense granular appearance and signify glomerular inflammation, and are also best seen in unspun urine. Both these findings support the need for further nephrological investigations. Epithelial-cell casts may be noted in the diuretic phase after acute tubular necrosis. Occasionally, hyaline casts may be noted in children with heavy proteinuria and these may appear waxy if lipid droplets are present.

Bacteria are usually easily seen in unstained urine, although careful examination is required when there are few bacteria present (see Chapter 11). Normal urine contains no bacteria. *Candida* spp. can easily be distinguished from coliforms; it is particularly important to search for hyphae as this suggests invasive fungal infection. Very occasionally, *Schistosoma* spp. may be noted.

Normal urine may contain calcium phosphate and calcium oxalate crystals. Other crystals arise from urinary cystine, uric acid and dihydroxyadenine, and each has a characteristic appearance.

Key points: Urine microscopy

- The morphology of red blood cells may help identify the origin of bleeding: dysmorphic cells indicate glomerular bleeding.

- Red-cell casts are pathognomonic of glomerular bleeding.

- White-cell casts signify glomerular inflammation.

- Bacteria are easily seen in unstained urine.

- Normal urine may contain calcium phosphate and calcium oxalate crystals.

Haematuria

Haematuria is a common presenting symptom of renal and urinary tract disorders, although population screening has revealed a 0.5–1.6% prevalence of asymptomatic microscopic haematuria in school-children [3,7]. Haematuria may or may not indicate serious underlying disease and it is therefore important to confirm the presence of haematuria and to document its severity and persistence. While the management of the child with haematuria and proteinuria or impaired renal function is not contentious, management of the child with isolated haematuria is the subject of continuing debate.

Children may present in various ways: as a result of an episode of macroscopic haematuria; as a result of urinary tract or other symptoms and the incidental finding of microscopic haematuria; as an incidental finding during routine urinalysis; or as a result of family screening after the identification of an index case. The mode of presentation has implications for the most likely diagnosis.

When eliciting a history, note should be made of generalized symptoms such as fever, lethargy, abdominal pain, oedema or urinary tract-specific symptoms such as dysuria, recurrence of bedwetting or frequency of micturition, which would suggest a urinary tract infection. Colicky loin pain preceding the onset of haematuria is suggestive of a renal or ureteric calculus and, in some instances, it may be possible to confirm the occasional passage of gravel in the urine. A history of a sore throat 10–14 days (or infective skin lesions 4–6 weeks) prior to the onset of haematuria is suggestive of a post-streptococcal nephritis, although other organisms may cause a similar illness (see Chapter 20). Particular note should be taken of any history of skin rashes, especially if the features were suggestive of a facial butterfly rash or if the rash was on sun-exposed areas, as in systemic lupus erythematosus, or if it had a purpuric characteristic as in Henoch–Schönlein purpura (see Chapter 21).

In considering the past medical history, specific enquiry should be made of any symptoms suggestive of arthritis. Although haematuria is a very unusual mode of presentation for a child with a coagulopathy, a history of easy bruising and delayed haemostasis may be relevant and will require investigation. A past history of trauma to the back may also be relevant, especially if the kidneys were known to have been involved.

A detailed family history is essential in the assessment of any child with haematuria, especially if first-degree relatives are known to have haematuria or renal impairment. Deafness and renal failure in male relatives is especially relevant and points to a possible diagnosis of Alport syndrome. A family history of autosomal dominant polycystic kidney disease is similarly relevant.

Physical examination is rarely useful in identifying the cause of haematuria, although the abdomen should be examined for renal enlargement, and the genitalia to exclude local trauma. Examination of the skin may identify a rash, and examination of the joints may provide evidence of an arthritis.

Macroscopic haematuria

Macroscopic haematuria is very uncommon in an unselected population of children, and has been reported to have an incidence of less than 0.2% [8]. In the majority, a diagnosis can readily be made from the history, physical examination and microscopy of urine. Urine infections account for the majority of cases, with perineal irritation and trauma accounting for many others (Table 1.3).

Viral infections such as adenovirus can cause acute haemorrhagic cystitis. Exercise-induced haematuria may be caused by the repeated impact of the posterior bladder wall against the bladder base or, with sustained exercise, as a result of glomerular afferent and efferent arteriolar vasoconstriction and a consequent rise in filtration pressure. Exercise-induced haematuria is not associated with renal disease. Hypercalciuria and hyperuricosuria are also reported to be associated with macroscopic haematuria, but the strength of this association has not been studied in a population-based study. Hypercalciuria may be noted in children with haematuria who also have a

Table 1.3 Aetiology of macroscopic haematuria in 150 children (Reproduced with permission from Paediatrics, Vol. 59, Page 558, Table 1, Copyright 1977 [8])

Cause	Number of children
Urine infection	
proven	39
suspected	35
Perineal irritation	16
Trauma	10
Acute nephritis	6
Coagulopathy	5
Stones	3
Tumour	1
Other	35

histological diagnosis, suggesting that hypercalciuria should only be considered as the cause of haematuria when other diagnoses have been excluded (see Table 1.4) [9]. Around 25% of renal tumours present with macroscopic haematuria, but there are usually other signs, in particular a palpable mass. Bladder tumours in children are much more likely to present with disorders of micturition rather than haematuria.

An algorithm outlining the initial investigation of a child presenting with macroscopic haematuria is shown in Fig. 1.1. Because of the likely potential causes, macroscopic haematuria should be investigated urgently. This can be done in primary care or in the district hospital setting. Early consultation should take place with a paediatric nephrologist if there is evidence of impaired renal function, proteinuria or hypertension at presentation. Where a clear diagnosis is made after the first stage of investigation, e.g. acute post-streptococcal glomerulonephritis (see Chapter 20), appropriate management may be instituted locally. Where complications or an atypical course ensues, or where there is uncertainty about the diagnosis, referral to a paediatric nephrologist should occur. Radiological investigation may reveal the presence of a renal structural abnormality or calculus. Here, referral to a paediatric urologist is recommended.

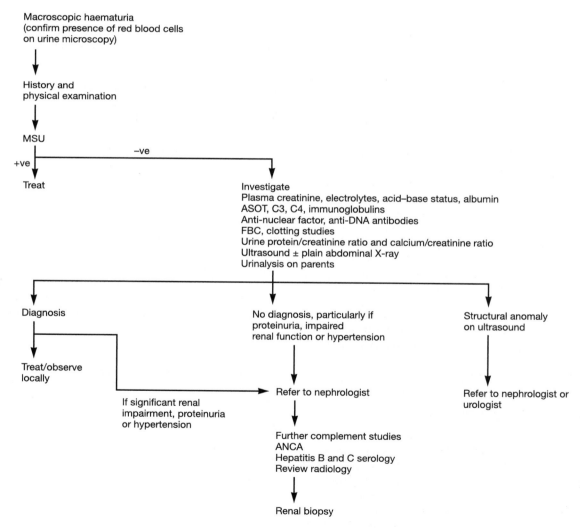

Fig. 1.1 A scheme for the investigation of a child presenting with macroscopic haematuria.

Table 1.4 Clinical features of 322 children undergoing renal biopsy for haematuria (Reproduced from Piqueras A. *et al*. Renal biopsy diagnosis in children presenting with haematuria. Pediatr Nephrol 1998 12 386–391 with permission from Springer-Verlag)

Clinical feature	IgAN	Alport syndrome	TMN	Misc. GN	Hilar vasculopathy	Normal
n	78	86	50	32	28	48
Male	61	50	18	14	23	32
MH	28%	1%	12%	22%	25%	38%
MH+mH	56%	26%	14%	31%	29%	31%
mH	16%	73%	74%	47%	46%	31%
No proteinuria	50%	36%	100%	75%	82%	85%
FH+	5%	87%	52%	25%	29%	15%
Hypercalciuria	1/22	ND	3/29	0/5	2/14	4/22

IgAN, IgA nephropathy; TMN, thin membrane nephropathy; GN, glomerulonephritis; MH, macroscopic haematuria; MH+mH, macroscopic haematuria with persistent microscopic haematuria; mH, persistent microscopic haematuria; FH+, positive family history; ND, not determined.

Following referral, the paediatric nephrologist may arrange further investigations, including a renal biopsy. Table 1.4 shows the histological diagnosis in 322 children biopsied at Birmingham Children's Hospital because of macroscopic or microscopic haematuria [9].

Key points: Macroscopic haematuria

- Urinary tract infection is the most common cause of macroscopic haematuria.

- Urgent investigation should be undertaken (Fig. 1.1).

- Exercise-induced haematuria is not associated with renal disease.

- Early consultation should take place with a paediatric nephrologist if there is evidence of impaired renal function, proteinuria or hypertension at presentation.

Microscopic haematuria

An algorithm for the management of the child with microscopic haematuria is shown in Fig. 1.2. Microscopic haematuria may be noted in the child with generalized symptoms (fever, lethargy, hypertension, oedema), symptoms not specific to the urinary tract (rash, purpura, arthritis, jaundice, respiratory, gastrointestinal) or symptoms related to the urinary tract (dysuria, urgency, frequency, enuresis). Fever,

illness, trauma and extreme exertion may all induce microscopic haematuria. Where the haematuria is related to a non-renal disease/cause it can be expected to disappear as the primary illness resolves. However, having demonstrated haematuria, it is important to document its resolution and to investigate further if haematuria persists, especially if it is accompanied by proteinuria. The conditions with renal involvement which may be readily diagnosed include post-infectious glomerulonephritis, urinary tract infection, familial haematuria (both benign and Alport syndrome), Henoch–Schönlein purpura, systemic lupus erythematosus, renal tumours, hypercalcuria [10] and urolithiasis. In most instances, microscopic haematuria associated with clinical symptoms will require referral to a paediatric nephrologist for further investigation and management.

The incidental finding of isolated microscopic haematuria is relatively common (0.5–4%), but varies because of different definitions used to diagnose haematuria. The incidence decreases in frequency as the stringency of the definition increases [3], indicating that the incidental finding of microscopic haematuria should prompt further testing on at least 3 or 4 occasions; many clinicians will issue parents with dipsticks and ask them to test their child's urine on a daily basis for 6–8 weeks to help ascertain whether the haematuria is persistent. Population studies have demonstrated that only approximately 30% of children continue to demonstrate persistent microscopic haematuria after 6 months, confirming that investigations should be delayed until after that time. Some clinicians choose to extend the period of observation to up to 2 years, although they stress the importance of regular follow-up to document

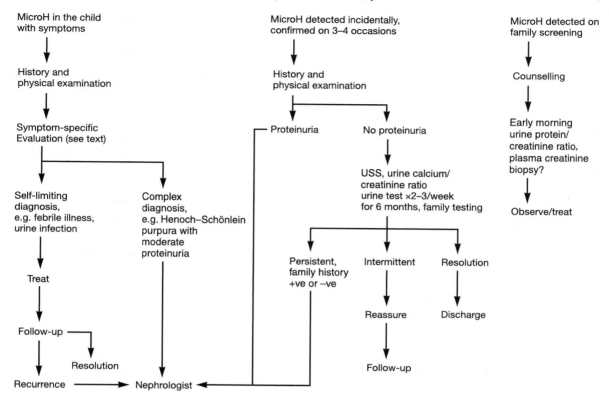

Fig. 1.2 A scheme for the management of the child with persistent microscopic haematuria (MicroH).

the continuing absence of proteinuria and to confirm that the nature of the haematuria is unchanged. The timing and value of renal biopsy remains contentious in this group of patients, although the views of families and children must be taken into account. A histological diagnosis should avoid unnecessary investigation such as cystoscopy and renal imaging later in life when haematuria is re-discovered during routine medical examinations. While much of the remainder of this chapter deals with specific renal diseases, it is important to recognize that most children do not have a worrying cause for their microscopic haematuria. Again, the detection of significant symptoms, impaired renal function, heavy proteinuria or hypertension should prompt early referral to a paediatric nephrologist.

Haematuria may be found as a result of family screening. In those instances in which a histological diagnosis has been made in a first-degree relative, counselling will be required and the family advised of the need for follow-up (see Chapter 16). This most

commonly occurs in Alport syndrome, with the need for long-term follow-up and genetic counselling. When haematuria is familial and a diagnosis of thin basement membrane nephropathy has been made in the index case, renal biopsy may still be indicated in other affected family members. The finding of thin basement membranes does not rule out a diagnosis of Alport syndrome and there are published cases of biopsy findings of thin basement membrane and Alport nephropathy in the same pedigree, suggesting that caution should be exercised when advising families on the merits of renal biopsy. The frequency of outpatient review for children with familial haematuria will vary by diagnosis, boys with Alport syndrome requiring annual measurement of blood pressure, growth, quantification of urinary protein and a hearing test while girls with Alport syndrome and children with thin basement membrane nephropathy require less frequent visits to measure blood pressure, growth and to quantify urinary protein.

Indications for renal biopsy in children with macroscopic and microscopic haematuria

Not all children with haematuria require a renal biopsy. It can be seen from Fig. 1.1 that a number of investigations should be undertaken prior to referral, but that children with persistent macroscopic haematuria of unknown aetiology require referral to a nephrologist for renal biopsy; children with a diagnosis of systemic lupus erythematosus (SLE) with renal involvement also require referral. The role of renal biopsy in the management of children found to have persistent microscopic haematuria is more contentious. However, children with persistent microscopic haematuria who have a systemic illness, significant proteinuria, impaired renal function, hypertension or a family history of haematuria may warrant renal biopsy.

Specific causes of haematuria

Alport syndrome and its variants

Alport syndrome is characterized by inherited nephritis with ultrastructural abnormalities of the glomerular basement membrane, sensorineural deafness, associated ocular defects and, much less commonly, large platelets. In familial cases, 80–90% of cases are X-linked dominant, with 10–20% being autosomal recessive and a very few cases reported to have an autosomal dominant mode of transmission.

New mutations are said to account for up to one-fifth of affected individuals [11,12].

Alport syndrome most commonly presents in childhood as a result of an episode of macroscopic haematuria or because of the incidental finding of microscopic haematuria, or because of family screening as a result of a diagnosis in an index case. The disease may be diagnosed in adulthood in patients presenting with microscopic haematuria and proteinuria, with or without hypertension and renal failure, and deafness. In the X-linked form, females usually have microscopic haematuria only and may be unaware of the risk to their male children.

Case 1

A 5-year-old boy presented with proteinuria and macroscopic haematuria associated with a sore throat and fever. His renal function, plasma albumin, C3, C4 and renal ultrasound scan were normal. Microscopic haematuria persisted and he continued to have macroscopic haematuria with intercurrent infections. By 7 months from presentation he required antihypertensive treatment for mild hypertension. His mother was noted to have haematuria and proteinuria during pregnancy and a renal biopsy was reported as being minimally abnormal with possible early focal segmental glomerulosclerosis (FSGS); electron microscopy was not undertaken. His maternal grandfather died having had an intracranial haemorrhage; he was reported to have kidney problems but had not been deaf. A renal biopsy was undertaken and a diagnosis of Alport syndrome was made. After 3 years of follow-up his renal function has remained normal, proteinuria has increased, he has developed hypoalbuminaemia and a raised plasma cholesterol, and his audiogram recently demonstrated a mild hearing loss preferentially affecting the higher frequencies. His 2-year-old brother did not have haematuria.

Points to note:

- Macroscopic haematuria coincided with intercurrent illnesses (including streptococcal infections), making post-infectious glomerulonephritis less likely.

- Mesangiocapillary glomerulonephritis was unlikely as C3 and C4 levels were normal at presentation.

- Alport syndrome in the mother could not be ruled out as her biopsy had been incompletely examined.

- Persisting proteinuria after resolution of the acute illness mandated renal biopsy.

Case 2

An 11-year-old boy presented to his family doctor with lethargy and was noted to have microscopic haematuria. His father had been investigated by a urologist for haematuria but no abnormality had been found and he was otherwise well. Occasional urine testing at home confirmed persistent microscopic haematuria but no proteinuria. When he was seen in the nephrology clinic his older brother was also reported to have microscopic haematuria, his father's haematuria had resolved and his mother had not tested her own urine. A first morning urine sample showed a protein/creatinine ratio of 46 mg/mmol (normal < 20 mg/mmol). A renal biopsy was undertaken and showed patchy thinning of the glomerular basement membrane, segments of thickening and splitting of the lamina densa with areas of rarefaction. A diagnosis of Alport syndrome was made.

Points to note:

- Familial haematuria, and even trivial proteinuria, warrants renal biopsy.
- All first-degree family members should be screened for haematuria.

Clinical and laboratory findings

Microscopic haematuria is persistent but episodes of macroscopic haematuria may be provoked by intercurrent viral illnesses and it is these episodes which often bring the child to medical attention. It is likely that microscopic haematuria is present from birth in the majority of boys, but may be intermittent in girls. Proteinuria may or may not be present in young boys but is commonly noted at diagnosis in older boys; heavy proteinuria at presentation predicts the development of deafness and end stage renal failure at an earlier age than in those who have mild proteinuria. Hypertension and renal impairment usually develop in the late teens or early twenties, although some males only develop end stage renal failure in their fourth decade. Girls usually have no proteinuria, but when it is present it is often mild or intermittent. Girls rarely develop end–stage renal failure.

Hearing loss develops in adolescent boys and usually pre-dates loss of renal function. The deafness is not congenital, is sensorineural and bilateral, and initially predominantly affects the higher frequencies. Girls rarely have deafness.

A number of ocular defects have been noted in Alport syndrome, affecting the lens, retina and cornea. The most common change is seen in the retina and is manifest as bilateral, densely packed pale granulations surrounding the fovea and affecting the macula [13]. A more obvious finding is that of anterior lenticonus, a conical protrusion on the anterior surface of the lens which is seen in older boys but not in infants [14]. Occasional corneal abnormalities have also been noted. As with all other clinical features, ocular abnormalities are much less common in girls.

Very rarely, oesophageal, tracheobronchial and genital leiomyomatosis has been associated with Alport syndrome [15].

The kidneys appear normal with all modalities of imaging, and in boys renal function is usually normal in the first decade and, as urinary protein losses are often slight, plasma albumin is normal. As boys become older, proteinuria rises into the nephrotic range and is associated with a fall in the plasma albumin, accompanied by a rise in plasma cholesterol and, in some instances, hypothyroidism.

Renal biopsy is diagnostic. In young children the appearances are usually normal by light microscopy, although with increasing age, mesangial matrix expansion, segmental sclerosis, interstitial foam cells and interstitial fibrosis may be noted. Immunostaining is non-contributory. Electron microscopy provides the diagnostic features of irregular thickening of the glomerular basement membrane, sometimes interposed with segments of thin and attenuated basement membrane; occasionally, thin basement membranes are the predominant or sole finding. The lamina densa is characteristically split and duplicated, giving a so-called 'basket weave' appearance [16]. The split lamina densa contains areas of lucency with electron-dense granules, and the epithelial surface of the basement membrane may be scalloped by hypertrophied podocytes. However, diagnosis may be difficult, even with good-quality ultrastructural examination, as the basement membrane abnormalities may be subtle and confined to short segments of the basement membrane. Furthermore, other disease processes, such as ischaemia, can cause basement membrane abnormalities. Some pathologists have used the absence of binding by an anti-glomerular basement membrane antibody to improve diagnosis, but this is not a technique that is widely available. If a diagnosis of Alport syndrome cannot confidently be made histologically in a family with a suggestive family history, other affected individuals should be biopsied to increase the likelihood of obtaining diagnostic histology. We have been unable to demonstrate any relationship between age and the extent of basement membrane changes, indicating that biopsies in young children can be diagnostic.

Management

The prognosis for males is poor as the majority can be expected to progress to end stage renal failure and deafness by the time they reach 30 years of age.

Regular clinic attendances are required to monitor the development of hypertension, hypercholesterolaemia, renal impairment and deafness. Although there is no curative therapy, many clinicians believe that most individuals with a progressively destructive renal disorder benefit from good blood pressure control and reduction of hypercholesterolaemia. A firm evidence base for this is, however, lacking. The use of angiotensin converting enzyme inhibitors or angiotensin receptor blockers may delay the progression to end stage renal failure by reducing hydrostatic glomerular damage resulting from the hyperperfusion and hyperfiltration consequent to reduced nephron mass brought about by the progression of the disease. This effect has been shown to be independent of any benefit from lowering blood pressure. Dialysis and transplantation are necessary once end stage renal failure has supervened. The development of anti-glomerular basement membrane nephritis in the transplanted organ is well recognized but is a very rare event, probably affecting less than 3% of renal transplants in patients with Alport syndrome [17]. Regular audiology review is essential once hearing is noted to be impaired, and hearing aids should be fitted and the child encouraged to make use of them, especially at school. Occasional ophthalmic reviews are necessary, but can be spaced at longer intervals.

Female carriers rarely develop the nephropathy but also require regular review to monitor blood pressure and urinary protein. A rising level of proteinuria should alert the clinician to the possibility of deafness and renal impairment developing with time.

Genetic counselling is an important part of the management of any family affected by Alport syndrome, particularly when discussing the significance of the disease to female carriers (see Chapter 16). As with all genetic conditions, it is the finding that younger siblings are also affected which parents find very difficult. In counselling the family about the disease and its long-term implications for an affected male the clinician needs to emphasize the importance of pursuing a normal lifestyle before renal impairment and deafness supervene, stressing the importance of achieving academic qualifications and physical fitness through full participation at school. None the less, parents often find it difficult to accept that their outwardly normal son will not have a normal adult life and often require frequent counselling after the diagnosis is made to help them understand and come to terms with the illness.

Pathogenesis

The ultrastructural abnormality noted in the glomerular basement membrane suggested a collagen defect. The demonstration that Alport kidneys did not bind antibody to the glomerular basement membrane suggested an absence or modification of basement membrane structural antigens. It was then shown that the non-collagenous peptides targeted by antibodies to glomerular basement membrane were absent in Alport kidneys, and this peptide was later shown to be the 28 kDa non-collagenous domain of the $\alpha 3$ chain of type IV collagen. Subsequent studies using other antibody preparations from Alport transplant recipients who developed anti-glomerular basement membrane nephritis showed that a 26 kDa non-collagenous peptide on the $\alpha 5$ chain of collagen IV could be identified.

The identification of the *COL4A5* gene at Xq22 quickly led to reports of mutations in Alport pedigrees [18]. Deletions or other major rearrangements have been noted, resulting in non-expression of the gene or an abnormal gene product, with a major effect on the organization of the collagen IV molecule and the basement membrane structure. Numerous small mutations throughout the gene have also been noted, with a resultant conformational change to the collagen IV molecule which could prevent the non-collagenous domain from making the required intermolecular crosslinks necessary to produce a normal basement membrane. However, most individuals with *COL4A5* mutations also demonstrate a lack of $\alpha 3$ and $\alpha 4$ collagen IV chains in the glomerular basement membrane, although they may demonstrate normal mRNA levels for these two proteins. The mechanism by which *COL4A5* mutations prevent the expression of the $\alpha 3$ and $\alpha 4$ chains is unknown, although it has been postulated that the mechanism may be through defective molecular assembly and subsequent proteolysis of the $\alpha 3$ and $\alpha 4$ chains.

There is evidence that the nature of the *COL4A5* mutation may influence the phenotype expressed. A recent study has shown that the probability of developing end stage renal failure before the age of 30 years is greater than 90% in males with large rearrangements or small mutations leading to premature stop codons, which have the effect of producing very abnormal or truncated proteins [19]. This same study showed a correlation between the type of *COL4A5* mutation and the onset of hearing loss and the development of lenticonus. In all cases of diffuse oesophageal leiomyomatosis a deletion was noted which removed the 5′ end of both the *COL4A5* and *COL4A6* genes. At the ultrastructural level, all patients with a large deletion of *COL4A5* had thickening of the glomerular basement membrane.

Autosomal recessive Alport syndrome

This variant has very similar clinical features to the X-linked form, with early end stage renal failure, deafness and ocular abnormalities, but the carriers may not have microscopic haematuria. Homozygotes have glomerular basement membrane ultrastructural changes indistinguishable from the X-linked type. Mutations have been noted in the *COL4A3* and *COL4A4* genes on chromosome 2q35–37. About 10–20% of Alport patients may have this mode of inheritance [20].

Autosomal dominant Alport syndrome

A few cases with this mode of inheritance have been reported; affected males have been found to have a better renal prognosis than those with X-linked inheritance, the median renal survival being 51 years in the former and 25 years in the latter. Father-to-son inheritance is characteristic [21].

Key points: Alport syndrome

- 80 to 90% of cases are X-linked dominant.

- The majority of affected males will progress to end stage renal failure and deafness by 30 years of age.

- Genetic counselling is an important part of the management of any family affected by Alport syndrome, particularly when discussing the significance of the disease to female carriers.

Benign familial haematuria

As the name suggests, this is defined by the familial occurrence of haematuria without significant proteinuria, progression to renal failure or hearing defect. The haematuria is often found incidentally in childhood, but may also be discovered for the first time in adulthood; it is usually microscopic but can be macroscopic, is persistent and the red cells may appear dysmorphic. Cases with hypercalciuria are usually

excluded from this diagnostic group. The inheritance is usually autosomal dominant [22,23]. Renal biopsy may demonstrate no abnormality by light or electron microscopy or immunostaining, or may reveal thin, attenuated glomerular basement membranes or deposits of C3 in the hilar vessels ('hilar vasculopathy').

The prognosis for children with this diagnosis is good. However, care must be exercised in making this diagnosis because of the difficulty in differentiating it from Alport syndrome, in which affected individuals also have persistent microscopic haematuria and attenuated glomerular basement membranes. It may not be possible to counsel accurately families in which only females are affected, as the case below illustrates.

Case 3

A 2-year-old girl presented with a urine infection and was found to have bilateral vesico-ureteric reflux. During the course of her follow-up she was noted to have microscopic haematuria, as did her mother, her maternal grandmother, her maternal aunt and her aunt's daughter. She did not have proteinuria. Her mother underwent renal biopsy and on electron microscopy was noted to have uniformly thin glomerular basement membranes. The child was lost to follow-up but returned, aged 6.5 years, with episodes of macroscopic haematuria associated with sore throats. In the clinic she was noted to have haematuria and proteinuria. A renal biopsy was undertaken and on electron microscopy this showed extensive thinning of the glomerular basement membrane with segments of focal thickening, splitting of the lamina densa and areas of rarefaction with electron-dense granules, confirming a diagnosis of Alport syndrome.

Points to note:

- The close temporal association of macroscopic haematuria with an intercurrent illness is against a diagnosis of post-streptococcal nephritis.

- Associated proteinuria is an indication for renal biopsy.

It is advisable that the diagnosis of benign familial haematuria is made with caution and affected individuals should be followed throughout childhood to monitor blood pressure and proteinuria. This periodic review can be undertaken by general paediatricians or general practitioners. In the absence of significant proteinuria, routine hearing tests are not required.

Thin basement membrane nephropathy

Although thin glomerular basement membranes are a common finding in cases of benign familial haematuria, these findings are also noted in cases of non-familial haematuria. The clinical course is variable, although most affected individuals do not develop significant proteinuria or renal failure. However, the finding of thin basement membranes on renal biopsy is not diagnostic and does not imply a benign condition, because the same appearances may be found in Alport syndrome and, if this finding is made in the context of familial haematuria, a diagnosis of Alport syndrome must be considered before any other possibility (Fig. 1.3). The recent advances in understanding the molecular biology of the collagen IV molecule has led to the finding of a *COL4A4* mutation in a pedigree previously thought to have thin basement membrane nephropathy, suggesting some individuals shown to have thin basement membranes on biopsy have autosomal recessive Alport syndrome. On the basis of these findings, it has been suggested that some individuals with benign familial haematuria may be heterozygotes for autosomal recessive Alport syndrome. The follow-up of children found to have thin basement membrane nephropathy is similar to that of children diagnosed to have benign familial haematuria.

IgA nephropathy

IgA nephropathy was first described by Berger and Hinglais in 1968 [24]. It is common at all ages but is most common during the second and third decades and has a male predominance. Familial cases have infrequently been reported. There are differing geographical incidences, IgA nephropathy accounting for 18–40% of all glomerulonephritides reported from Japan, France, Italy and Australia, while it only accounts for 2–10% in the USA, the United Kingdom

and Canada [25]. This differing incidence is not completely explained, but is probably influenced by racial and environmental factors, as well as the differing rates of urine testing in normal children and the readiness with which renal biopsy is undertaken when haematuria is found.

Clinical and laboratory findings

The clinical presentation is varied, but five broad syndromes have been identified at onset:

1. macroscopic haematuria;

2. asymptomatic microscopic haematuria and proteinuria;

3. acute nephritis (haematuria, proteinuria, hypertension and/or renal insufficiency);

4. nephrotic syndrome;

5. mixed nephritic–nephrotic syndrome.

The most common mode of presentation is with macroscopic haematuria, often precipitated by an intercurrent viral upper respiratory tract infection; the haematuria may be accompanied by loin pain. The interval between the precipitating infection and the onset of macroscopic haematuria is only 1–2 days, in comparison with the 2-week interval between a streptococcal infection and the onset of post-streptococcal nephritis. In contrast to Japanese children, only a minority of children in the United Kingdom have persistent microscopic haematuria as their sole urinary abnormality; the majority have recurrent macroscopic haematuria with persistent

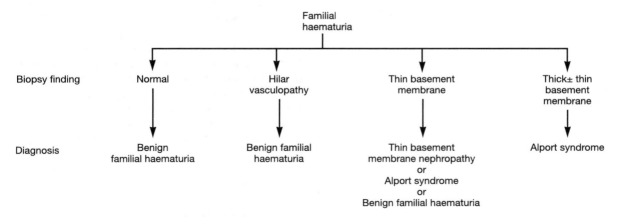

Fig. 1.3 Possible histological findings and final diagnosis in children with familial haematuria.

microscopic haematuria. It is helpful to define the pattern of haematuria, as children with Alport syndrome and thin basement membrane nephropathy usually have persistent microscopic haematuria, with only a minority having recurrent macroscopic haematuria. Those who present with a nephritic and/or nephrotic illness have the most severe glomerular damage, and hypertension and renal impairment is common in this group. A pure nephrotic presentation is unusual (<10%) but IgA nephropathy has been reported to develop in cases of steroid-responsive nephrotic syndrome. Very rarely, IgA nephropathy can lead to a rapidly progressive crescentic glomerulonephritis.

The diagnosis of IgA nephropathy can only be made with confidence by demonstrating deposits of IgA as the predominant immunoglobulin in the glomerular mesangium [26]. In less than 20% of children, plasma IgA may be elevated, suggesting the diagnosis [27]. However, this finding is not considered sufficiently diagnostic to avoid renal biopsy. Because the clinical features at presentation are not diagnostic, it is important to measure C3, streptococcal antibodies and antinuclear factor to exclude other causes.

Case 4

A 7-year-old boy presented with macroscopic haematuria at the time of a sore throat and a possible history of a similar episode 1 year previously. His antistreptolysin-O titre (ASOT) was elevated but C3, antinuclear antibody (ANA) and immunoglobulins were normal. He did not have proteinuria but was noted to have persistent microscopic haematuria for 6 months. Screening of the family was negative. On review in the nephrology clinic it was noted he had had an episode of Henoch–Schönlein purpura 3 months after his initial presentation with haematuria. A renal biopsy was undertaken and showed a diffuse increase in mesangial cellularity and matrix, and occasional areas of tubular atrophy were noted. Immunoperoxidase staining showed deposition of IgA, IgM and complement in the mesangium, confirming a diagnosis of IgA nephropathy.

Points of note:

- The close temporal association between a sore throat and the haematuria is against a diagnosis of post-streptococcal nephritis.

- The elevated ASO titre suggests a streptococcal infection but a normal C3 suggests post-streptococcal nephritis is unlikely.

- The relationship between IgA nephropathy and Henoch–Schönlein purpura is unclear, but this case demonstrates that both diseases may be manifest in one individual.

Renal biopsy findings are very variable and do not differentiate IgA nephropathy from Henoch–Schönlein purpura. In the mildest cases the glomeruli show trivial mesangial proliferation and appear almost normal by light microscopy. Where the biopsy has been undertaken early after presentation and the disease is more active there is usually more obvious mesangial cell proliferation, while biopsies undertaken later in the course of the disease demonstrate a predominant expansion of the mesangial matrix with lesser degrees of cellular proliferation [26]. Mesangial proliferation and expansion of matrix may be diffuse, affecting most glomeruli, or may be focal and segmental. Sequential biopsies demonstrate a resolution or diminution in the severity of mesangial proliferation but increasing matrix deposition, which may ultimately lead to glomerular sclerosis. A marked tubulo-interstitial inflammatory infiltrate is unusual in IgA nephropathy but, if present, may lead to interstitial fibrosis and tubular atrophy and declining renal function. Capsular adhesions and cellular epithelial crescents may also be noted early in the course of the disease, particularly if the clinical presentation is nephritic. As the disease becomes chronic, the cellular crescents become fibrotic and the adherent glomerular capillaries undergo sclerosis; while a small crescent may leave a small segmental scar of the glomerular tuft, large crescents may cause sclerosis of the entire tuft with loss of filtration.

Deposits of IgA can be demonstrated in the mesangial areas and along capillary walls, either by immunofluorescence or by immunoperoxidase staining; deposits of IgG and C3 may also be noted [26]. Diffuse mesangial deposits of IgA may be seen in several other diseases (e.g. Henoch–Schönlein purpura, systemic lupus erythematosus and some systemic diseases such as cystic fibrosis, coeliac disease and liver disease), so a diagnosis of IgA nephropathy can only be made after the exclusion of other diseases. Electron microscopy reveals deposits of electron-dense material in the mesangium and in the glomerular basement membrane below the endothelial cells which, on immunoelectron microscopy, are confirmed to contain IgA, C3 and IgG.

The histological similarities between IgA nephropathy and Henoch–Schönlein purpura suggest a close pathogenetic link between the two conditions. However, the two are clinically distinct, IgA nephropathy predominating in older children, adults and males, whereas Henoch–Schönlein purpura is seen mostly in young children without a marked gender predominance. Furthermore, the nephropathy in Henoch–Schönlein purpura is an acute glomerulonephritis, whereas IgA nephropathy tends to have a more chronic course (see Chapter 21).

The prognosis for childhood IgA nephropathy is better than for adults, but the clinical course is variable. Young children and those without macroscopic haematuria seem to have the best long-term outcome, while heavy proteinuria at onset suggests a poor outcome. Adults with diffuse mesangial proliferation appear to do worse than those who have focal proliferation or minor changes, while in children a high proportion of sclerosed glomeruli, crescents or capsular adhesions, tubulo-interstitial inflammation or fibrosis suggest a poor outcome. It remains uncertain if any treatment is appropriate for IgA nephropathy, although most clinicians would feel justified in treating those children with acute renal failure associated with a crescentic glomerulonephritis and an interstitial infiltrate with immunosuppression and possibly plasma exchange as well. The enthusiasm for prophylactic antibiotics or tonsillectomy to reduce the frequency of intercurrent throat infections in those with mild disease has not been shown to be justified and is rarely used today. The Japanese have used aggressive therapy with dipyridamole, prednisolone, azathioprine and heparin–warfarin, and have demonstrated a reduction in proteinuria and glomerular sclerosis, but this regime has not been adopted by paediatric nephrologists outside Japan [28]. More recently, an adult study showed that the use of a fish-oil preparation reduced the rate of decline in renal function, although protein excretion was unchanged [29]. It is unclear whether this therapy is suitable for children, particularly as large amounts of fish oil have to be taken and the associated smell would probably reduce compliance. The use of angiotensin converting enzyme inhibitors has been shown to reduce protein excretion and to preserve renal function, but should probably be reserved for those children with significant proteinuria and evidence of chronic glomerular damage; angiotensin receptor blocking agents are likely to have the same beneficial effects.

End stage renal failure as a result of IgA nephropathy is unusual in children, but its management is uncomplicated by the diagnosis. However, although renal transplantation is not contraindicated it is important to be aware that up to 50% of transplant recipients demonstrate a recurrence of mesangial IgA deposits; these are usually asymptomatic and it is unusual for graft failure to occur. In contrast, recurrence of Henoch–Schönlein purpura has been reported to cause graft failure.

Pathogenesis

The pathogenesis of IgA nephropathy is unknown. It has been shown that the mesangial IgA in IgA nephropathy belongs to the IgA_1 subclass, may be of bone marrow origin and is in a polymeric form. Studies have also demonstrated impairment of hepatic IgA_1 clearance, possibly because of defective glycosylation of the protein. Unfortunately, none of the progress that has been made in understanding the fundamental abnormalities of IgA in IgA nephropathy has resulted in elucidation of the pathogenesis of the disease or improved treatment strategies to reduce IgA deposition or inflammation.

Key points: IgA nephropathy

- Usually presents with macroscopic haematuria 1–2 days following an upper respiratory tract infection.

- The majority of affected children will also have persistent microscopic haematuria.

- The prognosis is better than for adults: young children and those without macroscopic haematuria have the best long-term outcome.

Proteinuria

The association between renal disease and proteinuria was described by Richard Bright more than 150 years ago. This section reviews the numerous causes for proteinuria but focuses on separating the proteinuric subject who has a serious aetiology for this urinary abnormality from the patient with a benign cause.

Renal handling of proteins

Filtration of proteins

The glomerular basement membrane provides both a mechanical and a charge barrier to the passage of plasma proteins into the glomerular filtrate. Nevertheless, some plasma proteins cross this barrier in concentrations that are related to the protein's size, charge, deformability and concentration in the plasma [30]. In health, the mechanical barrier to filtration virtually excludes the larger plasma proteins such as globulins from entering the glomerular filtrate. Smaller proteins such as albumin are filtered in concentrations as high as 20 mg/L which translates into a filtered load of up to 3.5 g/day. Small proteins, such as the peptide hormones, insulin or growth hormone, or derivatives of immunoproteins such as β_2-microglobulin, can penetrate the glomerular barrier with relative ease and their concentration in the glomerular filtrate may be 50% or more of that in the plasma. The relative impermeability of the glomerulus to albumin and other proteins which are negatively charged at pH 7.4 is due, in part, to glycosaminoglycans which are present in each layer of the basement membrane and which are also negatively charged.

Alterations to glomerular capillary flow can increase albumin entry into the glomerular filtrate. These effects are functional, not pathological, since restoration of blood flow to normal promptly reverses the leaky state of the glomerular capillary wall.

Tubular reabsorption

Almost all of the smaller proteins that enter the glomerular filtrate are reabsorbed in the proximal convoluted tubules by a process of endocytosis, which operates at well below maximum rates in health so that normal urine contains negligible quantities of the peptide hormones or immunoglobulin fragments even though they are readily filtered. Metabolism by the kidney represents an important regulatory process for many of these proteins.

The proximal convoluted tubules also reabsorb, by a second process of endocytosis, most of the larger plasma proteins that are filtered. None of these proteins are returned intact into the body's protein pool. They are partially digested in endocytic vacuoles, with the catabolic products being returned to the circulation. This transport system operates at, or close to, its maximum rate in health.

Protein secretion

Forty per cent of normal urinary protein is of tissue rather than plasma origin. It is composed of a heterogeneous group of proteins, primarily glycoproteins. Some of these are derived from cells lining the urinary tract and have the potential of being important diagnostic indicators [31]; others are from non-renal tissues such as the accessory sex glands. The major protein in this group is uromucoid or Tamm–Horsfall

protein, which is excreted in amounts of 30–60 mg/day in the adult. This large glycoprotein is a major constituent of urinary casts and is added to the urine, primarily in the thick ascending limb of the loop of Henle and at more distal sites.

Measurement of proteinuria

Screening techniques

Dipstick methods. Most proteinuria is first identified by a dipstick urinalysis. The simplicity and accuracy of this technique has increased the frequency with which it is used (see previous section on Dipsticks). Nevertheless, the method has limitations (see Table 1.2).

Quantification of proteinuria

Laboratory methods. Quantification of proteinuria is important in determining whether the patient requires a more extensive evaluation or to follow a patient's progress. Numerous methods are available [32]. Each has advantages and disadvantages. Unfortunately, results will vary depending on the method used, so the clinician must be cautious when comparing data from different laboratories.

The typical laboratory method in widespread use today utilizes a turbidometric method modified for use in a clinical analyser. Turbidometric assays (based on the principle that proteins are insoluble at an acid pH) are simple, convenient and cost effective; benzethonium chloride is used to precipitate urinary protein. They are accurate when the urine contains a relatively high protein concentration but tend to underestimate protein concentrations at lower levels (<20 mg/l).

Normal proteinuria

Healthy subjects have small amounts of protein in their urine. Under normal conditions, approximately 60% of this protein is derived from plasma protein. This results from a balance between the amount of these proteins filtered and the amount reabsorbed. Albumin predominates and constitutes about 40% of the total urinary protein, with another 15% being globulins. Numerous other proteins have been identified and include a variety of immunoproteins, peptides, enzymes, hormones and partially degraded plasma proteins. The proportions of the different proteins in urine can vary. For example, after severe exercise proteinuria may increase several-fold due to increased albuminuria, so that after exercise albumin may represent as much as 80% of total urinary protein.

Normal values for proteinuria

Dipsticks will detect protein concentrations as low as 0.15 g/l (trace); 1+ approximates 0.3 g/l; 2+, 1 g/l; 3+, 3 g/l; and 4+, 20 g/l. Unfortunately, dipsticks do not always indicate whether proteinuria is normal or pathological in amount. They may give a false-positive result when the urine is concentrated and the proteinuria is normal in amount; conversely they may give a false-negative result when the urine is dilute and the protein excretion rate is moderately increased. However, values of 3+ or 4+ almost always indicate the presence of pathological amounts of proteinuria.

'Normal' values for urinary protein excretion have not been established for children of different ages. There are practical reasons for this. Values are affected by the conditions under which the urine was collected, for example whether the child exercised or was at rest during the collection period; by the method used to measure protein concentration; by the age and sex of the patient; and whether a 12- or 24-hour urine sample was used, since proteinuria is higher during the day than during the night. The biggest problem, however, is to obtain complete and accurately timed urine collections, especially in younger children.

Published recommendations for 'normal' urine protein values in children have ranged from 60 to 240 mg/m^2 body surface area/day. At least one authority uses a single upper limit of normal value of 150 mg/day since he is not convinced that protein excretion is related to body size. The higher values allow for some of the practical difficulties associated with urine collection, such as the subject participating in vigorous activities during part of the collection. This would increase the level of proteinuria during the activity.

Our guideline is that if the urine is collected with the patient at rest and afebrile, urinary protein excretion should not exceed 60 mg/m^2/day. This value agrees well with the normal protein excretion rates in adults of up to 100 mg/day and applies to all age ranges, except during the first months of life when normal proteinuria typically is increased to as high as 240 mg/m^2/day [33]. We believe that the use of more liberal values has potential for error and recommend that if urine protein excretion is to be quantitated, the urine should be collected with the patient at rest when the lower 'normal' value applies.

For practical reasons, we obtain accurately timed overnight urine collections of approximately 12 hours'

duration. The protein excretion rate is then extrapolated to a 24-hour value by using the appropriate correction factor. For example, if the urine collection was obtained over an 11.5-hour period, the urine protein excretion rate would be multiplied by 24/11.5 to obtain a 24-hour value.

We do not think that there is any practical advantage in expressing urinary protein excretion per hour or per unit of body weight, as advocated by some.

Urinary protein/creatinine ratios

It is readily apparent that obtaining accurate 12- or 24-hour urine collections can be inconvenient and difficult to accomplish, so that quantitating proteinuria can be fraught with problems. In addition, changes in levels of proteinuria can be affected by glomerular filtration rate (GFR). A marked reduction in GFR will decrease filtered load of protein and can reduce proteinuria markedly. Attempts have been made to control for this by factoring urine protein excretion by GFR measured from the same urine sample. This is not practical for routine clinical use, however.

In an attempt to avoid these problems, single-void urine samples have been evaluated as a semi-quantitative estimate of proteinuria [34,35]. For this purpose, the concentration of both protein and creatinine are measured in the urine sample and protein concentration is factored by creatinine concentration, the urine protein/creatinine ratio. This technique has the advantages of not requiring timed urine samples and of not having to be corrected for body size. It assumes that creatinine excretion is directly related to body mass and is relatively constant throughout the day [36]. Many studies have found that values for urine protein/creatinine ratios measured in random urine samples correlate well with measurements of protein excretion in 24-hour urine collections from the same patients. It remains debated, however, whether random samples obtained during normal daytime activities or early morning samples are superior [35,37].

Most normal subjects will have values for urinary protein to creatinine ratios below 10 mg/mmol. This upper limit for normal correlates well with a protein excretion of 60 mg/m^2/day. Using a Coomassie blue dye-binding method to measure protein, a very extensive study showed that after age 2 years a ratio of less than 25 mg/mmol should be considered normal; in children aged 6–24 months, normal values may be as high as 50 mg/mmol; and even higher values can be found in normal infants less than 6 months in age. Values between 25 mg/mmol and 100 mg/mmol represent mild proteinuria, 100–500 mg/mmol indicate moderate proteinuria and those in excess of 500 mg/mmol are found with heavy proteinuria. The International Study of Kidney Disease in Children (ISKDC) definition of nephrotic proportion proteinuria, 40 mg/m^2/h, which many consider to be a somewhat low value, equates with a value of 250 mg/mmol.

There are two situations where urine protein/creatinine ratios can be misleading. Since creatinine production and excretion is related to muscle mass, children with severe malnutrition or other conditions associated with low muscle mass will have a decreased renal excretion of creatinine and a relatively elevated urine protein/creatinine ratio. Secondly, high ratios may be obtained in children with orthostatic proteinuria despite normal 24-hour protein excretion unless great care is taken to ensure that the sample is collected first thing in the morning immediately after adopting the upright position. Thus we believe that measuring urinary protein to creatinine ratio is of more value when monitoring the progress of proteinuria than in the initial evaluation of proteinuria. Our preference is to obtain both an overnight 12-hour protein excretion value and a urine protein/creatinine ratio in the investigation of proteinuria, and then to follow the patient's progress by serial measurements of the urine protein/creatinine ratio with urine samples being obtained under similar conditions at each follow-up visit.

Key points: Normal proteinuria

- Published recommendations for normal urine protein values in children have ranged from 60 to 240 mg/m^2/day.

- Our guideline is that if the urine is collected with the patient at rest and afebrile, urine protein excretion should not exceed 60 mg/m^2/day.

- The urine protein/creatinine ratio correlates well with measurements of protein excretion in 24-hour urine collections.

- Most normal subjects will have urinary protein/creatinine ratios below 10 mg/mmol; this correlates with a protein excretion of 60 mg/m^2/day.

- Other studies have shown the upper limit of normal to be 25 mg/mmol in children over 2 years old. In children aged 6–24 months, normal values may be as high as 50 mg/mmol; and even higher values van be found in normal infants less than 6 months old.

Measurement of specific urine proteins

Albumin/microalbuminuria

It has been found that some subjects will have modest increases in urinary albumin excretion even though values remain below those typically associated with clinical proteinuria and below the level of detection by conventional dipstick analysis. This phenomenon is referred to as microalbuminuria. By definition, this refers to albumin excretion rates from 20 to 200 μg/min (30–300 mg/day) in the adult. The main purpose of detecting microalbuminuria is to help identify those patients with diabetes mellitus, either insulin dependent or non-insulin dependent, who are at risk of progressing to macroalbuminuria and developing diabetic nephropathy. This is discussed further in Chapter 21.

In adult practice, microalbuminuria is usually diagnosed on the basis of a timed urine collection, although, because of difficulties in obtaining accurately timed urine collections in children, more practical approaches to identify microalbuminuria have been studied. Albumin excretion rates and urine albumin/creatinine ratios in normal children have been reported [38], and it is generally accepted that a urine albumin/creatinine ratio above 2.5 mg albumin/mmol creatinine is indicative of microalbuminuria (see Chapter 21).

The introduction of dipsticks which can measure low concentrations of albumin as well as creatinine concentrations has facilitated screening for subjects with microalbuminuria. When the dipsticks are read by the appropriate analyser, it provides semi-quantitative values for both of these concentrations and calculates the albumin/creatinine ratio within a minute.

β$_2$-Microglobulin

Elevated urinary concentrations of certain low molecular weight proteins can be a most sensitive indicator of even mild damage to the renal proximal tubule, and can identify injury induced by nephrotoxic drugs, such as aminoglycoside antibiotics, or by heavy metals, such as mercury, or damage due to interstitial nephritis.

One of these proteins that has been studied extensively is β$_2$-microglobulin. Its concentrations can be measured easily, either by radioimmunoassay or by enzymatic methodology, using commercially available kits. This small protein is freely filtered by the glomerulus and almost totally reabsorbed and degraded by the proximal tubules. Even subtle damage to the proximal tubule will result in decreased reabsorption of β_2-microglobulin, with increased excretion of the protein in the urine [39].

Urine β_2-microglobulin concentrations should not exceed 0.4 mg/l after 3 months of age. The level may be as high as 4.0 mg/l in the normal newborn child. Elevated levels indicate the presence of tubular injury or disease.

Protein selectivity

Nephelometry permits analysis of urinary protein by molecular size and enables calculation of protein selectivity. This index can help to define the underlying cause in a patient with nephrotic syndrome. Patients with glomerulonephritis tend to have *non-selective* proteinuria with relatively high clearances of globulins and other large proteins; those with minimal change nephrotic syndrome (MCNS) have *selective* proteinuria composed primarily of albumin. Unfortunately, there is considerable overlap in results, so that one cannot draw too firm conclusions from measurements of selectivity, and the technique has been almost entirely abandoned in routine clinical practice.

Prevalence of proteinuria

Studies of large populations of children have found that the prevalence of proteinuria varies from under 1% to more than 10%. As illustrated in Fig. 1.4, proteinuria occurs more often in girls than in boys and prevalence increases with age. Other studies confirm these findings. For example, another large study from the USA documented proteinuria in 0.94% of girls and 0.33% of boys [7]. A screening programme involving 560 000 children in Japan found the prevalence of proteinuria to be 0.08% in children attending elementary school and 0.37% in those attending junior high school [40]. The definition of proteinuria also affects its prevalence. Whereas 5.6% of 12-year-old schoolgirls had 10 mg/dl of protein in two out of three urine samples, only 0.2% of these same subjects had protein levels of 100 mg/dl or more in all three samples (Fig. 1.4) [7].

It is readily apparent that proteinuria is intermittent in the majority of proteinuric children. For example, one study analysed four urine samples from each of 8954 school children between 8 and 15 years. Proteinuria was documented to occur in at least one sample from 10% of the children. Only 0.1% of the

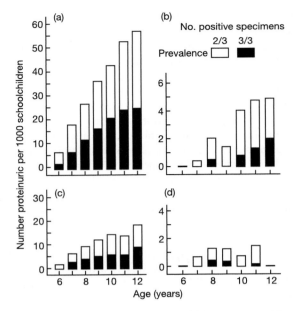

Fig. 1.4 Prevalence of proteinuria in school-aged children showing the influence of age, sex, level of proteinuria, and frequency at which proteinuria was documented in (a) and (b) girls; (c) and (d) boys. With proteinuria of (a), (c) 10 mg/dl and (b), (d) 100 mg/dl. (From the data of Dodge *et al.* [7] from *Clinical Paediatric Nephrology* 2/e by R.J. Postlethwaite. Reprinted by permission of Elsevier Science Ltd.)

population had all four urine samples positive for protein [41].

Classification of proteinuria

Proteinuria may be isolated or may be found in conjunction with other evidence for renal disease (e.g. haematuria, impaired renal function, hypertension). Isolated proteinuria may be further categorized into benign or fixed (reproducible) forms (Table 1.5).

Isolated proteinuria: benign forms

Functional.　This common form of proteinuria is usually associated with physiological stress, such as that seen with strenuous exercise or exposure to cold; it can also occur in conjunction with febrile illnesses or with congestive heart failure. It may be seen in up to 10% of patients admitted to hospital with acute illness.

Functional proteinuria occurs as a result of changes in renal haemodynamics, leading to increased glomerular filtration of plasma proteins. There is no abnormality in either renal function or structure. The proteinuria typically resolves after the precipitating

Table 1.5 Causes for isolated proteinuria

Artefact
    False-positive test, e.g. alkaline urine
    Contamination of urine, e.g. vaginal secretions
Benign
    Functional
    Idiopathic
        Transient
        Intermittent
    Orthostatic (postural)
        Transient
        Fixed (reproducible)
Persistent/non-benign
    Persistent isolated
    Disease related (see Table 1.6)

Key points: Functional proteinuria

- Proteinuria may be associated with physiological stress, such as strenuous exercise, exposure to cold, febrile illness or congestive cardiac failure.

- Such proteinuria typically resolves after the precipitating event has ameliorated.

---

event has ameliorated. Prognosis is good and progressive renal disease is not associated with this form of proteinuria.

Idiopathic transient proteinuria. This form of benign proteinuria is also common in children, adolescents and young adults. The patients are asymptomatic and the proteinuria is usually detected on routine urine screening, perhaps for athletic participation or as part of a physical examination. The urine sediment should be normal and there should be no other evidence for renal disease, such as hypertension. Repeat urine testing should document the transient nature of the proteinuria. Again, prognosis is excellent, the proteinuria being assumed to be due to temporary changes in renal haemodynamics.

Idiopathic intermittent proteinuria. This is characterized by the presence of protein in some, usually about 50%, but not all randomly collected urines. It occurs independent of body position and should not be associated with other urinary abnormalities,

decrease in renal function or hypertension. A renal biopsy study of 51 young adults with such proteinuria demonstrated normal or minimal histological changes in 40%. The remaining patients showed some glomerular changes, including hypercellularity and even sclerosis. However, 40 years of follow-up in these patients showed a favourable prognosis, especially if the proteinuria disappeared after a few years. The risk of renal insufficiency in these patients appears to be no greater than that in the general population.

Postural proteinuria. Often referred to as orthostatic proteinuria, patients with this entity exhibit proteinuria when they assume the upright position but not when they are recumbent. This latter point is most important since patients with renal disease typically exhibit increased proteinuria in the upright position but the proteinuria persists, even when they are recumbent.

Postural proteinuria is seen most commonly in adolescents and in males. Typically, it is transient or variable in nature, since not every challenge results in proteinuria. In about 15–20% of cases it is fixed and reproducible. Even in these cases, the orthostatic proteinuria decreases in amount with age and eventually disappears. The majority of patients with postural proteinuria excrete less than 2 g protein/24 hours, although urinary protein concentrations in excess of 10 g/L have been documented in subjects with the classical orthostatic pattern [42].

The mechanisms responsible for orthostatic proteinuria remain unclear. Alterations in renal or glomerular haemodynamics, renal vein entrapment and an immune-mediated renal parenchymal process have all been postulated to play a role [42].

Postural proteinuria was believed to be benign until a systematic study of young males with fixed orthostatic proteinuria demonstrated that 45% of the subjects had subtle alterations in glomerular architecture and that 8% had more severe morphological evidence of renal disease. Fortunately, a 20-year follow-up of these subjects has indicated that they had a good outcome despite the earlier biopsy findings [43]. None of the subjects had any evidence of significant or progressive renal disease, all had normal renal function, the incidence of hypertension in this population was normal and many of the subjects no longer showed significant proteinuria. Thus, all available evidence indicates that orthostatic proteinuria as an isolated finding is benign.

Key points: Postural (orthostatic) proteinuria

- Seen most commonly in adolescents and males.

- Typically transient or variable in nature.

- Decreases in amount with age and eventually disappears.

- Twenty-year follow-up studies have reported a good outcome, with no increased incidence of renal failure or hypertension.

Persistent isolated proteinuria. The presence of persistent proteinuria not related to posture and not accompanied by other evidence for renal disease presents a difficult management problem. Renal biopsies from such patients have revealed a wide array of findings. Many patients will have normal renal histology or mild effacement of the podocytes, as in minimal change nephrotic syndrome. It is not uncommon for the proteinuria to resolve following a trial of steroids (see below). Even if the proteinuria persists, these patients typically have a good prognosis.

Of more concern are the patients who have more severe glomerular changes. These may range from glomerular hypercellularity to segmental glomerulosclerosis or interstitial fibrosis. The presence of such findings increases the likelihood of progressive renal damage, nevertheless many such patients will continue to be proteinuric without any deterioration of renal function. There are few long-term follow-up data for patients who fall into this category, and they need to be followed closely.

Disease-related proteinuria

Patients who have persistent proteinuria associated with additional evidence of renal disease, such as microscopic haematuria, are the ones most likely to have significant pathology in the kidney or urinary tract. In the vast majority of cases, this form of proteinuria is of glomerular origin. However, non-glomerular mechanisms can cause marked proteinuria too. Thus, proteinuria can be classified logically according to the pathophysiological mechanism responsible, as shown in Table 1.6.

Table 1.6 Causes for disease-related proteinuria: classified by mechanism

Renal disease
  Glomerular causes (increased protein filtration)
    Glomerular damage to basement membranes, e.g. acute or chronic glomerulonephritis, diabetes mellitus
    Loss of glomerular anion, e.g. minimal change or congenital nephrotic syndrome
    Increased glomerular permeability
    Altered renal haemodynamics, e.g. end stage renal failure, post-nephrectomy hyper-reninaemia; diabetes mellitus (early stages)
  Tubular causes (decreased protein reabsorption)
    Hereditary disease, e.g. Fanconi syndrome, Lowes syndrome, galactosaemia; acquired diseases, e.g. vitamin D intoxication; analgesic abuse
    Heavy metal poisoning
    Acute tubular necrosis
  Secretory proteinuria
    Renal tubules, e.g. Tamm–Horsfall proteinuria (neonates)
    Lower urinary tract, e.g. prostatitis
    Other accessory sex gland
Other diseases
  Overflow proteinuria
    Normal renal function, e.g. albuminuria after repeated infusions or transfusions; small proteins or protein fragments, e.g. myeloma or macroglobulinaemia
  Histuria
    Kidney-specific antigens, e.g. rapidly progressive glomerulonephritis, analgesic abuse
    Other antigens, e.g. collagen disorders; neuroblastoma, urothelial carcinoma; melanoma
  Other
    Stress, e.g. fever, exposure to cold
    Heart disease, e.g. heart failure

Glomerular mechanisms

Any disease which damages the glomerular basement membrane increases glomerular permeability to plasma proteins. The increased filtered load of protein overwhelms the tubular reabsorption of protein so that proteinuria ensues. The damage to the glomerular barrier permits both albumin and larger globulin molecules to enter the urine, so the proteinuria is defined as being 'non-selective'. Any of the acute or chronic glomerulonephritides cause proteinuria by this mechanism.

A second major mechanism for glomerular proteinuria is loss, or reduction, of the glomerular charge barriers which, in health, contribute to the low permeability of the glomeruli to negatively charged selected proteins such as albumin. The classical cause for this kind of proteinuria is minimal change nephrotic syndrome. It is also seen in congenital nephrotic syndrome of the Finnish variety. The proteinuria is 'selective', consisting almost entirely of albumin.

A reduction in nephron mass results in increased glomerular permeability and in increased proteinuria from the residual nephrons, which undergo hyperfiltration injury. This mechanism probably accounts for the increased proteinuria observed in renal transplant donors and in those with single kidneys. It may be responsible for the proteinuria observed in some patients with progressive lesions associated with nephron loss, such as cystic kidney disease.

Any increase in filtration fraction will increase plasma protein concentrations at the distal end of the glomerular capillaries to a level above threshold. This could explain the proteinuria observed in patients with high levels of angiotensin.

It has been suggested that an increased transglomerular passage of protein may be responsible for producing permanent glomerular damage and contribute to the development of glomerulosclerosis. If this thesis is proven, treatments to reduce proteinuria *per se* (as well as treating the underlying disease) could assume an even greater importance in the future.

Non-glomerular mechanisms

Since the proximal convoluted tubule normally reabsorbs most of the filtered protein, it is not unexpected that any damage to this segment of the nephron can result in proteinuria. Typically, the amount of protein in the urine resulting from *tubular damage* is not marked, but cases have been reported in which such proteinuria was sufficient to result in the nephrotic syndrome. Examples of diseases which may induce tubular proteinuria are shown in Table 1.6.

The increased excretion of tissue proteins into the urine may result in proteinuria too, and is referred to as *secretory proteinuria*. In the neonatal period, losses of Tamm–Horsfall protein account for the higher levels of proteinuria typically seen at this age. Some of the proteinuria observed with the passage of renal stones and with urinary tract infections may result from irritation of the lower urinary tract and the increased secretion of tissue proteins from the ureter and bladder. Inflammation of the accessory sex glands may also cause secretory proteinuria by increased addition to the urine of tissue proteins.

Overflow proteinuria results when the plasma level of a protein exceeds the renal threshold for that protein. This can occur even when kidney function is normal. The protein may or may not be a normal constituent of the blood. For example, plasma albumin concentration may increase sufficiently to cause albuminuria after repeated transfusion of either albumin or whole blood. Alternately, in adults with multiple myeloma the appearance in the plasma of Bence Jones protein will result in loss of that protein in the urine and in clinically detectable proteinuria. Similarly, the release of free haemoglobin into the plasma causes the rapid appearance of this protein in the urine, probably because the haemoglobin tetramer dissociates readily into smaller dimers. The haemoglobin is identified as protein when turbidometric methods are used to measure proteinuria. This can represent a diagnostic problem if proteinuria and haemoglobinuria occur simultaneously, for example when haemolysis and renal disease coexist. In such situations, urinary protein electrophoresis can be most useful since haemoglobin migrates as a β_2-globulin. Other tests to quantitate haemoglobin in the urine are also available.

In the future, *histuria*, or loss of certain antigenic tissue proteins in the urine, may provide important diagnostic information about non-renal diseases. Although the amount of protein lost is not sufficient to be readily identified by screening methods, the topic is referred to here because of its potential importance. Non-specific antigens may be found in diseases that cause damage to basement membrane or collagen. Tissue-specific antigens have been described with urothelial carcinoma, melanoma and neuroblastoma.

Consequences of proteinuria

Proteinuria does not necessarily result in altered levels of protein in the plasma. The liver has considerable reserve capacity for increased production of new proteins and often can compensate for urinary losses. If proteinuria is heavy and protracted and exceeds the patient's ability to synthesize new protein, it will result in hypoproteinaemia and, on occasion, in the nephrotic syndrome.

Evaluation of the proteinuric subject

Since isolated proteinuria is most often a benign condition, it is neither necessary nor appropriate to undertake an extensive evaluation of all children who have a positive test for protein in their urine. The cost would be prohibitive, the returns small and a great deal of unnecessary anxiety would be generated in children and their families. The challenge facing the physician is to identify the small subgroup of children in whom proteinuria is the presenting abnormality of a serious renal disease. The following outline presents a step-by-step approach to address this task (Fig. 1.5). The first three steps can be accomplished at the patient's initial encounter with the

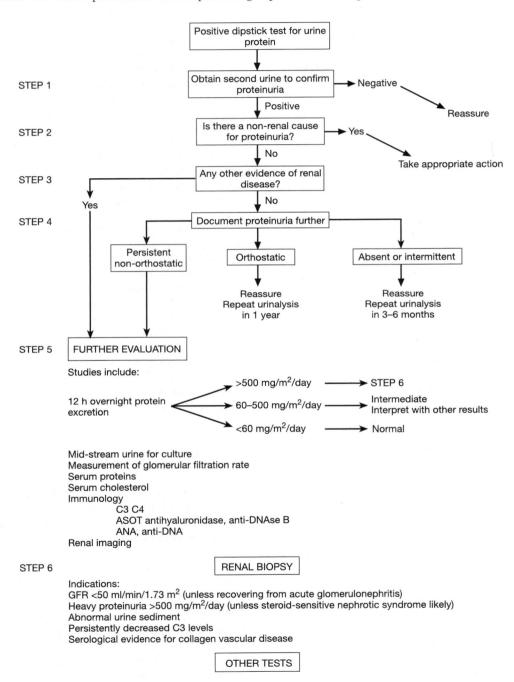

Fig. 1.5 Evaluation of proteinuria. From Clinical Paediatric Nephrology 2/e by R.J. Postlethwaite. Reprinted by permission of Elsevier Science.

physician; steps 4–6 require a return visit or admission to the hospital.

Step 1: Exclude false-positive results

Common reasons for false-positive results are given in Table 1.2. Agents used for cleaning the genitalia and detergents in urine containers are particularly important sources of error. If it is possible that the test was positive for one of these reasons, a repeat urine should be tested. If it is negative, reassure the family; if positive, move to step 2.

Step 2: Exclude non-renal causes of proteinuria

As detailed previously, proteinuria can arise in response to stress, as a result of overflow proteinuria or from non-renal diseases, such as congestive cardiac failure. If none of these conditions exist, move to step 3.

Step 3: Determine whether the patient has any other evidence of a disease of the kidney or urinary tract

History.   A history of oedema, haematuria, polyuria, nocturia, dysuria or colicky abdominal pain may be elicited. Proteinuria may have been demonstrated at a previous examination. There may be a family history of renal failure or deafness.

Examination.   Examination may reveal growth failure, hypertension, oedema, anaemia, renal tenderness or enlargement, or evidence of renal osteodystrophy.

Urinalysis.   Urinalysis may show a concentrating defect. With chronic renal failure, the kidney can neither concentrate nor dilute the urine appropriately so that the urine specific gravity is or close to 1.010. A fresh urine sample should be examined for abnormalities of sediment. Microscopic haematuria is the most common indicator of a glomerular lesion in a proteinuric patient, and the existence of haematuria with proteinuria carries a poorer prognosis than does proteinuria alone. Urine should be examined for blood, both with dipstick and microscopy.

If the history, physical examination and urinalysis are all negative, then one should proceed to step 4. If any of the results in this stage suggest the presence of disease of the urinary tract, especially if haematuria

is found, the patient requires a more detailed evaluation, as outlined in step 5.

Step 4: Further documentation of the proteinuria

The family is provided with a supply of dipsticks and instructed in their use. The urine is tested twice a day for 1 week. The two urine samples to be checked each day are the first sample passed in the morning as soon as the patient arises, and the last sample of the day voided just before the patient retires to bed. It is important that the patient remains supine throughout the night so that the early morning urine sample consists of urine formed when the patient was recumbent; in contrast, the evening samples represent urine formed when the patient was upright and active. These records may show:

1. *Intermittent proteinuria.* None, or only a few, of the samples are positive for protein. There is no evidence that such proteinuria is associated with severe or progressive renal disease. The patient and family are reassured, but as a precaution a complete urinalysis is repeated in 3–6 months' time.

2. *Orthostatic proteinuria.* The morning samples are negative for protein; varying concentrations of protein are present in the evening samples. The patient and family are reassured and given an optimistic prognosis. The urine is rechecked in 1 year to ensure that the initial studies were not misleading.

3. *Persistent proteinuria.* All urine samples contain protein, even though the levels may vary. This does not necessarily imply the presence of severe renal disease, but is does require that the patient is investigated in more detail, as outlined in step 5.

If the family is unable to carry out the dipstick tests in a reliable fashion, two further early morning urine samples are brought to the physician to be tested for protein. If both of these are negative, the patient is reassured but a further sample is tested in 3–6 months. If either of these tests is positive, the protein excretion rate is measured in a 12-hour urine sample collected overnight with the patient at rest. If the value is below $60\,mg/m^2/day$ (i.e. $<30\,mg/m^2$ in the 12-hour collection period) the family is reassured. Patients with higher values should be studied and counselled as outlined in step 5. This approach is based on the finding that only persistent proteinuria is associated with a significant increase in urine protein excretion in a 12-hour urine collected with the patient supine.

Step 5: The initial further evaluation of patients with isolated persistent proteinuria or those with proteinuria and other evidence for renal disease

Any patient who reaches this stage of study warrants a thorough evaluation. Too often, when a patient has been subjected to a less detailed series of tests than those outlined below, the physician is not able to make authoritative recommendations or to provide adequate reassurance. This is quickly sensed by the family, who lose confidence in the physician and request a second opinion. The recommended tests and their rationale are summarized below.

Urine collection. If not already obtained, an overnight urine sample with the patient supine should be collected to quantitate the proteinuria. Values below 60 mg/m^2/day are normal. Levels above 500 mg/m^2/day are cause for concern and usually indicate the need for a more advanced evaluation, as outlined in step 6. Intermediate values can only be interpreted in conjunction with the remaining test results. In addition, a random urine sample is obtained for measurement of the protein to creatinine ratio. This is done to obtain a baseline value only. It is not to be used in determining the management of the patient at this stage.

Urine culture. In at least one series of children with proteinuria, occult urinary tract infections were the most common cause for proteinuria. Thus, collection of a clean-catch urine sample should be a routine part of the evaluation.

Measurement of glomerular filtration rate. A reduction in GFR usually is one of the most important indicators that a renal biopsy is required. Plasma creatinine measurements provide useful information from which GFR can be estimated (see Chapter 28) and are measured as part of routine evaluation. In many patients, this data should be supplemented by a more precise measure of GFR using one of the clearance methods discussed in Chapter 28. Such measurements can help in determining the need for renal biopsy or provide a useful baseline value which helps in determining whether a patient is responding to prescribed treatment. The measurement of GFR and

plasma creatinine simultaneously at the initial evaluation permits subsequent monitoring of the patient's renal function by measurements of the latter test only. Repeat clearances are necessary only if the blood values indicate that a change in GFR has occurred.

Changes in GFR must always be considered when interpreting a finding of reduced urinary protein excretion on follow-up. A decrease in GFR due to progression of a renal disease may result in a decrease in proteinuria secondary to a decrease in the amount of protein filtered. Sometimes this can be so dramatic that it results in amelioration of the nephrotic syndrome. It may be misinterpreted as improvement rather than progression of the disease if changes in GFRs are not monitored.

Key points: Glomerular filtration rate

- Changes in GFR must always be considered when interpreting a finding of reduced urinary protein excretion on follow-up. A decrease in GFR due to progression of a renal disease may result in a decrease in proteinuria. This may be misinterpreted as improvement rather than progression of the disease if changes in GFR are not monitored.

Blood chemistries. Proteinuric subjects do not necessarily have altered plasma protein concentrations. Hypoproteinaemia usually indicates that the patient has had heavy proteinuria for a significant period of time. Such a finding may be an important indicator for a renal biopsy. Thus, total serum protein and serum albumin levels are measured. Serum cholesterol is measured to determine the presence or absence of hyperlipidaemia, which is seen in the nephrotic syndrome.

Immunology/serology. Both the third and fourth components of complement (C3 and C4) should be measured. Decreased values of complement provide indirect evidence for the presence of post-streptococcal glomerulonephritis, active systemic lupus erythematosus and other rarer pathologies (see Chapters 20 and 21). Additional tests may be required after these baseline values are available. Antistreptolysin-O (ASO) and antihyaluronidase titres, antinuclear antibodies (ANA) and anti-DNA antibodies are measured also, again to provide indirect evidence for glomerulonephritis as an underlying cause. The tests are performed even in patients with isolated proteinuria. The first two tests provide evidence for a preceding streptococcal infection, but do not indicate whether or not the strain was nephritogenic. Systemic lupus erythematosus may present in such a variety of ways that it is worth looking for serological evidence of a collagen vascular disease in any patient with either isolated proteinuria or haematuria, or with a combination of these abnormalities.

Radiology. The purpose of radiological investigation in this scenario is to identify an anatomical abnormality of the kidneys or urinary tract. Ultrasonography provides an excellent non-invasive screening test that will document most abnormalities. Rarely, excretory urography may be required to identify subtle abnormalities, especially those involving the renal pelvis or calyces.

If all of the results of the studies in step 5 are normal, it is most unlikely that the patient has a serious renal disease responsible for the proteinuria. In reassuring the family, it should be emphasized that proteinuria will disappear in many such children, and in others proteinuria may persist for protracted periods without any evidence for progressive renal failure developing. The patient is typically seen again in 3 months' time, at which outpatient visit urinalysis should be performed, along with repeat measurement of plasma creatinine and electrolytes and urine protein/creatinine ratio. This visit also gives an opportunity to answer the many questions which the family has thought about in the interval. If these repeat test results are satisfactory, it provides another opportunity to give further reassurance. The patient's progress is then monitored twice during the subsequent year and thereafter at yearly intervals.

If any of the screening test results are abnormal, the subsequent approach to the patient's management represents a matter of judgement, based on the magnitude of the abnormality. Such recommendations are usually made by a paediatric nephrologist. If the documented abnormalities at this stage of study are relatively minor, the patient is usually observed and the abnormal study or studies repeated in 1 or more month's time, before making a decision about further investigation. If, on the other hand, the abnormal finding is cause for concern, further evaluation is appropriate. The more common considerations in this advanced testing are analysed in step 6.

Step 6: More advanced evaluation of selected patients: approach and interpretation

Renal biopsy. Not all proteinuric patients warrant a renal biopsy. Indeed, there is a current trend to obtain a renal histological diagnosis in fewer patients. This is based on the argument that the biopsy does not influence management of many of the patients. We do not agree totally with this argument. Knowledge of the underlying disease process may not affect the immediate recommended therapy, but it can be most beneficial in discussing prognosis with the family. Thus, our guidelines for renal biopsy are more liberal than some found elsewhere.

The urinalysis findings are important when determining the need for a biopsy. Renal histology is more likely to be diagnostic when proteinuria is associated with urinary sediment abnormalities than when either proteinuria or haematuria are isolated abnormalities. Other test results also provide important indications for the need for a histological diagnosis. A reduction in GFR of approximately 50% or more typically indicates the need for a biopsy. The exception is the patient recovering from acute postinfectious glomerulonephritis, when it usually is safe to give the patient at least a month to demonstrate recovery before performing a biopsy.

The heavier the proteinuria, the more likely a tissue diagnosis will be established from the biopsy. Thus, we usually recommend biopsy for patients with heavy proteinuria, especially that in excess of $500\,mg/m^2/day$. Again, there is an exception. Patients with uncomplicated idiopathic nephrotic syndrome do not require a renal biopsy at presentation and should be treated empirically with a course of oral prednisolone: a biopsy should, however, be performed if there are atypical features at presentation or if the patient is prednisolone unresponsive (see Chapter 19).

Other potential indications for a renal biopsy include a persistent decrease below normal in C3 levels or serological evidence for a collagen vascular disease. The severity or type of renal involvement in systemic lupus erythematosus (SLE) does not always correlate with the findings on urine sediment. Thus, the absence of haematuria or red-cell casts does not exclude a serious form of glomerulonephritis due to SLE (see Chapter 21).

Occasionally the family of a proteinuric child can be reassured only if the renal histology is known. This can be an important indicator for performing a renal biopsy.

Trial of steroids. As described above and elsewhere (Chapter 19), the majority of children presenting with nephrotic syndrome are treated empirically with a course of corticosteroids. We have additionally cared for several children who had isolated proteinuria which persisted for several years. Mild hypoalbuminaemia was the only associated abnormality. The renal biopsy showed no histological abnormality other than a moderate degree of fusion of podocytes. A trial of steroids was followed by a protracted or apparently permanent remission of proteinuria in approximately half of these cases.

Tubular disorders. If it is suspected from the history or from the findings of eosinophils in the urine that proteinuria results from an interstitial nephritis or from some other disease process that modifies proximal tubular function, measurement of the urinary excretion of β_2-microglobulin (β_2M) can be most helpful. The normal fractional excretion of β_2M is less than 0.5%. With tubular disorders, values may increase to more than 50%. Similar high values are not seen with glomerular disease, even when renal function is markedly decreased. From a practical viewpoint, urine concentrations of β_2M correlate well with the fractional excretion of this protein. A urine β_2M concentration above 1 mg/l strongly suggests proximal tubule dysfunction.

Other tests. The presence of a urinary tract infection or abnormalities on the excretory urogram may indicate the need for more extensive evaluation of the lower urinary tract. The existence of severe hypertension may justify further study, too. Similarly, evidence of tubular dysfunction may warrant an evaluation to determine the cause and whether other abnormalities of tubular function exist.

Conclusions

It is important to re-emphasize that the majority of patients with isolated proteinuria do not have progressive renal disease. However, once it is determined that a proteinuric patient warrants further study, we recommend that this investigation be thorough. This is especially so since the degree of proteinuria correlates with outcome as well as with the rate of progression of the underlying renal disease [44]. It has been suggested that the passage of protein into the glomerular filtrate may result in further glomerular injury. Thus, current efforts are concentrating on

ways to reduce proteinuria, using drugs such as inhibitors of angiotensin converting enzyme or of prostaglandin synthesis [45].

At the end of the studies, the physician must be able to answer in an authoritative manner the multitude of questions that will be posed by the typical family. If the results of the tests indicate no cause for concern, reassurance should include a discussion about 'folk-remedies' and some of the common misconceptions advised by well-meaning but usually poorly informed friends or relatives. For example, a proteinuric patient who had had a partial evaluation one year earlier was referred to the author. The physician had not been able to assuage the family's fear and the child was kept on bed rest for a year on the advice of a friend who told them such bed rest would reduce the degree of proteinuria. Complete evaluation indicated no cause for concern and the patient was able to return to a normal lifestyle.

References

1. Kitagawa T. Lessons learned from the Japanese nephritis screening study. Pediatr Nephrol 1988 2 256–263
2. Birch DF, Fairley KF, Becker GJ, Kincaid-Smith P. Colour Atlas of Urine Microscopy. Chapman and Hall Medical London 1994
3. Vehaskari VM, Rapola J, Koskimies O, Savilahti E, Vilska J, Hallman N. Microscopic haematuria in schoolchildren: epidemiology and clinicopathologic evaluation. J Pediatr 1979 95 676–684
4. Birch DF, Fairley KF. Haematuria: glomerular or nonglomerular? Lancet 1979 ii 845–846
5. Stapleton FB. Morphology of urinary red blood cells: A simple guide in localizing the site of haematuria. Pediatr Clin North Am 1987 34 561
6. Fassett RG, Horgan BA, Mathew TH. Detection of glomerular bleeding by phase-contrast microscopy. Lancet 1982 i 1432–1434
7. Dodge WF, West EF, Smith EH, Bunce H. Proteinuria and hematuria in schoolchildren: epidemiology and early natural history. J Pediatr 1976 88 327–347
8. Ingelfinger JR, Davis AE, Grupe WE. Frequency and etiology of gross haematuria in a general pediatric setting. Pediatrics 1977 59 557–561
9. Piqueras AI, White RHR, Raafat F, Moghal NE, Milford DV. Renal biopsy diagnosis in children presenting with haematuria. Pediatr Nephrol 1998 12 386–391
10. Stapleton FB, Roy S, Noe NH *et al.* Hypercalciuria in children with haematuria. N Engl J Med 1984 310 1345
11. Alport AC. Hereditary familial congenital haemorrhagic nephritis. Br Med J (Clin Res) 1927 1 504–506
12. Flinter F. Alport's syndrome. J Med Genet 1997 34 326–330

13. Perrin D, Junger P, Grunfeld JP *et al*. Perimacular changes in Alport's syndrome. Clin Nephrol 1980 13 163–167

14. Gubler MC, Levy M, Broyer M *et al*. Alport's syndrome: a report of 58 cases and a review of the literature. Am J Med 1981 70 493–505

15. Garcia-Torres R, Guarner V. Leiomiomatosis del esophago, traqueo bronquial y genital asociada con nefropatia hereditaria tipo Alport: un nuevo sindrome. Rev Gastroenterol Mex 1983 48 163–170

16. Churg J, Sherman RL. Pathologic characteristics of hereditary nephritis. Arch Pathol 1973 95 374–379

17. Pirson Y, Goffin E, Cosyns J-P, Noel L-H, Squifflet J-P. Recurrent and de novo anti-GBM disease in the kidney graft. In Recurrence of the Disease in the Renal Graft. Cochat P, Ed. Paris, John Libbey Eurotext, 2001

18. Barker DF, Hostikka SL, Zhou J *et al*. Identification of mutations in the COL4A5 collagen gene in Alport syndrome. Science 1990 247 1224–1227

19. Jais JP, Knebelmann B, Giatras I *et al*. X-linked Alport syndrome: natural history in 195 families and genotype-phenotype correlations in males. J Am Soc Nephrol 2000 11 649–657

20. Knebelmann B, Benessy F, Buemi M *et al*. Autosomal recessive inheritance in Alport syndrome. J Am Soc Nephrol 1993 4 263

21. Flinter FA, Cameron JS, Chantler C *et al*. Genetics of classic Alport's syndrome.Lancet 1988 2 1005–1007

22. Rogers PW, Kurtzman NA, Bunn SM *et al*. Familial benign essential haematuria. Arch Intern Med 1973 131 257–262

23. Aarons I, Smith PS, Davies RA *et al*. Thin basement membrane nephropathy. A clinicopathological study. Clin Nephrol 1989 32 151–158

24. Berger J, Hinglais N. Les depots intercapillaire d'IgA-IgG. J Urol Nephrol (Paris) 1968 74 694–695

25. White RHR, Yoshikawa N, Feehally J. IgA nephropathy and Henoch–Schonlein nephritis. In Pediatric Nephrology. Barratt TM, Avner ED, Harmon WE, Ed. Lippincott Williams and Wilkins Baltimore 691–706

26. Churg J, Bernstein J, Glassock RJ. Renal Disease: Classification and Atlas of Glomerular Disease 2nd Edn. New York, Igaku-Shoin 1995 86

27. Yoshikawa N, Ito H, Nakamura H. IgA nephropathy in children from Japan. Child Nephrol Urol 1989 9 191–199

28. Yoshikawa N, Ito H, Sakai T *et al*. A controlled trial of combined therapy for newly diagnosed severe childhood IgA nephropathy. J Am Soc Nephrol 1999 10 101–109

29. Donadio JJ, Bergstralh EJ, Offord KP *et al*. A controlled trial of fish oil in IgA nephropathy. Mayo Nephrology Collaborative Group. N Engl J Med 1994 331 1194–1199

30. Robson AM. Proteinuria and the nephrotic syndrome. In The Kidney and Body Fluids in Health and Disease 2nd Edn. Klahr S, Ed. New York, Plenum Medical Book Company 1984 369–398

31. Ginevri F, Mutti A, Ghiggeri GM, Alinovo R, Ciardi MR, Bergamaschi E, Verrina E, Gusmano R. Urinary excretion of brush border antigens and other proteins in children with vesico-ureteric reflux. Pediatr Nephrol 1992 6 30–32

32. Buffone GJ. Specific protein measurements in pediatric laboratory medicine. In Pediatric Clinical Chemistry. Hicks JM, Boecky RL, Ed. Philadelphia, WB Saunders, 1984 447–481

33. Brem AS. Neonatal haematuria and proteinuria. Clin Perinatol 1981 8 321–332

34. Ginsberg JM, Chang BS, Matarese RA, Garella S. Use of single voided urine samples to estimate quantitative proteinuria. N Engl J Med 1983 309 1543–1546

35. Houser M. Assessment of proteinuria using random urine samples. J Pediatr 1984 104 845–848

36. Barratt TM, McLaine PN, Soothill JF. Albumin secretion as a measure of glomerular dysfunction in children. Arch Dis Child 1970 45 496–501

37. Yoshimoto M, Tsukahara H, Saito M, Hayashi S, Haruki S, Fujisawa S, Sudo M. Evaluation of variability of proteinuria indices. Pediatr Nephrol 1990 4 136–139

38. Davies AG, Postlethwaite RJ, Price DA, Burn JL, Houlton CA, Fielding BA. Urinary albumin excretion in school children. Arch Dis Child 1984 59 625–630

39. Tomlinson PA. Low molecular weight proteins in children with renal disease. Pediatr Nephrol 1992 6 565–571

40. Murakami M, Yamamoto H, Ueda Y, Murakami K, Yamauchi K. Urinary screening of elementary and junior high school children over a 13-year period in Tokyo. Pediatr Nephrol 1991 5 50–53

41. Vehaskari VM, Rapola J. Isolated proteinuria: analysis of a schoolage population. J Pediatr 1982 101 661–668

42. Vehaskari VM. Mechanism of orthostatic proteinuria. Pediatr Nephrol 1990 4 328–330

43. Springberg PD, Garrett LE, Thompson AL, Collins NF, Lordon RE, Robinson RR. Fixed and reproducible orthostatic proteinuria: results of a 20-year follow-up study. Ann Intern Med 1982 97 516–519

44. Walser M. Progression of chronic renal failure in man. Kidney Int 1990 37 1195–1210

45. Hebert LA, Wilmer WA, Falkenhain ME, Ladson-Wofford SE, Nahman NS, Rovin BH. Renoprotection: one or many therapies? Kidney Int 2001 1211–1226

2 | Disorders of fluid and electrolyte balance

T. James Beattie

Introduction

Disturbances of fluid and electrolyte balance are a frequent occurrence in paediatric practice, and present in a wide variety of clinical scenarios, varying from the previously well infant who develops acute viral gastroenteritis to the child in the intensive care unit with multiple organ failure.

The evaluation of a patient with a fluid and electrolyte problem is first and foremost clinical and laboratory parameters should always be regarded as complementary. Unfortunately, there is a natural tendency to correlate changes in plasma sodium (P_{Na}), with changes in total body sodium, e.g. a low P_{Na} is automatically assumed to indicate sodium deficiency. However, both extracellular fluid (ECF) depletion and expansion may occur with a low, normal or elevated P_{Na}, and the interpretation of changes in P_{Na} requires a parallel evaluation of ECF volume and, in particular, assessment of effective intravascular volume.

In practice, it is the combination of serial clinical examination, which should include weight recording, serial biochemical data and the response of both to intervention that allows successful management.

Distribution and composition of body fluid compartments

Osmotic forces are important in determining the distribution of water between the intracellular (ICF) and ECF compartments. Since cell membranes are fully permeable to water, osmotic equilibrium is maintained and the volume of each compartment is determined by the concentration of the principal osmotically active solute. Potassium is the principal solute for the ICF, sodium for the ECF and plasma proteins for the intravascular compartment. This differential composition is maintained by cell membrane pump activity and by molecular size and charge. Solutes such as urea and glucose (except in certain pathological states, particularly diabetic ketoacidosis [DKA]) have little influence on transcellular water movement.

It follows that changes in the body content of sodium chloride lead to parallel changes in ECF volume, i.e. sodium chloride retention results in ECF volume expansion while depletion leads to ECF volume contraction. The effects of ECF volume depletion are usually shared between the intravascular and interstitial fluid (ISF) compartments. However, plasma volume may be contracted while total ECF volume is increased, with the excess sequestered as oedema. Conversely, sodium retention secondary to renal disease usually leads to expansion in both plasma and ISF compartments, thus oedema may be present in both plasma volume expanded and contracted states.

Central to the evaluation of disturbances in sodium and water balance, is the assessment of ECF volume and, in practice, the accuracy of this evaluation reflects the experience of the clinician [1]. The signs of ECF volume contraction are usually divided into those signs of reduced ISF volume (dehydration) and those signs of reduced effective intravascular volume (hypovolaemia) (Table 2.1).

Role of urinary sodium and chloride concentration

Measurement of random urinary sodium (U_{Na}) and chloride (U_{Cl}) concentration is useful, particularly in patients with signs of ECF depletion and also as confirmation of hypovolaemia in patients with ECF expansion, e.g. cardiac and hepatic failure and nephrotic syndrome. U_{Na} and U_{Cl} usually vary in parallel and are typically less than 20 mmol/l at any level of renal function if hypovolaemia is the only problem, although somewhat higher levels do not exclude the diagnosis since there may also be a high rate of water reabsorption. The corollary is that values above 20 mmol/l suggest normal or increased intravascular volume [2].

However, in certain circumstances patients with ECF volume depletion may have a higher than expected U_{Na}. This most often occurs in metabolic alkalosis due to vomiting, and in this setting the

Table 2.1　Symptoms and signs of ECF volume contraction

	Body weight loss[a]		
	5% (3%)	10% (6%)	15% (9%)
Symptoms	Thirst	Restlessness/lethargy	Confusion/coma
Signs of reduced interstitial fluid (dehydration)			
Colour	Pale	Grey	Mottled
Mucous membranes	Dry	Parched	Cracked
Eyes		Sunken	Very sunken
Skin turgor		Diminished	Loss
Fontanelle	Flat	Depressed	Sunken
Signs of reduced intravascular volume (hypovolaemia)			
Pulse		Tachycardia	Tachycardia/low volume pulse
CRT		>3 s	>5 s
BP		Normal/low	Low/unrecordable
Urine output		Oliguria	Anuria

[a] Percentages outwith parentheses indicate estimates for infancy and those within are estimates beyond infancy.
BP, blood pressure; CRT, capillary refill time.

need to excrete bicarbonate in the urine as sodium bicarbonate, in order to correct the alkalosis may lead to a high U_{Na} despite the presence of ECF volume depletion. In contrast, there is no stimulus for urinary chloride wasting and the U_{Cl} will be appropriately low, reflecting both the true ECF volume status and the associated hypochloraemia. Other circumstances in which ECF depletion may be accompanied by a U_{Na} (and U_{Cl}) above 20 mmol/l are salt wasting states associated with renal or adrenal insufficiency and following diuretic therapy.

Fractional excretion of sodium

An alternative to random measurement of urinary sodium is the calculation of fractional excretion (FE_{Na}), i.e. the fraction of filtered sodium that is excreted in the urine. FE_{Na} directly evaluates renal sodium handling and is therefore not affected by urine volume. It is calculated as follows:

FE_{Na} (%) = ($U_{Na} \times$ plasma creatinine/$P_{Na} \times$ urine creatinine) $\times$ 100.

FE_{Na} is the most accurate screening test to differentiate pre-renal disease that is volume responsive from acute tubular necrosis, the two most common causes of acute renal failure (Chapter 22). In this setting, where the glomerular filtration rate (GFR) is very low, the FE_{Na} is usually less than 1% in the presence of volume-responsive pre-renal disease. However, it should be appreciated that in a number of specific types of acute renal insufficiency, e.g. congestive cardiac failure, severe liver disease and

acute glomerulonephritis, a FE_{Na} below 1% does not indicate a volume-responsive component [3].

In addition, FE_{Na} is more difficult to evaluate in patients with a relatively normal GFR, since there is no absolute value for the FE_{Na} in hypovolaemia and, in practice, a value of less than 0.1–0.2% is required. This apparent discrepancy relates to the importance of the filtered sodium load (GFR $\times P_{Na}$), the more important determinant of which is GFR, on the level of FE_{Na} that is indicative of hypovolaemia. The following case scenarios illustrate this principle:

- Case 1: GFR ~ 100 ml/min (150 l/day), P_{Na} 140 mmol/l, filtered sodium load 21 000 mmol/day. If hypovolaemia is present, the FE_{Na} required to produce a U_{Na} less than 20 mmol/day (or <20 mmol/l on a random sample) is less than 0.1%.

- Case 2: GFR ~ 10 ml/min (15 l/day), P_{Na} 140 mmol/l, filtered sodium load 2100 mmol/day. If hypovolaemia is the only problem, the FE_{Na} required to produce a U_{Na} less than 20 mmol/day (20 mmol/l on a random sample) is less than 1%.

These examples demonstrate the difficulty in using FE_{Na} as an indicator of hypovolaemia and unless the value is very low, i.e. less than 0.1–0.2%, the approximate GFR must be *known* in order to determine whether sodium is being conserved appropriately.

In the context of hypovolaemia and salt overload/poisoning (see later), the interpretation of U_{Na} and FE_{Na} is critically dependent on assessment of ECF volume. In most clinically important circumstances, U_{Na} and FE_{Na} parallel each other and are most diagnostically beneficial if very low or high. In these circumstances, it is highly unlikely that there would be a contradiction between the two parameters.

Urinary electrolyte concentrations need to be interpreted with care, since both spot samples and timed collections generally reflect the management immediately preceding sample collection, e.g. intravenous fluid and/or bicarbonate and diuretic therapy, irrespective of ECF volume or plasma electrolytes. Once the bolus effect has passed, however, U_{Na} and U_{Cl} reflect effective intravascular volume.

Plasma osmolality

The plasma osmolality (P_{osm}) is determined by the concentration of the different solutes in the plasma which, in normal circumstances, are predominantly sodium salts (chloride and bicarbonate), glucose and urea, and is measured by freezing-point depression. This technique measures the solute content of the water contained in the specimen of plasma, but provides no information about the tonicity or effective osmolality, since it measures all solutes whether permeant or impermeant. However, the contribution of urea and glucose (outside DKA) to tonicity of the plasma, and therefore ECF, is minimal.

When the water content of the plasma is normal (93%) the P_{osm}, and by deduction the ECF osmolality, may be approximated by the following formula, which has been shown to fall within 5–10 mosm/kg of the measured value:

calculated $P_{osm} = [2 \times$ plasma sodium (mmol/l)] + plasma glucose (mmol/l) + plasma urea (mmol/l) [4].

If some additional solute other than a sodium salt, glucose or urea is present in the plasma, the difference between the measured and calculated osmolalities, i.e. the osmolal gap, will be more than 10 mosm/kg. The osmolal gap is important in the evaluation of the patient with an increased anion-gap acidosis (Chapter 3), who may have ingested a low molecular weight but permeant toxin, such as methanol or ethylene glycol. In addition, an increased osmolal gap is seen in association with hyponatraemia, when an impermeant solute is present, resulting in a net transfer of water from the ICF to the ECF (see below).

Urine osmolality versus specific gravity

The urine osmolality (U_{osm}) is a measure of concentration of urine and is determined primarily by the level of

Key points: General principles of fluid and electrolyte balance

- Serial clinical evaluation of a patient with a fluid and electrolyte problem is paramount and laboratory parameters are complementary.

- Random urinary sodium and chloride concentrations are typically <20 mmol/l in hypovolaemia and >20 mmol/l with normal or increased intravascular volume.

- An unexpectedly high urine sodium concentration can occur in the presence of ECF depletion when there is:
  – metabolic alkalosis;
  – salt-wasting states (renal or adrenal insufficiency, following diuretic therapy).

- An alternative to random urinary sodium is the fractional excretion of sodium (FE_{Na}).

- With low GFR a FE_{Na} <1% suggests volume-responsive pre-renal disease.

- In certain types of acute renal failure (ARF) a FE_{Na} < 1% *does not indicate volume responsiveness* (congestive cardiac failure, severe liver disease, acute glomerulonephritis).

- FE_{Na} is more difficult to evaluate in patients with a relatively normal GFR as there is *no absolute value for FE_{Na} in hypovolaemia*.

- Urinary electrolyte concentrations, both random and timed, need to be interpreted with care as they may reflect the management immediately preceding sample collection.

- The osmolal gap, i.e. measured – calculated plasma osmolality, is important in the assessment of hyponatraemia and metabolic acidosis.

- The urine osmolality (U_{osm}) is of practical benefit in the evaluation of hyponatraemia and hypernatraemia.

- Generally the U_{osm} can be predicted from the specific gravity (SG). This correlation is lost when there are appreciable quantities of larger molecules in the urine, e.g. glucose and radio-contrast media.

antidiuretic hormone (ADH). In patients with normal renal function, U_{osm} can range from a minimum of 50 mosm/kg to a maximum of 1200 mosm/kg. Variations in the U_{osm} play a central role in the regulation of the P_{osm} and P_{Na}. These relationships allow the U_{osm} to be of practical benefit in the differential diagnosis of both hyponatraemia and hypernatraemia.

The U_{osm} is determined by the number of particles in the urine, in contrast to specific gravity (SG) which is a measure of the weight of the solution compared to that of an equal volume of distilled water. SG is determined by both the number and size of particles in the urine and, in most circumstances, varies in a relatively predictable way with the U_{osm}, with the SG rising by 0.001 for approximately every 40 mosm/kg increase in U_{osm}. The SG may be converted into U_{osm} by multiplying the last two figures of the SG by 40. Thus, a U_{osm} of 280 mosm/kg (equivalent to that of plasma) is usually associated with a SG of 1.007.

This relationship between U_{osm} and SG is altered when there are appreciable quantities of larger molecules in the urine, such as glucose and radiocontrast media. In these settings the SG may reach 1.030–1.050, falsely suggesting a concentrated urine despite a U_{osm} that may only be 300 mosm/kg. In circumstances in which the urine is maximally dilute, there is a close correlation between the U_{osm} and SG as there are no causes of falsely low SG measurements.

Hyponatraemia

Hyponatraemia is by definition a P_{Na} of less than 130 mmol/l and reflects a deficiency of sodium relative to water; however, total body sodium may be low, normal or high. Pure sodium deficiency is very rarely observed at any age, the occurrence and association with a fluid deficit being the norm and, in practice, hyponatraemia is equally, or more likely to be due to water retention. The two mechanisms that result in hyponatraemia are:

- loss of sodium in excess of water;
- gain of water in excess of sodium.

Steps in assessment

These are summarized in Fig. 2.1.

Step 1: Ensure that the venous blood sample has not been improperly drawn

For example, at a site proximal to a hypotonic saline or dextrose infusion.

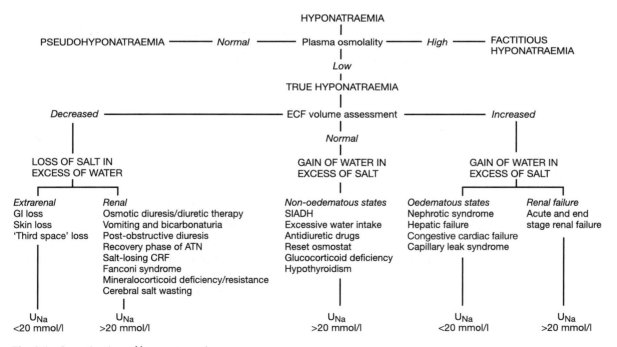

Fig. 2.1 Investigation of hyponatraemia.

Step 2: Measure the P_{osm} and osmolal gap to establish that true hyponatraemia is present

Factitious hyponatraemia occurs as a result of a fluid shift between the ICF and ECF compartments due to the presence of abnormal, relatively impermeant solutes in the ECF compartment. Examples of such solutes are glucose in excess, mannitol, sorbitol and maltose. In factitious hyponatraemia, the measured P_{osm} is high despite the low P_{Na} and, with the exception of hyperglycaemia, the osmolal gap will be greater than 10 mosm/kg.

Pseudohyponatraemia is associated with a normal P_{osm} and an increased osmolal gap may occur if there is a reduction in the fraction of plasma water. In normal subjects, the plasma water is approximately 93% of the plasma volume, with fats and proteins accounting for the remaining 7%. The plasma water fraction may fall below 80% in patients with marked hyperlipidaemia or hyperproteinaemia and if the technique of flame photometry, which measures electrolyte concentration in whole plasma, is used, the P_{Na} is artefactually reduced. If the protein or lipid is extracted and the estimation repeated, the P_{Na} concentration will be normal and the osmolal gap will disappear. Most laboratories now use ion-selective electrodes or other techniques that measure the plasma water electrolyte concentration directly, and thus in most circumstances the above problem should no longer arise.

In *true hyponatraemia* both the calculated and measured P_{osm} will be subnormal (<280 mosm/kg) and the osmolal gap less than 10 mosm/kg.

Step 3: Assess ECF volume

In order to allow further evaluation, an accurate assessment of ECF volume status and, in particular, of effective intravascular volume status, is essential. This should be complemented by measurement of the urine sodium concentration.

Extrarenal loss of sodium in excess of water (Table 2.2 and Fig. 2.1) will give rise to signs of dehydration/hypovolaemia. If renal function is normal, the

Table 2.2   Causes of hyponatraemia

Factitious hyponatraemia	ascites
(P_{osm} high and osmolal gap > 10)	pancreatitis
Hyperglycaemia	muscle trauma
Impermeant solutes:	Renal loss (U_{Na} > 20 mmol/l)
Mannitol	Osmotic diuresis
Sorbitol	Diuretic therapy
Maltose	Vomiting and bicarbonaturia
Pseudohyponatraemia	Post-obstructive diuresis
(P_{osm} normal and osmolal gap > 10)	Recovery phase of ATN
Hyperlipidaemia	Salt-losing CRF
Hyperproteinaemia	Fanconi syndrome and RTA
True hyponatraemia	Mineralocorticoid deficiency/resistance
(P_{osm} low and osmolal gap < 10)	Cerebral salt wasting
Loss of sodium in excess of water	Gain of water in excess of sodium
Extrarenal loss (U_{Na} < 20 mmol/l)	Non-oedematous states (U_{Na} > 20 mmol/l)
Gastrointestinal loss:	SIADH
diarrhoea	Excessive water intake
vomiting	Glucocorticoid deficiency
aspiration	Hypothyroidism
fistula	Antidiuretic drugs
stoma	Reset osmostat
Skin loss:	Oedematous states (U_{Na} < 20 mmol/l)
heat stress	Nephrotic syndrome
cystic fibrosis	Hepatic failure
adrenal insufficiency	Cardiac failure
'Third space' loss:	'Capillary/vascular leak' syndrome
thermal injury	Renal failure (U_{Na} > 20 mmol/l)
intestinal obstruction	

P_{osm}, plasma osmolality; U_{Na}, urinary sodium; ATN, acute tubular necrosis; CRF, chronic renal failure; RTA, renal tubular acidosis; SIADH, syndrome of inappropriate ADH secretion.

appropriate response will be the production of a small volume of urine with a U_{Na} of less than 20 mmol/l and U_{osm} greater than 800 mosm/kg.

All of the conditions listed in Table 2.2 under extrarenal losses may result in isotonic fluid losses, i.e. equivalent losses of sodium and water, but in this circumstance the P_{Na} will remain within normal limits (130–150 mmol/l) and the urine biochemical findings will remain unchanged, i.e. the U_{Na} will be less than 20 mmol/l.

Hyponatraemic states are increasing in incidence and may account for around 25% of infants with diarrhoeal dehydration. The clinical signs of dehydration/hypovolaemia may present with a corresponding smaller fluid deficit than with isotonic fluid loss. As well as the effect on ECF volume, the fall in ECF sodium concentration leads to a drop of ECF osmolality and, if hypotonic fluid replacement is given, symptomatic water intoxication (see below) may occur despite the presence of a fluid deficit [5].

Renal salt-losing states will similarly give rise to signs of dehydration/hypovolaemia. U_{Na} remains high (>20 mmol/l) and urine volume will be maintained until a relatively late stage, thereby exacerbating the loss of salt and water. In patients with a metabolic alkalosis secondary to prolonged vomiting, bicarbonaturia may result in a U_{Na} greater than 20 mmol/l; however, in this circumstance the U_{Cl} will be discrepant, at less than 20 mmol/l. The association of hyponatraemia and significant hyperkalaemia should always suggest the possibility of adrenal insufficiency or mineralocorticoid resistance. The syndrome of *cerebral salt wasting* (CSW) leads to renal salt wasting due to defective tubular reabsorption, probably mediated by a brain natriuretic hormone. CSW may be associated with subarachnoid haemorrhage, CNS infection, head injury, intracranial tumours and both open and closed neurosurgical procedures. In contrast to the *syndrome of inappropriate ADH secretion* (SIADH) (see below), which can present with identical changes in electrolyte balance, the hyponatraemia in CSW is secondary to volume depletion and is associated with hypouricaemia. However, differentiating between these two conditions may be difficult and in the absence of clinical signs of hypovolaemia central venous pressure recording is necessary [6].

The other major mechanism of true hyponatraemia is *gain of water in excess of sodium* (Table 2.2 and Fig. 2.1). This is further subdivided into situations in which the ECF is normal or reduced. SIADH is the paradigm of a *non-oedematous state with true hyponatraemia*. In this condition the primary underlying mechanism is retention of water. As water (unlike sodium) is freely permeant, the water is distributed equally between the ICF and ECF compartments. The expansion of the ICF compartment has a much greater clinical effect because of the increase in intracerebral water, resulting in neurological complications. These supervene before the water retention is sufficient to produce clinically apparent oedema. Additionally, the maintained ECF volume results in an appropriate renal response with excretion of sodium, so that, typically, as SIADH develops the U_{Na} is greater than 20 mmol/l.

Physiological regulation of ADH secretion involves both osmotic and non-osmotic stimuli. In certain clinical conditions, continued secretion of ADH in the presence of ECF hypo-osmolality may either be appropriate, in the presence of non-osmotic stimuli (e.g. diminished effective intravascular volume), or inappropriate, if no obvious stimuli are present. Since the original description of the syndrome of inappropriate ADH secretion (SIADH), it has become clear that in some of the conditions in which it has been described (Table 2.3), notably malignant disease, ectopic production of ADH is responsible. In others, the mechanism remains unclear and the subject of ongoing debate [7].

In SIADH, an increase in the ECF volume and reduction in osmolality fails to suppress ADH

Table 2.3 Causes of the syndrome of inappropriate ADH secretion

CNS disorders
  Infection
  Malignancy, primary or secondary
  Trauma
  Hypoxic–ischaemic encephalopathy
  Vascular accidents
  Guillain–Barré syndrome
  Cerebral malformation
Pulmonary disorders
  Infection, acute and chronic
  Malignancy
  Cystic fibrosis
  Positive-pressure ventilation
Post-surgery
  Anaesthetic or premedication
  Abdominal, cardiothoracic and neurosurgery
Miscellaneous
  Acute intermittent porphyria
  Leukaemia
  Lymphoma

secretion and, if normal fluid intake is maintained, hyponatraemia develops. This sequence of events will continue until a new equilibrium is achieved, when restoration of aldosterone secretion and decrease in collecting duct permeability serve to limit the sodium loss and water retention respectively.

Unfortunately, the term SIADH is frequently abused in clinical practice, since many examples of hyponatraemia have an alternative explanation. It is therefore important that the following diagnostic criteria are adhered to:

- Hyponatraemia and hypo-osmolality.

- An inappropriately elevated U_{osm}. In the presence of reduced P_{osm}, a maximally dilute urine (osmolality < 100 msom/kg) should be expected. A U_{osm} above this level should be viewed as inappropriate in the presence of reduced P_{osm}.

- U_{osm} may therefore be isotonic or hypotonic compared with plasma and still be considered inappropriately high in the context of this syndrome.

- Evidence of an increase in body water. This is perhaps best characterized as an absence of signs and symptoms of dehydration/hypovolaemia in the presence of hyponatraemia, rather than the presence of overt oedema or a hyperdynamic circulation.

- Absence of other conditions which cause retention of free water and hyponatraemia, e.g. renal, hepatic or cardiac failure, or adrenal, pituitary and thyroid dysfunction.

- The absence of other known stimuli of ADH secretion, e.g. pharmacological, thermal injury, pain and nausea.

- Decrease in haematocrit, plasma albumin, plasma urea and creatinine concentrations as a consequence of increased ECF volume and GFR.

- Urinary sodium excretion, as in normal subjects, is a reflection in sodium intake and U_{Na} is usually greater than 20 mmol/l and shows a normal response to sodium restriction.

SIADH may be acute or chronic in evolution and the neurological symptoms rarely present until the P_{Na} falls below 120 mmol/l, but, importantly, they may develop at higher levels of P_{Na} if the rate of fall is rapid. The early signs are lethargy and irritability, with later signs of stupor, disorientation and convulsions being indicative of raised intracranial pressure.

Compulsive water drinking sufficient to produce hyponatraemia is rare in childhood but is occasionally seen in adolescents with emotional or psychiatric disturbance. *Other examples of excessive water intake* occur with the use of hypotonic intravenous and oral fluid and enema therapy and following the absorption of water through the respiratory tract in patients treated with nebulized gas therapy or in a humidified atmosphere. As with SIADH, the retained water is distributed between the ICF and ECF compartments so that oedema and/or hyperdynamic circulation is rarely seen. In severe cases the neurological symptoms are similar to those of SIADH. Urine volume is increased in an attempt to eliminate the excess water intake and is maximally dilute ($U_{osm} < 100$ mosm/kg). Urinary sodium excretion will reflect sodium intake and the U_{Na} is also affected by the high urine flow.

A number of *antidiuretic drugs* are capable of causing hyponatraemia secondary to water retention (Table 2.4).

Chronic asymptomatic hyponatraemia may occasionally be seen in children with chronic infection and malnutrition. In these patients the level of ECF osmolality at which ADH is released is less than 285 mosm/kg [8] (*reset osmostat*). Since these patients respond appropriately to both salt and water loading, specific therapy is not indicated.

Table 2.4 Drugs associated with hyponatraemia

Promote ADH release
Chlorpropamide
Clofibrate
Carbamazepine
Vincristine
Vinblastine
Cyclophosphamide
Opiates
Histamine
Isoprenaline
Nicotine
Colchicine
Barbiturates
Potentiate ADH action
Chlorpropamide
Tolbutamide
Phenformin
Impair renal water excretion independent of ADH
Oxytocin
Thiazide diuretics
NSAID

Hyponatraemia may occur in patients with *gluco-corticoid deficiency* secondary to impaired diluting capacity even in the absence of mineralocorticoid deficiency, and in *hypothyroidism* secondary to impaired distal nephron sodium delivery and non-osmotic release of ADH.

In *oedematous states*, such as nephrotic syndrome, and in hypoproteinaemia secondary to malnutrition, the reduction in plasma oncotic pressure allows a movement of fluid from the intravascular into the ISF compartment. This reduction in effective intravascular volume leads to the activation of the three 'hypovolaemic' hormones, angiotensin II, noradrenaline and ADH, resulting in a decrease in renal sodium and water excretion. This may be viewed as an attempt to correct the hypovolaemia but, because of the reduced plasma oncotic pressure, the sodium and water retention leads to an expansion of the ECF and the production of oedema. In congestive cardiac failure and hepatic insufficiency, the effective intravascular volume is reduced due to a reduced cardiac output and peripheral vasodilatation, respectively. In these contexts, the increase in plasma ADH levels tends to correlate with the severity of the disease, making the presence of hyponatraemia an important prognostic sign.

The *'capillary or vascular leak' syndrome* is seen in patients who have undergone prolonged cardio-pulmonary bypass, ECMO, liver transplantation or other surgical procedures, and in acute sepsis in which cardiac output, renal perfusion and capillary integrity are compromised. These patients often require large volumes of intravenous fluid in an attempt to maintain intravascular volume and urine output, resulting in oedema and hypoproteinaemia in the absence of proteinuria.

Provided the renal function is normal, the U_{Na} will be less than 20 mmol/l and U_{osm} greater than 800 mosm/kg in oedematous states and in the capillary leak syndrome.

Salt and water retention may occur in both *acute* and *end stage renal failure*. In the presence of a hypo-osmolar intake, more water than sodium will be retained, resulting in hyponatraemia. Retention of sodium and water results in expansion of the ECF, so that oedema and a hyperdynamic circulation dominate the clinical picture. The urine volume is reduced and the U_{Na} is greater than 20 mmol/l. The U_{osm} will be similar to the P_{osm} that should be maintained despite the hyponatraemia, because of the elevation in plasma urea.

Key points: Assessment of hyponatraemia

- Hyponatraemia occurs when there is either a loss of sodium in excess of water or a gain of water in excess of sodium.

- Clinical assessment of ECF volume is essential in the evaluation of hyponatraemia, since total body sodium may be normal, increased or decreased.

- Hyponatraemia due to extrarenal loss of salt in excess of water characteristically results in a U_{Na} concentration of <20 mmol/l.

- All the causes of extrarenal loss of salt in excess of water can also result in isotonic losses, when the P_{Na} will be normal but the U_{Na} will be <20 mmol/l.

- U_{Na} > 20 mmol/l in the presence of signs of dehydration/hypovolaemia suggests a renal salt-losing state.

- The exception to this rule is metabolic alkalosis, e.g. due to prolonged vomiting, where the U_{Na} may be >20 mmol/l but the U_{Cl} will be discrepant at <20 mmol/l.

- The association of hyponatraemia and significant hyperkalaemia suggests adrenal insufficiency or mineralocorticoid resistance.

- Hyponatraemia due to gain of water in excess of sodium is the other major mechanism of true hyponatraemia. This is further subdivided into:
  – non-oedematous states with true hyponatraemia (SIADH is the paradigm);
  – oedematous states including renal failure.

- The label of SIADH is often applied erroneously to situations in which there are alternative explanations for hyponatraemia, and strict diagnostic criteria should be applied.

Management of hyponatraemic states

Management of renal and extrarenal losses of salt and water

When considering therapy of extrarenal losses of salt and water and renal salt-losing states, it is important to consider the extent of the fluid (Table 2.1) and sodium deficit. The sodium deficit, in mmoles, may be approximated in the following manner: $(140 - P_{Na}) \times 0.65 \times$ body weight (kg).

The main issues relating to fluid and electrolyte therapy in hyponatraemic (and isonatraemic) dehydration are: firstly, whether the replacement should be oral or intravenous; secondly, the duration of the rehydration period; and finally, whether colloid solutions, including human albumin, should continue to be used in resuscitation regimes.

Parenteral fluid and electrolyte replacement has been popular and, to some extent, remains so despite the abundant evidence that oral rehydration therapy (ORT) with glucose/electrolyte solutions is a safe and effective alternative [9]. The rationale for the composition of ORT solutions is that glucose promotes the active transport of electrolytes, the absorption of which theoretically increases in efficiency as the ratio of carbohydrate to sodium approaches 1:1.

The WHO solution (sodium 90 and glucose 110 mmol/l) was designed for use in developing countries where the risk of bacterial diarrhoea, and therefore of high stool electrolyte loss, is much higher. In the United Kingdom, where viral diarrhoea, which is associated with a lower stool electrolyte concentration, is more common, commercial ORT solutions have a sodium and glucose content of 50–60 and 90–110 mmol/l, respectively.

Recent evaluation of ORT solutions of reduced osmolality (sodium 60 and glucose 84 mmol/l) has shown that these may be preferable to the conventional WHO solution in non-cholera diarrhoea in developing countries [10]. In addition, there is good evidence that cereal, e.g. rice-based solutions, tend to produce more rapid resolution of diarrhoea and should be the ORT of choice in cholera.

Provided the infant is not shocked and is able to tolerate oral or nasogastric fluids, 50 ml/kg (3–5% weight loss) or 100 ml/kg (6–10% weight loss) of an ORT solution with a sodium content of 60–90 mmol/l, with allowances for ongoing losses, should be administered over a period of 4–6 hours. If the infant is clinically hydrated at that point, half-strength milk feeds (10 mmol/l sodium) should be introduced at 120 ml/kg/day, again with an additional allowance for ongoing losses. If not, the above regime is repeated, based on the current deficit.

As clinical evidence of hypovolaemia develops early in hyponatraemic dehydration, a resuscitation phase is not uncommonly required. In this event, intravenous 0.9% saline or Ringer's solution at a volume of 20 ml/kg should be given over 30 min and repeated twice if necessary. In those who do not improve significantly with this volume of fluid, and in patients with pre-existing renal, cardiac or pulmonary disease, early establishment of central venous pressure measurement is advisable. If the possibility of a hypoadrenal state is considered, intravenous hydrocortisone should be given.

If large volumes of saline are used acutely in resuscitation, hyperchloraemic metabolic acidosis may develop as a consequence of dilution of ECF bicarbonate. This may be prevented by the use of Ringer's solution, although in the context of a significant pre-existing metabolic acidosis, e.g. DKA or underlying hepatic dysfunction, infusion of Ringer's solution may exacerbate the acidosis because of impaired conversion of lactate to bicarbonate.

When the resuscitation phase has been completed, ORT should be introduced but, if continuing intravenous replacement is deemed necessary, the remaining deficit should be replaced with 0.9% saline and the maintenance fluid should be appropriate to the age of the child (Table 2.5). Throughout the period of rehydration, routine clinical monitoring is important, in particular of urine output and weight, and intravenous potassium replacement should only be given when urine output is satisfactory.

The duration of the fluid and sodium deficit correction period in hyponatraemic and isonatraemic dehydration following correction of shock, has traditionally been 24 hours. However, clinical experience with 'rapid rehydration', i.e. deficit correction over 6 hours by ORT as above, is favourable, particularly in the treatment of diarrhoeal dehydration [11].

The issue of the safety and efficacy of crystalloid versus colloid solutions in resuscitation remains

Table 2.5 Maintenance fluid and electrolyte requirements

	Weight (kg)	Daily requirement
Water	3–10	100 ml/kg
	11–20	1000 ml plus 50 ml/kg for each additional kg above 10 kg
	>20	1500 ml plus 20 mg/kg for each additional kg above 20 mg
Sodium, potassium and chloride	3–10	2.5 mmol/kg
	11–30	2 mmol/kg
	>30	1.5 mmol/kg

contentious and the existing data, suggesting an increased risk of mortality with the use of various colloid solutions to treat hypovolaemia following trauma and surgery and in thermal injury, have to be interpreted with caution [12]. At present, since there is no clear consensus, clinicians should assess the risk/benefit ratio of colloid in individual clinical circumstances and perhaps continue to use a judicious mix of both types of fluid according to their own experience, remembering that the main priority in hypovolaemia is rapid restoration of circulating volume.

Key points: Management of hyponatraemia due to renal and extrarenal losses of salt and water

- Unless the child is shocked, there is abundant evidence that oral rehydration therapy (ORT) is safe and effective.

- ORT solution with a sodium concentration of 60–90 mmol/l should be used.

- In children with hypovolaemia, 20 ml/kg of 0.9% saline or Ringer's solution should be given intravenously (i.v.) over 30 minutes and repeated on two occasions if necessary.

- In those who do not improve with this volume of fluid, and in patients with pre-existing renal, cardiac or pulmonary disease, central venous pressure measurement is advisable.

- When successful resuscitation has been achieved, i.v. or orally, ORT should be introduced to correct the deficit (and provide for maintenance fluids and ongoing losses) over 24 hours.

- More rapid rehydration (over 6 hours) has proved safe and effective, particularly in diarrhoeal dehydration.

- Potassium replacement should only be commenced when a satisfactory urine output is established.

- There is no consensus about the safety of colloid in resuscitation, and clinicians should assess the risk/benefit ratio in individual cases, remembering that the main priority is rapid restoration of circulating volume.

Management of water retention in the presence of elevation of ADH levels

The management of water retention in the presence of an elevation in ADH is dependent on the severity of the neurological symptoms. The basis of therapy is the creation of a negative water balance at the same time as attempting to manage the underlying disease process. In the asymptomatic patient, water should be restricted to 25% of daily maintenance requirements (Table 2.5). If water restriction is unsuccessful, intravenous loop diuretic therapy should be used to increase free water excretion. Sodium and potassium losses in the urine should be measured and replaced within the restricted fluid regime.

When symptoms of water intoxication, particularly headache, lethargy, confusion or altered conscious level, are present, the objective is to institute a rapid but controlled correction of the cerebral overhydration. This may be accomplished by increasing the tonicity of the ECF with the use of hypertonic saline in combination with loop diuretic therapy. Sodium chloride—10 ml/kg of 3% (513 mmol/l) and 6 ml/kg of 5% (855 mmol/l)—will increase the P_{Na} by 10 mmol/l. The infusion rate should be designed to increase the P_{Na} by 1–2 mmol/l/h (1–2 ml/kg/h of 3% solution), depending on the severity of the neurological symptoms, the aim being to increase the P_{Na} to 120–125 mmol/l [13]. Further correction to a normal P_{Na} should then be achieved by continuing fluid restriction. If the neurological symptoms are severe, e.g. convulsions and/or coma, 3% sodium chloride may be safely infused at a rate of 4–6 ml/kg/h [14]. If SIADH is felt to warrant prolonged therapy, certain pharmacological agents could be considered, e.g. lithium or demeclocycline.

Attention has been focused in recent years on the possible relationship between the treatment of patients with hyponatraemia due to water retention and the neurological outcome. Concern exists that some patients, particularly those with chronic hyponatraemia, i.e. longer than 48 hours' duration, do well initially but may suddenly develop significant neurological deterioration leading to death or permanent sequelae [14]. The brain histology in fatal cases shows both central pontine myelinolysis and demyelination of the extrapontine myelin-bearing neurons. In the typical case behavioural change, fluctuating levels of consciousness and convulsions are the prodromal signs. Despite some experimental data supporting the relationship of this complication to the rapidity of correction of hyponatraemia, there are a few clinical data, especially in children, to support this concept.

However, in view of the possibility that rapid correction of hyponatraemia predisposes to demyelination, it is appropriate that correction is handled carefully in symptomatic patients with chronic hyponatraemia or if the duration is unclear. The rate of correction should be 1–2 mmol/l/h, depending on the severity of the neurological symptoms, until the P_{Na} has increased by 10% or about 10 mmol/l, and thereafter at a rate not exceeding 1 mmol/l/h or 15 mmol/l/24 h, until a P_{Na} of 120–125 mmol/l has been achieved [13].

In refractory congestive cardiac failure, fluid restriction in combination with an angiotensin converting enzyme (ACE) inhibitor and a loop diuretic may correct the P_{Na}. However, despite these benefits, ACE inhibitors may be poorly tolerated in patients with advanced congestive cardiac failure, leading to symptomatic hypotension and further elevation in plasma urea and/or hyperkalaemia.

Guidelines on the management of salt and water retention in renal failure are given in Chapter 22.

Key points: Management of water retention in the presence of elevation of ADH levels

- Management is dependent on the severity of the neurological symptoms.

- In the asymptomatic patient water should be restricted to 25% of maintenance.

- If this is not successful, intravenous loop diuretic should be used.

- If there are symptoms of water intoxication, hypertonic saline and loop diuretics should be used to raise P_{Na} by 1–2 mmol/l/h.

- If symptoms are very severe, 3% sodium chloride can be infused at 4–6 ml/kg/h.

- If prolonged SIADH is anticipated, lithium or demeclocycline may be useful.

Key points: Management of hyponatraemia due to gain of water in excess of salt

- Treatment is primarily salt and water restriction and diuretic therapy.

- In hypoproteinaemic states 20% albumin may be indicated.

- In capillary leak syndrome:
  – diuretics tend to aggravate the hypovolaemia;
  – use of low-dose mannitol (2–4%) may allow establishment of stable diuresis;
  – if this is unsuccessful, haemofiltration should be considered.

- In refractory congestive cardiac failure, fluid restriction in combination with an ACE inhibitor and a loop diuretic may correct the P_{Na}, but may lead to symptomatic hypotension.

Management of hyponatraemia due to gain of water in excess of salt

Hyponatraemia in the presence of clinically obvious fluid overload should be treated primarily by salt and water restriction and diuretic therapy. In hypoproteinaemic states, in order to preserve the intravascular volume a concomitant infusion of 20% albumin may be advisable.

In the capillary/vascular leak syndrome, the use of diuretics, e.g. furosemide, bumetanide, ethacrynic acid and metolazone, tend to aggravate the hypovolaemia and the use of low-dose mannitol (2–4%) in the maintenance or replacement fluid may allow the establishment of a stable diuresis with less need to expand the ECF with further colloid or crystalloid solutions. If this is unsuccessful, haemofiltration should be considered (see Chapter 22).

Illustrative cases: hyponatraemia

Case 1

A 3-month-old female infant, who was the product of a 28-week twin pregnancy, presented with a 2-day history of cough, increasing tachypnoea and reluctance to feed. On admission the infant was pale, lethargic and had a respiratory rate of 80 per minute with marked substernal recession. In view of her tachypnoea she was given standard maintenance i.v. fluids. 12 hours following admission she developed recurrent apnoeic episodes. Investigations at this time were as follows:

Plasma:

sodium	110 mmol/l
chloride	86 mmol/l
bicarbonate	20 mmol/l
urea	2 mmol/l
creatinine	40 μmol/l

Arterial blood gases in air:

pH	7.19
Po_2	80 mmHg
Pco_2	65 mmHg
base deficit	−10

Urine:

osmolality	210 mosm/kg
sodium	50 mmol/l
potassium	40 mmol/l

Commentary This infant presented with a clinical picture consistent with acute bronchiolitis and was found to be respiratory syncytial virus (RSV) positive. Although initially the apnoeic episodes were thought to be due to impending respiratory failure, in retrospect these reflected generalized seizures secondary to hyponatraemia related to SIADH. She was intubated and ventilated and given an infusion of 3% sodium chloride, 2 ml/kg/h for 4 hours and 1 ml/kg/h for 8 hours, by which time the P_{Na} was 124 mmol/l. Intravenous frusemide (1 mg/kg) was given at the onset of, and midway through, the infusion and maintenance fluids were reduced by 50%. She was extubated after 5 days and on follow-up at the age of 12 months had evidence of neurodevelopmental delay and spastic diplegia.

The risk of SIADH in acute bronchiolitis appears to be greatest in young infants, below the age of 2 months, particularly if they have a history of pre-term delivery. In this group, elective fluid restriction and regular estimation of P_{Na} is advisable.

Case 2

A 3-week-old male infant presented with a 24-hour history of lethargy, irritability and reluctance to feed. He was a full-term normal delivery (birth weight 3.2 kg) and was breast fed. He had one healthy 17-month-old sibling and no significant family history. On examination his temperature was 39.3 °C and weight 2.98 kg. He was pale, mottled and irritable. Investigations on admission were as follows:

Haemoglobin	14.9 g/dl
White blood cells (WBC)	24.9 × 10⁹/l
	(polymorphs 50%)

Plasma:

sodium	115 mmol/l
potassium	5.5 mmol/l
chloride	84 mmol/l
bicarbonate	8 mmol/l
creatinine	350 μmol/l
glucose	7.2 mmol/l

Arterial:

pH	7.14
Pco_2	15 mmHg
base deficit	−19

CSF (bloodstained sample):

microscopy	WBC 5 × 10⁶/l (lymphocytes)
glucose	5.5 mmol/l
protein	1.5 g/l
urine microscopy	WBC 1000 × 10⁹/l

He was treated with intravenous cefotaxime and 0.45% saline and made a good symptomatic response. Urinary tract ultrasound (US) showed bilateral marked hydronephrosis and hydroureter and a thick-walled bladder. Subsequently, urine culture showed a significant growth of coliforms, and contrast cystography confirmed the diagnosis of posterior urethral valves.

Commentary This infant presented with urinary tract sepsis associated with a congenital obstructive uropathy and advanced renal insufficiency. The hyponatraemia was due to a combination of impaired free water clearance because of the low GFR and excess urinary sodium loss secondary to the obstructive uropathy and associated renal dysplasia. The plasma electrolyte profile improved with sodium chloride and bicarbonate supplementation and the plasma creatinine subsequently fell to 175 μmol/l on urethral catheter drainage prior to ablation of the urethral valves.

Case 3

A 5-week-old male infant was admitted to the paediatric intensive care unit following a prolonged period of cardiopulmonary bypass during surgery for complex congenital heart disease. He was initially haemodynamically unstable and required frequent boluses of blood products and 5% albumin solution to maintain his blood pressure. By day three he had developed significant oedema. Investigations are this point showed:

Plasma:

sodium	125 mmol/l
chloride	90 mmol/l
potassium	3.8 mmol/l
bicarbonate	23 mmol/l
urea	15 mmol/l
creatinine	100 μmol/l
albumin	22 g/l

Commentary This patient has a 'capillary or vascular leak' syndrome. This is seen following prolonged cardiopulmonary bypass, ECMO, liver transplantation and other major surgical procedures in which cardiac output, renal perfusion and capillary integrity are compromised. These infants require large infusions of ECF-like solutions and tend to develop hypoproteinaemia and severe oedema. Management involved the addition of 2–4% mannitol to the maintenance solution. The combined effect of raising the plasma oncotic pressure and the induction of a stable osmotic diuresis enabled regulation of his urine output with a reduced requirement for expansion of the ECF volume.

Hypernatraemia

Hypernatraemia is by definition a P_{Na} above 150 mmol/l and reflects a deficiency of water relative to sodium; however, total body sodium may be high, normal or low.

Since sodium is the principal ECF osmole, hyper-natraemia leads to hypertonicity of the ECF. The volume of the ECF compartment is therefore relatively well maintained and the ICF compartment bears the brunt of any fluid deficit. The classical signs of dehydration/ hypovolaemia are therefore relatively less evident for any given fluid deficit. The physiological response to hypernatraemia is firstly an increase in ADH secretion, which occurs when the P_{osm} increases above 285 mosm/kg. If the plasma tonicity remains high despite ADH secretion, the second and more important response, that of thirst, comes into play. The awake and alert patient will then increase his water intake in order to maintain normal ECF tonicity.

The two mechanisms that result in hypernatraemia (Table 2.6, Fig. 2.2) are:

- loss of water in excess of sodium;

- gain of sodium in excess of water.

Table 2.6 Causes of hypernatraemia

Loss of water in excess of sodium
Extrarenal water loss ($U_{osm} > 800$ mosm/kg)
  $U_{Na} < 20$ mmol/l
    Diarrhoea
    Vomiting
    Gastrointestinal fistulae
    Thermal injury
  U_{Na} variable
    Hyperventilation
    Pyrexia
Inadequate water intake
($U_{osm} > 800$ mosm/kg and U_{Na} variable)
Renal water loss ($U_{osm} < 800$ mosm/kg)
  U_{Na} variable
    Central and nephrogenic diabetes insipidus
  $U_{Na} > 20$ mmol/l
    Hyperglycaemia
    Osmotic/loop diuretic therapy
    Intrinsic renal disease
Gain of sodium in excess of water
  (U_{osm} variable and $U_{Na} > 75–100$ mmol/l)
Excess oral ingestion
  Erroneous/deliberate reconstitution of milk/nasogastric feeds
  Sea water ingestion
Excessive intravenous administration
  Sodium bicarbonate
  Hypertonic saline
  Sodium citrate
Saline enemas
Hypertonic dialysis
Mineralocorticoid excess
  Cushing's syndrome
  Conn's syndrome

Loss of water in excess of sodium

Extrarenal loss: The most common presentation of hypernatraemia in clinical practice is in association with a fluid deficit, the syndrome of 'hypernatraemic dehydration'. This picture is seen in acute viral gastroenteritis, although less frequently than isonatraemic and hyponatraemic dehydration, as well as in the osmotic diarrhoea induced by lactulose or charcoal/sorbitol used in the treatment of drug overdose. In gastroenteritis, although the diarrhoeal fluid is isosmotic, the electrolyte (sodium and potassium) concentration varies between 40 and 100 mmol/l, with organic solutes making up the remaining osmoles. Less commonly, hypernatraemia may occur as a result of increased insensible water loss through the lung in acute respiratory infection and in other febrile illnesses through increased insensible skin water loss.

When a hypernatraemic state develops, the pathogenetic mechanism differs from that of isotonic and hypotonic ECF constriction, in that water loss is proportionately greater than sodium loss. Because the ECF volume is relatively well maintained, signs of dehydration/hypovolaemia are less evident and shock is an infrequent occurrence. Classically the infant presents with a history of irritability and lethargy which, if untreated, progressively leads to diminished conscious level, hypertonia, convulsions and coma.

Neurological complications are the predominant risk factor in patients with hypernatraemia and are more likely if the P_{Na} is above 160 mmol/l. These are the result of two main mechanisms. Firstly, prior to institution of therapy, intracranial haemorrhage may occur when the osmolal gradient between the ICF and ECF develops rapidly, reflecting the fact that the brain acts as a single cell in response to osmotic changes in the ECF. Both intra- and extracerebral bleeding may occur, and thrombosis often follows and may extend the neurological insult [15].

The second neurological complication—that of cerebral oedema—occurs during therapy and again reflects the rapid fluid shifts which may occur across the blood–brain barrier. This complication develops because of the existence of intracellular 'idiogenic' osmoles, thought to be complexes of amino acids, particularly taurine. The relevance of these idiogenic osmoles relates to the attractiveness of the brain for water during rehydration and, if rehydration is uncontrolled, there is a significant risk of cerebral oedema. Idiogenic osmoles may develop as a result of intracellular dehydration or as a mechanism to protect

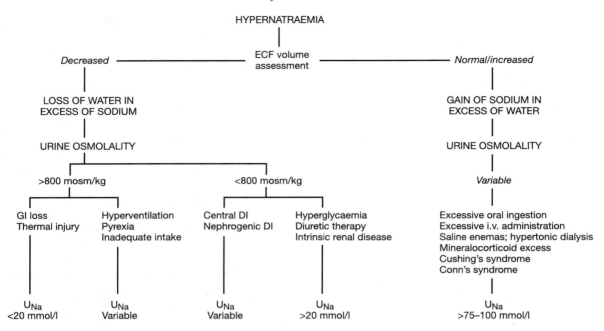

Fig. 2.2   Investigation of hypernatraemia.

cellular integrity. The latter suggestion is perhaps more appropriate, in that when the hypernatraemic state is chronic, brain water content returns to normal or near normal levels [16].

In hypernatraemic dehydration, the U_{Na} is less than 10–20 mmol/l and U_{osm} greater than 800 mosm/kg. Another biochemical feature is hypocalcaemia, which is rarely associated with frank tetany and is of obscure aetiology. In addition, hyperglycaemia is also a frequent occurrence in hypernatraemic states and, again, is of unknown aetiology but, importantly, does not require insulin therapy.

Inadequate water intake presents with the same clinical picture as excessive extrarenal loss of water in excess of sodium. Examples are infants exclusively breast fed in whom the volume of breast milk is inadequate, patients intolerant of oral fluids because of severe vomiting, comatose patients and patients with hypodipsia, either primary or secondary to a lesion affecting the thirst centre. In these patients the renal response will be appropriate, with production of a small volume of urine with a U_{osm} above 800 mosm/kg and a variable U_{Na}.

Uncontrolled renal water loss occurs due to impaired urinary concentrating ability in two circumstances. Firstly, where there is an absent/poor response to adequate ADH levels and, secondly, in

the absence/reduction of ADH secretion. In both these circumstances the U_{osm} is inappropriately low (<800 mosm/kg) in the face of a high P_{osm}.

Diabetes insipidus (DI) is a generic term applied to a number of disorders with similar clinical features (Table 2.7) [17]. Polyuria in the absence of osmotic diuresis and episodic hypernatraemia is the hallmark of these disorders. At all ages, polyuria, thirst and polydipsia are present, although these may not be obvious in the infant. In the older child, non-selective drinking, both day and night, and nocturia and nocturnal enuresis are present. Affected infants demonstrate irritability, frequent feed requirements, unexplained fever, constipation, failure to thrive and developmental delay. Infants are at significant risk of hypernatraemic dehydration, in contrast to older children, who are able to regulate their fluid intake.

Assessment of the above patients should include simple baseline plasma electrolytes, plasma calcium and urinary tract ultrasound. Assuming these investigations are normal, assessment of the urinary concentrating capacity by controlled water deprivation with or without DDAVP® is warranted. One of the major advantages of a water deprivation test is the recognition of partial defects in ADH secretion/action.

However, a water deprivation test is a potentially hazardous procedure and should under no

Table 2.7 Causes of diabetes insipidus

Central
  Idiopathic
  Cerebral malformation, e.g. septo-optic dysplasia,
    Bardet–Biedl syndrome
  Post head injury; intracranial surgery; hypoxic
    ischaemic encephalopathy
  Intracranial tumour or haemorrhage
  Granulomatous disease, e.g. tuberculosis, sarcoidosis,
    histiocytosis
  Intracranial infection, e.g. congenital CMV and
    toxoplasmosis, meningitis and encephalitis
  Lymphocytic neurohypophysitis
  Inherited
    Autosomal dominant
    Autosomal recessive (DIDMOAD syndrome)
Nephrogenic
  Inherited
    X-linked (V2 receptor gene defect)
    Autosomal recessive (aquaporin 2 gene defect)
  Renal disease
    Chronic renal insufficiency
    Obstructive uropathy
    Dysplasia
    Nephronophthisis
    Reflux nephropathy
    Sickle-cell nephropathy
    Fanconi syndrome
  Hypokalaemia
  Hypercalcaemia
  Drugs (lithium, demeclocycline)

CMV, cytomegalovirus; DIDMOAD, diabetes insipidus and mellitus, optic atrophy and deafness.

circumstances be undertaken in the presence of hypernatraemia and increased P_{osm}. In these circumstances DDAVP® should be administered at a dose of $0.5 \, \mu g/m^2$ by the intravenous, intramuscular or subcutaneous route or $5 \, \mu g/m^2$ intranasally. U_{osm} should be repeated in 4 hours and, if the response is adequate, the U_{osm} should be greater than 800 mosm/kg.

If the patient is adequately hydrated and has a normal P_{Na}, a careful water deprivation test should be carried out over 6–8 hours or until 3% of the body weight is lost, should this occur first. Each sample of urine passed within this period should be collected for measurement of volume and osmolality and if at any point the U_{osm} exceeds 800 mosm/kg, the test can be aborted. At the end of the deprivation period, the U_{osm} and P_{osm} should be estimated. If the U_{osm} is < 800 mosm/kg, DDAVP® should be given and a further U_{osm} and P_{osm} checked 4 hours later.

In central DI (CDI), secondary to a complete defect in ADH secretion, and in nephrogenic diabetes insipidus (NDI), there will be no significant change in U_{osm} during water deprivation, but the P_{osm} often rises to more than 300 mosm/kg. Following DDAVP®, the U_{osm} should be more than 800 mosm/kg in CDI but will remain unchanged in NDI. In partial CDI, the U_{osm} will be 300–800 mosm/kg but will show an adequate response to DDAVP®.

NDI refers to an ADH-resistant defect in urine concentration and may be either congenital or acquired (Table 2.7). Almost all patients with congenital NDI are males and have the X-linked dominant variety secondary to a mutation in the *AVPR2* gene and present in early infancy with marked symptomatology, although variation in clinical severity is seen. Female siblings may have a mild form of the disorder only demonstrable by fluid deprivation. There is also a rare autosomal recessive variety secondary to a mutation in the *AQP2* gene. Acquired NDI occurs more frequently and usually in the context of some form of intrinsic renal disease. A similar picture may be present in longstanding hypercalaemia or hypokalaemia and with certain drug therapy, e.g. lithium, demeclocycline.

Adolescents with compulsive water drinking present with polyuria and may demonstrate a suboptimal response to water deprivation and DDAVP® (U_{osm} 500–800 mosm/kg). Importantly, the P_{osm} in these patients remains normal during water deprivation, in contrast to patients with DI, and a period of treatment with DDAVP® and fluid restriction is required to re-establish a normal urine concentrating ability.

Other major causes of hypotonic fluid loss are diabetic ketoacidosis (DKA), hyperglycaemia associated with parenteral nutrition, and occasionally following therapy with osmotic and loop diuretics.

Hyperglycaemia in DKA has a variable effect on the P_{Na} as factors are present which can both lower and raise this parameter. By raising the P_{osm}, hyperglycaemia results in an osmotically driven shift of water from the ICF to the ECF, resulting in a dilution in P_{Na}. However, this direct effect of hyperglycaemia is counteracted by the hypotonic osmotic diuresis, which will tend to raise the P_{Na} and P_{osm} unless there is a comparable increase in water intake. The final P_{Na} will reflect the balance between these two mechanisms and although most patients with DKA are mildly hyponatraemic, the 'true' or 'corrected' P_{Na} may be calculated by using the following formula: corrected P_{Na} = measured P_{Na} + 2.5 mmol/l for every 5 mmol/l elevation in the plasma glucose [18]. By using this formula it can easily be appreciated that patients with DKA who have a measured P_{Na} within the normal range may have a corrected value of more than 150 mmol/l. These patients are extremely hyperosmolar and often have neurological symptoms such as diminished conscious level and seizures prior to therapy.

Gain of sodium in excess of water

Hypernatraemia in the absence of a fluid deficit is a rare clinical occurrence. Marked hypernatraemia (plasma sodium 175–200 mmol/l) and elevation in U_{Na} (>100 mmol/l) can develop after administration of an excessive amount of sodium. When such administration is iatrogenic, the clinical context is usually obvious, e.g. administration of sodium bicarbonate in the treatment of acidosis following cardiopulmonary arrest, following exchange transfusion when sodium citrate has been used as the anticoagulant and accidentally in dialysis against a high sodium dialysate. It has long been recognized, however, that salt administration by various routes is a presentation of Münchausen syndrome by proxy with a very high mortality [19]. Even if the salt administration is claimed to be accidental, e.g. preparing milk with salt rather than sugar, the action should be assumed to be deliberate and the possibility of serious abuse must always be considered. It is also clear that the presence of an existing illness, e.g. chronic renal failure, does not preclude deliberate salt poisoning, and in such circumstances the possibility of abuse should be considered, particularly if hypernatraemia is recurrent. Occasionally patients with conditions associated with mineralocorticoid excess, such as Cushing's and Conn's syndrome, present with hypernatraemia and oedema.

Management of hypernatraemic states

Management of hypernatraemic dehydration

The basic principles of fluid replacement in hypernatraemic dehydration do not differ from those in hypotonic or isotonic dehydration, i.e. calculation of fluid deficit based on admission body weight added to maintenance fluid requirement and any ongoing losses over the chosen period of rehydration. The main differences in the management of hypernatraemia are firstly that correction of the P_{Na} by the

intravenous route should be no more rapid than 15 mmol/l/day and secondly, that normal hydration should be achieved over a period of no less than 36–48 hours, and perhaps longer if the initial P_{Na} is above 170 mmol/l.

Key points: Assessment of hypernatraemia

- Hypernatraemia occurs when there is either a loss of water in excess of sodium or a gain of sodium in excess of water.

- Because the ECF volume is relatively well maintained, the classical signs of dehydration/hypovolaemia are less evident for any given fluid deficit.

- Clinical assessment of ECF volume is essential in the evaluation of hypernatraemia since total body sodium may be normal, increased or decreased.

- Extrarenal loss of water in excess of sodium most commonly occurs in hypernatraemic dehydration. The U_{Na} is <10–20 mmol/ and P_{osm} >800 mosm/kg.

- Inadequate water intake results in the same clinical and biochemical pattern as hypernatraemic dehydration.

- Uncontrolled renal water loss occurs with impaired urinary concentrating ability, either due to absent/poor response to ADH or to absent/reduced secretion of ADH. The U_{osm} is inappropriately low (<800 msom/kg) in the face of the high P_{osm}.

- Hypernatraemia due to gain of sodium in excess of water:
  – is rare;
  – U_{Na} > 100 mmol/l is highly suggestive of excess sodium intake;
  – non-accidental salt poisoning *must always be considered in hypernatraemia due to excess sodium intake*.

- The increased risk of neurological complications on presentation and during therapy of hypernatraemia should be appreciated.

However, experience with ORT in the management of diarrhoeal-induced hypernatraemic dehydration suggests that if the infant is not shocked and able to tolerate oral or nasogastric fluids, the WHO solution (sodium 90 mmol/l) is safe and effective, despite a somewhat faster fall in P_{Na} and shorter period of rehydration than with intravenous replacement [10]. In developed countries, an ORT with a sodium content of 60 mmol/l should be used and the initial volume, based on the estimated deficit, administered over 12 hours. If the infant is clinically hydrated at that point, half-strength milk feeds (10 mmol/l sodium) are introduced at 120 ml/kg/day; if not, the above regime is repeated, based on the current deficit.

In the presence of circulatory compromise, which is more likely with a P_{Na} above 160 mmol/l, 20 ml/kg of 0.9% saline or Ringer's solution should be given over 30 minutes, and repeated on two occasions if necessary. If intravenous therapy is continuing, provided there is no oliguria, the remaining deficit should be added to the maintenance fluid over a 48-hour period and the total volume given over this period as 0.18% sodium chloride solution in 5% dextrose. If the initial plasma sodium is above 170 mmol/l, it is safer to extend this period to 72 hours. In view of the coexisting potassium depletion, potassium as chloride may be added to the infusion fluid in the presence of adequate urine flow at a concentration of 30 mmol/l.

In the presence of a significant metabolic acidosis, the composition of the infusion may be altered to contain bicarbonate, e.g. a combination of 1 litre of 5% dextrose with 32 ml of 8.4% sodium bicarbonate is approximately equivalent to a 0.18% sodium solution. P_{Na} levels should be monitored every 6 hours and, if there is any deterioration in the neurological status, water intoxication should be suspected and the rate of infusion must be slowed and mannitol given if there is adequate urine output.

If oliguria is noted in the absence of circulatory impairment on initial assessment, the U_{Na} should be assessed to obtain confirmation of ECF volume depletion, in which case the U_{Na} should be less than 20 mmol/l and the other parameters consistent with pre-renal uraemia (see Chapter 22). In these circumstances a fluid challenge with 0.45% saline in 5% dextrose at a rate of 5–10 ml/kg/h for 4 hours should be given and, if urine output responds, intravenous fluids should be changed to 0.18% saline in 5% dextrose, and the remaining deficit and maintenance replaced over the following 48 hours [15].

If oliguria persists, a further complication of the hypernatraemic state, that of renal venous thrombosis, should be suspected [20]. This is usually associated with the presence of either frank or microscopic haematuria, thrombocytopenia and clinical and/or ultrasonographic evidence of renal enlargement. In the presence of continued oliguria, careful replacement should be carried out under central venous pressure monitoring, and renal replacement therapy should be considered since peritoneal dialysis, haemodialysis and haemofiltration are effective in lowering the P_{Na}.

Key points: Management of hypernatraemic dehydration

- The main differences in the management of hypernatraemic dehydration are:
  - the P_{Na} should be reduced by not more than 15 mmol/day;
  - normal hydration should be achieved over 36–48 hours and perhaps 72 hours if the initial P_{Na} is >170 mmol/l.

- ORT in diarrhoeal-induced hypernatraemic dehydration is safe in children who are not shocked, despite a faster fall in P_{Na}.

- Circulatory collapse should be corrected by 0.9% saline or Ringer's solution 20 ml/kg over 30 minutes, and repeated if necessary.

- Bicarbonate should be added to the infusion if there is significant metabolic acidosis.

- Persistent oliguria when circulatory impairment has been corrected indicates:
  - acute renal failure;
  - renal venous thrombosis.

Management of diabetes insipidus

The mainstay of treatment of central DI is desmopressin (DDAVP®), a two-amino-acid substitute of ADH which has potent antidiuretic but no vasopressor activity [17]. Desmopressin may be administered orally by tablet, intra-nasally, in a liquid form or metered dose spray, or parenterally. There are wide variations in the dose required to control diuresis. Daily requirements for the oral preparation, which has only 5–10% of the potency of the nasal form, vary from 0.1 to 1 mg. The dose range for the intra-nasal preparations in children older than 1 year is 2–40 µg/day, and for the parenteral preparation, 0.1–1 µg/day, all in two or three divided doses. A low dose should be used initially and titrated upwards as necessary. As little as 0.5 µg of the nasal solution given twice daily may suffice in small infants. This dose can be diluted from a standard desmopressin solution and administered in a 1 ml syringe.

The management of CDI in infants and small children, and in children with adipsia or hypodipsia, is challenging and requires close involvement and clear instruction of the carers. This is best done initially during a period of inpatient observation, during which the dose of DDAVP® and a target fluid intake is established, based on regular weight recording and measurements of P_{Na}. In practice, nasogastric or gastrostomy tube placement allows the target fluid intake to be achieved consistently.

Hyponatraemia secondary to an inability to excrete a water load is an important potential risk in patients on DDAVP® replacement, as they effectively have non-suppressible ADH. This should be taken into account during periods of illness, particularly if managed by intravenous fluid replacement, and in this circumstance aqueous vasopressin which has a short half-life (4–6 hours) may be considered, but the disadvantage of this preparation is the associated pressor activity. In partial CDI drugs that potentiate the release of ADH, e.g. chlorpropamide and carbamazepine, and as in NDI, thiazide diuretics and non-steroidal anti-inflammatory drugs (NSAIDs), may be of benefit in combination with hormonal therapy.

In NDI the optimal management consists of the establishment of a target fluid intake as above in combination with sodium restriction (1 mmol/kg/day), and diuretic therapy with a thiazide diuretic, e.g. hydrochlorothiazide (2–4 mg/kg/day) and the potassium-sparing diuretic, amiloride (20 mg/1.73 m²/day), both in two or three divided doses. Occasionally, particularly in young children, amiloride may produce nausea and, in this context, the combination of hydrochlorothiazide and an NSAID, e.g. indomethacin (2 mg/kg/day), may be necessary in the short term.

Key points: Management of diabetes insipidus

- Central diabetes insipidus (CDI):
  - desmopressin (DDAVP®) and a target fluid intake are the mainstay of treatment;
  - management in infants and young children requires close monitoring
  - hyponatraemia due to an inability to excrete a water load is a risk in patients on DDAVP® and should be considered during periods of illness;
  - in partial CDI, drugs that potentiate the release of ADH (e.g. chlorpropamide and carbamazepine) and the drugs used in NDI may be helpful.

- Nephrogenic diabetes insipidus (NDI) is best managed by:
  - a target fluid intake;
  - diuretic therapy with a combination of a thiazide diuretic and a potassium-sparing diuretic;
  - addition of a NSAID may be necessary in the short term.

Fluid and electrolyte management in diabetic ketoacidosis

The main concern in the management of patients with DKA, particularly those who have 'corrected' P_{Na} above 150 mmol/l, is the prevention of cerebral oedema. Reversal of the hyperglycaemia with insulin will sequentially lower the P_{osm} and allow water to move from the ECF to the ICF, resulting in an increase in P_{Na} by 2.5 mmol/l for every 5 mmol/l reduction in plasma glucose. Thus, a patient with a normal initial measured P_{Na} is likely to become hypernatraemic during therapy with insulin and isotonic saline.

Children with DKA are at higher risk of developing cerebral oedema than adults, but the mechanism by which cerebral oedema occurs is incompletely understood [21]. The combination of insulin and relatively dilute replacement fluid may lower the plasma glucose concentration by 10 mmol/l/h (10 mosm/kg/h). This rapid reduction in P_{osm} can promote osmotic water movement into the brain as in hypernatraemic dehydration, and there is good evidence that a fall or absence of the above predicted rise in measured P_{Na}, coincident with the fall in plasma glucose following

Key points: Management of diabetic ketoacidosis

- The main concern is the prevention of cerebral oedema.

- The aetiology of this is unclear, but it is children with 'corrected' $P_{Na} > 150$ mmol/l who are most at risk.

- Reduction in plasma glucose would be predicted to increase the P_{Na} by 2.5 mmol/l for every 5 mmol/l reduction in plasma glucose. *Absence of this predicted rise in P_{Na} correlates with the development of cerebral oedema.*

- The rate of fall of the P_{osm} should be limited and adjusted depending on the 'corrected' P_{Na}. The duration of rehydration should be similarly modelled.

- Potassium chloride should be added to the replacement solution as soon as urine output is established.

- All patients should be monitored carefully for signs of cerebral oedema.

- If signs develop early, treatment with 20% mannitol and reduction in fluid replacement may prevent neurological damage.

treatment, correlates strongly with the development of cerebral oedema [22].

The optimal treatment regimen remains uncertain, in part because it is not understood why only a small number of patients develop neurological symptoms, but it is nevertheless prudent to minimize the rate of fall in P_{osm} by varying the replacement fluid and duration of rehydration dependent on the 'corrected' P_{Na}. When the 'corrected' plasma sodium is less than 150 mmol/l, 0.9% saline should be used until the plasma glucose has fallen to 15 mmol/l and substituted thereafter by 0.45% saline in 5% dextrose, the aim being to achieve a rehydration period of 48 h. Potassium chloride (40 mmol/l) should be added to the replacement solution as soon as urine output has been established.

In patients with 'corrected' plasma sodium values above 150 mmol/l an alternative to 0.9% saline, when urine flow has been established, is 0.45% saline with potassium chloride (40 mmol/l), which is equivalent to 0.7% saline. In addition, the duration of

rehydration in patients with 'corrected' P_{Na} of 150–160 mmol/l, should be 48–60 h, and 60–72 h in those with a 'corrected' P_{Na} of more than 160 mmol/l. All patients should be monitored carefully for the development of signs of cerebral oedema, such as severe headache or decreased conscious level. Early treatment with 20% mannitol, 0.5–1 g/kg (2.5–5 ml/kg), over 15 min, combined with a 50% reduction in intravenous fluid replacement, may prevent irreversible neurological damage in this setting.

Management of hypernatraemia due to salt excess

The hypernatraemia in this setting will correct spontaneously if renal function is normal, since the excess sodium will be excreted rapidly in the urine. This process may be facilitated by inducing a sodium and water diuresis with a loop diuretic and replacing the urine output solely with water. Too rapid a correction of P_{Na} should be avoided if a patient is symptomatic. However, this group of patients is less likely to develop cerebral oedema during correction, since the hypernatraemia is generally very acute, leaving little time for cerebral adaptation. For reasons that are not clearly understood, severe hypernatraemia is often better tolerated in children than in adults.

In patients with concurrent renal insufficiency or oliguria the use of peritoneal or haemodialysis is recommended.

Illustrative cases: hypernatraemia

Case 1

A 10-year-old, mentally retarded boy was admitted with a history of increasing somnolence. He had undergone a right hemispherectomy 6 months previously for intractable seizures. Investigations on admission were as follows:

Haemoglobin	13 g/dl
WBC	14×10^9/l
Platelet count	250×10^9/l
Plasma:	
sodium	165 mmol/l
chloride	130 mmol/l
bicarbonate	80 mmol/l
urea	22 mmol/l
creatinine	180 μmol/l
glucose	9.5 mmol/l

Commentary This boy presenting with hypernatraemia, had a calculated and measured plasma osmolality in excess of 330 mosm/kg. The history of intracranial surgery was relevant and the presumptive diagnosis was that of central diabetes insipidus. Urine osmolality taken on admission was 200 mosm/kg, which, in the face of hypernatraemia, is subnormal. He was managed by careful intravenous fluid replacement and given a test dose of 20 μg of intranasal DDAVP®. A urine osmolality taken 4 hours later was 850 mosm/kg, confirming the diagnosis. He was discharged on regular DDAVP®.

Case 2

An 18-month-old, previously well child presented with a 10-day history of general malaise, anorexia and polyuria. On admission she was drowsy but rousable (Glasgow coma scale 9) and showed signs of clinical dehydration, but was not shocked. Initial investigations were as follows:

Plasma:
sodium	145 mmol/l
potassium	5.5 mmol/l
bicarbonate	10 mmol/l
urea	25 mmol/l
creatinine	105 μmol/l
glucose	45 mmol/l

Arterial:
pH	7.15
base deficit	−16
P_{CO_2}	23

Initial fluid management involved intravenous 0.9% saline until urine output was established and at that point switched to 0.45% saline with potassium chloride (40 mmol/l) and the rehydration period calculated over a 72-hour period.

By 12 hours of beginning an insulin infusion (0.05 U/kg/h), the plasma glucose had fallen to 29 mmol/l and the plasma sodium had risen to 157 mmol/l, but thereafter stabilized and fell to 149 mmol/l by 36 hours (plasma glucose 15 mmol/l) and to 139 mmol/l by 60 hours. Her neurological status returned to normal by 36 hours.

Commentary The main feature in the initial clinical and biochemical assessment of this child was the finding of extreme hyperosmolality (calculated $P_{osm} > 330$ mosm/kg). The 'corrected' plasma sodium of 165 mmol/l revealed the extent of the underlying hypernatraemia and, in view of this, the deficit and maintenance fluids were calculated over a 72-hour period. The initial rise in the measured plasma sodium reflected the fall in plasma glucose, but the subsequent fall was appropriately slow in order to reduce the risk of cerebral oedema.

Case 3

A 2-year-old girl with a 5-day history of increasing irritability and unsteadiness was brought to the Accident and Emergency Department by her father. On admission she was moderately dehydrated (6% body weight loss) but not shocked, drowsy and rather unkempt, and her weight was significantly below the third percentile for her age. Further examination revealed several crusted lesions on the right side of her chest wall and on the dorsum of her right foot. Investigations on admission were as follows:

Plasma:
sodium	190 mmol/l
potassium	3.5 mmol/l
chloride	135 mmol/l
bicarbonate	22 mmol/l
urea	39 mmol/l
creatinine	100 μmol/l
glucose	21 mmol/l
Plasma osmolality	470 mosm/kg

Urine:
sodium	145 mmol/l
chloride	120 mmol/l
osmolality	1190 mosm/kg

In view of the presentation of hypernatraemic dehydration, the deficit and maintenance fluid regime was calculated over a 72-hour period and given as 0.18% saline in 5% dextrose, with potassium chloride 30 mmol/l when urine flow was established. She made a complete recovery and her subsequent plasma electrolyte profile remained consistently normal.

Commentary Although her mother claimed that she had restricted her fluid intake to 'help with toilet training', the diagnosis of deliberate salt poisoning was supported by the very high U_{Na} in a clinically dehydrated child who showed an otherwise very appropriate renal response to a fluid deficit as evidenced by the U_{osm} and the U/P ratios of osmolality and urea.

Further supportive evidence of non-accidental injury (NAI) was the presence of skin lesions suggestive of cigarette burns and the poor weight gain.

Disorders of potassium balance

Introduction

Potassium is the principal intracellular cation, and is important in the regulation of a variety of cell functions. Disorders of potassium balance and distribution, especially those of rapid onset, are of clinical importance because of the effect on resting membrane potential of nerve and muscle cells. The distribution of potassium between the ICF and ECF compartments is maintained in the face of variation of intake by a number of control mechanisms, but primarily by cell membrane pump activity, which is influenced by acid–base status, ECF tonicity and hormonal (insulin, mineralocorticoid) and adrenergic (both α and β) activity [23].

The kidney is the major excretory organ for potassium, but is less effective in responding to wide variations in intake than with sodium. Urinary potassium is derived predominantly from distal nephron secretion, since over 90% of the potassium filtered by the glomeruli is reabsorbed. Potassium secretion reflects total body potassium as well as potassium intake and is enhanced by increased delivery of sodium and water to the distal nephron as well as by increased mineralocorticoid activity and ECF alkalosis.

Ideally, assessment of urinary potassium excretion should be by a timed, preferably 24-hour collection; however, provided the patient is not hypovolaemic or polyuric, a random urinary potassium (U_K) of more than 20 mmol/l in the presence of hypokalaemia generally indicates renal potassium wasting [24]. Additional data in support of renal potassium wasting are a fractional excretion of potassium of more than 40% (normal: 10–30%) and a urinary sodium/ potassium ratio of less than 1 (normal: 1–3.5) [23].

Hyperkalaemia and hypokalaemia may result from alterations in either total body potassium or in the distribution of potassium between ECF and ICF compartments. The growing child maintains a state of positive potassium balance, unlike the adult who has a zero balance, and the relative conservation of potassium early in life is associated with higher plasma levels (Table 2.8) [25].

Table 2.8 Plasma potassium concentration in newborns, infants and children (mean ± standard deviation)

Age	Plasma K concentration (mmol/l)
Newborn[a]	
30–32	6.5 ± 0.5
33–35	5.6 ± 0.2
36–38	5.3 ± 0.3
39–41	5.1 ± 0.2
Infants[b] (*n* = 14)	
1–12 months	5.0 ± 0.5
Children[b] (*n* = 22)	
2–20 years	4.3 ± 0.4

[a] Gestational age in weeks; measurements obtained at 1 week of age (from Sulyok *et al.* [25]).
[b] From G.J. Schwartz and L.G. Feld (unpublished observations).

Hypokalaemia

Summaries of the investigation and causes of hypokalaemia are given in Fig. 2.3 and Table 2.9.

Hypokalaemia associated with total body potassium deficiency

Inadequate intake

The majority of patients with hypokalaemia will have a deficiency in total body potassium. This may result from inadequate intake in association with physiological renal and gastrointestinal loss that is accentuated if the sodium content of the diet is high. Hypokalaemia and total body potassium deficiency is commonly seen in protein calorie malnutrition and may also be seen in infants fed incorrect formulae and in adolescents who use low-calorie, liquid protein diets for rapid weight loss.

Extrarenal loss

The most common cause of hypokalaemia in children is secondary to acute or chronic gastrointestinal loss. Potassium concentration in lower intestinal fluid is relatively high (50–80 mmol/l), in contrast to the concentration of potassium in gastric secretions (5–10 mmol/l). The main conditions leading to gastrointestinal loss are therefore acute and chronic diarrhoea, and losses from lower gastrointestinal fistulae and stomas. In the infant and young child, and in the adolescent, deliberate or surreptitious use of laxatives may also be relevant. In these settings, the hypokalaemia is usually accompanied by a metabolic

---

Key points: Potassium homeostasis

- Potassium is the principal intracellular cation.

- Distribution of potassium between the ICF and ECF is maintained primarily by the cell membrane pump. This is influenced by:
  - acid/base status;
  - ECF tonicity;
  - hormones (insulin and mineralocorticoid);
  - α- and β-adrenergic activity.

- The kidney is the major excretory organ for potassium but is less effective in responding to wide variations in intake than with sodium.

- In the absence of polyuria or hypovolaemia, a $U_K > 20$ mmol/l in the presence of hypokalaemia generally indicates renal potassium wasting.

- The growing child, unlike the adult, maintains a positive potassium balance and this is associated early in life with a higher plasma potassium level.

- Both hyperkalaemia and hypokalaemia can result from alterations in either the total body potassium or distribution of potassium between ECF and ICF.

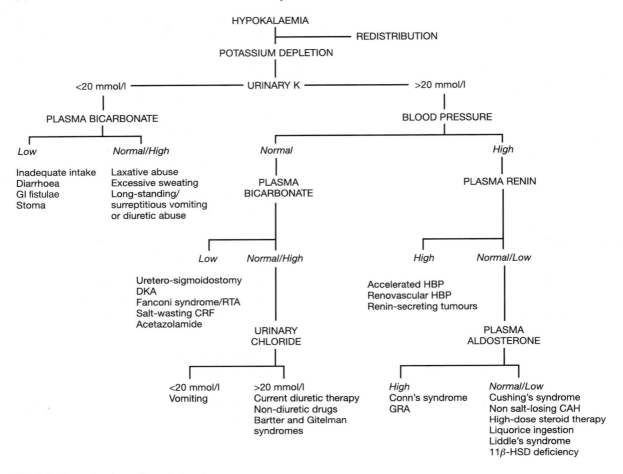

Fig. 2.3 Investigation of hypokalaemia.

acidosis due to the associated loss of bicarbonate in the stool.

Excessive sweating may induce potassium deficiency through a combination of exocrine gland loss and secondary hyperaldosteronism due to ECF volume contraction. Patients with cystic fibrosis are at risk of this complication and may present with a pseudo-Bartter's syndrome.

Renal potassium wasting with normal blood pressure

Renal potassium wasting with a metabolic alkalosis, in the presence of normal blood pressure, is most often seen in patients with recurrent vomiting [26]. Since the potassium concentration in gastric secretions is low, potassium depletion in this setting is primarily due to increased urinary loss. The associated metabolic

alkalosis results in an increase in the filtered bicarbonate load that exceeds the renal reabsorptive threshold. The net effect of increased delivery of sodium and water to the distal nephron and the hypovolaemia-induced release of aldosterone results in a significant increase in potassium secretion. There is also inappropriate sodium wasting and only the demonstration of a U_{Cl} of less than 20 mmol/l points to the presence of ECF depletion. The urinary potassium wasting seen with vomiting is typically most prominent in the first few days, thereafter the renal bicarbonate reabsorptive capacity increases with a consequent reduction in urinary bicarbonate and electrolyte losses.

A similar picture is seen in long-term diuretic use or abuse and in Bartter's and Gitelman's syndromes, but in this context, the U_{Cl} will be above 20 mmol/l (see Chapter 5). Occasionally, however, a patient with surreptitious vomiting, often with bulimia or diuretic

Table 2.9 Causes of hypokalaemia

*Hypokalaemia associated with total body
potassium deficiency*
Inadequate intake ($U_K < 20$ mmol/l)
Extrarenal loss ($U_K < 20$ mmol/l)
  Low plasma bicarbonate
    Diarrhoea
    GI fistulae
    GI stomas
  Normal/high plasma bicarbonate
    Laxative abuse
    Excessive sweating, e.g. cystic fibrosis
    (Long-standing/surreptitious vomiting or diuretic abuse)
Renal loss ($U_K > 20$ mmol/l)
  With normal BP
    Low plasma bicarbonate
      ureterosigmoidostomy
      diabetic ketoacidosis
      Fanconi syndrome and RTA
      salt-wasting chronic renal failure
      acetazolamide
    Normal/high plasma bicarbonate
      vomiting
      diuretic therapy
      non-diuretic drug therapy
      Bartter and Gitelman syndromes
  With hypertension
    Low/normal plasma renin
      High plasma aldosterone
        Conn's syndrome
        glucocorticoid remediable hyperaldosteronism
        thermal injury
      Low/normal plasma aldosterone
        Cushing's syndrome
        non-salt-losing CAH
        high-dose corticosteroid therapy
        Liddle's syndrome
        11β-hydroxysteroid dehydrogenase deficiency
        liquorice ingestion
    High plasma renin
      accelerated hypertension
      renovascular hypertension
      renin-secreting tumours
Redistribution hypokalaemia
  Metabolic/respiratory alkalosis
  Hypokalaemic periodic paralysis
  Insulin administration
  Drugs/toxins

BP, blood pressure; CAH, congenital adrenal hyperplasia; RTA, renal tubular acidosis; U_K, urinary potassium.

abuse, may present with a metabolic alkalosis and a low U_K and U_{Cl}. In the latter circumstance, detection of diuretic metabolites in the urine is diagnostic.

Certain non-diuretic drug therapies, e.g. penicillin, carbenicillin, cisplatin and amphotericin B, may be associated with an increase in U_K and U_{Cl}. Other causes of renal potassium wasting with normal blood pressure are DKA, salt-wasting chronic renal failure, the use of carbonic anhydrase inhibitors, e.g. acetazolamide, and a variety of renal tubular diseases, e.g. Fanconi syndrome and renal tubular acidosis.

Renal potassium wasting with hypertension

The presence of primary mineralocorticoid excess (aldosterone and, to a much lesser extent, deoxycorticosterone) should be suspected in any patient with the combination of hypertension, unexplained hypokalaemia and metabolic alkalosis [26]. However, the degree of hypokalaemia may be relatively subtle and a number of these patients may have a normal plasma potassium. The further evaluation of these patients should include estimation of plasma renin and aldosterone, and urinary aldosterone.

An elevation in the plasma aldosterone is a primary manifestation of glucocorticoid remediable hyperaldosteronism (GRA) and Conn's syndrome. Clinical features of mineralocorticoid excess with a normal plasma aldosterone occur in Cushing's syndrome and in the rare disorders of non-salt-losing congenital adrenal hyperplasia secondary to 11β- and 17α-hydroxylase deficiency, Liddle's syndrome

---

Key points: Hypokalaemia with total body potassium deficiency

- The majority of patients with hypokalaemia will have a deficiency of total body potassium.

- Hypokalaemia due to inadequate intake is accentuated if the sodium content of the diet is high.

- The most common cause of hypokalaemia in children is extrarenal loss in acute or chronic gastrointestinal disease.

- Renal potassium wasting with metabolic alkalosis and a normal blood pressure is most often seen in patients with recurrent vomiting.

- Hypertension, metabolic alkalosis and hypokalaemia suggest primary mineralocorticoid excess.

and 11β-hydroxysteroid dehydrogenase (11β-HSD) deficiency. More frequently, high-dose corticosteroid therapy may mimic the features of mineralocorticoid excess and a similar picture is seen in patients who ingest large quantities of natural liquorice which contains glycyrrhizic acid, a potent inhibitor of 11β-HSD.

Excess renin production may occur as a secondary feature in accelerated hypertension, renal artery stenosis and may be associated with certain tumours, e.g. Wilms' and haemangiopericytoma.

Redistribution hypokalaemia

Hypokalaemia may occur without a deficiency in total body potassium. This is most commonly seen in the context of either acute metabolic or respiratory alkalosis. The intracellular shift of potassium is precipitated by a fall in extracellular hydrogen ion concentration. Hypokalaemic periodic paralysis is a rare disorder characterized by intermittent attacks of muscle weakness and may be familial with autosomal dominant inheritance or acquired in patients with thyrotoxicosis. In the familial disease, the abnormal gene has been localized to a calcium channel in skeletal muscle. Plasma potassium concentration falls during the attack and returns to normal during the recovery phase. Episodes are precipitated by a high carbohydrate and low potassium diet, exercise and infection, and may also be alcohol induced.

Glucose administration and glucose and insulin given together induce a shift of potassium from the ECF to the ICF compartments. The clinical setting in which this may be seen is in the management of DKA, and the effect is used in the therapy of hyperkalaemia (Chapter 22).

Catecholamines, acting via the β$_2$-adrenergic receptor, promote potassium entry into cells, primarily by increasing sodium/potassium ATPase activity. As a result, transient hypokalaemia can be caused in any setting where there is stress-induced release of adrenaline, as with any acute illness. Similarly, theophylline intoxication and the administration of a β-adrenergic agonist, such as salbutamol, terbutaline or dopamine, may lead to an acute fall in plasma potassium by more than 0.5–1 mmol/l.

Hypokalaemia has been described in patients who have acute chloroquine intoxication, and in those who ingested food contaminated with soluble barium salts.

Key points: Redistribution hypokalaemia

- In this condition total body potassium is normal but there is an intracellular shift of potassium.

- Most commonly seen in either metabolic or respiratory alkalosis.

- Episodic redistribution is the underlying problem in hypokalaemic periodic paralysis. This may be:
  – familial (autosomal dominant);
  – acquired in thyrotoxicosis.

- A number of drugs, including glucose and insulin, induce a shift of potassium from the ECF to the ICF.

Clinical features of hypokalaemia

The effects of hypokalaemia depend on the extent and duration of associated total body potassium deficiency and the rapidity of onset. The symptoms and signs are mainly the result of the effect on skeletal, cardiac and smooth muscle and renal tubular function. Clinical features may therefore be a combination of polyuria and polydipsia secondary to an ADH-unresponsive urinary concentration defect, muscle weakness and paralytic ileus. Characteristic ECG changes occur, e.g. lowering or inversion of the T wave and exaggeration of the U wave, often producing an impression of QT lengthening (Fig. 2.4). Bradyarrhythmias may develop, especially if hypokalaemia develops with concomitant digoxin therapy. Further manifestations of hypokalaemia and potassium deficiency are glucose intolerance and neuropsychiatric symptoms, e.g. depression and confusional states.

Management of hypokalaemia

In hypokalaemic states, potassium supplementation should take place in association with treatment of the primary condition. In mild to moderate deficiency, either the encouragement of a potassium-rich food intake or the use of oral potassium supplementation with the chloride or bicarbonate salt is sufficient. In conditions associated with metabolic acidosis, e.g. renal tubular acidosis, the citrate salt should be used.

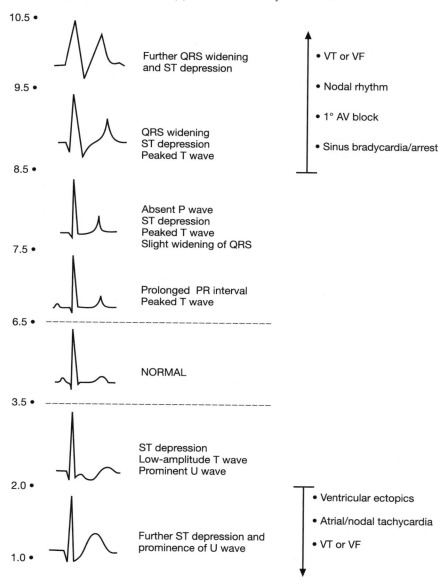

Fig. 2.4 Plasma potassium and ECG abnormalities (modified from Williams *et al.* [27] reproduced with permission from Lippincott Williams and Wilkins).

Alternatively, the use of a commercial ORT solution, which has a potassium concentration of 15–20 mmol/l, is usually adequate for replacement purposes.

In severely depleted patients with neuromuscular symptoms and/or ECG abnormalities, intravenous supplementation is necessary but great care should be taken since the rate of potassium uptake by the cell is limited. A dose of 1 mmol/kg given over 30 minutes should reverse ECG changes if these are present. Thereafter intravenous supplementation should be limited to 0.25 mmol/kg/h, with a potassium concentration of no greater than 60 mmol/l in the replacement fluid. This should be carried out in conjunction with ECG monitoring and frequent monitoring of the plasma level. Potassium chloride is the usual salt for intravenous use and should be the only one used in alkalotic states.

Potassium supplementation may be indicated in redistribution hypokalaemia despite the absence of a total body deficit, and in familial hypokalaemic periodic paralysis, acetazolamide may be of value.

Key points: Clinical features and management of hypokalaemia

- The effects of hypokalaemia depend on the rapidity, extent and duration of potassium deficiency.

- The clinical features are mainly the result of the effects on skeletal, cardiac and smooth muscle and renal tubular function.

- Mild to moderate deficiency can be corrected orally with high potassium foods and/or potassium chloride or potassium bicarbonate.

- If there are neuromuscular and/or ECG abnormalities, intravenous supplementation is necessary. This requires very careful monitoring (see the text for details).

- Potassium chloride is the usual salt for intravenous use and should be the only one used in alkalotic states.

- Acetazolamide may be of value in familial periodic paralysis.

Illustrative cases: hypokalaemia

Case 1

An 8-year-old girl was referred with a history of increasingly frequent headaches and was found to have a blood pressure of 160/110 (95th centile values: 114/76). On clinical examination she had evidence of multiple café au lait spots and axillary freckling and an epigastric abdominal bruit. Examination of her fundi revealed grade III hypertensive change and an ECG and echocardiogram showed left ventricular hypertrophy. The initial plasma biochemical picture was as follows:

Plasma:

sodium	140 mmol/l
potassium	3 mmol/l
chloride	105 mmol/l
bicarbonate	28 mmol/l
urea	5 mmol/l
creatinine	50 μmol/l

Urine:

potassium	40 mmol/l

Abdominal ultrasound and $^{99}Tc^m$ DMSA scan showed normal-sized kidneys with no parenchymal defect. Subsequent investigations included an elevated plasma renin and low/normal plasma aldosterone.

Commentary This previously well child with presumed neurofibromatosis type I presented with significant hypertension and hypokalaemia with an elevated plasma renin but low/normal plasma aldosterone. In view of the clinical history, examination and biochemical findings, the diagnosis of renovascular hypertension was suspected. She subsequently underwent magnetic resonance angiography and was shown to have bilateral main renal artery stenosis.

Case 2

A 2-year-old boy presented with a history of failure to thrive, polydipsia and long-standing constipation. Investigations on admission were as follows:

Plasma:

sodium	133 mmol/l
potassium	2.2 mmol/l
bicarbonate	16 mmol/l
urea	8 mmol/l
creatinine	75 μmol/l
calcium	2.2 mmol/l
phosphate	0.6 mmol/l

Urine:

sodium	50 mmol/l
potassium	60 mmol/l
chloride	45 mmol/l

Commentary The combination of hypokalaemia, metabolic acidosis and hypophosphataemia strongly suggests the presence of a generalized tubulopathy or Fanconi syndrome. This was confirmed with the finding of generalized aminoaciduria on a semiquantitative urinary amino acid chromatogram, and the specific diagnosis of nephropathic cystinosis was made by the finding of an elevated white cell cystine level (see Chapter 5).

Case 3

A 7-month-old female infant known to have significant gastro-oesophageal reflux, presented with marked failure to thrive. There was no history of diarrhoea and she was on no medication. Investigations on admission were as follows:

Plasma:

sodium	122 mmol/l
potassium	1.7 mmol/l
chloride	76 mmol/l
bicarbonate	28 mmol/l
urea	10 mmol/l
creatinine	67 μmol/l

Urine:

sodium	65 mmol/l
potassium	70 mmol/l
chloride	55 mmol/l

Capillary blood:

pH	7.6
base excess	+10

Commentary In view of the fact that she was known to have a severe gastro-oesophageal reflux, the main differential diagnoses were recurrent vomiting, or alternative explanations for the hypokalaemic metabolic alkalosis, e.g. Bartter's syndrome or non-accidental diuretic administration.

The elevated urinary chloride is helpful in this regard as this effectively eliminates recurrent vomiting as a diagnosis. The prolonged use or abuse of diuretic therapy is indistinguishable from Bartter's syndrome as both may lead to the above biochemical picture. In practice, the only way to distinguish these two conditions is by detection of diuretic metabolites in the urine. This assay was negative.

Hyperkalaemia

Pseudohyperkalaemia

Pseudohyperkalaemia refers to those conditions in which elevation of the plasma potassium concentration is due to potassium movement out of the cells during or after the blood specimen has been drawn. The main reason is mechanical trauma during venepuncture, resulting in the release of potassium from red cells and a characteristic reddish tint of the plasma due to the release of haemoglobin. Similar circumstances occur when the capillary route is used for blood sampling. It may also occur in hereditary spherocytosis and in familial pseudohyperkalaemia, in which there is increased temperature-dependent leakage of potassium out of the red blood cells after specimen collection. Potassium also moves out of white cells and platelets and although this is not clinically important in patients with normal peripheral white cell and platelet counts, the measured serum potassium concentration may be as high as 9 mmol/l in patients with marked leucocytosis or thrombocytosis as may occur in myeloproliferative disease. The presence of pseudohyperkalaemia should be suspected when there is no apparent cause for an elevated plasma potassium concentration in the asymptomatic patient.

True hyperkalaemia

The aetiology of hyperkalaemia secondary to potassium retention is best considered in relation to the GFR [28], which may be estimated by using the Schwartz formula (Chapter 28). The investigation and causes of hyperkalaemia are summarized in Fig. 2.5 and Table 2.10.

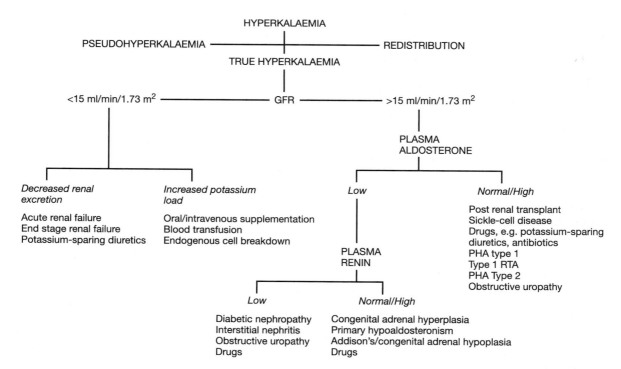

Fig. 2.5   Investigation of hyperkalaemia.

Table 2.10 Causes of hyperkalaemia

Pseudohyperkalaemia
Improper collection or handling of blood sample
In vitro haemolysis
Leucocytosis or thrombocytosis
True hyperkalaemia
GFR < 15 ml/min/1.73 m^2
  Decreased renal excretion
    Acute renal failure
    End stage renal failure
    Potassium-sparing diuretics
  Increased potassium load
    Oral/intravenous supplementation
    Blood transfusion
    Endogenous cell breakdown
GFR > 15 ml/min/1.73 m^2
  Low plasma aldosterone
    Low plasma renin
      diabetic nephropathy
      interstitial nephritis
      obstructive uropathy
      drugs, e.g. ciclosporin, tacrolimus, NSAIDs,
        β-adrenergic and calcium channel
        blockers
    Normal/high plasma renin
      congenital adrenal hyperplasia
      primary hypoaldosteronism
      Addison's/congenital adrenal hypoplasia
      drugs, e.g. ACEI, ARB
  Normal/high plasma aldosterone
    Post renal transplantation
    Sickle-cell disease
    Drugs, e.g. potassium-sparing diuretics, antibiotics
    PHA Type 1
    Type 1 RTA
    PHA Type 2 (Gordon's syndrome)
    Obstructive uropathy
Redistribution hyperkalaemia
Metabolic/respiratory acidosis
Hyperkalaemic periodic paralysis
Mineralocorticoid and insulin deficiency
Drugs/toxins

ACEI, angiotensin converting enzyme inhibitors; ARB, angiotensin receptor antagonists; GFR, glomerular filtration rate; NSAIDS, non-steroid anti-inflammatory drugs; PHA, pseudohypoaldosteronism; RTA, renal tubular acidosis.

Glomerular filtration rate less than 15 ml/min/1.73 m^2

Potassium loading is far more likely to induce hyperkalaemia if the renal function is significantly impaired and may occur with excessive oral or intravenous administration, gastro-intestinal bleeding, the use of old blood for transfusion and when massive cell breakdown occurs in thermal injury, extensive crush injury, massive intravascular haemolysis or spontaneous/chemotherapeutic-induced tumour lysis [29]. However, all of these circumstances may lead to significant hyperkalaemia in patients with normal or mildly impaired renal function.

Glomerular filtration rate greater than 15 ml/min/1.73 m^2

A combination of hyperkalaemia and a normal or minimally elevated plasma creatinine, generally indicates the presence of impaired urinary potassium excretion secondary to aldosterone deficiency/resistance and/or a reduction in distal nephron sodium and water delivery. The action of aldosterone at the level of the distal nephron may be evaluated by the transtubular potassium gradient (TTKG) using the formula:

$$TTKG = \frac{[\text{Urine K (mmol)}/(U/P_{osm})]}{\text{Plasma K (mmol/l)}}.$$

Values in children vary from 4.1 to 10.5 (median 6.0) and in infants from 4.9 to 15.5 (median 7.8) [30]. An increase in TTKG suggests dietary excess and a decrease suggests aldosterone deficiency/resistance.

Salt wasting and hyperkalaemia with relatively normal renal function, a low plasma aldosterone and high renin level should suggest the presence of adrenal insufficiency, either congenital or acquired. Similar findings may occur with the use of angiotensin converting enzyme inhibitors (ACEI) and angiotensin receptor antagonists (ARB) and in primary hypoaldosteronism. The finding of salt wasting and hyperkalaemia in the presence of a normal/increased plasma aldosterone indicates end organ resistance and is seen after renal transplantantation, in sickle-cell disease, with the use of potassium sparing diuretics and some antibiotics, e.g. trimethoprim and pentamidine and in pseudohypoaldosteronism (PHA) Type 1. Some patients with Type 1 (distal) renal tubular acidosis present with a combination of metabolic acidosis and hyperkalaemia. Although this maybe an isolated presentation, it is more commonly seen in sickle-cell nephropathy and in obstructive uropathy.

Rarely, a combination of sodium and potassium retention may occur with Gordon's syndrome (PHA Type 2) and in obstructive uropathy. Finally, patients with mild to moderate chronic renal insufficiency, usually secondary to diabetic nephropathy, interstitial nephritis, obstructive uropathy or sickle-cell disease or with the use of various drugs, e.g. ciclosporin, tacrolimus, β-adrenergic and calcium channel blockers and NSAIDs, may develop the syndrome of hyporeninaemic hypoaldosteronism.

Redistribution hyperkalaemia

The most common situation in which distribution of potassium is disturbed is metabolic acidosis. The shift of potassium from ICF to ECF is precipitated by an increase in the ECF hydrogen ion concentration. In DKA, the effect of metabolic acidosis is enhanced by insulin deficiency and the glycaemic-induced bulk flow of potassium-rich fluid from the cell to the ECF. A similar transmembrane potassium shift may be seen following a rapid infusion of mannitol. Mineralocorticoid deficiency also inhibits transmembrane potassium movement, as does therapy with β-adrenergic blockers and angiotensin converting enzyme inhibitors. Arginine, used in growth hormone provocation tests, has been reported to induce hyperkalaemia in patients with chronic renal failure. Familial hyperkalaemic periodic paralysis is an autosomal dominant disorder in which episodes of weakness or paralysis are usually precipitated by cold exposure, exercise or ingestion of small amounts of potassium. The primary abnormality in this condition appears to be a mutation in the gene for the α subunit of a skeletal muscle cell sodium channel. Other rare causes of hyperkalaemia due to translocation of potassium from the ICF to the ECF include digoxin overdose and the administration of succinylcholine to patients with thermal injury, extensive trauma or neuromuscular disease.

Clinical features of hyperkalaemia

Generally speaking, mild elevation in the plasma potassium concentration is not associated with clinical signs or symptoms. With a more significant increase, the patient may exhibit muscle weakness, but the main features of significant hyperkalaemia are visible on ECG monitoring (Fig. 2.4). The first abnormality appears with a plasma level of 6.5 mmol/l, and is that of prolongation of the PR interval and peaking of the T wave. A further increase in the plasma level leads to widening of the QRS complex and the depression of the ST segment. The risk of a major arrhythmia is significant above 8.5 mmol/l, but arrhythmias may occur at lower levels in the presence of acidosis and hypoxia.

The priority in the treatment of hyperkalaemia (Chapter 22) is dictated by the presence of major ECG abnormalities. Management of hyperkalaemia in chronic renal insufficiency and in conditions associated with impaired renal excretion, is based on dietary restriction in combination with loop diuretic therapy, and/or bicarbonate supplementation and/or 9α-fludrocortisone. Some patients with hyperkalaemic periodic paralysis benefit from treatment with a β-adrenergic agonist, e.g. salbutamol, that enhances cellular potassium uptake.

Key points: Hyperkalaemia

- Elevated plasma potassium in an asymptomatic patient with no apparent cause suggests pseudohyperkalaemia.

- Hyperkalaemia may result from an increase in total body potassium or from maldistribution between the ECF and ICF compartments.

- Hyperkalaemia from potassium retention is far more likely with a GFR $<$ 15 ml/min/1.73 m^2.

- Hyperkalaemia in the presence of a GFR $>$ 15 ml/min/1.73 m^2 generally indicates impaired potassium excretion secondary to aldosterone deficiency or resistance and/or a reduction in distal nephron sodium and water delivery.

- The action of aldosterone at the level of the distal nephron may be evaluated by the transtubular potassium gradient (TTKG).

- Salt wasting and hyperkalaemia with relatively normal renal function, a low plasma aldosterone and high renin level suggests adrenal insufficiency (or the use of ACEI or ARB drugs).

- The above picture but with normal/increased aldosterone suggests end organ resistance to aldosterone, e.g. PHA Type 1.

- Sodium and potassium retention can occur with PHA Type 2 and in obstructive uropathy.

- Hyporeninaemic hypoaldosteronism is associated with certain specific causes of mild to moderate chronic renal failure.

- Redistribution hyperkalaemia:
  – is most commonly seen in metabolic acidosis;
  – in DKA, insulin deficiency and hyperglycaemia enhance the effects of acidosis;
  – mineralocorticoid deficiency and certain drugs can cause this problem;
  – familial hyperkalaemic paralysis is an autosomal dominant condition.

- The priority in managing hyperkalaemia is dictated by the presence of major ECG abnormalities (see Chapter 22).

Illustrative cases: hyperkalaemia

Case 1

A male infant, born by SVD at term, was admitted to the SCBU on day 5 with a history of poor feeding. On examination he was lethargic, mildly dehydrated and non-virilized. He was started empirically on intravenous antibiotics after cerebrospinal fluid (CSF), blood and urine cultures were taken, which were subsequently sterile. His condition abruptly deteriorated on day 7. Investigations at that point revealed:

Plasma:

sodium	118 mmol/l
potassium	9.2 mmol/l
chloride	87 mmol/l
bicarbonate	12 mmol/l
urea	14 mmol/l
creatinine	56 μmol/l
cortisol	1140 nmol/l
	(normal range < 720 nmol/l)
17α-hydroxyprogesterone	< 5 nmol/l
	(normal range < 30 nmol/l)
renin	66 ng/ml/h
	(normal range < 15 ng/ml/h)

Commentary A combination of hyponatraemia, extreme hyperkalaemia, metabolic acidosis and a normal plasma creatinine strongly suggests adrenal insufficiency, mineralocorticoid deficiency or resistance. The presence of a normal plasma cortisol and 17α-hydroxyprogesterone level eliminates the commoner salt-losing forms of congenital adrenal hyperplasia. The key investigation here is the plasma aldosterone value, which was recorded at >20 000 pmol/l (normal 1000–5000 pmol/l), confirming the diagnosis of pseudohypoaldosteronism. Subsequent investigation revealed an elevated sweat sodium and chloride consistent with multiple receptor type PHA.

Case 2

An 18-month-old girl with no significant past history presented with a 5-day history of bloody diarrhoea and a generalized clonic convulsion on the day of admission. She had not passed urine in the 24-hour period prior to admission. On admission she was pale, mildly oedematous and had a blood pressure of 120/90. Investigations carried out on admission were as follows:

Plasma:

sodium	128 mmol/l
potassium	6.9 mmol/l
urea	40 mmol/l
bicarbonate	12 mmol/l

creatinine	450 μmol/l
Haemoglobin	8.5 g/dl
Platelet count	40 × 10⁹/l

Commentary This child has the classic presentation of acute renal failure secondary to diarrhoea-associated haemolytic uraemic syndrome. The degree of hyperkalaemia reflects the acute reduction in GFR over the preceding 24–48 hours and is exacerbated by the associated metabolic acidosis. Prior to the institution of peritoneal dialysis she was treated with intravenous sodium bicarbonate 2 mmol/kg and calcium resonium 1 g/kg. After a period of oliguria and dialysis dependency of 7 days, renal function progressively improved and ultimately returned to normal.

Case 3

A 6-month-old infant with complex cyanotic congenital heart disease was admitted for assessment and control of increasing cardiac failure. Therapy on admission was captopril, spironolactone and furosemide. Investigations on admission were as follows:

Haemoglobin	19.4 g/dl
Plasma:	
sodium	130 mmol/l
chloride	75 mmol/l
potassium	6.7 mmol/l
bicarbonate	26 mmol/l
urea	19 mmol/l
creatinine	100 μmol/l

Commentary This child had a reduced effective intravascular volume secondary to advanced cardiac failure resulting in a low GFR and enhanced, non-osmotic release of ADH. Hyperkalaemia is a recognized complication of the use of ACEI, particularly if there is coexisting hypovolaemia. In addition, potassium-sparing diuretics are likely to induce hyperkalaemia if the GFR is low for any reason.

The spironolactone and captopril were discontinued and she was treated with an infusion of dobutamine which resulted in both clinical and biochemical improvement. The mainstay of subsequent management was fluid restriction which was difficult in view of the intense neuro-humoral stimulation of thirst.

References

1. MacKenzie A., Barnes G. and Shann F. Clinical signs of dehydration in children. Lancet 1989; 2:605–607.
2. Kamel K.S., Ethier J.H., Richardson R.M.A., Bear R.A. and Halperin M.L. Urine electrolytes and osmolality: when and how to use them. Am. J. Nephrol. 1990; 10:89–102.
3. Steiner R.S. Interpreting the fractional excretion of sodium. Am. J. Med. 1984; 77:699–702.

4. Gennari F.J. Serum osmolality: uses and limitations. N. Eng. J. Med. 1984; 310:102–105.

5. Finberg L. The changing epidemiology of water balance and convulsions in infant diarrhoea. Am. J. Dis. Child. 1986; 40:524–528.

6. Albanese A., Hindmarsh P., Stanhope R. Management of hyponatraemia in patients with acute cerebral insults. Arch. Dis. Child. 2001; 85:246–251.

7. Haycock G.B. The syndrome of inappropriate secretion of anti-diuretic hormone. Pediatr. Nephrol. 1991; 9:375–381.

8. Robertson G.L., Aycinena P. and Zerbe R.L. Neurogenic disorders of osmoregulation. Am. J. Med. 1982; 72(2):339–353.

9. AAP. Provisional Committee on Quality Improvement, Sub-committee on Acute Gastroenteritis. Practice parameter: Management of acute gastroenteritis in young children. Pediatrics 1996; 97:424–430.

10. International Study Group on Reduced Osmolarity ORS Solutions: Multicentre evaluation of reduced osmolarity oral rehydration salts solution. Lancet 1995; 345:282–285.

11. Holliday M.A., Friedman A.L. and Wassner S.J. Extracellular fluid restoration in dehydration: A critique of rapid versus slow. Pediatr. Nephrol. 1999; 13:292–297.

12. Cochrane Injuries Group Albumin Reviewers: Human albumin administration in critically ill patients: systematic review of randomised controlled trials. BMJ 1998; 317:235–240.

13. Kumar S. and Berl T. Sodium. Electrolyte quintet. Lancet 1998; 352:220–228.

14. Soupart A. and Decaux G. Therapeutic recommendations for the management of severe hyponatraemia: Current concepts on pathogenesis and prevention of neurological complications. Clin. Nephrol. 1996; 46:149–154.

15. Finberg L. Hypernatraemic (hypertonic) dehydration in infants. N. Eng. J. Med. 1973; 289:196–198.

16. Trachtman H., Barbour R., Sturman J.A. and Finberg L. Taurine and osmoregulation: Taurine is an osmoprotective molecule in chronic hypernatraemic dehydration. Pediatr. Res. 1988; 23(1):35–39.

17. Baylis P.H. and Cheetham T. Diabetes insipidus. Arch. Dis. Child. 1998; 79:84–89.

18. Hillier T.A., Abbott R.D. and Barrett E.J. Hyponatraemia: Evaluating the correction factor for hyperglycaemia. Am. J. Med. 1999; 106:399–402.

19. Meadow R. Non-accidental salt poisoning. Arch. Dis. Child. 1993; 68:448–452.

20. Arneil G.C. and Beattie T.J. Renal venous thrombosis. In: Edelmann C.M. Jr (Ed.) Pediatric Kidney Disease 2nd Edition. Boston, Little Brown 1992:1905–1915.

21. Silver S.M., Clarke E.C., Schroeder B.M. and Sterns R.H. Pathogenesis of cerebral oedema after treatment of diabetic ketoacidosis. Kidney Int. 1997; 51:1237–1241.

22. Harris G.D., Fiordalisi I., Harris W.L., Mosovich L.L. and Finberg L. Minimizing the risk of brain herniation during treatment of diabetic ketoacidosis: a retrospective and prospective study. J. Pediatr. 1990; 117(1):22–31.

23. Schwartz. G.J. Potassium and acid base. In: Barratt T.M., Avner E.D. and Harmon W.E (Eds) Pediatric Nephrology 4th Edition. Lippincott Williams and Wilkins 1998:155–189.

24. Dalton R.N. and Haycock G.B. Laboratory investigation. In: Barratt T.M., Avner E.D. and Harmon W.E. (Eds) Pediatric Nephrology 4th Edition. Lippincott Williams and Wilkins 1998:343–364.

25. Sulyok E., Meneth M. and Tenyl I. Relationship between maturity, electrolyte balance and the renin angiotensin aldosterone system in newborn infants. Biol. Neonate 1979; 35:60–65.

26. Gennari F.J. Hypokalaemia. N. Eng. J. Med. 1998; 339(7): 451–458.

27. Williams G.S., Klenk E.L. and Winters R.W. Acute renal failure in pediatrics. In: Winters R.W. (Ed.) The Body Fluids in Pediatrics. Boston, Little Brown 1973:523–557.

28. DeFronzo R.A. and Smith J.D. Clinical disorders of hyperkalaemia. In: Narins R.G. (Ed.) Clinical Disorders of Fluid and Electrolyte Metabolism 5th Edition. New York, McGraw-Hill 1994:697–754.

29. Weiner I.D. and Wingo C.S. Hyperkalaemia: a potential silent killer. J. Am. Soc. Nephrol. 1998; 9:1535–1543.

30. Rodriguez-Soriano J., Ubetagoyena M. and Vallo A. Transtubular potassium concentration gradient: a useful test to estimate renal aldosterone bioactivity in infants and children. Pediatr. Nephrol. 1990; 4:105–110.

3 | The approach to a child with metabolic acidosis or alkalosis

Robert J. Postlethwaite

Discussions of metabolic acidosis are almost invariably dominated by complex arguments about the differentiation between ever-changing types of renal tubular acidosis. This might be of interest to professional nephrologists but not to most other practitioners. While not wishing to underplay the importance of this group of conditions, the children are rarely acutely unwell with life-threatening illness and there is usually time to establish the diagnosis. In contrast, extrarenal metabolic acidosis may be due to, among other causes, inborn errors of metabolism [1,2] and either accidental or non-accidental poisoning [3]. Prompt identification of extrarenal acidosis in these circumstances may be literally life saving, both by virtue of allowing for the institution of appropriate management [1–4] and by facilitating effective child protection measures in the case of non-accidental poisoning. Furthermore, extrarenal metabolic acidosis is a very important management problem in sick children, particularly in intensive care [5], and thus the identification and characterization of metabolic acidosis is a fundamental skill that all paediatricians must possess.

Metabolic alkalosis receives less attention and frequently is not dangerous [6]. It can, however, be a diagnostic problem [7–9]. In some settings metabolic alkalosis may contribute to mortality and morbidity and should be treated aggressively. Renal tubulopathies are discussed in Chapter 5.

This chapter will present a practical approach to the identification and evaluation of metabolic acidosis and alkalosis. Theoretical principles are introduced where they are crucial to understanding the investigation algorithms. There is no discussion of respiratory acidosis or alkalosis.

Metabolic acidosis

Metabolic acidosis can be defined as a disorder associated with a low arterial pH and serum bicarbonate concentration.

Initial assessment of metabolic acidosis

The initial assessment of metabolic acidosis is summarized in Fig. 3.1.

Step 1(a): Measure the serum anion gap

Sodium is the principal measured cation and chloride and bicarbonate the principal measured anions. The serum anion gap (SAG), which is accounted for by a number of unmeasured anions (predominantly negatively charged proteins), is calculated using equation 3.1:

$$SAG = Na^+ - (Cl^- + HCO_3^-) \qquad (3.1)$$

If the metabolic acidosis is due to accumulation of hydrochloric acid, this is buffered by bicarbonate (eqn 3.2), i.e. bicarbonate is replaced by chloride on an equimolar basis so there is no change in the SAG. It is important to remember that loss of bicarbonate, e.g. from the gut, is equivalent to gain of hydrogen ion and will provoke the same consequences.

$$HCl + NaHCO_3 \rightarrow NaCl + H_2CO_3 \rightarrow CO_2 + H_2O \qquad (3.2)$$

This disorder is called *hyperchloraemic acidosis*, because of the rise in the plasma chloride concentration.

The outcome is different if the accumulated acid is not hydrochloric acid but hydrogen ion with some other anion (e.g. lactic acid, labelled 'L' in eqn 3.3):

$$HL + NaHCO_3 \rightarrow NaL + H_2CO_3 \rightarrow CO_2 + H_2O \qquad (3.3)$$

As before, bicarbonate is replaced by the new anion, L. L differs from chloride because it is not routinely measured, whereas the sodium is. Thus there is an increase in the anion gap. Increased *anion-gap acidosis* is due to the accumulation of an acid other than hydrochloric acid as a result of endogenous production or exogenous administration.

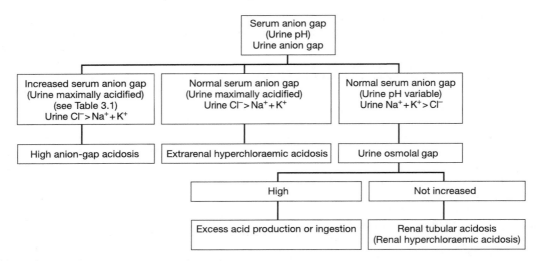

Fig. 3.1 Initial assessment of metabolic acidosis.

There are a number of methodological problems with the estimation of the SAG. For example, it will be lower in the presence of hypoalbuminaemia. The autoanalyser used to measure chloride significantly affects the estimate [10]. Thus the anion gap should be considered as only an approximation, with a normal value of 12 ± 2 mmol/l. These figures are confirmed by recent data in neonates where an SAG above 16 mmol/l was highly predictive of lactic acidosis [5]. Thus SAG greater than 16 mmol/l is suggestive of acidosis due to increased acid production or ingestion, and the higher the SAG, the more likely is this conclusion. However, there is overlap with lower values, which makes interpretation difficult [5].

Step 1(b): Estimate renal acid output

In the presence of metabolic acidosis, the healthy kidney will maximize the excretion of acid. Estimating the renal output of acid is, therefore, useful in confirming the presence of increased acid load.

One obvious way to estimate renal acid output is to measure the urine pH (U_{pH}). However, the renal capacity to excrete free hydrogen ions (which is indicated by the U_{pH}) is limited, varies with maturity, and an acid urine (but not a maximally acidified urine) occurs in renal tubular acidosis. For all these reasons, the measurement of U_{pH} is of limited value in the assessment of acidosis (hence it appears in brackets in Fig. 3.1). If the U_{pH} is measured, it must be done with a pH meter, rather than a dipstick, which is far too

Table 3.1 Maximal urine acidification following acute acid load as a function of age

Age	Urine pH (mean $\pm$ SD)
Preterm (1–3 weeks)[11]	6.0 (0.1)
Preterm (4–6 weeks)[11]	5.2 (0.4)
Preterm (3–4 months)[12]	5.2 (0.2)
Term (1–3 weeks)[11]	5.0 (0.2)
Term (1–16 months)[13]	4.9 (0.1)
7–12 years[13]	4.9 (0.2)

inaccurate, and the value must be compared with age-appropriate values (see Table 3.1).

The net urine excretion of acid is defined conventionally by equation 3.4 [14].

Renal net acid excretion

$$= U_{\text{titratable acid excretion}} + U_{NH_4^+} - U_{HCO_3^-} \qquad (3.4)$$

The renal ability to excrete ammonium (NH_4^+) is much greater than the ability to excrete free hydrogen ions. Urinary ammonium is, therefore, a much more sensitive indicator of a renal response to an increased acid load [15]. Urinary ammonium is not measured routinely, but can be estimated from the urine anion gap (UAG) [16–18]. UAG is calculated in the same way as SAG (eqn 3.5).

$$UAG = (U_{Na^+} + U_{K^+}) - U_{Cl^-} \qquad (3.5)$$

Unlike SAG, bicarbonate does not appear in this equation because it is usually completely reabsorbed. The major unmeasured cation is ammonium. Other unmeasured urinary anions include phosphate, sulphate and organic acids. Generally, the unmeasured anions exceed the unmeasured cations so that there is a urinary anion gap, often referred to as a positive UAG (Urine $Na^+ + K^+ > Cl^-$). In the presence of acidosis, urinary ammonium will increase. This combines with chloride to produce ammonium chloride. As can be seen from equation 3.5, this will increase urine chloride, but as ammonium is not measured there is no measured increase in cations. Thus in acidosis there will be a urinary cation gap ($Cl^- > Na^+ + K^+$). This is often referred to as a negative urinary anion gap [14–18]. This terminology is cumbersome and potentially confusing. To think in terms of urine anion gap or cation gap or perhaps more simply urinary ($Na^+ + K^+ > Cl^-$) or ($Cl^- > Na^+ + K^+$) is possibly less confusing. *Urine $Cl^- > Na^+ + K^+$ suggests increased urinary ammonium and is characteristic of a normal renal response to acidosis.*

Thus in increased SAG acidosis the urine should be maximally acidified and urine $Cl^- > Na^+ + K^+$. This is also helpful to evaluate overlap situations or situations where the SAG is artefactually low, when a urine response suggestive of increased acid load should be present.

This initial evaluation identifies three patterns (Fig 3.1)

- increased serum anion gap with appropriate renal response to acid load: *high anion gap acidosis*;
- normal serum anion gap with appropriate renal response to acid load: *extrarenal hyperchloraemic acidosis*;
- normal serum anion gap but failure to acidify urine ($Na^+ + K^+ > Cl^-$: *further evaluation required (Fig. 3.1).*

In this latter situation, the UAG may be misleading [16, 17, 19]. There are two main reasons for this:

1. If a patient is volume depleted with a urine sodium concentration less than 25 mmol/l the consequent increased chloride reabsorption will limit the excretion of ammonia as ammonium chloride. The kidney will not, therefore, be able to produce a normal response to an acid load, so that the urinary anion gap will remain positive ($Na^+ + K^+ > Cl^-$). Thus the urinary picture will suggest renal tubular acidosis despite the primary problem being volume depletion due, for example, to diarrhoea. This should not cause a major problem because the acidosis will resolve and the renal handling

of acid will normalize when the volume deficit is corrected.

2. If there is an increase in unmeasured urinary anions, there will be an increase in measured urinary cations such as sodium and potassium to maintain electroneutrality. This will counterbalance the increase in urinary chloride as a consequence of ammonium chloride excretion. Thus the UAG may remain positive ($Na^+ + K^+ > Cl^-$) despite significant ammonium excretion. In these circumstances measurement of the *urine osmolal gap* is helpful.

Step 2: Measure urine osmolal gap

Osmotic effects are colligative, they depend on the number of particles in the solution. Sodium and potassium (and their associated anions, predominantly chloride), urea and glucose are the main determinants of urine (and serum) osmolality. Thus the urine (or serum) osmolality can be calculated from equation 3.6:

$$Osmolality = 2 (Na^+ + K^+) + urea + glucose \qquad (3.6)$$

Note: ($Na^+ + K^+$) is multiplied by 2 because there will be equimolar concentrations of anions which exert an equal effect on the urine osmolality. All measurements are in mmol/l.

The urine osmolality can also be measured and the urine osmolal gap calculated by equation 3.7:

urine osmolal gap

$$= measured\ urine\ osmolality - calculated\ urine\ osmolality \qquad (3.7)$$

If there is some other salt in the urine exerting a significant effect on the urine osmolality, there will be an increased urine osmolal gap. In acidosis, the urine osmolal gap will largely represent ammonium salts. *A urine osmolal gap greater than 40 mosm/kg suggests significant ammonium excretion* [19]. Ketoacids in diabetic ketoacidosis and hippurate following toluene ingestion are examples of this situation.

This further step in evaluation of acidosis will identify two further types of acidosis (Fig. 3.1). Excess acid production or ingestion is not really a separate type, but an example of high anion-gap acidosis or extrarenal hyerchloraemic acidosis in which the SAG and/or UAG have been misleading. The final type is that of renal tubular acidosis.

High anion-gap acidosis

In this circumstance there is either an endogenous or an exogenous load of acid (Table 3.2). Clinical features and age of the patient usually give a good clue

Table 3.2 Causes of increased anion-gap metabolic acidosis

Inborn errors of metabolism, e.g. organic acidaemias
Lactic acidosis
    Type A—tissue under perfusion and/or hypoxia
    Type B—in the absence of hypotension and hypoxia
        Inborn errors of metabolism
        Salicylates
        Metformin/phenformin
        Isoniazid
        Ethanol
        Ethylene glycol
        Methanol
        Cyanide
        Liver disease
Ketoacidosis
    Diabetes mellitus
    Starvation
Renal failure
Toxins and drugs
    Toluene

---

as to whether or not the acid load was likely to be endogenous or exogenous.

Inborn errors of metabolism are a group of inherited disorders that can present in the newborn period or early childhood with an overwhelming illness associated with a marked metabolic acidosis [1,2]. The disorder may be one of amino-acid metabolism, e.g. maple syrup urine disease, or organic acid metabolism, e.g. methyl-malonic or proprionic acidaemia.

Typical symptoms include lethargy, poor feeding, apnoea or tachypnoea, vomiting, hypotonia, seizures and coma/encephalopathy. These clinical signs are very non-specific and the key to diagnosis is a high index of suspicion by the clinician. A history of a previous neonatal death in a sibling and consanguinity are helpful clues. Typically the infant is normal at birth and symptoms usually develop towards the end of the first week, after milk feeds have been established. The presence of massive ketonuria is an unusual finding in the newborn period and should always suggest the possibility of an inborn error of metabolism. Rarely, inborn errors of metabolism may present with recurrent acidosis in older children [4].

With some disorders the urine has a characteristic odour, e.g. maple syrup in maple syrup urine disease or 'sweaty feet' in isovaleric acidaemia.

Plasma amino acid and urine amino and organic acid analyses should be carried out by a laboratory experienced in the diagnosis of these disorders. While awaiting results, dietary protein should be restricted and adequate calories supplied as carbohydrate and lipid emulsions. Once diagnosis is established, the offending metabolite can be reduced by dialysis or haemofiltration, or rendered harmless by transportation into the cells by using a glucose and insulin infusion similar to that used in the treatment of hyperkalaemia.

Lactic acidosis is an important cause of severe metabolic acidosis. It has been proposed that lactic acidosis be separated into two major types [20].

Type A lactic acidosis is characterized by disorders in which there is tissue under perfusion or hypoxia, such as profound hypotension or sepsis. It is very common in intensive care situations [5,21].

Type B lactic acidosis occurs in the absence of hypoperfusion or hypoxia. It can occur in inborn errors of metabolism such as glycogen storage disease type I or defects in pyruvate metabolism. It also occurs with drug ingestions; indeed, the presence of a severe metabolic acidosis in a previously healthy child should raise the possibility of accidental or deliberate ingestion of drugs and toxins. In childhood, the classic example is due to salicylates, which disrupt the Krebs' cycle and oxidative phosphorylation, leading to a marked metabolic acidosis due to lactate accumulation. The other major effect of salicylates on the respiratory centre, leading to respiratory alkalosis, is much less evident in children as compared to adults. The finding of a positive urinary Phenistix® is a clue to diagnosis, and the excretion of harmful metabolites can be enhanced by a forced alkaline diuresis.

Ethanol inhibits hepatic gluconeogenesis and causes underutilization of lactate by the liver, leading to lactic acidosis which can be severe in children, especially if there is pre-existing liver disease. Phenformin, metformin, and isoniazid are other drugs that can produce lactic acidosis. Breakdown products of methyl alcohol and ethylene glycol also precipitate lactic acidosis secondary to a disruption of mitochondrial function due to a direct toxic effect.

In clinical practice, the distinction between Type A and Type B lactic acidosis is often not clear-cut, with patients showing features of both.

The primary goal in the therapy of lactic acidosis is correction of the underlying disorder. The role of alkali therapy is controversial. However, haemodynamic instability is common with severe acidosis (pH < 7.1). Alkali therapy may cause hypernatraemia and/or volume overload. Dialysis or haemofiltration is then indicated. It is essential to avoid the use of lactate-containing replacement fluids.

The identification of *diabetes mellitus* or *starvation* as a cause of increased anion-gap acidosis should not present many problems.

In *renal failure*, because of the variable accumulation of metabolites, an acidosis with either a normal or increased anion gap can occur.

Poisons (e.g. toluene) can also present as increased anion-gap acidosis.

Extrarenal hyperchloraemic acidosis

The causes of extrarenal hyperchloraemic acidosis are summarized in Table 3.3. The small bowel, biliary and pancreatic secretions contain about five times as much bicarbonate as plasma. Any condition leading to severe diarrhoea, artificial drainage or fistula will lead to a considerable loss of bicarbonate. Compensatory hyperchloraemia maintains a normal anion gap. These conditions, particularly acute diarrhoeal diseases, are a very common cause of acidosis but rarely cause a diagnostic problem. The only severe diarrhoeal illness not associated with bicarbonate loss is congenital chloride diarrhoea (see below).

Table 3.3 Extrarenal hyperchloraemic acidosis

Diarrhoeal disease
Small bowel, biliary or pancreatic drainage
Gastrointestinal–ureteral connections, e.g. bowel
  augmentation cystoplasty
(Carbonic anhydrase inhibitors/deficiency)

Urine in contact with the colon for any length of time will exchange chloride for bicarbonate and hence cause loss of bicarbonate. This was a considerable problem when ureterosigmoidostomy was a common form of urinary diversion. This problem largely disappeared when cutaneous urinary diversions were fashionable, but with the advent of bowel augmentation cystoplasty it is beginning to appear again [22].

Carbonic anhydrase inhibitors (such as acetazolamide) or deficiency produce a similar picture of acidosis but the urine pH will be above 6.5.

Renal hyperchloraemic acidosis

An algorithm for further evaluation of renal tubular acidosis (RTA) is given in Fig. 3.2. The first point to note is that a urine pH below 5.5 can be achieved in some forms of RTA. This apparent paradox is explained by equation 3.4. Bicarbonate loss in the urine is equivalent to gain of hydrogen ion and is, therefore, included in the formula to express net acid loss. If the predominant problem in RTA is loss of bicarbonate (e.g. proximal renal tubular acidosis), once bicarbonate falls below the reduced renal threshold it will be reabsorbed and disappear from the urine. If the other mechanisms of acid excretion are intact, a urine pH lower than 5.5 can then be achieved.

Proximal renal tubular acidosis (PRTA, RTA Type II) is caused by an impairment of resorption of bicarbonate by the proximal tubule and characterized by a decreased renal bicarbonate threshold. It results in

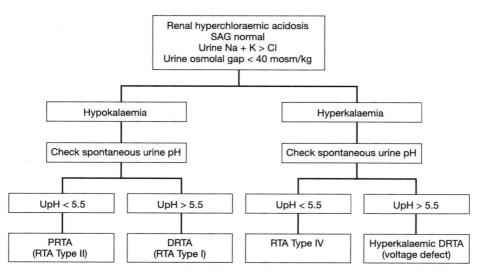

Fig. 3.2 Renal hyperchloraemic acidosis.

urinary bicarbonate wasting and metabolic acidosis (blood pH 7.20–7.35) with a low plasma bicarbonate (12–15 mmol/l). The bicarbonate wasting can be revealed by bicarbonate loading. Administration of a bicarbonate load (3 mmol/kg) will result in urinary loss of bicarbonate (fractional excretion of $HCO_3^- > 10$–15%). Fractional excretion is calculated by equation 3.8:

$$\text{Fractional excretion of } HCO_3^- = \frac{U_{HCO_3^-} \times P_{Cr}}{P_{HCO_3^-} \times U_{Cr}} \times 100 \ (3.8)$$

A characteristic finding in PRTA is hypokalaemia. The development of hypokalaemia is the result of renal potassium wasting caused by the increased aldosterone levels as a consequence of increased distal delivery of sodium. Distal tubular acidification is intact; thus when bicarbonate is below threshold, the urinary pH can be reduced below 5.5 and adequate amounts of ammonium can be produced. For this reason rickets, hypercalciuria and nephrocalcinosis do not occur.

The usual presenting features include failure to thrive, poor growth and vomiting. There are a large number of causes of PRTA (Table 3.4). Isolated PRTA is rare and much more commonly PRTA is associated with other tubular disturbances, as in Fanconi's syndrome (see Chapter 5).

Table 3.4 Causes of proximal renal tubular acidosis

Primary
  Sporadic
    Transient childhood [23]
    Persistent (adult onset) [24]
  Genetic [25]
  Carbonic anhydrase deficiency [26]
Secondary
  Hereditary multiple proximal tubular dysfunction
    (Fanconi syndrome)—see Chapter 5
  Associated with other metabolic disorders
    Hyperparathyroidism
    Vitamin D deficiency and dependency
    Leigh's syndrome
    Metachromatic dystrophy
    Osteopetrosis
    Pyruvate carboxylase deficiency
    Lowe's syndrome
    Mitochondrial myopathies
  Miscellaneous, including
    Cyanotic heart disease, particularly Fallot tetralogy
    Renal cystic disease
    Nephrotic syndrome
    Hereditary nephritis
    Renal transplant

Management consists of alkali supplements in the form of bicarbonate, citrate or lactate (2–20 mmol/kg/day of alkali may be required) [27]. The losses are very variable and, additionally, as the serum bicarbonate rises and exceeds the renal threshold, increasing amounts of bicarbonate are lost in the urine. Thus only partial correction is generally possible, but this is sufficient to relieve symptoms and restore growth.

Distal renal tubular acidosis (DRTA, RTA Type I) is caused by an impairment of distal acidification and is characterized by an inability to lower the urine pH maximally under acid load. Further evaluation can be achieved with acid loading [28], urine to blood carbon dioxide tension [29,30], and frusemide challenge [27,29,30]. The reduced excretion of titrable acid and ammonium are a consequence of the primary defect. In general, bicarbonate resorption is normal but, because of the elevated urine pH, a certain fraction of bicarbonate escapes resorption, although the fractional excretion of bicarbonate is less than 5%. Unlike those with PRTA, these patients are always in a state of persistent positive acid balance which requires buffering against bone buffers to prevent severe systemic acidosis and gives rise to bone disease, hypercalciuria, nephrocalcinosis, renal calculi and renal concentrating defect. Renal potassium wasting also ensues by a number of different mechanisms.

The clinical features are the same as those of PRTA with the addition of bone disease, polyuria/polydipsia and renal colic because of the abnormalities in calcium metabolism. The causes of DRTA are given in Table 3.5.

Management consists of correction of the acidosis. This can be achieved with administration of alkali, equal in amount to daily acid production (usually 1–2 mmol/kg/day), which results in complete correction of the acidosis and resolution of the bone disease and hypercalciuria. Nephrocalcinosis persists and might lead to continuing polyuria. In the long term,

Table 3.5 Causes of distal renal tubular acidosis

Primary (persistent classical syndrome)
  Genetic
  Sporadic
Secondary
  Hypercalciuria and nephrocalcinosis
  Associated with genetically transmitted diseases
  Autoimmune disorders
  Drugs or toxins
  Other renal disease
  Endocrine disease

hypokalaemia is corrected by alkali administration, but initially can be aggravated by alkali administration. Therefore the hypokalaemia should be at least partially corrected before the acidosis is corrected. Subsequently, administration of alkali as citrate or bicarbonate with one-third to one-half as the potassium salt will aid resolution of the hypokalaemia. As there is often increased bicarbonate loss in younger children, and in view of their rapid growth, higher rates of alkali replacement are usually given (4–15 mmol/kg/day).

RTA Type IV (hyperkalaemic DRTA) is in a sense misnamed. It arises from either aldosterone deficiency or unresponsiveness of the distal tubule to aldosterone (pseudohypoaldosteronism). Acidosis is only one element of the metabolic derangement evoked in these patients [31]. It is seen in hypo- or pseudohypoaldosteronism, probably most commonly as transient pseudohypoaldsteronism in urinary tract infection (UTI) and/or urinary obstruction [32]. It is also a feature of renal parenchymal disease, particularly when this affects the interstitium (e.g. obstructive uropathy, reflux nephropathy, interstitial nephritis). In these conditions, it gives rise to hyperkalaemia disproportionate to the degree of glomerular impairment. It is distinguished from RTA Type I by the hyperkalaemia. Measurement of plasma renin and aldosterone is helpful. Both will be extremely high in pseudohypoaldosteronism, either as a primary defect or secondary to renal parenchymal disease. In hypoaldosteronism the renin will be extremely high with low, normal or marginally elevated aldosterone. The problems associated with hyopaldosteronism should resolve with administration of mineralocorticoids. Correction of acidosis, sodium loading, thiazide diuretics and loop diuretics may all have an impact on pseudohypoaldosteronism. In the extreme hyperkalaemia seen in acute pseudohypoaldosteronism in UTI/obstruction, dramatic reduction in the plasma potassium is achieved by sodium loading [32].

Hyperkalaemic DRTA (voltage defect) is a further variant of hyerkalaemic RTA. It is beyond the scope of this text, and original articles should be consulted for details [31].

Management of severe metabolic acidosis

The mainstay of treatment of acid–base disorders has to be the treatment of the underlying conditions. Occasions arise where treatment with a buffer is required, either as emergency management of an acute clinical state or as chronic management of a tubular disorder not amenable to specific correction.

Immediate treatment of an acute acidotic state is indicated in the presence of a deteriorating clinical condition while the underlying disorder is being treated, or to maintain a reasonable haemodynamic state while treatment is started for the underlying condition. This usually only applies to situations where the blood pH is below 7.10. There are good theoretical reasons for not correcting less severe acidosis that is not, in itself, life threatening. Acidosis causes vasodilation and correction with bicarbonate causes vasoconstriction. Thus in the acutely sick patient, administration of bicarbonate leads to a worsening of the peripheral circulation, allowing a persistence of anaerobic metabolism and lactic acid production in the tissues. Good oxygenation with vasodilatation is a much more appropriate and successful course of action. This is made more pertinent by experimental evidence showing that administration of bicarbonate worsens intracellular acidosis by the formation of carbonic acid in the cytoplasm of the cells [33].

The usual buffer used to correct acidosis is sodium bicarbonate (see Table 3.6). THAM (trometamol) combines with carbonic acid to form hydroxy-THAM and bicarbonate. It has no advantage over sodium bicarbonate, although it is often used as it has a non-sodium base, on the mistaken assumption that this will avoid volume overload. Giving cations in the form of THAM is no different to giving cations in the form of sodium. A disadvantage of THAM is the strong alkalinity of the solution, which proves highly irritant.

The actual amount of buffer to give is at best a guess. An approximate formula which is widely used for total correction of acidosis is:

amount of base in mmol
$$= 0.3 \times \text{base deficit} \times \text{body weight (kg)} \qquad (3.9)$$

Table 3.6 Commonly available buffers

Sodium bicarbonate 8.4%[a]: 1 ml = 1 mmol
Sodium bicarbonate 4.2%: 1 ml = 0.5 mmol
THAM (trometamol) 7.2%: 1 ml ~ 1 mmol sodium
  bicarbonate

[a] It is generally recommended that sodium bicarbonate 8.4% solutions should be diluted to 4.2% before peripheral intravenous administration.

Total correction is rarely, if ever, indicated. In addition, the relationship between plasma bicarbonate and pH is far from linear, small increments in bicarbonate leading to large shifts in pH for initial pH values less than 7.20. In the severely acidotic patient, initial therapy aimed at raising the plasma bicarbonate by 5 mmol/l will have a marked effect on pH even if the initial bicarbonate is less than 10 mmol/l.

Assuming an effective volume of distribution of bicarbonate of 50% of body weight, to raise the bicarbonate by 5 mmol/l involves giving an initial dosage of 2.5 mmol/kg. Using this formula, with subsequent repetition if necessary, is more appropriate than total or half-correction using the formula stated earlier (3.9) and avoids large, potentially harmful swings in pH.

Metabolic alkalosis

Metabolic alkalosis is probably more common than realized, but generally presents no diagnostic or management problem as the cause is obvious—usually diuretic administration or vomiting. More rarely it presents as a diagnostic problem, with the differential diagnosis including tubulopathies such as Bartter's syndrome and surreptitious administration of emetics, laxatives and diuretics.

Metabolic alkalosis can be defined as a primary elevation of plasma bicarbonate (>30 mmol/l) with corresponding rise in arterial pH (>7.40). If the pH is below 7.4 with raised bicarbonate, the likely problem is a compensated respiratory acidosis.

The causes of metabolic alkalosis are listed in Table 3.7, but these are not sufficient on their own to produce a metabolic alkalosis as the renal capacity to excrete bicarbonate is so great that the excess of bicarbonate would be excreted rapidly. Thus to sustain the high plasma bicarbonate another factor has to be present which limits renal excretion of bicarbonate. One or more of the factors listed in Table 3.8 must additionally be present to allow for the development of metabolic alkalosis.

The interplay of the various factors in chloride depletion, such as those which occur in pyloric stenosis, is shown in Fig. 3.3. Impaired bicarbonate secretion, reduced glomerular filtration rate, increased sodium bicarbonate reabsorption, hypokalaemia with secondary rise in ammonium and hydrogen ion excretion all contribute to the genesis and maintenance of the alkalosis.

Table 3.7   Causes of metabolic alkalosis

Gastrointestinal hydrogen ion loss
Renal hydrogen ion loss
Intracellular shift of hydrogen ion
Alkali administration
Contraction alkalosis

Table 3.8   Factors responsible for net bicarbonate resorption in metabolic alkalosis

Effective circulating volume depletion
Chloride depletion and hypochloraemia
Hypokalaemia

Another related issue is the use of urinary sodium in alkalosis. The measurement of the urine sodium concentration is often used to distinguish between volume depletion (<25 mmol/l) and euvolaemia (>40 mmol/l). There are problems in alkalosis, where the need to retain sodium is counteracted by the need to excrete bicarbonate and high urine sodium concentration might ensue despite the presence of volume depletion [35,36]. The same constraints do not apply to chloride excretion, so that a urine chloride concentration below 25 mmol/l is a better guide to the presence of volume depletion in alkalosis than the urine sodium concentration. This is particularly important because assessment of volume status and response to chloride administration are the crucial steps in evaluation of metabolic alkalosis (Fig. 3.4).

Most of the causes of chloride-responsive metabolic alkalosis are clinically obvious and present no problem in diagnosis (Table 3.9). Intestinal secretions typically contain a relatively high bicarbonate concentration and hence loss of intestinal secretions results in acidosis. However, in some cases of diarrhoea, metabolic alkalosis results [37]. This is characteristic in congenital chloride diarrhoea and in laxative abuse in adults [38,39]. Surreptitious vomiting in adults is another cause of metabolic alkalosis [40]. This reminds one to think of child abuse in a child with unexplained metabolic alkalosis. Surreptitious administration of diuretics has been described [41]. Vomiting and/or diarrhoea are some of the most common presenting features in fabricated and induced illness in children (Münchausen syndrome by proxy abuse) [42]. Such presentations are often due to laxative or emetic abuse and could present with metabolic alkalosis. Cystic fibrosis presenting as alkalosis because of chloride loss in the sweat should not be forgotten [43].

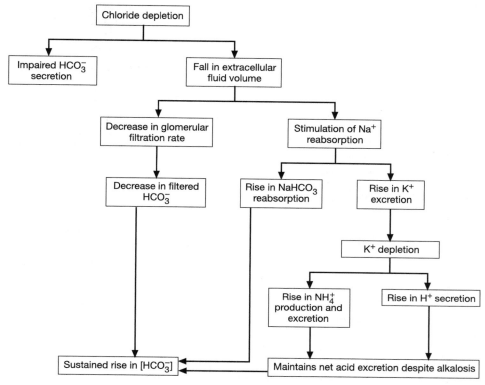

Fig. 3.3 Pathophysiology of chloride-responsive metabolic alkalosis (reproduced with modifications from [34] with permission from Mosby Inc.).

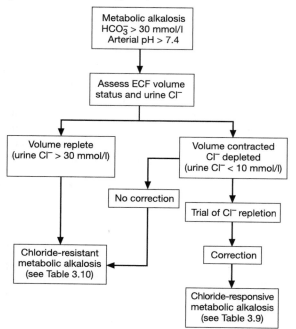

Fig. 3.4 Evaluation of metabolic alkalosis.

Table 3.9 Causes of chloride-responsive metabolic alkalosis

Acid loss from the stomach
Vomiting
Nasogastric suction
Diuretic administration
Chloride-depleting diarrhoea
Congenital chloride diarrhoea
Laxative abuse
Other
Cystic fibrosis

The causes of chloride-resistant metabolic alkalosis are given in Table 3.10. Further evaluation depends on the clinical features, particularly the blood pressure and measurement of renin and aldosterone [44] (see Fig. 3.5). Bartter's and Gitelman's syndromes are discussed in Chapter 5.

Management of severe metabolic alkalosis

Severe metabolic alkalosis, i.e. plasma bicarbonate greater than 50 mmol/l, is a rare occurrence. Changes

Table 3.10 Causes of chloride-resistant metabolic alkalosis

Mineralocorticoid excess
  Primary hyperaldosteronism
  Cushing syndrome
  ACTH-secreting tumour
  Renin-secreting tumour
  Adrenogenital syndromes
  Fludrocortisone treatment
Apparent mineralocorticoid excess
  Liquorice
  Liddle's syndrome
  11β-Hydroxysteroid dehydrogenase deficiency
  High-dose glucocorticoids
Impairment of Cl-linked Na^+ reabsorption
  Bartter's syndrome
  Gitelman's syndrome
  Severe K^+ deficiency

in the peripheral and central nervous systems are similar to those in hypocalcaemia, with mental confusion, predisposition to seizures, paraesthesiae, muscle cramps and cardiac arrhythmias. This situation is usually only seen in patients with long-term loss of gastric secretions, excessive diuretic therapy or hyperadrenalism due to neoplasia. In such patients, corrective measures are slow and often take quite some time to correct the degree of alkalosis. The most important aspect of therapy is saline repletion. As long as renal function is good, potassium chloride infusion in a dosage of 3 mmol/kg/day is useful in the treatment of alkalosis associated with the loss of gastric secretions. More rapid correction can be achieved with ammonium chloride 5.35% solution (1 mmol/ml), infused using the same formula as for the correction of metabolic acidosis. The use of acetazolamide or other acids is not advised.

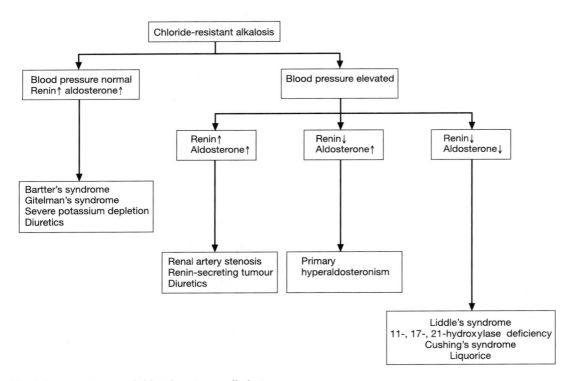

Fig. 3.5 Investigation of chloride-resistant alkalosis.

References

1. Burton BK. Inborn errors of metabolism in infancy: a guide to diagnosis. Pediatrics 1998; 102, E69.
2. Wraith JE. Diagnosis and management of inborn errors of metabolism. Arch Dis Child 1989; 64, 1410–1415.
3. Kreisberg RA, Wood BC. Drug and chemical-induced metabolic acidosis. Clin Endocrinol Metab. 1983; 12: 391–411.
4. Shetty AK, Craver RD, Harris JA, Schmidt-Sommerfield E. Delayed diagnosis of fatal medium-chain acyl-CoA dehydrogenase deficiency in a child. Pediatr Emerg Care 1999; 15, 399–401.

5. Lorenz JM, Kleinman LI, Markarian K, Oliver M, Fernandez J. Serum anion gap in the differential diagnosis of metabolic acidosis in critically ill newborns. J Pediatr 1999; 135, 751–755.

6. Plamer BF, Alpern RJ. Metabolic alkalosis. J Am Soc Nephrol 1997; 8, 1462–1469.

7. Bartholow C, Whittier FC, Rutecki GW. Hyopkalaemia and metabolic alkalosis: algorithms for combined clinical problem solving. Compr Ther 2000; 26, 114–120.

8. Schurman SJ, Shoemaker LR. Barrter and Gitelman syndromes. Adv Pediatr 2000; 47, 223–248.

9. Van't Hoff WG. Molecular developments in renal tubulopathies. Arch Dis Child 2000; 83, 189–191.

10. Winter SD, Pearson R, Gabow PA, *et al.* The fall of the serum anion gap. Arch Intern Med 1990; 150, 311–313.

11. Svenningsen NW. Renal acid–base titration studies in infants with and without metabolic acidosis in the postneonatal period. Pediatr Res 1974; 8, 659–672.

12. Schwartz GJ, Haycock GB, Edelmann CM Jr, *et al.* Late metabolic acidosis: a reassessment of the definition. J Pediatr 1979; 95, 102–107.

13. Edelmann CM Jr, Rodriguez-Soriano J, Boichis H, *et al.* Renal bicarbonate reabsorption and hydrogen ion excretion in infants. J Clin Invest 1967; 46, 1309–1317.

14. Manz F, Kalhoff H, Remer T. Renal acid excretion in early infancy. Pediatr Nephrol 1997; 11, 231–243.

15. Carlisle EJ, Donnelly SM, Halperin ML. Renal tubular acidosis (RTA): recognize the ammonium defect and pHorget the urine pH. Pediatr Nephrol 1991; 5, 242–248.

16. Batlle DC, Hizon M, Cohen E, Gutterman C, Gupta R. The use of the urinary anion gap in the diagnosis of hyperchloraemic acidosis. N Engl J Med 1988; 318, 591–599.

17. Halperin ML, Vasuvattakul S, Bayoumi A. A modified classification of metabolic acidosis. A pathophysiological approach. Nephron 1992; 60, 129–133.

18. Rose BD. Clinical physiology of acid–base and electrolyte disorders, 4th edn. New York, McGraw-Hill, 1994; 551–553.

19. Meregalli P, Luthy C, Oetliker OH, Bianchetti MG. Modified urine osmolal gap: an accurate method for estimating the urinary ammonium concentration? Nephron 1995; 69: 98–101.

20. Madias N. Lactic acidosis. Kidney Int 1986; 29, 752–774.

21. Oriot D, Nasimi A, Berthier M, *et al.* Lactate and anion gap in asphyxiated neonates. Arch Dis Child Fetal Neonatal Ed 1997; 76, F15–20.

22. Repassy DL, Becsi A, Tamas G, Weninger T. Metabolic consequences of orthotopic ileal neobladder. Acta Chir Hung 1999; 38, 321–328.

23. Nash MA, Torrado AD, Griefer I, *et al.* Renal tubular acidosis in infants and children. J Pediatr 1972; 80, 736–748.

24. York SE, Yendt ER. Osteomalacia associated with renal bicarbonate loss. Can Med Assoc J 1966; 94, 1329–1342.

25. Brenes LG, Brenes JN, Hernandez MM. Familial proximal renal tubular acidosis. A distinct clinical entity. Am J Med 1977; 63, 244–252.

26. Donckerwolke RA, Van Steckelenberg GJ, Tiddens HA. A case of bicarbomate-losing renal tubular acidosis with defective carboanhydrase activity. Arch Dis Child 1970; 45, 403–412.

27. Dubose TD. Hyperkalemic hyperchloremic metabolic acidosis: pathophysiologic insights. Kidney Int 1997; 51, 591–602.

28. Edelmann CM Jr, Boichis H, Rodriguez-Soriano J, *et al.* The renal response of children to acute ammonium chloride acidosis. Pediatr Res 1967; 1, 452–460.

29. Battle DC. Segmental characterization of defects in collecting tubule acidification. Kidney Int 1986; 30, 546–554.

30. Rodriguez-Soriano J, Vallo A, Castillo G, *et al.* Pathophysiology of primary distal renal tubular acidosis. Int J Pediatr Nephrol 1985; 6, 71–78.

31. Rodrigeuz-Soriano J, Vallo A. Renal tubular hyperkalaemia in childhood. Pediatr Nephrol 1988; 2, 498–509.

32. Schoen EJ, Bhatia S, Ray GT, Clapp W, To TT. Transient pseudohypoaldosteronism with hyponatremia-hyperkalemia in infant urinary tract infection. J Urol 2002; 167, 680–682.

33. Ritter JM, Doktor HS and Benjamin N. Paradoxical effect of bicarbonate on cytoplasmic pH. Lancet 1990; 335, 1243–1246.

34. Gennari FJ. Metabolic alkalosis. In: Jacobson HR, Striker GF, Klahr S (eds). The principles and practice of nephrology, 2nd ed. St Louis, Mosby, 1995; 832–941.

35. Sherman RA, Eisinger RP. The use (and misuse) of urinary sodium and chloride measurements. JAMA 1982; 247, 3121–3124.

36. Kassirer JP, Schwartz WB. The response of normal man to selective depletion of hydrochloric acid. Factors in the genesis of persistent gastric alkalosis. Am J Med 1966; 40, 1–8.

37. Perez GO, Oster JR, Rogers A. Acid–base disturbances in gastrointestinal disease. Dig Dis Sci 1987; 32, 1033–1044.

38. Holmberg C. Congenital chloride diarrhoea. Clin Gastroenterol 1986; 15, 583–602.

39. Bytzer P, Stokholm M, Andersen I, *et al.* Prevalence of surreptitious laxtive abuse in patients with diarrhea of uncertain origin. Gut 1989; 30, 1379–1384.

40. Mitchell JE, Seim HC, Colon E, Pomeroy C. Medical complications and management of bulimia. Ann Intern Med 1987; 107, 71–77.

41. D'Avanzo M, Satinelli R, Tolone C, Bettinelli A, Bianchetti MG. Concealed administration of frusemide simulating Bartter syndrome in a 4.5-year-old boy. Pediatr Nephrol 1995; 9, 749–750.

42. Postlethwaite RJ, Eminson DM, Vail A. Why study case reports? Gathering evidence about the physical intrusiveness and outcome of Munchausen syndrome by proxy. Arch Dis Child In Press 2002.

43. Kennedy JD, Dinwiddie R, Daman-Willems C, *et al.* Pseudo-Bartter's syndrome in cystic fibrosis. Arch Dis Child 1990; 65, 786–787.

44. Bartholow C, Whittier FC, Rutecki GW. Hypokalaemia and alkalosis: algorithms for combined clinical problem solving. Comp Ther 2000; 26, 114–120.

4 | Disorders of mineral metabolism and nephrolithiasis

Caroline Jones and Zulf Mughal

This chapter discusses the regulation of calcium, phosphorus, magnesium and vitamin D metabolism and disorders that arise when there is pathology of their control mechanisms. The renal handling of these cations is one of the factors involved in the pathogenesis of nephrolithiasis, which is discussed later in the chapter. Renal osteodystrophy is discussed in Chapter 23.

Regulation of serum calcium concentration

Parathyroid hormone and the calcium-sensing receptor

In the plasma, calcium exists in three different forms: 50% as ionized (the biologically active form), 45% bound to plasma proteins (mainly albumin), and 5% complexed to anions, such as phosphate and citrate. The normal concentration of ionized calcium is critical for many important biological functions, such as nerve conduction, muscle contraction, blood coagulation, hormone secretion and cellular differentiation. Automated analysers will perform a mathematical calculation to give serum calcium corrected for albumin. This, however, is an approximated figure and in some clinical conditions direct measurement of ionized calcium is useful. Metabolic acidosis reduces protein binding and therefore increases ionized calcium. Treatment of the acidosis before correction of hypocalcaemia, for example in acute renal failure, will result in a fall in ionized calcium and may cause tetany or cardiac arrest.

The extracellular fluid (ECF) calcium concentration is maintained within tight limits (2.2–2.7 mmol/l total or 1.0–1.5 mmol/l ionized) by parathyroid hormone (PTH), 1,25-dihydroxyvitamin D_3 $(1,25(OH)_2D_3)$ and calcitonin. These hormones

regulate calcium transport in the kidney, bone and gastrointestinal tract.

Parathyroid hormone enhances renal calcium reabsorption and increases the rate of calcium resorption from bone. PTH also promotes the renal conversion of 25-hydroxyvitamin D_3 to 1,25-dihydroxyvitamin D_3. This is the biologically active metabolite of vitamin D which stimulates gastrointestinal calcium absorption. The increase in plasma calcium reduces synthesis and secretion of PTH.

Parathyroid cells and renal tubules express a cell-surface calcium-sensing receptor (CaSR) that enables these cells to detect and respond to small changes in the extracellular calcium concentration [1]. An increase in serum calcium concentration activates the CaSR, leading to decreased secretion of PTH and inhibition of renal calcium reabsorption. A decrease in serum calcium concentration results in inactivation of this receptor and has an opposite effect. The CaSR is also involved in renal water handling. Water reabsorption is enhanced by vasopressin, which inserts the water channel, aquaporin-2, into the cell membranes of the collecting duct. The CaSR is found in the same apical endosomes in the collecting duct that contain aquaporin-2. The reduction in renal tubular concentrating ability that occurs with hypercalciuria may result from a reduction in the availability and/or activity of these water channels. The increase in urinary flow reduces the luminal calcium concentration and may have a potential role in reducing the risk of nephrocalcinosis and renal stone formation in hypercalcaemic conditions [1,2].

The gene for the CaSR is located on chromosome 3q13.3–q21 and several mutations have been found that lead to inactivation (loss of function) and activating (gain of function) of the CaSR. Heterozygous inactivating mutations of the CaSR give rise to familial hypocalciuric hypercalcaemia (FHH) [3,4]. Subjects with this autosomal dominant disorder have asymptomatic mild elevation of serum calcium concentration but a low urinary excretion of calcium. Homozygous inactivating mutations in the CaSR result in neonatal severe hyperparathyroidism (NSHP) [3,4]. This is a rare condition characterized by severe hypercalcaemia, markedly elevated PTH concentration and a demineralized skeleton. NSHP is fatal unless treated by total parathyrodectomy. Conversely, patients with activating mutations of the CaSR have autosomal dominant hypocalcaemia with hypercalciuria [3,4]. Increased activity of the mutant CaSRs in the renal collecting duct results in impaired urinary concentration and, in these patients, polyuria and polydipsia develop when the serum calcium concentration is normal. The majority of these patients have asymptomatic 'hypocalcaemia'. However, a few patients will require treatment with calcium 1α-hydroxycholecalciferol (alfacalcidol) in order to alleviate the symptoms of hypocalcaemia. This must be undertaken with great care as the combined effects of hypercalciuria and dehydration may make subjects with this condition particularly susceptible to nephrocalcinosis and renal impairment.

As mentioned in Chapter 23, secondary hyperparathyroidism associated with renal osteodystrophy is often difficult to control, even with optimal medical management. Development of calcimimetic agents that act on the CaSR to lower plasma levels of PTH provide a novel therapeutic approach to treatment of the secondary hyperparathyroidism that accompanies chronic renal failure [5].

1,25-Dihydroxyvitamin D$_3$

Calcium is absorbed in the gastrointestinal tract by both active and passive mechanisms. $1,25(OH)_2D_3$ stimulates active calcium absorption in the duodenum and proximal jejunum by increasing the synthesis of the intestinal vitamin D-dependent calcium-binding protein, calbindin D9K. Passive transport of calcium occurs throughout the small intestine. The rate of absorption is directly proportional to the intraluminal concentration of calcium. $1,25(OH)_2D_3$ also stimulates osteoclastic activity and mobilization of calcium from bone.

Calcitonin

Calcitonin inhibits osteoclastic bone resorption and therefore its production is reduced by hypocalcaemia. In humans, its physiological importance remains unclear as bone mineral metabolism is unperturbed in athyreotic patients who produce very low levels of calcitonin and in patients with medullary carcinoma of the thyroid who produce very high levels of calcitonin.

Key points: Regulation of serum calcium

- Plasma calcium exists in three different forms: ionized (50%), bound to plasma proteins (45%) and complexed to anions (5%).

- Metabolic acidosis reduces protein binding and increases ionized calcium.

- ECF calcium concentration is maintained within tight limits by parathyroid hormone (PTH), 1,25-dihydroxyvitamin D$_3$ ($1,25(OH)_2D_3$) and calcitonin.

- Parathyroid cells and renal tubules express a cell-surface calcium-sensing receptor (CaSR) that enables these cells to detect and respond to small changes in the extracellular calcium concentration.

- CaSR is also involved in renal water handling.

- The CaSR gene is located on chromosome 3q13.3–q21 and several mutations have been found that lead to inactivation (loss of function) and activation (gain of function).

- Calcium is absorbed in the gastrointestinal tract by both active and passive mechanisms.

- $1,25(OH)_2D_3$ stimulates active calcium absorption in the duodenum and proximal jejunum.

- Calcitonin inhibits osteoclastic bone resorption and therefore its production is reduced by hypocalcaemia.

Regulation of serum magnesium homeostasis

Magnesium is the fourth largest cation within the body and is crucial for many functions, including normal enzyme function, replication and transcription of DNA, cellular energy metabolism, membrane stabilization, nerve conduction, ion transport and calcium channel activity. Of the total serum magnesium, approximately 30% is protein bound, 55% is ionized and 15% is complexed. The maintenance of extracellular fluid magnesium concentration is mainly dependent on gastrointestinal absorption and renal excretion. Hypocalcaemia is typically present in severe hypomagnesaemia. Most patients with hypocalcaemia and hypomagnesaemia have a low or normal plasma PTH, suggesting impaired synthesis or secretion of PTH. Treatment with magnesium results in a rise in PTH and, as a consequence, correction of hypocalcaemia.

Urinary magnesium excretion and hypermagnesuria

Up to 70% of filtered magnesium is reabsorbed in the loop of Henle. Hypermagnesaemia inhibits loop absorption and the reverse occurs during hypomagnesaemia. This is regulated by the Ca^{2+}/Mg^{2+} sensing receptor. Other factors which influence magnesium resorption include PTH, calcitonin, glucagon, vasopressin, magnesium restriction, and acid–base balance. Population data on magnesium excretion in healthy children are available but urinary magnesium should be interpreted in context with dietary magnesium and serum magnesium.

Increased urinary magnesium may be related to a primary defect in renal tubular magnesium reabsorption or secondary to reduced tubular reabsorption of sodium. Increased urinary flow, as in diabetes mellitus, volume overload, the diuretic phase of acute tubular necrosis and post–obstructive nephropathy, also results in increased magnesium losses. Hypercalcaemia and hypercalciuria reduce tubular magnesium reabsorption. Increased renal losses also occur with phosphate

depletion and the correction of chronic systemic acidosis. Increased tubular magnesium losses are observed in proximal renal tubular acidosis and other tubulo-interstitial disorders.

Hypercalcaemia

Hypercalcaemia develops when the rate of calcium entry into the extracellular fluid exceeds the capacity of the kidneys for its excretion. It occurs when there is increased absorption of calcium from the gastrointestinal tract, increased release of calcium from the skeleton or decreased excretion of calcium from the kidneys. The causes of hypercalcaemia in childhood are listed in Table 4.1. A detailed description of these conditions, which occur infrequently in the general paediatric setting, is beyond the scope of this chapter.

Regardless of the aetiology, symptoms of hypercalcaemia are similar. Infants have non-specific symptoms, including feeding difficulties, vomiting, constipation, hypotonia and failure to thrive. Older children may present with muscle weakness and neuropsychiatric symptoms. Activation of the CaSR in the kidney caused by hypercalcaemia leads to impaired renal concentrating ability, which results in polydipsia and polyuria. This may lead to dehydration and fever. Chronic hypercalcaemia and accompanying

Table 4.1 Causes of hypercalcaemia in childhood

Increased intestinal calcium absorption
  Williams syndrome (syndrome of distinctive facial
    features, developmental delay, supravalvular or
    peripheral pulmonary stenosis and hypercalcaemia
    during early childhood. Over 90% have microdeletion
    of the elastin gene, 7q11.23)
  Idiopathic infantile hypercalcaemia
  Vitamin D intoxication
  Vitamin A intoxication
  Granulomatous disorders, e.g. sarcoidosis
Decreased renal calcium excretion
  Primary hyperparathyroidism
  Autosomal dominant familial hypocalciuric
    hypercalcaemia
  Thiazide diuretics
Increased bone resorption
  Immobilization
  Primary hyperparathyroidism
  Malignancy
Uncertain mechanism
  Hypophosphatasia
  Subcutaneous fat necrosis
  Blue diaper syndrome
  Dietary phosphate deficiency

Key points: Regulation of serum magnesium

- Of the total serum magnesium, approximately 30% is protein bound, 55% is ionized and 15% is complexed.

- Hypocalcaemia is typically present in severe hypomagnesaemia.

- Up to 70% of filtered magnesium is reabsorbed in the loop of Henle.

- Increased urinary magnesium may be related to a primary defect in renal tubular magnesium reabsorption or secondary to reduced tubular reabsorption of sodium.

hypercalciuria may predispose to nephrocalcinosis and nephrolithiasis.

Principles of treatment of hypercalcaemia

Treatment of symptomatic hypercalcaemia includes general supportive measures to lower plasma calcium concentration and specific treatment of the underlying cause.

Hydration and sodium diuresis

In severe hypercalcaemia, dehydration occurs as a result of impaired ability to concentrate urine, nausea and vomiting. Intravenous isotonic saline (1–1.5 times the daily fluid allowance) can be used to rehydrate the patient. This results in an increase in urinary sodium, which is coupled to an increase in urinary calcium. This sodium diuresis can be enhanced with a loop diuretic (e.g. frusemide, 1 mg/kg/12 hours). Thiazide diuretics must be avoided since they impair urinary calcium excretion and may exacerbate the problem. Increased urinary losses of water, potassium, sodium, phosphate and magnesium need to be replaced.

Mobilization

Patients should avoid immobilization, which increases bone resorption and aggravates hypercalcaemia. This is particularly important in adolescents.

Reduction of gastrointestinal calcium absorption

Reduction of dietary calcium and vitamin D intake is effective in treating hypercalcaemia in conditions where there is increased intestinal calcium absorption, including idiopathic infantile hypercalcaemia and Williams syndrome. Oral prednisolone (2 mg/kg/day, maximum dose 60 mg/day) reduces intestinal calcium absorption in vitamin D toxicity and ectopic synthesis of 1,25-dihydroxyvitamin D_3 (e.g. in sarcoidosis).

Inhibition of bone resorption

Subcutaneous synthetic or salmon calcitonin (4 to 8 units/day) inhibits bone resorption. The calcium-lowering response of calcitonin may be reduced during prolonged and continuous administration. The bisphosphonates are a group of drugs which inhibit osteoclastic bone resorption. They are effective in the treatment of hypercalcaemia secondary to malignancy and in conditions causing increased bone resorption. Intravenous pamidronate disodium (1 mg/kg/day,

maximum dose 60 mg) can be infused over 4 hours and is usually administered daily until serum calcium concentration normalizes. Side-effects of pamidronate disodium include post-infusion fever, myalgia and reversible leucopenia.

Dialysis

Peritoneal or haemodialysis against a low-calcium dialysis solution is highly effective in lowering plasma calcium concentration. This measure is reserved for life-threatening hypercalcaemia.

Hypocalcaemia

The causes of hypocalcaemia in childhood are shown in Table 4.2. Hypocalcaemia may occur as a consequence of an inadequate calcium supply, following an acute increase in plasma phosphate concentration, impaired PTH secretion and end organ resistance to PTH (e.g.

Table 4.2 Causes of hypocalcaemia in childhood

Inadequate calcium supply
  Early neonatal hypocalcaemia—abrupt fall in placental
    calcium supply at birth
  Severe malabsorption (short bowel syndrome)
  'Hungry bone syndrome'—post-parathyroidectomy or
    after rapid healing of severe vitamin D deficiency rickets
Decrease in ionized calcium concentration
  Chelation
  Respiratory or metabolic alkalosis
Phosphate overload
  Excessive phosphate intake (e.g. ingestion of unmodified
    cow's milk in the neonate)
  Acute and chronic renal failure
  Crush injuries and rhabdomyolysis
Hypoparathyroidism
  Transient—from suppression of fetal parathyroid
    glands secondary to maternal hypercalcaemia
  DiGeorge syndrome—congenital agenesis or hypoplasia
    of parathyroid glands. Associated with distinctive
    facial features, developmental delay, congenital heart
    disease, thymic aplasia and T-cell
    dysfunction. The majority of patients have a
    microdeletion of 22q11.21–q11.23
  HDR syndrome (hypoparathyroidism, deafness, and
    renal dysplasia)
  Autoimmune polyglandular endocrinopathy—associated
    with mucocutaneous candidiasis and Addison's disease
  Post-thyroidectomy or parathyrodectomy
  Haemosiderosis, e.g. thalassaemia major
Resistance to parathyroid hormone
  Pseudohypoparathyroidism
  Hypomagnesaemia

---

pseudohypoparathyroidism). Hypomagnesaemia leads to resistance of the action of PTH on bone and kidney. Therefore the clinical manifestations of hypomagnesaemia are frequently those of hypocalcaemia.

In neonates, symptoms of hypocalcaemia include jitteriness, stridor, apnoea, tetany and convulsions. An older child with mild hypocalcaemia may complain of numbness and tingling sensation in the circumoral region, fingers and toes. Latent tetany can be elicited by Chevostek's sign. This is twitching of the facial muscles in response to gentle tapping over the branches of the facial nerve anterior to the earlobe, but below the zygomatic arch. Symptoms of severe hypocalcaemia include muscle cramps, tetanic carpopaedal spasm, laryngospasm and convulsions. Cardiovascular manifestations include hypotension, heart failure and arrhythmias. An ECG will show prolonged Q–T interval in children with reduced ionized serum calcium concentration.

Parathyroid hormone resistance

Parathyroid hormone resistance is characterized by hypocalcaemia, hyperphosphataemia and elevated plasma PTH concentration. It is secondary to end organ resistance to PTH. Patients with pseudohypoparathyroidism type 1 have absent urinary cAMP and do not have a phosphaturic response to exogenous PTH administration. Phenotypic features include short stature, round face, short metacarpals and metastatic calcification. The majority of these patients have a loss of function mutation in the gene encoding for Gsα protein within the cell walls.

Hypomagnesaemia

Magnesium deficiency leads to end organ renal and skeletal refractoriness to the effects of PTH.

Hypomagnesaemia usually arises as a result of increased gastrointestinal or renal losses (Table 4.3).

Treatment of hypocalcaemia

Intravenous 10% calcium gluconate solution (0.2 ml/kg) should be given to infants with symptomatic hypocalcaemia. This is infused over 10 minutes as rapid injection can cause cardiac arrhythmias. Placement of the intravenous catheter in a large vein avoids extravasation into the subcutaneous tissues, which may lead to tissue necrosis and permanent scarring. Once the patient is asymptomatic, a maintenance infusion of 10% calcium gluconate (0.2–1 mmol/kg/day) or oral calcium supplements (50–75 mg/kg/day of elemental calcium in four divided doses) can be prescribed. For older children and adolescents the maximum dose of oral calcium supplements is 2 g/day.

In infants, intramuscular 50% magnesium sulphate solution (0.2 ml/kg) is used to treat hypocalcaemia secondary to magnesium deficiency. Two injections, 12 hours apart, are sufficient for most cases of neonatal hypocalcaemia. Patients with primary defects of magnesium metabolism require long-term treatment with oral magnesium supplements.

1,25-dihydroxycholecalciferol (calcitriol) and 1α-hydroxycholecalciferol (alfacalcidol) are used to treat chronic hypocalcaemia resulting from hypoparathyroidism and pseudohypoparathyroidism. Calcitriol is started at the initial oral dose of 15 ng/kg (maximum dose 1.5 μg/day) or alfacalcidol at the initial starting dose of 25 ng/kg (maximum dose is 2 μg/day). Alfacalcidol can be administered as a single dose, whereas calcitriol has a shorter half-life and should be administered twice daily. The aim of the treatment is to maintain the plasma calcium concentration in the low normal range

Table 4.3 Causes of hypomagnesaemia in childhood

Gastrointestinal losses	
Primary hypomagnesaemia	Genetic defect of intestinal magnesium absorption
Secondary hypomagnesaemia	Infants of diabetic mothers, diarrhoea, malabsorption, ileostomy
Renal losses	
Primary hypomagnesaemia	Primary renal tubular magnesium wasting
	Gittleman's syndrome
Secondary hypomagnesaemia	Hypercalcaemia and hypercalciuria
	Osmotic diuresis (diabetes, mannitol)
	Thiazide and loop diuretics, alcohol, aminoglycosides, cisplatin, amphotericin B, cyclosporin, pentamidine
	Diuresis following acute renal failure or post-obstructive nephropathy
	Phosphate depletion

(2.0–2.25 mmol/l). In the absence of PTH, or resistance to its biological action, renal tubular calcium absorption is reduced, and therefore at high-normal plasma calcium concentrations hypercalciuria and nephrocalcinosis may occur.

Key points: Hypercalcaemia and hypocalcaemia

- Regardless of the aetiology, symptoms of hypercalcaemia are similar:
  - infants have non-specific symptoms;
  - older children present with muscle weakness and neuropsychiatric symptoms;
  - activation of CaSR in the kidney leads to impaired renal concentrating ability, which results in polydipsia and polyuria.

- Treatment of hypercalcaemia includes:
  - general supportive measures to lower plasma calcium concentration;
  - specific treatment of the underlying cause.

- The clinical manifestations of hypomagnesaemia are frequently those of hypocalcaemia:
  - in neonates, symptoms of hypocalcaemia include jitteriness, stridor, apnoea, tetany and convulsions;
  - an older child with mild hypocalcaemia may complain of numbness and tingling sensation in the circumoral region, fingers and toes;
  - latent tetany can be elicited by Chevostek's sign.

- Treatment of hypocalcaemia:
  - intravenous 10% calcium gluconate solution (0.2 ml/kg) should be given to infants with symptomatic hypocalcaemia;
  - in infants, intramuscular 50% magnesium sulphate solution (0.2 ml/kg) is used to treat hypocalcaemia secondary to magnesium deficiency;
  - patients with primary defects of magnesium metabolism require long-term treatment with oral magnesium supplements;
  - vitamin D metabolites are used to treat chronic hypocalcaemia resulting from hypoparathyroidism and pseudohypoparathyroidism.

The regulation of phosphorous metabolism

The normal plasma level of inorganic phosphate is essential for normal cell function and skeletal mineralization. In contrast to calcium, the plasma phosphate concentration is not tightly controlled and is influenced by age, sex and dietary intake. The amount of dietary phosphate absorbed from the gut is relatively constant, although it is enhanced by $1,25(OH)_2D_3$. The plasma concentration of phosphate is regulated primarily by renal tubular reabsorption of filtered phosphate. This is decreased by PTH, phosphate overload and in inherited or acquired renal tubular disorders. Other common causes of increased urinary phosphate losses include osmotic diuresis, polyuria after treatment of obstructive uropathy or the diuretic phase of acute renal failure and renal transplantation. The tubular dysfunction associated with ifosfamide and cisplatin is usually dose dependent and is manifested by hypercalciuria, hyperphosphaturia, hypermagnesuria and generalized aminoaciduria. Other drugs that may lead to a tubulopathy include toluene (glue sniffing), gentamicin and heavy metals. Renal tubular reabsorption is increased by dietary phosphate deprivation, $1,25(OH)_2D_3$, growth hormone, insulin-like growth factor-I and insulin.

In assessing phosphate handling by the kidney, it is important to take account of the filtered load of phosphate as well as of the amount of phosphate reabsorbed by the tubules. A 24-hour urinary phosphate measurement alone is insufficient as it does not take into account the filtered load of phosphate. The simplest measurement of renal phosphate handling is the percentage of tubular reabsorption of phosphate (TRP), which is easily calculated from the phosphate and creatinine concentrations of random urine and plasma samples.

$$\text{TRP\%} = 1 - \frac{[U_{PO_4}] \times [P_{Cr}]}{[P_{PO_4}] \times [U_{Cr}]} \times 100$$

where
$[U_{PO_4}]$ = urine phosphate concentration (mmol/1);
$[P_{PO_4}]$ = plasma phosphate concentration (mmol/l);
$[U_{Cr}]$ = urine creatinine concentration (mmol/l); and
$[P_{Cr}]$ = plasma creatinine (mmol/l).

Normally, more than 85% of the filtered load of phosphate is reabsorbed, but it approaches 100% during dietary phosphate deprivation. Alternatively, the renal tubular phosphate threshold maximum of phosphate per unit volume of glomerular filtrate (T_{MPO_4}/GFR) can be determined from the plasma phosphate concentration and TRP, using the Walton and Bijvoet normogram [6].

Key points: Regulation of phosphorous metabolism

- The plasma phosphate concentration is not tightly controlled and is influenced by age, sex and dietary intake.

- The plasma concentration of phosphate is regulated primarily by renal tubular reabsorption of filtered phosphate.

- In assessing phosphate handling by the kidney, it is important to take account of the filtered load of phosphate as well as of the amount of phosphate reabsorbed by the tubules.

Rickets

Rickets is the term applied to impaired mineralization at the epiphyseal growth-plate, resulting in deformity and impaired linear growth of long bones [7]. The clinical features of rickets are dependent on the underlying cause. Rickets may be classified as vitamin D-related, secondary to low dietary calcium and those due to hypophosphataemia. These aetiological factors may be inherited or acquired. The causes and biochemical characteristics are summarized in Table 4.4.

Vitamin D metabolism and function

Dietary vitamin D may be supplied in the diet as either vitamin D_3 (cholecalciferol), which is derived from 7-dehydrocholesterol, or from the plant sterol ergosterol as vitamin D_2 (ergocalciferol). These two forms will be referred to as vitamin D when it is not necessary to distinguish between them. Vitamin D absorbed from the diet enters the bloodstream in the form of chylomicrons. In the skin, 7-dehydrocholesterol is converted to vitamin D_3, through the intermediate pre-vitamin D_3, by the action of ultraviolet B (UVB) radiation in sunlight. Vitamin D_3 formed in the skin is removed from subcutaneous tissues by the

serum vitamin D binding protein. From either source, the vitamin is transported to the liver for hydroxylation at the 25 position. Vitamin D and 25-hydroxyvitamin D [25(OH)D] may be redistributed into body tissues, especially fat and muscle, from where they are mobilized slowly. This physico-chemical phenomenon enables vitamin D synthesized in the previous summer to provide a continuing, though diminishing, source during the following winter. This is important at higher latitudes where there is insufficient UVB to permit vitamin D synthesis in the winter months.

Circulating 25(OH)D is hydroxylated by the 1α-hydroxylase enzyme in the kidney to the active hormonal metabolite 1,25-dihydroxyvitamin D [1,25(OH)$_2$D] [8]. The production of 1,25(OH)$_2$D is enhanced by PTH and also by low concentrations of either calcium or phosphate. To limit the concentration of 1,25(OH)$_2$D, both 25(OH)D and 1,25(OH)$_2$D are hydroxylated by a renal enzyme at the 24 position. The hydroxylation of vitamin D at the 25-, 24- and 1 position all involve a specific cytochrome P450 oxidase (CYP27, CYP24, and CYP27B1, respectively), a flavoprotein and a ferredoxin. These form an electron transfer chain to hydroxylate the vitamin D substrate.

1,25(OH)$_2$D functions as a steroid hormone, regulating the expression of target genes through the intranuclear vitamin D receptor (VDR). Genes upregulated by 1,25(OH)$_2$D include those in the intestinal mucosa concerned with calcium transport, e.g. calbindin D9K [9]. Lack of 1,25(OH)$_2$D will result in defective calcium absorption. Inadequate concentrations of 1,25(OH)$_2$D are also reflected in bone function [10]. Osteoblasts have VDRs and express genes which are regulated by 1,25(OH)$_2$D, including alkaline phoshatase, osteocalcin, and osteopontin. 1,25(OH)$_2$D also regulates the function of genes outside the calcium homeostatic system. Many cells possess VDRs and 1,25(OH)$_2$D may modulate cellular differentiation and proliferation and immune-related processes.

Vitamin D-related rickets

Vitamin D deficiency

Vitamin D-deficiency rickets results from inadequate synthesis of 1,25(OH)$_2$D. This is usually secondary to a lack of the precursor, as in nutritional or privational rickets and in liver and gastrointestinal diseases, which are associated with fat malabsorption. In renal

Table 4.4   Types of rickets, causes and biochemical findings

Type	Basic cause	Serum biochemical changes
VITAMIN D RELATED		
Acquired		
Nutritional and Privational	Lack of vitamin D in diet and/or inadequate exposure to sunlight. Insufficient 1,25$(OH)_2$D for absorption of adequate calcium from diet and for normal skeletal mineralization	Calcium low or normal, phosphate low, alk phos high, PTH high, 25(OH)D low, and 1,25$(OH)_2$D high/normal/low (see text)
Malabsorptive disorders	Malabsorption of vitamin D and also possibly calcium	As above
Inherited		
Pseudovitamin D deficiency (PDDR, VDDR type I)	Mutations in the 25-hydroxyvitamin D-1α-hydroxylase genes. Insufficient 1,25$(OH)_2$D for absorption of adequate calcium from diet and for normal skeletal mineralization	Calcium low, phosphate low, alk phos high, PTH high, 25(OH)D normal, and 1,25$(OH)_2$D low
Hypocalcaemic vitamin D resistant (HVDRR, VDDR type II)	Mutations in the vitamin D receptor (VDR) gene. Inability of cells to respond to 1,25$(OH)_2$D	Calcium low, phosphate low, alk phos high, PTH high, 25(OH)D normal, and 1,25$(OH)_2$D very high
CALCIUM DEFICIENCY	Insufficient calcium in diet	Calcium low, phosphate normal, 25(OH)D normal, and 1,25$(OH)_2$D high
HYPOPHOSPHATAEMIC		
Acquired		
Fanconi's syndrome[a]	Renal tubular damage leading to increased renal loss of phosphate	Calcium normal, phosphate low, PTH normal, 25(OH)D normal, 1,25$(OH)_2$D variable, acidosis
Oncogenic	Overproduction by tumour of FGF23. This results in increased renal loss of phosphate and inadequate synthesis of 1,25$(OH)_2$D	Calcium normal, phosphate low, PTH normal, 25(OH)D normal, 1,25$(OH)_2$D low
Inherited		
X-linked hypophosphatemia	Mutations in the *phex* gene causing increased renal loss of phosphate plus inadequate synthesis of 1,25$(OH)_2$D	Calcium normal, phosphate low, PTH normal, 25(OH)D normal, 1,25$(OH)_2$D inappropriately normal
Autosomal dominant hypophosphatemic rickets	Missense mutations in the FGF23 (12p13.3) gene	Calcium normal, phosphate low, PTH normal, 25(OH)D normal, 1,25$(OH)_2$D inappropriately normal
Hypercalciuric hypophosphatemic rickets		Calcium normal, phosphate low, PTH low, 25(OH) D normal, 1,25$(OH)_2$ D high
RENAL OSTEODYSTROPHY		
Renal disease[b]	Raised serum phosphate, secondary hyperparathyroidism and impaired synthesis of 1,25$(OH)_2$D	Calcium normal or decreased, phosphate increased, PTH increased, 25(OH)D usually normal low 1,25$(OH)_2$D

[a] Fanconi's syndrome encompasses a wide range of conditions, including some that are inherited.
[b] Renal osteodystrophy is a complex bone disorder, which is discussed in detail in Chapter 23.

osteodystrophy 1,25$(OH)_2$D deficiency is secondary to impaired synthesis (Table 4.4).

In the nineteenth century, during the period of urbanization that accompanied the Industrial Revolution, there was a marked increase in the prevalence of rickets in northern Europe. Atmospheric pollution reduced UVB radiation reaching the ground. The incidence of rickets has declined following improved social and environmental awareness.

Vitamin D-deficiency rickets is now a rare disease. In the United Kingdom rickets remains an important public health problem among children of Indo-Asian and Middle Eastern immigrants. Cases of privational rickets have also been reported recently in the USA and Canada [11,12]. In this group, the aetiology of vitamin D deficiency includes limitation of ultraviolet radiation due to skin pigmentation or sunshine avoidance for religious and cultural reasons, and vegetarian diets. Prolonged total breast-feeding without vitamin D supplements also contributes to the problem [13]. It is important that clinicians do not overlook this once-traditional source of rickets in a mistaken belief that vitamin D deficiency has been eradicated

The normal diet cannot supply the recommended daily intake of 7–10 µg/day of vitamin D (280–400 i.u.). In many European countries, supplementation of foodstuffs with vitamin D is limited, and therefore solar exposure is responsible for providing most of the body's vitamin D. An epidemiological model regarding the development of privational rickets in the British Indo-Asian population has been published [14]. In this paper the authors conclude that the prevalence and severity of rickets are related to the extent of vegetarianism in the diet. Conversely, an omnivorous diet that includes meat exerts a protective effect which cannot be attributed to the vitamin D content of the meat consumed.

Pseudovitamin D-deficiency rickets (PDDR)

This was previously known as vitamin D-dependent rickets type I (VDDR type I). Prader first described this rare autosomal recessive disorder in which affected individuals have rickets, hypocalcaemia, tooth enamel hypoplasia, secondary hyperparathyroidism and greatly reduced serum levels of $1,25(OH)_2D$ despite normal concentrations of $25(OH)D$ [15]. Symptoms are reversed by treatment with $1,25(OH)_2D_3$, or 1α-hydroxyvitamin D_3 ($1\alpha(OH)D_3$). The disease is now believed to result from a defect in the $P450_c1$ component of the renal 1α-hydroxylase. The gene coding for $P450_c1$ (CYP27B1) is on chromosome 12q13.1–13.3 and maps to the disease locus of PDDR [16]. During the past 2 years, mutations in the gene from various cell types have been identified in PDDR patients [17–19]. Different point mutations have been described, but an interesting 7 bp duplication has been recorded in patients from Japan, Canada, and the United Kingdom. This mutation changes the structure of the critical haem-binding region of the cytochrome and leads to a premature stop codon [19,20]. All the P450 mutations reported so far are inactivating and lack 1α-hydroxylase activity. The clinical syndrome must, therefore, be assumed to arise from a failure to express the 1α-hydroxylase in the kidney. The lack of functional 1α-hydroxylase activity has been demonstrated in macrophages [20] and keratinocytes from PDDR patients [21].

Hereditary vitamin D-resistant rickets (HVDRR) (VDDR type II)

This extremely rare autosomal recessive condition is also known as VDDR type II. The inherited defects are in the VDR gene, which is located on chromosome 12q, in the same region as the gene coding for 1α-hydroxylase. In HVDRR the VDR-mediated actions of $1,25(OH)_2D$ are eliminated or reduced, even though supranormal concentrations of the hormone are present in the circulation. The high circulating levels of $1,25(OH)_2D$ are secondary to hypocalcaemia and low 24-hydroxylase activity. A range of mutations affecting the ligand-binding domain of the receptor and the DNA-binding region are described. Clinical manifestations include rickets and hypocalcaemia and some children also have alopecia. This suggests that the VDR may play a role in the development of the hair follicle. A recently published review summarizes the mutations and relates them to the clinical phenotypes [22]. The lack of VDR also results in underexpression of the gene coding for 24-hydroxylase [23]. This may contribute to the raised serum $1,25(OH)_2D$ levels observed in HVDRR as 24-hydroxylase initiates the catabolic pathway of $1,25(OH)_2D$.

Clinical features of vitamin D-related rickets

Vitamin D-deficiency rickets is a disorder of the growing child and is therefore manifested during infancy and the adolescent growth spurt. Clinical features vary with severity and the age of onset of rickets. Florid skeletal deformities are more common in infancy (Fig. 4.1). Infants with rickets usually develop deformities of their weight-bearing limbs. A crawling child develops deformities in the forearms, whereas a walking toddler develops bow legs (genu varum) or knock knees (genu valgum). Other features of rickets include growth retardation, frontal bossing of the skull, swelling of the wrists, knees, and ankles. Rachitic rosary is the name given to the 'bumps' at the anterior ends of the ribs, which is secondary to expansion of the costo-chondral junctions, and Harrison's sulcus refers to a deformity of the soft rib cage, which is caused by an inward diaphragmatic pull. The

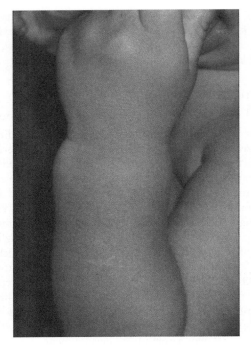

Fig. 4.1 A swollen wrist in a toddler with vitamin D-deficiency rickets.

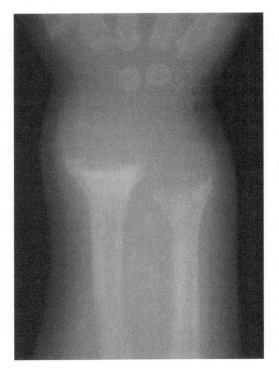

Fig. 4.2 Radiograph of the wrist, showing classical changes of rickets: cupping, widening, and fraying of the distal ends of the radius and ulna.

forward projection of the sternum produces the 'pigeon chest' deformity. Dentition may be delayed and development of tooth enamel impaired. Irritability, considered secondary to bone pain, is a common feature in rachitic infants. Muscle weakness associated with vitamin D deficiency leads to hypotonia and developmental delay of the motor milestones.

Adolescents with rickets usually present with vague symptoms such as aches and pains in the lower limbs, which are precipitated by walking or playing games. They also complain of muscle weakness, and the proximal myopathy may cause difficulty in climbing stairs. Frequently, musculoskeletal symptoms in these youngsters are attributed to 'growing pains' and are inappropriately treated with analgesics. Muscle cramps and tetany are more likely to occur at this age than in infants with rickets. The positive Chvostek's sign indicates latent tetany due to a low serum concentration of ionized calcium. Florid signs of rickets are rare in adolescents. Deformities such as bow legs may develop with long-standing vitamin D deficiency. Pelvic deformities that occur at this age can lead to difficult childbirth or obstructed labour.

Radiological features

The characteristic radiological signs of rickets include cupping, widening and fraying of the metaphyses, with generalized osteopenia (Fig. 4.2).

Biochemical findings

In the early stages of vitamin D deficiency, plasma calcium concentration is low with a normal plasma phosphate concentration. Hypocalcaemia leads to secondary hyperparathyroidism, which, in turn, results in an increase in plasma $1,25(OH)_2D$ concentration, normalization of plasma calcium concentration and a decrease in serum phosphate concentration. At this stage plasma $25(OH)D$ concentration is low and the concentration of $1,25(OH)_2D$ is normal or high. This biochemical state is maintained at the expense of the resorptive action of PTH on bone. Long-standing vitamin D deficiency eventually leads to recurrence of hypocalcaemia. Plasma alkaline phosphatase activity is raised above the upper limits of normal for the age and there may be generalized aminoaciduria.

Key points: Vitamin D-related rickets

- $1,25(OH)_2D$ functions as a steroid hormone regulating the expression of target genes through the intranuclear vitamin D receptor (VDR).

- Vitamin D-deficiency rickets:
  - is now a rare disease but it is important that it is not overlooked;
  - remains an important public health problem among children of Indo-Asian and Middle Eastern immigrants in the United Kingdom;
  - cases of privational rickets have also been reported recently in the USA and Canada.

- Pseudovitamin D-deficiency rickets (PDDR):
  - is an autosomal recessive disorder;
  - results from a defect in the $P450_c1$ component of the renal 1α-hydroxylase, and hence serum $1,25(OH)_2D$ levels are greatly reduced.

- Hereditary vitamin D-resistant rickets (HVDRR):
  - is an autosomal recessive disorder;
  - the VDR-mediated actions of $1,25(OH)_2D$ are eliminated or reduced, even though supranormal concentrations of the hormone are present in the circulation.

- Clinical features of vitamin D-related rickets:
  - all these conditions result in a similar clinical picture;
  - vitamin D-deficiency rickets is a disorder of the growing child and is therefore manifested during infancy and the adolescent growth spurt;
  - clinical features vary with severity and the age of onset of rickets;
  - the characteristic radiological signs include cupping, widening, and fraying of the metaphyses with generalized osteopenia.

- Treatment:
  - oral vitamin D_2 or D_3 in therapeutic doses is the treatment of vitamin D-deficiency rickets;
  - PDDR is usually cured with physiological doses of $1,25(OH)_2D$ or alfacalcidol;
  - there is no satisfactory treatment for HVDRR.

Biochemical features of PDDR and HVDRR are similar to those in vitamin D deficiency rickets except that plasma $1,25(OH)_2D$ concentration is low in PDDR and high in HVDRR.

Treatment

Oral vitamin D_2 or D_3 in therapeutic doses (1500–3000 i.u./day) for 6–8 weeks is the treatment of vitamin D-deficiency rickets. Healing of rickets is monitored by a fall in plasma alkaline phosphatase activity, normalization of plasma calcium, phosphate, and PTH concentrations. Radiological and clinical improvement is also observed. Supplemental sources of vitamin D are important to prevent rickets in children with insufficient exposure of the skin to sunlight. In most countries the recommended prophylactic dose of vitamin D is between 300 and 400 i.u./day.

PDDR is usually cured with physiological doses of calcitriol or alfacalcidol. At present, there is no satisfactory treatment of patients with HVDRR. Some patients have benefited from long-term treatment with nocturnal calcium infusions [24].

Rickets due to dietary calcium deficiency

In certain parts of Africa, rickets in children has been attributed to a very low dietary intake of calcium [25]. These children have normal serum concentrations of 25(OH)D but elevated levels of $1,25(OH)_2D$. Calcium supplements alone lead to healing of rickets [26].

Rickets secondary to chronic hypophosphataemia

Hypophosphataemic rickets is characterized by a low rate of tubular reabsorption of phosphate and the absence of secondary hyperparathyroidism.

Familial hypophosphataemic rickets (XLH)

The majority of patients with familial hypophosphataemic rickets have an X-linked dominant mode of inheritance (XLH). Most patients have been shown to have mutations in the *PHEX* gene (phosphate-regulating gene with homologies to endopeptidases on the X chromosome). This gene has been localized to the Xp22.1 position on the short arm of the X chromosome [27]. The product of the *PHEX* gene is a type II membrane glycoprotein, the physiological function of which is to activate the putative phosphate-regulating hormone called 'phosphatonin' [28].

Affected children develop genu varum at the time of weight bearing. The child often walks with a waddling gait due to coxa vara, and/or an 'in-toeing' gait secondary to medial tibial torsion. Short stature with disproportionate shortening of the lower limbs is an important clinical feature in an untreated child. In contrast to vitamin D-deficiency rickets, hypotonia, myopathy, and tetany are absent in patients with XLH. Patients with this condition often develop spontaneous dental abscesses in the absence of dental caries. Premature fusion of the cranial sutures may lead to distortion of the skull shape and occasionally raised intracranial pressure. As shown in Fig. 4.3, clinical manifestations of XLH can be variable, even within family members with the same *PHEX* gene mutation.

Radiological features are usually worse in the lower limbs, showing thick cortices and coarse trabeculae. The cupping, widening, and fraying of metaphyses is usually less marked than that seen in vitamin D-deficiency rickets.

The primary defect in this condition is defective proximal renal tubular phosphate transport, which leads to excessive renal phosphate wastage and chronic hypophosphataemia. Subjects with XLH characteristically have a low tubular reabsorption of phosphate (<85%) or a reduced T_{MPO_4}/GFR against a background of low serum phosphate concentration. Plasma concentrations of 25(OH)D and 1,25(OH)$_2$D are usually within the normal range. Hypophosphataemia is a potent stimulator of the renal 1α-hydroxylase enzyme, which is responsible for the conversion of 25(OH)D to 1,25(OH)$_2$D. In patients with XLH, plasma 1,25(OH)$_2$D concentrations are inappropriately low in the face of chronic hypophosphataemia. This suggests either defective production or increased degradation rate of 1,25(OH)$_2$D in this condition. In summary, in XLH the main changes in biochemistry include:

(1)   low serum phosphate concentration for the age of the child (hypophosphataemia);

(2)   increased renal phosphate wastage;

(3)   normal serum 25(OH)D concentration;

(4)   an inappropriately low concentration of 1,25(OH)$_2$D in the face of hypophosphataemia;

(5)   normal serum calcium concentration;

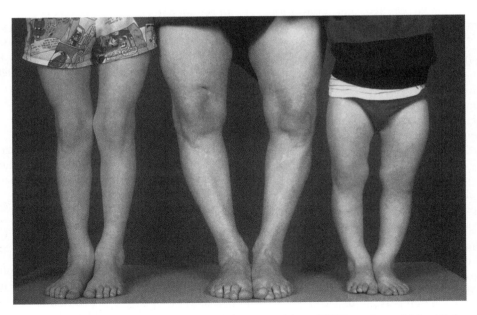

Fig. 4.3   Clinical features of X-linked familial hypophosphataemic rickets (XLH) can be variable. All three members of this family had biochemical features of XLH and the same nonsense mutation in exon 8 of the *PHEX* gene. The mother, in the middle, bears scars on her legs from unsuccessful surgery carried out during childhood to correct her bowed legs. Her eldest son, standing on the left, presented with short stature but without lower-limb deformities. Her youngest son, standing on the right, developed bowed legs and he walked with a waddling gait. All three of them have suffered from multiple spontaneous dental abscesses.

(6) absence of secondary hyperparathyroidism in untreated patients; and

(7) elevated age-adjusted serum alkaline phosphatase activity.

Treatment

Currently, the treatment of this condition is with oral phosphate supplements and calcitriol or alfacalcidol. Phosphate supplements are administered as neutral phosphate tablets in doses of 1–4 g/day, in four to six divided doses. Joulie's solution, which contains 30.4 mg of inorganic phosphate per millilitre solution, can be given to infants and toddlers. Common but transient side-effects of phosphate therapy include abdominal pain and diarrhoea. The concomitant use of calcitriol or alfacalcidol enhances intestinal phosphate and calcium absorption. This helps to prevent secondary hyperparathyroidism, which invariably occurs with phosphate therapy alone. Alfacalcidol may be preferred as it is administered once a day. Treatment with alfacalcidol is started at a dose of 25 ng/kg/day and can be increased gradually to 50 ng/kg/day (maximum dose 2 µg/day) until there is biochemical and radiological evidence of the healing of rickets. Careful monitoring of treatment is required to avoid secondary hyperparathyroidism, hypercalcaemia, hypercalciuria, and nephrocalcinosis. Elevated plasma PTH concentration suggests either overtreatment with phosphate or undertreatment with alfacalcidol. If there is hypercalciuria or hypercalcaemia, alfacalcidol or calcitriol should be temporarily stopped until urine calcium excretion and serum calcium concentration have returned to normal. These agents should then be reintroduced at 75% of the previous dose.

Despite adequate medical treatment, some patients are left with residual skeletal deformities. These may require surgical correction with bilateral tibial and femoral osteotomies, when growth has ceased. Treatment should be stopped at 1 week before elective surgery, to prevent hypercalcaemia secondary to postoperative immobilization, and later reintroduced once the patient is ambulant. These patients have a high risk of spontaneous dental abscess formation and require regular dental care.

Future developments in determining the precise function of the *PHEX* gene will lead to improved understanding of renal phosphate metabolism and the development of a rational therapy for XLH patients.

Hypophosphataemic rickets with hypercalciuria

This is an autosomal recessive condition [29]. Unlike XLH, plasma concentrations of $1,25(OH)_2D$ are elevated in response to low plasma phosphate concentrations. These patients therefore have increased intestinal calcium absorption, which results in increased urinary calcium excretion. Treatment with oral phosphate supplements alone results in healing of rickets and normocalciuria. Unlike XLH, these patients have muscle weakness.

Fanconi's syndrome (see Chapter 5)

This term refers to a heterogeneous group of conditions characterized by proximal tubular dysfunction, resulting in renal phosphate wastage, hypokalaemia, renal tubular acidosis, aminoaciduria, and glycosuria. The management of hypophosphataemic rickets in this situation is identical to that recommended for XLH.

Tumour-induced hypophosphataemic rickets

Hypophosphataemic rickets may be associated with benign fibrous or mesenchymal tumours and with other conditions, such as the linear sebaceous nevus syndrome [30]. It is likely that these tumours secrete a hormone which causes increased renal phosphate loss and reduced $1,25(OH)_2D$ synthesis [31,32]. These changes are caused by the over production of fibroblast growth factor-23 by the tumours. Excision of the tumour leads to dramatic cure of the bone disease.

An approach to a toddler with suspected rickets

History and examination

Although there are many causes of rickets, by far the most common clinical dilemma occurs in differentiating the toddler with vitamin D-deficiency rickets from the one with familial hypophosphataemic rickets (XLH). Rickets is often suspected when a toddler presents with bilaterally bowed legs. Most toddlers go through the stage of having bow legs, but this 'physiological bowing' is easily differentiated from pathological bowing by measuring the distance between upper tibial medial condyles. The measurement is taken with the child standing erect and the medial malleoli in contact. In healthy children the gap should be less than 5 cm.

Key points: Rickets secondary to hypophosphataemia

- Hypophosphataemic rickets is characterized by a low rate of tubular reabsorption of phosphate and the absence of secondary hyperparathyroidism.

- Familial hypophosphataemic rickets:
  - the majority of patients have an X-linked dominant mode of inheritance (XLH);
  - the gene has been localized to the Xp22.1 position on the short arm of the X chromosome;
  - short stature with disproportionate shortening of the lower limbs is an important clinical feature in an untreated child;
  - in contrast to vitamin D-deficiency rickets, hypotonia, myopathy, and tetany are absent;
  - spontaneous dental abscesses in the absence of dental caries are common;
  - premature fusion of the cranial sutures may occur;
  - the cupping, widening, and fraying of metaphyses is usually less marked than that seen in vitamin D-deficiency rickets;
  - treatment consists of oral phosphate supplements and calcitriol or alfacalcidol;
  - careful monitoring of treatment is required to avoid secondary hyperparathyroidism, hypercalcaemia, hypercalciuria, and nephrocalcinosis;
  - despite adequate medical treatment, some patients are left with residual skeletal deformities.

- Hypophosphataemic rickets with hypercalciuria:
  - is an autosomal recessive condition distinguished from XLH by elevated $1,25(OH)_2D$ levels;
  - treatment with oral phosphate alone results in healing of the rickets and correction of the hypercalciuria;

- The management of hypophosaphataemic rickets in Fanconi's syndrome is identical to that recommended for XLH.

- Tumour-associated hypophosphataemic rickets is cured by excision of the tumour.

A detailed medical history is always important. A history of residence in northern latitudes, where parents are of dark skin and wear concealing clothing for religious or cultural reasons and have breast-fed their child for more than 6 months without giving vitamin D supplements points to a diagnosis of vitamin D-deficiency rickets. A history of malabsorptive symptoms is also important, as this can also lead to calcium and/or vitamin D-deficiency rickets.

A positive family history with an X-linked dominant mode of inheritance points to the possibility of XLH. If the father is affected, then all his daughters will also be affected. If the mother is affected, then there is a 50% chance that her offspring, regardless of gender, will be affected. A family history may also be found in pseudovitamin D-deficiency rickets and hereditary vitamin D-resistant rickets (see above).

Height, head circumference, and weight should be measured in all patients. Children with vitamin D-deficiency rickets and XLH tend to be small for their age. Vitamin D-deficient patients tend to have frontal bossing of the skull, which may also be very soft (craniotabes), with parietal flattening. Children with XLH might have distortion of the skull secondary to craniosynostosis. Sparse hair or alopecia is often seen in children with hereditary vitamin D-resistant rickets. Skeletal deformities, such as visible and palpable enlargement of the ends of the long bones and costochondral junctions (rachitic rosary) and Harrison's sulcus, are more evident in children with vitamin D-deficiency rickets. In XLH, swelling of the metaphyses is usually confined to the lower-limb bones. Walking is often delayed in vitamin D deficiency, owing to proximal muscle myopathy. Children with both these conditions often walk with a waddling gait. Dentition is usually delayed in children with vitamin D-deficiency rickets. Careful examination of the teeth may show dental enamel hypoplasia. In contrast, children with XLH tend to have normal-looking teeth but are plagued with painful dental abscesses, which eventually lead to premature dental loss. Occasionally latent hypocalcaemic tetany in children with vitamin D-deficiency rickets can be elicited by the Chvostek's sign.

Investigations

In addition to cupping and fraying of the metaphyses that are seen in children with vitamin D-deficiency, pseudovitamin D-deficiency rickets, hereditary vitamin

D-resistant rickets and XLH, children with the latter condition often tend to have a very coarse trabecular pattern. Biochemical differentiation is usually straightforward (Table 4.4).

Renal calculi

Crystal formation is dependent upon the supersaturation of a solution by the formation product. This occurs if there is an increased concentration of the ions causing the crystals, which in urine may be calcium, phosphate, oxalate, and uric acid, or a decrease in urinary volume. Crystal formation is increased by alterations in urinary pH, which decrease the solubility of certain products, and by decreased concentration of inhibitors of crystal formation, including citrate, magnesium, nephrocalcinin, and glycosaminoglycans. Once the first crystal has been formed, growth occurs by the addition of further crystals, which in turn will obstruct urinary flow, leading to increased formation of crystals.

Epidemiology

The reported incidence and aetiological factors of renal calculi in children vary according to the geographical region and socio-economic climate. The prevalence of paediatric urolithiasis in developed countries had fallen following improved socio-economic conditions, but currently is increasing. This may be explained by an increase in diagnosis secondary to improved diagnostic techniques.

Endemic calculi

There has been a general reduction in endemic stones with improved socio-economic conditions. Bladder stones were once common in the Far East and Turkey and are considered to be secondary to a diet rich in cereals and rice, which are metabolized to oxalate. Bladder stones, composed predominantly of ammonium acid urate, are common in India, North Africa, and the Middle East. They are considered to be secondary to an acidic, purine-rich and phosphorus-poor diet, in combination with low fluid intake and gastrointestinal infections.

Infective stones

In the United Kingdom and other European countries, the incidence of renal calculi secondary to infection is between 1 and 2 per million population per annum

[33]. In some studies, urinary infection is considered to be the main cause of renal calculi, accounting for 60–80% [34]. Typically, *Proteus* sp. infection is associated with infective renal calculi, but other organisms which can produce urease, releasing ammonia from urea, include *Pseudomonas* sp., *Klebsiella* sp., *Esherichia coli* and *Staphylococcus* sp. These organisms produce an alkaline medium favouring the precipitation of calcium phosphate and magnesium ammonium phosphate (struvite). These stones can increase in size and form staghorn calculi, filling the pelvicalyceal system. Stone fragments are usually soft.

To prevent persistent or recurrent infection these stones require complete removal. Complete removal also avoids ill-health, pyonephrosis, and destruction of renal tissue.

Infective stones may be observed in patients with anatomical urological abnormalities which result in urinary stasis. A metabolic screen is likely to be normal in a child with a *Proteus* infection and a struvite stone. Urine infection is often the presenting clinical symptom in a young child with a renal stone and an underlying metabolic abnormality.

Stones associated with urinary stasis

Congenital malformations of the renal tract, for example congenital megacalyces, megaureter, pelvi–ureteric junction obstruction and tubular ectasia, cause urinary stasis, which encourages crystal aggregation. Risk factors for stone formation in patients with ileal loops include residual loop residues, hyperchloraemic acidosis, and ureteral dilatation causing stasis.

Renal calculi are a common presenting feature of medullary sponge kidney and are considered to be secondary to hypercalciuria, an alkaline urine, and urinary stasis in the ectatic tubules.

Metabolic calculi

Improved screening in children with urolithiasis is likely to explain the changes seen in the reported prevalence of nephrolithiasis due to metabolic abnormalities. The likelihood of finding a metabolic abnormality is increased if there is a positive family history, nephrocalcinosis, sterile urine, recurrent stone disease, and other clinical features such as failure to thrive, polyuria, and rickets. General ill-health, a catabolic state, and immobilization may cause false-positive results during a metabolic evaluation. To avoid this, screening for a metabolic disorder should occur after the stone has been removed.

The most common metabolic abnormality in children with renal stone disease is hypercalciuria, but other important metabolic abnormalities include disorders of oxalate, cystine, urate, and citrate metabolism. Calcium stones are observed in conditions where there is hypercalciuria, hyperoxaluria, hyperuricosuria, or hypocitraturia. The incidence of calcium-rich stones is high in South America and low in African-American children, who have a lower excretion of calcium.

Initial investigations to diagnose a metabolic abnormality include plasma creatinine, urea, albumin, calcium, phosphate, magnesium, bicarbonate, chloride, urate, and PTH. Urinary calcium, phosphate, sodium, creatinine, citrate, oxalate, and the metabolites glycolate and glycerate should be measured from a 24-hour collection. More than one urine collection may be required because of the daily variations in the urinary excretion of solutes. Age, diet, ethnicity, geographical region, and laboratory reference ranges should be considered when these results are interpreted. A spot urine to screen for cystinuria and hyperuricosuria is recommended. If a sterile urine has a urinary pH below 5.5, this excludes a diagnosis of distal renal tubular acidosis.

The difficulties in collecting 24-hour urine samples in children are well known. The reliability of a urine collection can be estimated from the timing recorded on the collection and, in conditions with stable renal function, from the urinary creatinine excretion. A urine collection can be regarded as adequate if the 24-hour urinary creatinine is $175\,\mu mol/kg \pm 40\%$. If 24-hour collections are unsuccessful, and to avoid urethral catheterization in younger children, a spot urine can be used to screen for increased urinary excretion of calcium and oxalate. The time of day and relation to meals should be noted in interpreting these results.

If the stone is captured from the urine or following surgical treatment, it should be sent for biochemical analysis and culture. Further investigations can then be tailored accordingly. Frequently, the composition of renal stones may be mixed, indicating that different mechanisms are responsible for the production of these stones. Struvite and calcium oxalate, or calcium oxalate and uric acid, are examples of mixed stones. Struvite stones are often formed around other stones, usually calcium oxalate. In these instances treatment of the metabolic condition is required to prevent

further stone formation after the infected stone has been removed.

Key points: Renal calculi

- There has been a general reduction in endemic stones with improved socio-economic conditions.

- In the United Kingdom and other European countries the incidence of renal calculi secondary to infection is reported to be between 1 and 2 per million population per annum and accounts for 60– 80% of renal calculi.

- Congenital or acquired abnormalities of the urinary system cause urinary stasis and predispose to stone formation.

- With metabolic stones:
  - the most common metabolic abnormality is hypercalciuria;
  - other important metabolic abnormalities include disorders of oxalate, cystine, urate, and citrate metabolism;
  - if 24-hour collections are unsuccessful, a spot urine can be used to screen for increased urinary excretion of calcium and oxalate;
  - if the stone is captured from the urine, or following surgical treatment, it should be sent for biochemical analysis and culture.

Hypercalciuria

Approximately 60% of the plasma calcium is filtered by the glomerulus, of which 99% is reabsorbed by the renal tubules. The proximal tubule reabsorbs approximately 70% of the filtered load, primarily by passive transport in parallel with the reabsorption of sodium and water.

Calcium excretion is affected by race, with lower values reported in Black compared to White people from the same geographical region [35]. Geographical influences, including climate, exposure to sunlight, mineral composition of drinking water, and nutritional differences, in combination with genetic factors influence urinary calcium excretion. Urinary calcium excretion is also age related, with higher values in infants compared to older children [36].

Dietary calcium and sodium, the timing of urine collections in relation to meals, and mobility influence measurements of urinary calcium excretion.

Urinary calcium excretion should be measured from a 24-hour urine sample collected in an acidified container to avoid precipitation of calcium. To avoid the difficulties of a 24-hour urine collection, the urinary calcium/urinary creatinine ratio (U_{Ca}/U_{Cr}) in a spot urine from either a first morning or a second fasting urine sample, or a sample following a calcium-enriched meal, can be used as a measure of calcium excretion [37,38]. However, some children may have a high UCa/UCr but a normal 24-hour urinary calcium, and vice versa.

Hypercalciuria in childhood is defined as a 24-hour urinary calcium above 4 mg/kg/day (0.1 mmol/kg/day) [37] or a second fasting U_{Ca}/U_{Cr} above 0.74 mmol/mmol (0.24 mg/mg) [37,38]. As urinary calcium is influenced by many factors, including diet, race, and geographical placement, it is not surprising that the upper limit of normal varies in different population studies [39,40].

A useful definition is that which has biological significance in a specific population, rather than the 95th percentile. Current literature provides age-specific reference values for 24-hour urine samples and spot urine samples in healthy children, but does not provide longitudinal data as to whether these children are at risk of nephrolithiasis. In children who are investigated for conditions such as renal calculi or macroscopic haematuria, a urinary calcium towards the upper limit for that population is likely to be a contributing factor to their clinical condition. Other factors that require consideration in these patients include reduced urinary flow, urinary stasis, and a reduction in the inhibitors of crystal formation, including citrate. In these children, a second urine collection should be performed to confirm the diagnosis of hypercalciuria, including a measurement of urinary sodium excretion, which is a measure of dietary sodium. Dietary sodium, calcium, protein, vitamin C and vitamin D are reported to increase urinary calcium excretion, and therefore a dietary history should also be collected. This information is useful before recommending any dietary modifications.

The clinical significance of increased calcium excretion in an asymptomatic child is not yet fully understood, and future research will determine if these children are at risk of renal calculi or osteoporosis.

Pathogenesis of hypercalciuria

Normocalcaemic hypercalciuria

Idiopathic hypercalciuria is one of the most common causes of normocalcaemic hypercalciuria. Other causes include distal renal tubular acidosis, furosemide, hyperalimentation, hypophosphataemia, juvenile rheumatoid arthritis, renal tubular disorders, and medullary sponge kidney.

Idiopathic hypercalciuria. The difficulties in classifying idiopathic hypercalciuria into renal or absorptive subtypes have led to a change in classification according to the pathogenesis of hypercalciuria. The calcium load test was described initially to differentiate absorptive from renal hypercalciuria and guide treatment, but is no longer recommended as a routine screening test. Hypercalciuria is now classified as either genetically or environmentally induced. The mode of inheritance for patients with idiopathic calcium stone disease is likely to be polygenic, with clinical expression being modified by sex or environmental factors. An autosomal dominant pattern of inheritance has been postulated for familial hypercalciuria [41]. The underlying pathogenesis may be secondary to renal tubular abnormalities, including reduced tubular phosphate reabsorption [42]; abnormal handling of salt [43]; abnormal synthesis and metabolism of 1,25-dihydroxyvitamin D and the vitamin D receptor [44]; and increased prostaglandin E_2 production [45].

Idiopathic hypercalciuria should be considered in a patient with macroscopic or microscopic haematuria and sterile pyuria. Urinary incontinence [46] and the urinary frequency/dysuria syndrome have also been described in patients with idiopathic hypercalciuria [47]. Children with idiopathic hypercalciuria are reported to have a lower trabecular bone mineral density, but the clinical significance of this is not yet known.

Avoiding dehydration and restricting salt intake may be sufficient to prevent further stone formation in the majority of children. Restricting dietary sodium also has the potential benefit of reducing the risk of hypertension and increasing bone mineral density [48]. It is not yet known if this effect is maintained over prolonged periods, and dietary compliance may be difficult to achieve in the paediatric population.

Dietary calcium restriction or sodium cellulose phosphate, which reduces calcium absorption, is not recommended for children with normocalcaemic hypercalciuria, due to the potential risk of reducing bone mineralization. Sodium cellulose phosphate reduces cation–oxalate complexes and increases calcium oxalate absorption.

Citrate chelates calcium in the urine and oral potassium reduces calcium excretion and increases renal phosphate retention, which in turn reduces calcitriol production and intestinal calcium absorption [49,50]. Oral potassium citrate can be prescribed as a solution or powder, but citrate is unpalatable and other side-effects include diarrhoea, indigestion, nausea, and mucosal ulceration in the upper gastrointestinal tract.

Thiazide diuretics increase tubular calcium reabsorption. This effect is dependent on sodium intake and increasing the dietary intake of sodium reduces the hypocalciuric influence of thiazides. The side-effects of thiazide diuretics include hypokalaemia, increased tubular phosphate losses, hyperuricaemia, and glucose intolerance. Thiazide diuretics may also adversely influence lipid metabolism and therefore their use should be restricted to patients who do not respond clinically to sodium restriction and potassium citrate.

Further research into the pathogenesis of idiopathic hypercalciuria will enable us to tailor treatment accordingly.

Hypercalciuria associated with other renal tubular disorders.   Hypercalciuria may be one of the biochemical features observed in other renal tubular or tubulo–interstitial disorders, including proximal or distal renal tubular acidosis, Bartter's syndrome and familial hypomagnesaemia-hypercalciuria.

Dent's disease is an X-linked familial defect of the proximal tubule, characterized by hypercalciuria, low-molecular weight proteinuria, nephrocalcinosis and, in some instances, rickets and progressive renal failure. The recent cloning of the gene responsible for Dent's disease, which codes for the chloride channel CIC-5, has highlighted the importance of the CIC chloride channel family in the renal tubular handling of calcium [51].

Isolated familial hypomagnesaemia is a rare condition and is secondary to congenital impairment of tubular reabsorption of magnesium. Familial hypomagnesaemia-hypercalciuria is manifested by symptoms of hypocalcaemia including tetany, convulsions, and nephrocalcinosis, the latter causing polyuria, progressive renal insufficiency, and hypertension. Ocular abnormalities, including nystagmus, macular coloboma, and chorioretinitis, are also well described. Familial hypomagnesaemia-hypercalciuria hypermagnesuria is considered to be due to a mutation in *PCLN-1* on chromosome 3q27. Paracellin-1 is a a tight

junction protein, which regulates the paracellular transport of magnesium. Familial hypomagnesaemia-hypercalciuria hypermagnesuria can be differentiated from Gitelman's syndrome by the presence of a metabolic alkalosis, hypokalaemia, and hypocalciuria in the latter.

Hypercalcaemic hypercalciuria

In most children with hypercalcaemia, hypercalciuria is also observed. Treatment of the underlying condition reduces the urinary calcium. Hypercalciuria is not present in patients with familial benign hypocalciuric hypercalcaemia and helps to differentiate this condition from hyperparathyroidism. In this condition urinary calcium excretion is in the low normal range and is therefore inappropriate as these patients are hypercalcaemic.

Figure 4.4 is an algorithmn that may be helpful in the initial investigation of children with hypercalciuria. Further investigations may be required in some cases.

Key points: Hypercalciuria

- Calcium excretion is affected by race, geography, diet, and age.

- A useful definition of hypercalciuria is that which has biological significance in a specific population, rather than the 95th percentile.

- Idiopathic hypercalciuria is:
  – one of the most common causes of normo-calcaemic hypercalciuria;
  – now classified as either genetically or environmentally induced, rather than renal or absorptive;
  – avoiding dehydration and restricting salt intake is sufficient to prevent further stone formation in the majority of children;
  – dietary calcium restriction or sodium cellulose phosphate are not recommended, due to the potential risk of reducing bone mineralization.

- Other causes of normocalcaemic hypercalciuria include distal renal tubular acidosis, frusemide, hyperalimentation, hypophosphataemia, juvenile rheumatoid arthritis, renal tubular disorders, and medullary sponge kidney.

- Hypercalciuria occurs in most children with hypercalcaemia.

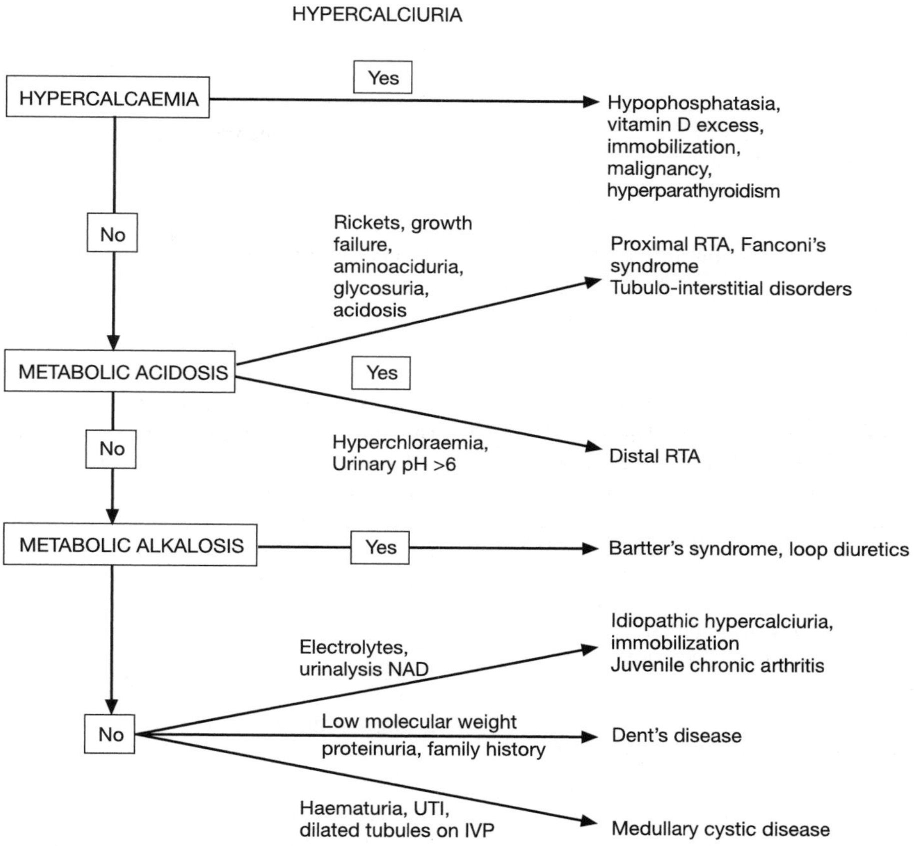

HYPERCALCIURIA

Fig. 4.4 Algorithmn for the investigation of hypercalciuria.

Cystinuria

Cystine stones, which are radiopaque but less dense than calcium stones, may occur in children at all ages. Cystine stones are usually larger than calcium stones and have smooth contours. They account for approximately 2% of childhood renal calculi. This condition should be screened for in children with renal calculi and in infants with bladder or renal calculi.

Oxalosis

Primary hyperoxaluria type 1

Primary hyperoxaluria type 1 (PH1) is an autosomal recessive disorder and is caused by a deficiency in activity of the peroxisomal hepatic enzyme alanine-glyoxylate aminotransferase (AGT). In approximately 30% of cases the enzyme is present but is mistargeted from the peroxisomes to the mitochondria and is unable to function [52,53]. This leads to an overproduction and accumulation of oxalate, which is excreted via the kidneys as urinary oxalate and urinary glycolate. There is no clinical correlation between the degree of enzyme activity and the clinical presentation [54]. The *AGXT* gene is located on chromosome 2q37.3 and although at least 25 mutations have been identified so far, the mutation has not yet been identified in approximately one-third of patients [55].

Reports from the United Kingdom and France suggest that the incidence is between 1 in 60 000 and 1 in 120 000 [56,57]. The disease is most common in Tunisia and accounts for 13% of end stage renal disease (ESRD) paediatric patients [56]. It is likely that this reported incidence is an underestimate due to difficulty in diagnosis.

Clinical presentation

The genetic heterogenicity may explain some of the differences in clinical presentation, which are divided according to age and clinical severity into three types. The infantile form is associated with early nephrocalcinosis and rapid progression to end stage renal disease. The childhood/adolescent form is associated with recurrent urolithiasis and progressive renal failure. In adults, the occasional passage of a renal stone may be the only clinical manifestation. Siblings may have a different clinical course despite an identical mutation [58].

Children may present initially with symptoms secondary to stone formation, including abdominal pain, haematuria, and urinary tract infection. As the GFR falls there is reduced renal clearance of oxalate, leading to systemic oxalosis. This occurs before ESRD [59]. Oxalate is then deposited in other tissues, including bone (the major compartment for oxalate deposition), joints (synovitis), retina, heart (cardiomyopathy, conduction defects), vessels (disseminated occlusive vascular lesions, limb gangrene, arteriovenous fistula, thrombosis), skin (ulcerating subcutaneous calcium oxalate calcinosis, livedo reticularis), and nerves (peripheral nephropathy, mononeuritis multiplex) [52].

Diagnosis

The difficulty in diagnosing PH1 means that it may often be missed or delayed. Twenty-four hour urine samples or spot urine samples for urinary oxalate and the metabolites glycolate and glycerate should be collected into containers containing hydrochloric acid to prevent oxalate crystallization and ascorbate conversion to oxalate. Plasma oxalate samples should be separated immediately after venepuncture, before freezing, as *in vitro* oxalate samples may be generated from ascorbate and certain medications. The patient should not be on vitamin C supplements as this can falsely increase plasma oxalate values (see reference 57 for normal urine and plasma values). AGT catalytic activity or immunoreactive AGT protein can be assayed from a freshly frozen liver biopsy.

Prenatal diagnosis from DNA analysis of chorionic villi or amniocytes is possible if DNA can be obtained from an affected family member and the parents.

Treatment

Treatment should be early and aggressive to reduce secondary oxalate deposition. The aim should be to keep urinary oxalate excretion below 0.4 mmol/l by a high fluid intake (>2 litres/m^2/day). Oral citrate (100–150 mg/kg/day) can be given as it reduces calcium oxalate precipitation. Diuretics increase urinary volume but should be used with caution as frusemide increases urinary calcium excretion [55].

Restriction of dietary oxalate has little influence on the disease [52]. Pyridoxine sensitivity may be observed in 10–40% of patients. An initial starting dose is 3–5 mg/kg, and this can be increased up to 15 mg/kg [57]. Response to pyridoxine and other conservative measures can be assessed by measurement of urinary oxalate and glycolate, the measurement of calcium oxalate supersaturation, or the calculation of a crystalluria score [55].

Conventional dialysis does not prevent further tissue oxalate accumulation and therefore ideally transplantation should occur before the onset of end stage renal failure, to reduce the amount of extrarenal oxalate tissue deposition.

In patients with pyridoxine-insensitive primary hyperoxaluria, isolated renal transplantation is not recommended because extrarenal oxalate deposition continues to occur and oxalate accumulates in the grafted kidney, leading to shortened graft survival. Combined liver and kidney transplantation both replaces the deficient enzyme, reducing oxalate synthesis, and also replaces the damaged kidney. The renal graft is at risk of nephrocalcinosis and recurrent calculi as oxalate is released from the body stores. In some centres isolated renal transplantation pre-ESRD is considered for patients who have a living-related renal donor and either have pyridoxine-responsive PH1 or PH2 [60,61].

Isolated liver transplantation before the onset of end stage renal failure reduces both the risk of tissue oxalate deposition and of nephrolithiasis in the later-grafted kidney [62]. The problems associated with this approach may be the increased risk of infection and a higher risk of rejection if two separate donors are used.

As primary hyperoxaluria is a monogenic disease which does not involve the central nervous system, gene therapy may be considered in the future. At present the scientific knowledge to transfect a sufficient number of liver cells to prevent excess oxalate production from the non-transfected cells is not available.

Primary hyperoxaluria type 2 (PH2)

Primary hyperoxaluria type 2 (PH2) is considered to be secondary to cytosolic glyoxalate reductase/D-glycerate

Key points: Oxalosis

- Primary hyperoxaluria type 1 (PH1):
  - is an autosomal recessive disorder due to a deficiency in the activity of the peroxisomal hepatic enzyme alanine-glyoxylate aminotransferase;
  - this leads to an overproduction and accumulation of oxalate, which is excreted via the kidneys as urinary oxalate and urinary glycolate;
  - the *AGXT* gene is located on chromosome 2q37.3;
  - the incidence in the United Kingdom and France is 1 : 60 000 to 1 : 120 000;
  - the disease is most common in Tunisia and accounts for 13% of ESRD paediatric patients;
  - the clinical presentation is divided according to age and clinical severity into three types:
    - an infantile type characterized by early nephrocalcinosis and rapid progression to ESRD;
    - a childhood/adolescent type with recurrent urolithiasis and progressive renal failure;
    - an adult type in which the occasional passage of a renal stone may be the only clinical manifestation;
    - siblings may have a different clinical course despite an identical mutation;
    - as the GFR falls there is reduced renal clearance of oxalate, leading to systemic oxalosis;
  - treatment should be early and aggressive to reduce secondary oxalate deposition;
  - combined liver and kidney transplantation both replaces the deficient enzyme, reducing oxalate synthesis, and also replaces the damaged kidney.

- In primary hyperoxaluria type 2 (PH2) the clinical course is less severe than PH1 and systemic involvement is rare.

- Hyperoxaluria is observed in patients with malabsorption syndromes.

presentation is 15 years [55]. Urolithiasis leads to ESRD in adulthood in approximately 12% of patients. Diagnosis is dependent on the elevated excretion of urinary oxalate and L-glycerate and deficiency of GR/HGD, which is present in the liver and leucocytes.

Supportive treatment includes the use of a high fluid intake and urinary inhibitors of crystallization.

Other enzymatic abnormalities have been detected in patients with primary hyperoxaluria that cannot be explained by either a deficiency in AGT or GR/HGD activity [56].

Enteric/secondary hyperoxaluria

Hyperoxaluria is observed in patients with malabsorption syndromes. Oxalate absorption is increased if there is a reduction in the available calcium to bind to oxalate following calcium-restricted diets, or if calcium is bound to fatty acids as in malabsorption syndromes. It is more common in patients with pancreatic involvement where the influence of fatty acids on the sequestration of calcium is increased. Bile salts and fatty acids are also considered to damage the colonic mucosa and increase its permeability to oxalate. The reduction of dietary oxalate and vitamin C, which is a precursor of oxalate, may be of some benefit. Oral calcium may form crystals with oxalate in the gut and reduce its absorption, although it may result in hypercalciuria. Oral citrate or bicarbonate can also be considered.

Disorders of purine metabolism

The precipitation of uric acid is encouraged by acid urine, reduced urinary volume with dehydration, a purine-rich diet, and hyperuricaemia. Uric acid stones account for 5–10% of renal calculi and may be observed in conditions of overproduction, for example following induction chemotherapy in patients with leukaemia or lymphoma. Generous intravenous fluid allowances and allopurinol are usually given to avoid acute renal failure. Hyperuricaemia may be absent in these instances as the kidney can increase tubular secretion of uric acid before there is an observed increase in serum uric acid.

Laxative abuse is associated with the formation of ammonium acid urate calculi and is considered to be secondary to volume depletion, intracellular acidosis, and increased ammonia excretion.

dehydrogenase (GR/HGD) deficiency [55]. The gene has been located to chromosome 9q11.p11 [63]. This is a rare condition but is likely to be under-reported.

The clinical course is less severe than PH1 and systemic involvement is rare. The median age at

Uric calculi secondary to gout are rarely seen in children. Uric acid calculi are found in patients with Lesh–Nyhan syndrome (hypoxanthine guanine phosphoribosyl transferase deficiency). This is a disorder characterized by choreoathetosis, self-mutilation, mental retardation, and hyperuricaemia. Hyperuricosuria is observed occasionally in type I glycogen storage disease.

Uric acid stones may be observed with hypouricaemia in conditions where there is a generalized tubular leak, or in isolated renal hypouricaemia [64].

A deficiency in the enzyme adenine phosphoribsyl transferase causes dihydroxyadenine stones. These stones are more common in males of Mediterranean background. Allopurinol is used to treat this condition [65].

Medical treatment for uric acid stones includes alkalinization of urine with sodium bicarbonate, sodium citrate, or potassium citrate, and maintaining a high urinary flow. Allopurinol should also be considered.

Xanthine oxidase converts xanthine to uric acid. A deficiency in this enzyme and acid urine encourages the formation of radiolucent xanthine calculi. Xanthinuria is a rare condition but is suggested by an orange/brown sediment in the urine [66].

Citrate

Citrate forms soluble complexes with calcium and therefore decreases stone formation. Metabolic acidosis and hypokalaemia reduce urinary citrate excretion. Hypocitraturia is considered to be a urinary excretion below 300 mg of citrate/gram of creatinine (175 μmol/mmol) in girls and below 125 mg (75 μmol/ mmol) in boys [67].

Miscellaneous conditions

Nephrolithiasis occurs in children with inflammatory bowel disease and cystic fibrosis. Stone formation in children with inflammatory bowel disease is a result of multiple factors, including steroid treatment with associated hypercalciuria, low urinary volume as a result of salt and water depletion, and bowel dysfunction which results in altered oxalate metabolism. Salt and water loss leading to extracellular volume depletion and intracellular acidosis in combination with acidic urine is involved in the pathogenesis of ammonium acid urate calculi.

Urolithiasis and nephrocalcinosis are well recognized in patients with cystic fibrosis [68,69]. Hyperoxaluria secondary to malabsorption or a change in intestinal bacterial colonization may explain the presence of calcium oxalate stones. Hyperuricosuria has also been documented and may be related to the high energy/high protein diets that these patients are advised to take.

Clinical features of renal calculi

A typical history of renal colic is uncommon in childhood. Loin pain is described in approximately 50% of children and is more often a presenting feature in older children and adolescents. Urinary tract infection is often the presenting symptom in pre-school children. Macroscopic or microscopic haematuria is frequently documented in both age groups. Children with a metabolic abnormality are more likely to form multiple stones and have a tubulo-interstitial nephropathy causing anuria.

Radiopaque renal calculi may be visible on a plain abdominal film, although an ultrasound scan is considered to be more sensitive in diagnosing renal calculi and nephrocalcinosis, and will also demonstrate radiolucent calculi. Computed tomography is useful in cases where there is discrepancy between the ultrasound and abdominal film, and is considered to be the most sensitive radiological technique for diagnosing renal calculi. The distal ureter is often difficult to visualize on ultrasound and an intravenous pyelogram (IVP) may be useful if a ureteric calculus is suspected.

Bladder calculi

In developed countries bladder calculi are rarely found in children with normal bladders but may be found in up to 50% of children with augmented bladders. The aetiology of these calculi is multifactorial, including foreign-body reactions, metabolic abnormalities, infection, and intestinal mucus. The stones that develop in augmented bladders are primarily composed of phosphate, with calcium, magnesium, and ammonium as the cation, indicating that chronic infection may be a major factor. Mucus may predispose to recurrent infection by providing a protective environment for bacteria. It may also obstruct bladder emptying, either in the outflow tract or during catheterization.

Complete bladder emptying during catheterization reduces the risk of chronic infection. Antibiotic prophylaxis is likely to result in bacterial resistance and therefore its use remains controversial. Urinary tract infections with systemic symptoms should be treated promptly. There may also be a case for using potassium citrate to correct some of the metabolic abnormalities. These stones are typically too large to pass via the urethra or catheter and require surgical removal.

Treatment of renal calculi

Medical treatment is dependent on the underlying condition. Patients are encouraged to avoid episodes of dehydration. Urinary tract infections should be identified and treated promptly. Children with renal obstruction should be referred urgently to a paediatric urologist. A number of different surgical techniques may be used to treat renal calculi.

Extracorporeal shock-wave lithotripsy

With this technique a shock wave that traverses through a liquid exerts compressive and tensile forces on the stone, causing fragmentation. The need for anaesthesia is dependent on the age of the child and the intensity of the shock wave, as the procedure may be painful.

Calculi composed of uric acid and calcium oxalate disintegrate easily but cystine and calcium phosphate calculi do not. This technique is particularly suitable for radiopaque stones in the renal pelvis and upper ureter. The upper limit for stone size suitable for extracorporeal shock-wave lithotripsy (ESWL) has not been clearly defined in children, but in some centres stones up to 15 mm have been treated successively with ESWL. Stones usually above 3 cm in diameter require percutaneous nephrolithotomy or open surgery. Relative contraindications to ESWL include bleeding diathesis, oliguric renal failure, obstruction secondary to a congenital anomaly and significant orthopaedic deformities, which may cause difficulty in localizing the stone.

If stone fragments cause obstruction, they must be dealt with surgically to avoid infection. Temporary subcapsular and intrarenal haematomas have been identified by CT or MRI scanning, but long-term studies indicate that ESWL does not influence renal growth or function.

Percutaneous nephrolithotomy

Percutaneous nephrolithotomy may be appropriate in patients with relative contraindications to ESWL or with stones considered too large for ESWL. Postoperative complications include ureteral avulsion, bleeding, extraperitoneal or intraperitoneal extravasation, and fistula formation. The success of this technique is approximately 70% but is increased to 90% if the procedure is repeated or combined with ESWL.

Ureteroscopy

This is usually considered as first-line therapy for distal ureteric calculi and is also useful for mid-ureteric calculi. This technique is not usually required for ureteric stones below 5 mm, which usually pass spontaneously. This technique is limited by the age and size of the child as the surgical instruments are designed for adults.

Open surgery

Open surgery may be the preferred technique in removing stones that are too large or not amenable to be treated with ESWL. This is still considered the preferred technique in patients with renal calculi and PUJ obstruction.

Percutaneous nephrostomy

This procedure is appropriate for a child presenting with anuric renal failure secondary to bilateral renal obstruction or obstruction of a single functioning kidney. Once the obstruction has been relieved and the patients clinical and biochemical status has been stabilised then the definitive surgical procedure can be undertaken.

A clinical approach to a child with renal calculi

The initial evaluation of a child with renal calculi should include a detailed medical history, including asking about any family history of urolithiasis, haematuria, and renal failure, and a dietary history with particular attention to fluid intake, vitamin, and

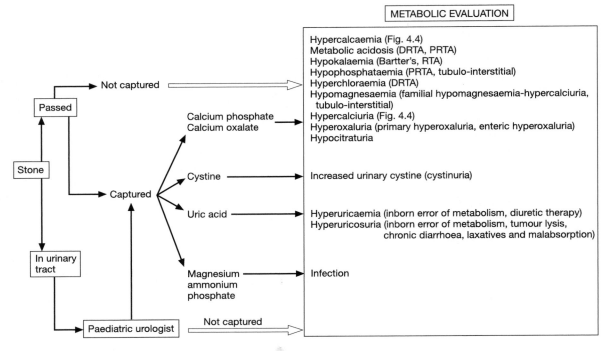

Fig. 4.5 Algorithm for the investigation of renal calculi.

mineral supplementation. An underlying metabolic abnormality may be suggested by symptoms of thirst, polyuria, anorexia, muscle cramps, abdominal, or bone pain. The physical examination should include an evaluation of growth and development, bone structure, and blood pressure.

The information shown in Fig. 4.5 can be obtained from routine biochemistry, a 24-hour urine collection, or spot urine sample. If a stone is available for analysis, then the metabolic evaluation can be tailored accordingly.

Nephrocalcinosis

Nephrocalcinosis refers to an increase in calcium content within the cortex or medulla of the kidney. Nephrocalcinosis may be focal and related to a damaged part of the kidney and is then referred to as dystrophic calcification. Focal calcification may also occur in abnormal vasculature or if there is an underlying infection, such as tuberculosis. Calcification may also occur in tumours, for example nephroblastoma.

Diffuse nephrocalcinosis is usually a consequence of a metabolic disorder and is observed in patients with distal renal tubular acidosis, hyperoxaluria, idiopathic hypercalciuria and other genetic renal tubular disorders, including Dent's disease and Bartter's syndrome. The likelihood of finding an underlying metabolic disorder is increased in patients with a positive family history, history of consanguinity, failure to thrive, poor growth, rickets, reduced renal function, and younger age at presentation.

Nephrocalcinosis is well described in preterm neonates with a reported incidence of 12–64% [70,71]. The variation in incidence reflects differences in the clinical characteristics of the patient group. Immaturity, low birth weight, diuretic therapy, inadequate dietary phosphate and duration of oxygen therapy are reported risk factors for neonatal nephrocalcinosis. The causes of nephrocalcinosis are listed in Fig. 4.6.

Clinical presentation and diagnosis

Nephrocalcinosis is usually diagnosed on ultrasound scan, which may have been requested following

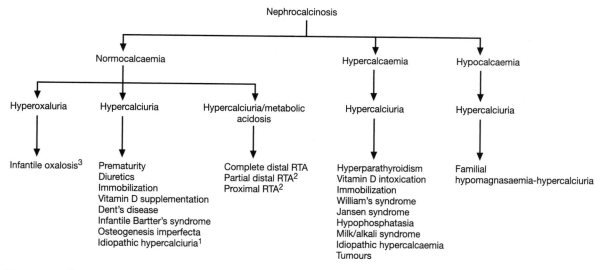

Fig. 4.6 Differential diagnosis of nephrocalcinosis. 1, Usually associated with renal calculi. 2, Nephrocalcinosis and renal calculi are rare in PRTA. A common feature of DRTA due to hypercalciuria, an alkaline urine and reduced urinary citrate. 3, Hyperoxaluria can coexist with hypercalciuria.

biochemical abnormalities suggesting a renal tubular disorder, or in a child with failure to thrive, hypotonia, or rickets. In some neonatal units an ultrasound scan may be a routine investigation in preterm infants.

On ultrasound, hyperechoic medullary pyramids are suggestive of calcification. Acoustic shadowing confirms calcification but may not be observed if the echogenic foci are less than 3 mm in diameter. Renal vessels, including arcuate and branch arteries, produce linear echoes. These vessels may later calcify and be difficult to differentiate from hyperechogenic foci within the renal pyramids.

In the neonate, medullary fibrosis, autosomal recessive polycystic kidney disease, and infection of the renal medulla with cytomegalovirus or *Candida albicans* may also cause echogenic renal medullary pyramids. In these situations, a renal CT scan can determine if the hyperechoic areas are secondary to calcification. Transient hyperechoic areas are also apparent in neonates following renal insufficiency and are considered to represent protein precipitation in the renal tubules.

Nephrocalcinosis may cause a tubulo-interstitial nephropathy and children present with clinical symptoms secondary to renal acidification defects, reduced urinary concentrating ability, poor growth and development, or rickets. In some of the inherited conditions, including oxalosis, Dent's disease, neonatal

Bartter's syndrome and familial hypomagnesaemia–hypercalciuria, this may progress to renal insufficiency and ESRD.

There are limited reports on the long-term effects of nephrocalcinosis in the preterm infant. Unlike most renal tubular disorders, in which nephrocalcinosis may be persistent or progressive, current literature suggests that there is resolution of renal calcification with increasing age and discontinuation of diuretic therapy. The influence on renal tubular and glomerular function is considered to be small.

Key points: Nephrocalcinosis

- Diffuse nephrocalcinosis is usually as a consequence of a metabolic disorder.

- Nephrocalcinosis is common in preterm neonates, occurring in 12–64%.

Assessment of bone mass in children

Renal osteodystrophy (see Chapter 23) is the most common bone disease seen in children with chronic renal failure. Osteoporosis, a condition characterized by reduced bone mass and disruption of bone architecture leading to fractures, may occur in children with chronic conditions requiring long-term treatment with corticosteroids. Techniques that measure *in vivo* bone mass and density have improved the assessment of insidious bone loss or the response to treatment in children and adolescents with such disorders. The most commonly used techniques that are used to measure bone mass in children will be discussed briefly. A detailed discussion of the techniques, indications, and interpretations of bone mass measurement is beyond the scope of this chapter.

Bone is highly specialized rigid tissue, which provides the structural integrity for the entire body. It allows for mobility and withstands voluntary load-bearing activities of the skeleton without fracturing. During childhood and adolescence, growth involves an increase in skeletal length, alteration in the shape and volume of bones (modelling) as well as accumulation of skeletal mass (bone mineral content). Growth of long bones ends with epiphyseal closure, but additional bone mineral content continues during a period of consolidation. To maintain its structural integrity, bone continuously remodels itself through removal of the old and fatigued bone and replacement with new bone. Remodelling also allows the skeleton to adapt its strength to prevailing mechanical forces and provides a source of calcium ions to exchange with the extracellular fluid.

The mechanical properties of a bone depends on the amount of mineral content, the material quality (elasticity), its three-dimensional shape and size, and the amount of fatigue damage in it. Three-dimensional shape and size are important independent determinants of bone strength. Thin and narrow bones with normal bone mineral content and density are weaker than bigger and wider bones.

An ideal technique for the assessment of bone mass and density measurement in children should be able to measure these parameters of bone strength accurately and safely without the need for sedation. Such a technique should also permit separate assessment of both trabecular and cortical bone in the axial and appendicular skeleton. Age-, gender-, and ethnic-specific normal values should be available. At present a single technique, which fulfils all of these requirements and also determines fatigue damage *in vivo*, is unavailable.

Dual-energy X-ray absorptiometry

Dual-energy X-ray absorptiometry (DXA), with its short scan time, very low radiation dose, high precision and accuracy, and ability to assess bone mass at both the axial and appendicular sites is particularly suitable for measuring bone mineral content and density in children. DXA measures bone mineral content (BMC g/cm) and bone mineral 'density' (BMD g/cm^2). Bone mineral density is calculated by dividing BMC by the scan area and is referred to as the 'areal bone mineral density' (aBMD).

Volumetric bone density is defined as the amount of BMC per unit volume of bone tissue (g/cm^3). The posterior–anterior DXA scan does not measure the depth of the bone and is unable to measure the bone volume that is required for the estimation of volumetric BMD. Areal BMD density is influenced by differences in bone size. Large bones with the same actual density as smaller bones will have a greater measured aBMD. Interpretation of aBMD is difficult in children due to age-related changes in skeletal size. Short stature and pubertal delay in chronic illness make interpretation even more complex. A number of approaches have been proposed for reducing the dependence of aBMD on growth parameters. One approach involves dividing the BMC of a bone site by its estimated volume [72]. Mølgaard *et al.* [73] use three steps to estimate the total body BMC of a child: assessment of (1) height for age, (2) bone area for height, and (3) BMC for bone area, using gender-specific normative data. These three steps correspond to three different causes of reduced bone mass: short bones, narrow bones, and light bones. Prentice *et al.* [74] reported a statistical model to calculate predictive or size-adjusted BMC, taking into account the influence of age, bone area, height, weight and pubertal status.

Quantitative computed tomography

Quantitative computed tomography (QCT) allows selective measurement of volumetric density (g/cm^3) of cortical and trabecular bone. QCT is therefore a particularly useful technique in a growing child [75]. The equipment required is expensive and the radiation dose is relatively high (approximately 10–15 times the whole-body DXA dose). Recently, peripheral quantitative computed tomography (pQCT) scanners have become available for the assessment of the BMD of appendicular bones, e.g. the radius and the tibia.

Key points: Assessment of bone mass in children

- Renal osteodystrophy is the most common bone disease seen in children.

- Osteoporosis may occur in children with chronic conditions requiring long-term treatment with corticosteroids.

- Techniques that measure *in vivo* bone mass and density have improved the assessment of insidious bone loss or the response to treatment in children and adolescents with such disorders.

- Dual-energy X-ray absorptiometry (DXA) is particularly suitable for measuring bone mineral content and density in children.

- Quantitative computed tomography (QCT) allows selective measurement of volumetric density (g/cm^3) of cortical and trabecular bone and is therefore a particularly useful technique in a growing child.

- Broadband ultrasonic attenuation and the velocity of ultrasound passing through the calcaneum, tibia, patella and fingers are being evaluated as radiation-free assessment of bone status in children.

These scanners are cheaper than the conventional whole-body QCT machines and the radiation dose is considerably lower (approximately same as spinal BMD measurement by DXA). pQCT also measures the cross-sectional area of the bone, which is a more important determinant of bending and torsional bone strength, than its mineral content and density.

Quantitative ultrasound

In post-menopausal women with osteoporosis, the attenuation of broadband ultrasound waves passing through the calcaneum have been shown to predict the vertebral and hip fracture risk independently of bone mineral density. Currently, broadband ultrasonic attenuation and the velocity of ultrasound passing through the calcaneum, tibia, patella and fingers are being evaluated as radiation-free assessment of bone status in children [76].

References

1. Herbert SC, Brown EM, Harris HW. Role of the Ca(2+)-sensing receptor in divalent mineral ion homeostasis. J Exp Biol 1997;200:295–302.
2. Sands JM, Naruse M, Baum M, Jo I, Hebert SC, Brown EM, Harris HW. Apical extracellula calcium/polyvalent cation-sensing receptor regulates vasopressin-elicited water permeability in rat kidney inner medullary collecting duct. J Clin Invest 1997; 99:1399–1405.
3. Brown E. Physiology and pathophysiology of the extracellular calcium-sensing receptor. Am J Med 1999;106:238–253.
4. Schienman SJ, Guay-Woodford LM, Thakker RV, Warnock DG. Mechanisms of disease: Genetic disorders of renal electrolyte transport. N Engl J Med 1999;340:1177–1187.
5. Coburn JW, Elangovan L, Goodman WG, Frazao JM. Calcium-sensing receptor and calcimimetic agents. Kidney Int Suppl 1999;73:S52–S58.
6. Walton RJ, Bijovet OLM. Nomograms for derivation of renal threshold phosphate concentration. Lancet 1975;II:309–310.
7. Dunn PM. Francis Glisson (1597–1677) and the 'discovery' of rickets. Arch Dis Child Fetal Neonatal Ed 1998;78:F154–F155.
8. Fraser DR, Kodicek E. Unique biosynthesis by kidney of a biologically active vitamin D metabolite. Nature 1970;228:764–766.
9. Johnson JA, Kumar R. Renal and intestinal calcium transport: Roles of vitamin D and vitamin D-dependent binding proteins. Semin Nephrol 1994;14:119–128.
10. Lian JB, Stein GS. Vitamin D regulation of osteoblast growth and differentiation. In Nutrition and Gene Expression. Berdanier CD, Hargrove JL (ed.). Boca Raton FL: CRC Press, 1993:391–429.
11. Pugliese MT, Blumberg DL, Hludzinski J, Kay S. Nutritional rickets in suburbia. Am Coll Nutr 1998;17:637–641.
12. Binet A, Kooh SW. Persistence of vitamin D-deficiency rickets in Toronto in the 1990s. Can J Public Health 1996; 87:227–230.
13. Mughal MZ, Salama H, Rimmer S, Russell S, Laing I, Mawer EB. Florid rickets associated with prolonged breastfeeding and maternal vitamin D deficiency. BMJ 1999;318:39–40.
14. Dunnigan MG, Henderson JB. An epidemiological model of privational rickets and osteomalacia. Proc Nutr Soc 1997;56:939–956.
15. Prader A, Illig R, Heierli E. Eine besondere form der primaren vitamin D resistenten rachitis mit hypocalcamie und autosomal-dominantem erbgany: die heridtare pseudo-mangel rachitis. Helv Paediatr Acta 1961;16:452–468.
16. St-Arnaud R, Messerlian S, Moir JM, Omdahl JL, Glorieux FH. The 25-hydroxyvitamin D 1-alpha-hydroxylase gene maps to the pseudovitamin D-deficiency rickets (PDDR) disease locus. J Bone Miner Res 1997;12:1552–1559.

17. Kato S, Yanagisawa J, Murayama A, Kitanaka S, Takeyama K. The importance of 25-hydroxyvitamin D3 1 alpha-hydroxylase gene in vitamin D dependent rickets. Curr Opin Nephrol Hypertens 1998;7:377–383.

18. Yoshida T, Monkawa T, Tenehouse HS, Goodyer P, Shinki T, Suda T, Wakino S, Hayashi M, Saruta T. Two novel mutations in French-Canadians with vitamin D dependency rickets type I. Kidney Int 1998;54:1437–1443.

19. Wang JT, Lin C-J, Burridge SM, Fu GK, Labuda M, Portale AA, Miller WL. Genetics of vitamin D 1α-hydroxylase deficiency in 17 families. Am J Hum Genet 1998;63:1694–1702.

20. Smith SJ, Rucka AK, Berry JL, Davies M, Mylchreest S, Paterson CR, Heath DA, Tassabehji M, Read AP, Mee AP, Mawer EB. Novel mutations in the 1-hydroxylase (P450c1) gene in three families with pseudovitamin D-deficiency rickets resulting in loss of functional enzyme activity in blood-derived macrophages. J Bone Miner Res 1999;14:730–739.

21. Fu GK, Lin D, Fu GK, Lin D, Zhang MYH, Bickle DD, Shackleton CHL, Miller WL, Portale AA. Cloning of human 25-hydroxyvitamin D-1α-hydroxylase and mutations causing vitamin D-dependent rickets type 1. Mol Endocrinol 1997;11:1961–1970.

22. Malloy PJ, Pike JW, Feldman D. The vitamin D receptor and the syndrome of hereditary 1,25-dihydroxyvitamin D-resistant rickets. Endocr Rev 1999;20:156–188.

23. Griffin JW, Zerwekh JE. Impaired stimulation of 25-hydroxyvitamin D-24-hydroxylase in fibroblasts from a patient with vitamin D-dependent rickets, type II. A form of receptor-positive resistance to 1,25-dihydroxyvitamin D3. J Clin Invest 1983;72:1190–1199.

24. Balsan S, Garabedian M, Larchet M, Gorski A, Cournot G, Tau C, Bourdeau A, Silve C, Ricour C. Long-term nocturnal calcium infusions can cure rickets and promote normal mineralisation in hereditary resistance to 1,25-dihydroxyvitamin D. J Clin Invest 1986;77:1661–1666.

25. Oginni LM, Worsfold M, Oyelami OA, Sharp CA, Powell DE, Davie MW. Etiology of rickets in Nigerian children. J Pediatr 1996;128:692–694.

26. Pettifor J M, Ross FP, Travers R, Glorieux F H, DeLuca HF. Dietary calcium deficiency: A syndrome associated with bone deformities and elevated serum 1,25-dihydroxyvitamin concentrations. Metab Bone Dis Rel Res 1981;2:301–306.

27. The HYP Consortiuum. A gene (PEX) with homologies to endopeptidases is mutated in patients with X-linked hypophosphatemic rickets. Nat Genet 1995;11:130–136.

28. Rowe PS. The role of the PHEX gene (PEX) in families with X-linked hypophosphatemic rickets. Curr Opin Nephrol Hypertens 1998;7:367–376.

29. Tieder M, Modai D, Samuel R, Arie R, Halabe A, Bab I, Gabizon D, Liberman UA. Hereditary hypophosphatemic rickets with hypercalciuria. N Engl J Med 1985;312:611–617.

30. Olivares JL, Ramos FJ, Carapeto FJ, Bueno M. Epidermal nevus syndrome and hypophosphatemia: Description of a patient with central nervous system anomalies and review of the literature. Eur J Pediatr 1999;158:103–107.

31. Nelson AE, Robinson BG, Mason RS, Oncogenic osteomalacia: Is there a new phosphate regulating hormone? Clin Endocrinol 1997;47:635–642.

32. Rowe PSN, Ong ACM, Cockerill FJ, Goulding JN, Hewison M. Candidate 56 and 58 kDa protein(s) responsible for mediating the renal defects in oncogenic hypophosphatemic osteomalacia. Bone 1996;18:159–169.

33. Ghazali S. Childhood urolithasis in the United Kingdom and Eire. Br J Urol 1975;47:109–116.

34. Diamond DA, Rickwood AMK, Lee PH, Johnston HB. Infection stones in children: A twenty-seven-year review. Pediatr Radiol 1994;43:525–527.

35. Bell NH, Yergey AL, Vieira NE, Oexmann MJ, Shary JR. Demonstration of a difference in urinary calcium, not calcium absorption in Black and White adolescents. J Bone Miner Res 1993;8:1111–1115.

36. Reusz GR, Dobos M, Byrd D, Sallay P, Miltényi M, Tulassay T. Urinary calcium and oxalate excretion in children. Pediatr Nephrol 1995;9:39–44.

37. Ghazali S, Barratt TM. Urinary excretion of calcium and magnesium in children. Arch Dis Child 1974;49:97–101.

38. Shaw NJ, Wheeldon J, Brocklebank T. Indices of intact serum parathyroid hormone and renal excretion of calcium, phosphate and magnesium. Arch Dis Child 1990;65:1208–1211.

39. DeSanto NG, Di Iorio B, Capasso G, Paduano C, Stamler R, Langman CB, Stamler J. Population based data on urinary excretion of calcium, oxalate, phosphate and uric acid in children from Cimitile (southern Italy). Pediatr Nephrol 1992;6:149–157.

40. Esbojörner E, Jones IL. Urinary calcium excretion in Swedish children. Acta Pediatr 1995;84:156–159.

41. Coe FL, Parks JH, Moore ES. Familial idiopathic hypercalciuria. N Engl J Med 1979;300:337–340.

42. Shen FH, Ivey JL, Sherrard DJ, Nielson RL, Haussler MR, Baylink DJ. Further evidence supporting the phosphate leak hypothesis of idiopathic hypercalciuria. Adv Exp Med Biol 1978;193:217–223.

43. Lemann J, Adams ND, Gray RW. Urinary calcium excretion in human beings. N Engl J Med 1979;301:535–541.

44. Broadus AE, Insogna KL, Lang R, Ellison AF, Dreyer BE. Evidence for disordered control of 1, 25 dihydroxyvitamin D production in absorptive hypercalciuria. N Eng J Med 1984;311:73–80.

45. Leonhardt A, Timmermanns G, Roth B, Seyberth HW. Calcium homeostasis and hypercalciuria in hyperprostaglandin E syndrome. J Pediatr 1992;120:546–554.

46. Vachvanichsanong P, Malagon M, Moore ES. Urinary incontinence due to idiopathic hypercalciuria in children. J Urol 1994;152:1226–1228.

47. Alon U, Warady BA, Hellerstein S. Hypercalciuria in the frequency–dysuria syndrome of childhood. J Pediatr 1990;116:103–105.

48. McGregor GA, Cappucio FP. The kidney and essential hypertension: a link to osteoporosis? J Hypertens 1993;11:781–785.

49. Lemann J Jr, Pleuss J, Gray R, Hoffman R. Potassium administration reduces and potassium deprivation increases urinary calcium excretion in healthy adults. Kidney Int 1991;39:973–983.

50. Jaeger P, Bonjour P, Karlmark B, Stanton B, Kirk RG, Duplinsky T, Giebisch G. Influence of acute potassium loading on renal phosphate transport in the rat kidney. Am J Physiol 1983;245:F601–F605.

51. Lloyd SE, Pearce SHS, Fisher SE, Steinmeyer K, Schwappach B, Scheinman SK, Harding B, Bolino A, Devoto M, Goodyer P, Rigden SP, Wrong O, Craig IW, Jentsch TJ, Thakker RW. A common molecular basis for three inherited kidney stone diseases. Nature 1996;379:445–449.

52. Barrat TM, Danpure CJ. Hyperoxaluria. In Paediatric Nephrology, (4th edn), Barrat TM, Avner ED, Harmon WE (ed.). Baltimore: Lippincott Williams and Wilkins, 1999:609–619.

53. Leiper JM, Danpure CJ. A unique molecular basis for enzyme mistrageting in primary hyperoxaluria type1. Clin Chim Acta 1997;266:39–50.

54. Danpure CJ, Rumsby G. Enzymology and molecular genetics of primary hyperoxaluria type 1: consequences for clinical management. In Calcium Oxalate in Biological Systems, Khan SR (ed.) Boca Raton: CRC Press, 1995:189–205.

55. Cochat P, Basmaison O. Current approaches to the management of primary hyperoxaluria. Arch Dis Child 2000;82:470–473.

56. Abstracts of 5th Workshop on Primary Hyperoxaluria, Kappel/Zurich, 12–13 March 1999. Nephrol Dial Transplant 1999;14:2784–2789.

57. Cochat P. Nephrology forum: Primary hyperoxaluria type 1. Kidney Int 1999;55:2533–2547.

58. Hoppe B, Danpure CJ, Rumsby G, *et al.* A vertical (pseudodominant) pattern of inheritance in the autosomal recessive disease primary hyperoxaluria type 1. Lack of relationship between genotype, enzymatic disease severity. Am J Kidney Dis 1997;29:36–44.

59. Hoppe B, Kemper MJ, Bokenkamp A, Langman CB. Plasma calcium-oxalate saturation in children with renal insufficiency and in children with primary hyperoxaluria. Kidney Int 1998;54:921–924.

60. Milliner DS, Wilson DM, Smith LH. Clinical expression and long-term outcomes of primary hyperoxaluria types 1 and 2. J Nephrol 1998,II S-1:56–59.

61. Marangella M. Transplantation strategies in type 1 primary hyperoxaluria: the issue of pyridoxine responsiveness. Nephrol Dial Transplant 1999; 14:301–303.

62. Cochat P, Scharer K. Should liver transplantation be performed before advanced renal insufficiency in primary hyperoxaluria type 1? Pediatr Nephrol 1993; 7:212–218.

63. Cramer SD, Ferree PM, Lin K, Milliner DS, Holmes RP. The gene encoding hydroxypyruvate reductase (GRHPR) is mutated in patients with primary hyperoxaluria typeII. Hum Mol Genet 1999;8:2063–2069.

64. Sperling O. Hereditory renal hypouricaemia. In The Metabolic and Molecular Basis of Inherited Disease, Scriver CR, Beaudet AL, Sly WS, Valle D (ed.). New York: McGraw Hill, 1995:3747–3762.

65. Greenwood MC, Dillon MJ, Simmonds HA, *et al.* Renal failure due to 2,8-dihydroxyadenine urolithiasis. Eur J Pediatr 1982;138:346–349.

66. Bradbury MG, Henderson M, Brocklebank JT, Simmonds HA. Acute renal failure due to xanthine stone. Pediatr Nephrol 1995;9:476–477.

67. Norman ME, Feldeman NI, Cohn RM, Roth KS, McCurdy DK. Urinary citrate excretion in the diagnosis of distal tubular acidosis. J Pediatr 1978;82:394–400.

68. Matthews LA, Doershuk CF, Stern RC, Resnick MI. Urolithiasis in cystic fibrosis. J Urol 1996;155:1563–1564.

69. Hoppe B, Hesse A, Brömme S, Rietschel E, Michalk D. Urinary excretion substances in patients with cystic fibrosis: risk of urolthiasis? Pediatr Nephrol 1998;12:275–279.

70. Jacinto JS, Houchang D, Modanlou MD, Crade M, Strauss AA, Bosu SK. Renal calcification incidence in very low birth weight infants. Pediatrics, 1988;81:31–35.

71. Short A, Cooke RWI. The incidence of renal calcification in preterm infants. Arch Dis Child 1991; 66:412–417.

72. Carter DR, Bouxsein ML, Marcus R. New approaches for interpreting projected bone densitometry data. J Bone Miner Res 1992;7:137–145.

73. Mølgaard C, Thomsen BL, Prentice A, Cole TJ, Michaelsen KF. Whole body bone mineral content in healthy children and adolescents. Arch Dis Child 1997;76:9–15.

74. Prentice A, Parsons TJ, Cole TJ. Uncritical use of bone mineral density in absorptiometry may lead to size-related artifacts in the identification of bone mineral determinants. Am J Clin Nutr 1994;60:837–842.

75. Gilsanz V, Roe TF, Mora S, Costin G, Goodmans WG. Changes in vertebral bone density in black and white girls during childhood and puberty. N Engl J Med 1991;325:1597–1599.

76. Mughal, MZ, Lorenc R. Assessment of bone status in children using quantitative ultrasound techniques. In Quantitative Ultrasound. Assessment of Osteoporosis and Bone Status, Njeh CF, Hans D, Fuerst T, Gluer CC, Genant HK (ed.) London: Martin Dunitz, 1999:309–323.

5 | *Renal tubular disorders*

William van't Hoff

Introduction

The renal tubule is responsible for the final regulation of the body's fluid, electrolyte and acid–base balance. Its principal function is the reabsorption of water and electrolytes in the glomerular ultrafiltrate, utilizing specialized transporters and channels. Tubular dysfunction, either congenital or acquired, can lead to profound electrolyte and volume disturbance. The proximal tubule is responsible for the majority of solute and water reabsorption including sodium, potassium, bicarbonate, phosphate, amino acids and low molecular weight proteins. Proximal tubule disorders may be isolated, involving only a single transporter (e.g. for glucose or for dibasic amino acids such as cystine) or generalized. The distal tubule is responsible for the final composition of urine, and specific transporters regulate sodium and potassium reabsorption and proton secretion. Distal tubular dysfunction is usually isolated to a specific transporter. Recent developments in molecular genetic research have led to a huge advance in our understanding of the pathogenesis of these disorders.

Most patients with genetic defects in tubular function present in the first years of life, often with rather non-specific symptoms, such as poor feeding, vomiting, and poor growth. Since the tubule has such an important role in fluid balance, symptoms of polyuria and polydipsia are often felt to indicate tubular dysfunction. In practice, even in children with severe and life-threatening problems, these features are often not appreciated by the child's carers, although they may be evident when careful fluid balance observations are made. Most children who 'drink too much' do not have a tubular disorder but have simply become accustomed to a large fluid intake (e.g. of fruit juices). In the assessment of a child with a suspected tubulopathy, a careful history of fluid intake and output is, however, helpful (how many cups of juice per day, any at night, any nocturia?). Details of the pregnancy (? polyhydramnios) and the age of onset of the problem should be noted. A history of vomiting is common, but constipation rather than diarrhoea is more often found (as a consequence of dehydration). In the clinical examination, it is important to pay special attention to growth, blood pressure and to check for rickets. Much information can be gained from the results of routine biochemical plasma and urine investigations. Further tests may include an assessment of urinary acidification and concentration, determination of specific proximal tubular markers, such as urinary levels of low molecular weight proteins (retinol binding protein, β_2-microglobulin) and enzymes (e.g. *N*-acetyl glucosaminidase), amino acids, and phosphate reabsorptive capacity. A renal ultrasound to determine the size and echogenicity (increased in nephrocalcinosis) of the kidneys should also be undertaken.

This chapter focuses on clinical cases of the more important renal tubulopathies, with an emphasis on the clinical approach to diagnosis. It is not intended to be either comprehensive or to detail the molecular and biochemical bases; further information may be found in the listed references. Renal tubular acidosis is discussed in Chapter 3.

Key points: Tubular disorders

- Most patients with genetic defects of tubular function present in the first years of life with non-specific symptoms.

- Most children who 'drink too much' do not have a tubular disorder.

- In the clinical examination, it is important to pay special attention to growth, blood pressure, and to check for rickets.

Case 1

A 6-month-old girl presents with failure to thrive, poor feeding, vomiting, and lethargy. Her weight and length are both below the 3rd centiles but the examination, including blood pressure, is otherwise normal. Preliminary biochemical investigations are as follows:

Blood:

sodium	133 mmol/l
potassium	2.4 mmol/l
bicarbonate	30 mmol/l
chloride	90 mmol/l
urea	4.5 mmol/l
creatinine	48 μmol/l
calcium	2.45 mmol/l
phosphate	1.75 mmol/l
albumin	39 g/l

Urine:

sodium	25 mmol/l
potassium	60 mmol/l
calcium	0.9 mmol/l
chloride	45 mmol/l
creatinine	1.5 mmol/l

These results demonstrate hyoponatraemia and hypokalaemia. Hyponatraemia may be due to salt loss (dehydration) or may be dilutional (water overload). Distinction between these will depend on clinical history and examination. However, the combination of hyponatraemia and hypokalaemia is very suggestive of combined and excessive losses of both sodium and potassium, usually due to vomiting or diarrhoea, less commonly due to renal tubular losses. Gastrointestinal losses should be evident, so that if there is no such history, a renal cause should be sought. Excessive losses of salt and potassium are frequently associated with a metabolic acidosis or alkalosis—in this case the bicarbonate was 30 and the chloride 90 mmol/l. A low plasma chloride would be seen in gastrointestinal or renal losses, the cause can be ascertained from measurement of the urine chloride, which will be low in cases of diarrhoea or vomiting and high in certain renal tubulopathies [1]. In this case the urine chloride is high (45 mmol/l), suggesting tubular loss.

Further assessment of renal tubular function is required. Proximal tubular dysfunction is unlikely since this nearly always leads to acidosis (extremely rarely, children with very severe proximal damage can dehydrate so much as to cause a contractual hypokalaemic alkalosis). Generalized proximal dysfunction is often associated with a low plasma phosphate. Other markers which should be checked include urinary amino acids and, if available, urinary tubular proteins (which were normal in this case). The above results demonstrate a urinary calcium/creatinine ratio of 0.60 which is normal (<0.74 mmol/mmol) but other children with this biochemical picture often have hypercalciuria, which can lead to nephrocalcinosis. A renal ultrasound is therefore an important investigation. The evidence leads to a diagnosis of a renal tubulopathy affecting the reabsorption of sodium, chloride, and potassium; this pattern is that of Bartter's syndrome. These excess losses are associated with marked polyuria and polydipsia, but this is not often reported as a presenting problem. The same scenario can be seen in patients on loop diuretics (such as furosemide) or in those abusing laxatives. In the latter cases, the urine chloride should be low, whereas with furosemide abuse, it should be high (although it may be lower than expected[1]). Bartter's syndrome is rare, but a more likely diagnosis in a young child. The converse is true for older patients, in whom urine toxicology should be considered.

Bartter's syndrome

Bartter's syndrome is a term used to describe a number of different genetic salt-losing tubulopathies occurring due to defective sodium, chloride, and potassium reabsorption. All are inherited in an autosomal recessive manner. The most severe form causes an affected fetus to be polyuric, leading to severe polyhydramnios, intrauterine growth retardation and premature delivery. Postnatally, these babies have very severe polyuria, electrolyte disturbance, and poor growth in the first weeks of life. In contrast to the case described above, there is marked hypercalciuria and nephrocalcinosis [2]. Very rarely, these severely affected babies can present with a transient metabolic acidosis and hyperkalemia, with a gradual evolution to a more classical biochemical disturbance [2]. Case 1, described above, is more typical of a milder form of the disorder, presenting in early childhood with poor growth, polyuria, and polydipsia. The outstanding biochemical abnormality is severe hypokalaemia (e.g. 2.0–2.5 mmol/l) secondary to increased urinary losses of salt and potassium. Urinary calcium loss is normal or only slightly elevated and nephrocalcinosis is not seen, in contrast to the more severe neonatal form. The evaluation is not complete unless the blood pressure is confirmed as normal, since an identical biochemical picture can be seen in patients with hyper-reninaemic hypertension, for instance secondary to renovascular disease or renal scarring. In these cases of hypertension, the elevated renin, and hence aldosterone, levels underpin the excess sodium reabsorption that elevates blood pressure with secondary potassium loss. In Bartter's syndrome, the prime defect is tubular loss of sodium and chloride, which leads secondarily to excessive losses of potassium in the distal tubule, associated with hyper-reninaemia and hyperaldosteronism. Measurement of renin and aldosterone in suspected cases of Bartter's syndrome may help, but elevated concentrations are non-specific. In previous years, when the molecular basis of the syndrome was not understood, there was emphasis placed on the abnormalities of prostaglandin production and ion transport (e.g. in erythrocytes). Such determinations are not readily available outside research centres.

The treatment of Bartter's syndrome involves replacement of fluid and electrolyte losses followed by administration of indomethacin, which reduces renal salt, water and potassium losses (principally by reducing glomerular filtration). Severely affected children may initially require saline rehydration, milder cases can simply be started on potassium chloride, ideally split into 3–4 doses. It is usually very difficult to achieve adequate potassium supplementation to restore the plasma level into the normal range, and most patients tolerate a potassium concentration of 2.5 mmol/l without the expected associated problems (e.g. dysrhythmias and muscle weakness). Indomethacin is usually started at a dose of 0.5–1.0 mg/kg/day, split into four divided doses, with stepwise increases in dose to a maximum of 2–4 mg/kg/day [2]. It should be given with food (or milk) and parents counselled that a small number of children may suffer gastro-duodenal irritation or frank ulceration. There are other rarer side-effects (including benign intracranial hypertension) and some authorities have concerns about chronic usage within the neonatal period.

Molecular basis of Bartter's syndrome

Although the basis of Bartter's syndrome was considered to be multifactorial, including an abnormal pressor response to angiotensin II, excessive production of prostaglandins or defects in renal tubular electrolyte transport, recent evidence supported only the latter theory. It was recognized that furosemide (a loop diuretic) could mimic the Bartter phenotype, whereas thiazide treatment could reproduce the features of a related disorder: Gitelman's syndrome. Furosemide acts by inhibiting the sodium–potassium–chloride co-transporter (Na–K–2Cl) located in the apical membrane of the thick ascending limb. Defects in NKCC2, the gene encoding this co-transporter, were found to be the underlying cause in some children with Bartter's syndrome [3]. Defective function of N–K–2Cl would lead to severe urinary losses of sodium, chloride, and water. These lead, in turn, to hyper-reninaemia, hyperaldosteronism and excessive potassium losses.

This molecular defect was identified in some, but not all, children with the severe neonatal form of Bartter's syndrome. Other patients with a similar phenotype have been found to have mutations in a gene (KCNJ1) which encodes ROMK, one of a family of inwardly rectifying potassium channels [4], involved in recycling potassium from the tubular cell back into the urinary lumen, thereby maintaining the efficient functioning of the Na–K–2Cl transporter [5]. Defects in ROMK would secondarily inhibit effective function of N–K–2Cl, thereby producing the features of Bartter's syndrome. In addition, calcium reabsorption in the thick ascending limb is linked to Na–K–2Cl transport, so that loss of function would explain the hypercalciuria and nephrocalcinosis seen in this neonatal form of Bartter's syndrome.

Most children with Bartter's syndrome have less severe symptoms and do not have hypercalciuria or nephrocalcinosis. Genetic analysis has shown that they do not have mutations affecting the Na–K–2Cl or ROMK channels. Some have mutations affecting the CLCNKB gene, coding for a renal chloride channel, CLC-Kb [6]. This channel is expressed in the basolateral membrane of the thick ascending limb and transports chloride from the tubular cell into the blood. Defective chloride reabsorption in the thick ascending limb would also lead to excessive urinary losses of sodium and secondarily of potassium, producing the hypokalaemic alkalosis. There are, however, families with Bartter's syndrome who do not have mutations in any of these three genes, suggesting that there are other channels or genes involved in the regulation of sodium chloride transport in the thick ascending limb.

Key points: Bartter's syndrome

- Autosomal recessive inheritance.

- Early childhood form typically presents with poor growth, polydipsia and polyuria.

- Hypokalaemia, hyponatraemia and alkalosis with increased urinary chloride excretion are the cardinal biochemical features.

- Hypercalciuria and nephrocalcinosis occur in the severe infantile form.

- Plasma magnesium level is normal, unlike in Gitelman's syndrome.

Case 2

A 5-year-old boy is admitted to hospital with a 3-day history of diarrhoea and vomiting. He is found to be dehydrated and his initial investigations are as follows:

Blood:

sodium	135 mmol/l
potassium	2.6 mmol/l
bicarbonate	29 mmol/l
urea	6.5 mmol/l
creatinine	67 μmol/l
calcium	2.42 mmol/l
magnesium	0.45 mmol/l
phosphate	1.30 mmol/l
albumin	48 g/l

Urine:

chloride	30 mmol/l
calcium/creatinine	0.05 mmol/mmol (normal 0.06–0.74)

He is rehydrated with intravenous 0.9% saline with potassium supplements and his symptoms resolve. At clinic review 4 weeks later, the plasma potassium has risen slightly to 3.0 mmol/l and the magnesium to 0.55 mmol/l. These data show a marked hypokalaemic alkalosis but, in contrast to Case 1, there is also profound hypomagnesaemia (normal level 0.65–1.0 mmol/l). Hypomagnesaemia can occur due to excessive losses from the gut (e.g. in diarrhoea) or from urine, due either to an inherited tubular defect or secondary to thiazide diuretics or other drugs (e.g. ciclosporin). As with Case 1, measurement of the urinary chloride may be helpful in distinguishing gastrointestinal from renal losses of magnesium in this patient. Determination of urinary calcium excretion and a renal ultrasound to check for the presence of nephrocalcinosis, are also important (see Chapter 4). This boy was found to have a high urine chloride, suggesting a renal tubular leak. Tests of proximal tubular function were normal, so the principal differential diagnosis lay between two genetic renal tubulopathies: hypomagnesaemia–hypercalciuria syndrome and Gitleman's syndrome. These are distinguished by differences in urinary calcium excretion: markedly elevated and causing nephrocalcinosis and nephrolithiasis in the first disorder and very low in Gitelman's syndrome, the diagnosis in this case [7].

Individuals affected by Gitelman's syndrome are often asymptomatic and the diagnosis is only suspected after plasma biochemistry, checked for another indication, is found to be abnormal. However, profound hypomagnesaemia, perhaps accentuated during an intercurrent illness, can lead to marked weakness and/or tetany. Treatment may not be required but, if necessary, patients should receive magnesium supplements [2,8]. The genetic basis for this syndrome is similar to that for Bartter's syndrome, involving defective tubular sodium–chloride transport. Patients have mutations in the *SLC12A3* gene, coding for the thiazide-sensitive sodium chloride co-transporter (NCCT) [9], which is expressed in the distal tubule. Defective function of NCCT leads to salt wasting, hypokalaemic alkalosis, and hyper-reninaemia. Excessive urinary magnesium loss, leading to hypomagnesaemia, may result from impaired distal tubular magnesium reabsorption, in turn secondary to the hypokalaemic alkalosis [10].

Case 3

A 10-month-old boy presents with a 4-month history of poor feeding, recurrent vomiting, poor growth, and weakness (delayed gross motor milestones). He is found to have a weight and height significantly below the 3rd centiles, appears 10% dehydrated and has swollen wrists, knees and ankles, consistent with rickets. The results of preliminary investigations are as follows:

Blood:

sodium	134 mmol/l
potassium	2.8 mmol/l
urea	5.0 mmol/l
creatinine	40 μmol/l
calcium	2.35 mmol/l
phosphate	1.05 mmol/l

These results are quite similar to those of Case 1: there is mild hyoponatraemia, marked hypokalaemia and, in addition, a low phosphate. As before, likely causes are excessive losses either due to vomiting, diarrhoea, or in the urine. In contrast to Case 1, where there was an alkalosis, in this child the bicarbonate is low (15 mmol/l), suggesting a metabolic acidosis. The plasma chloride is raised, at 108 mmol/l, so the anion gap, $Na - (Cl + HCO_3)$, is normal (i.e. 10–14 mmol/l). In the absence of symptoms suggesting gastrointestinal losses, a hyperchloraemic acidosis is likely to be due to renal tubular acidosis. The urine pH at a time of severe acidosis was 5.2, confirming a proximal renal tubular acidosis (RTA). In children, proximal RTA usually occurs as part of a generalized proximal tubular dysfunction associated with rickets (renal Fanconi's syndrome). The low plasma phosphate concentration in this child is consistent with generalized proximal tubular dysfunction in which there is hypophosphataemia due to phosphaturia, aminoaciduria, glycosuria, acidosis due to excessive bicarbonaturia and low molecular weight proteinuria. There are many causes of renal Fanconi's syndrome (see below) and the extent of the above abnormalities varies between different disorders (e.g. acidosis is much more severe in cystinosis than in Dent's disease). Once the diagnosis of renal Fanconi's syndrome is made, the child must be investigated to elucidate the cause.

Causes of renal Fanconi's syndrome

The differential diagnosis of the Fanconi syndrome involves a number of genetic (metabolic) disorders, predominant in childhood, and acquired causes including some nephropathies and several drugs (reviewed in Foreman 1999 [11]). The age of onset and associated features narrow further the diagnostic possibilities. Table 5.1 lists genetic causes in order of age of onset and Table 5.2 the more common acquired causes.

Cystinosis

Nephropathic cystinosis is an autosomal recessive disorder characterized by defective lysosomal cystine transport leading to excessive intracellular cystine accumulation [12]. Cystine accumulation affects predominantly the proximal tubule, leading to a severe Fanconi's syndrome and presenting usually in late infancy with poor feeding, excessive thirst, delayed growth, weakness, and rickets. All racial groups are affected, but Caucasians commonly have blond hair and a fair complexion. Clinical diagnosis can also be confirmed by slit-lamp demonstration of corneal cystine crystals. As well as general measures appropriate for any child with Fanconi's syndrome (rehydration, bicarbonate, electrolyte and vitamin D supplements), patients with cystinosis require therapy with a cystine-depleting agent (cysteamine) to reduce progressive glomerular damage which, if untreated, leads to end stage renal failure by 10 years [13]. Renal transplantation is successful but does not correct the disorder

Table 5.1 Genetic causes of renal Fanconi' syndrome

Onset	Disorder	Associated features	Diagnostic test
Neonatal	Galactosaemia	Liver dysfunction, jaundice, encephalopathy, sepsis	Red cell galactose 1-phosphate uridyl transferase
	Mitochondrial disorders	Usually multisystem dysfunction (brain, muscle, liver, heart)	Lactate/pyruvate (may be normal plasma lactate due to urinary losses), muscle enzymology
	Tyrosinaemia	Poor growth, hepatic enlargement and dysfunction	Plasma amino acids, urine organic acids (succinyl acetone)
Infancy	Fructosaemia	Rapid onset after fructose given, vomiting, hypoglycaemia, hepatomegaly	Hepatic fructose 1-phosphate aldolase B
	Cystinosis	Poor growth, may have blond/fair hair, rickets, corneal cystine crystals	Leucocyte cystine concentration, —nutation analysis (*CTNS*)
	Fanconi–Bickel syndrome	Failure to thrive, hepatomegaly, hypoglycaemia, rickets, severe glycosuria, galactosuria	Mutation analysis (*GLUT2*)
	Lowe's syndrome	Males (X-linked), cataracts, hypotonia, developmental delay	Clinical and molecular genetic diagnosis (*OCRL*)
Childhood	Cystinosis	As above	
	Dent's disease	Males (X-linked), hypercalciuria, nephrocalcinosis	Molecular diagnosis (*CLCN5*)
	Wilson's disease	Hepatic and neurological disease, Kayser–Fleischer rings	Copper, caeruloplasmin

Table 5.2 Acquired causes of renal Fanconi's syndrome

Drugs	Renal disorders	Other causes
Aminoglycosides (common)	Nephrotic syndrome (FSGS)	Multiple myeloma
Ifosfamide (common)	After renal transplantation	Heavy metals (lead, cadmium, mercury, uranium)
Outdated tetracyclines	Recovery phase of acute tubular necrosis	Toluene
Sodium valproate (rare)	Acute interstitial nephritis	Paraquat
6-Mercaptopurine (rare)		

and cystine continues to accumulate in non-renal tissues, causing multisystem dysfunction (delayed puberty, hypothyroidism, diabetes mellitus, myopathy, and central nervous system involvement) [12]. It is therefore essential for patients to continue their cysteamine therapy even after transplantation.

The cystinosis gene, CTNS, has been identified and found to code for a lysosomal membrane protein, cystinosin, presumed to be the cystine transporter [14]. Forty per cent of cystinosis patients have been found to be homozygous for a large 57 kb deletion involving the CTNS gene, and many others are heterozygously deleted [15]. This large deletion has only been identified in patients of northern European origin (found in 76% of such individuals) and can therefore be used as a diagnostic test. Patients who are heterozygous for the deletion, or who do not have the major deletion, can be screened using single-strand conformation polymorphism (SSCP) analysis covering the complete CTNS coding sequence and intron/exon boundaries [14]. Overall, using this strategy, mutations have been detected in 90% of cystinotic patient samples.

Key points: Cystinosis

- An autosomal recessive disorder characterized by defective lysosomal cystine transport, leading to excessive intracellular cystine accumulation.

- All racial groups are affected, but Caucasians commonly have blond hair and a fair complexion.

- Treatment consists of general measures to control Fanconi's syndrome and cysteamine.

- Renal transplantation is successful but does not correct the disorder and cystine continues to accumulate in non-renal tissues, causing multisystem dysfunction.

- The cystinosis gene, CTNS, has been identified and found to code for a lysosomal membrane protein, cystinosin, presumed to be the cystine transporter [14].

Tyrosinaemia type I

This is an autosomal recessive disorder due to a deficiency of fumaryl acetoacetase (FAH), which is involved in the degradation of tyrosine. FAH deficiency causes a build-up of toxic metabolites, in particular succinyl acetone and succinyl acetoacetate [16]. Children present in early infancy with a combination of severe liver disease and renal Fanconi's syndrome. The liver disease progresses to hepatic cirrhosis, with a major risk of hepatocellular carcinoma. Renal involvement is with severe Fanconi's syndrome with rickets and, in the long term, chronic renal failure. Recurrent episodes of polyneuropathy can also occur secondary to FAH-induced inhibition of porphobilinogen synthetase (akin to hepatic porphyria). In addition to supportive treatment of the liver and renal dysfunction, patients can be treated with NTBC [2-(2-nitro-4-trifluoromethylbenzoyl)-1,3-cyclohexanedione], which inhibits 4-hydroxyphenylpyruvate dioxygenase, at a step in the tyrosine pathway more proximal to FAH. NTBC therapy prevents the accumulation of succinyl acetoacetone and subsequent metabolic and clinical derangements [17,18].

Lowe's syndrome

The oculocerebrorenal syndrome of Lowe is an X-linked disorder, characterized by congenital cataracts, hypotonia, intellectual impairment, and renal Fanconi's syndrome [19]. Affected boys usually present with the cataracts, which are prenatal in onset, and then develop renal tubular dysfunction over the first year of life. Fanconi's syndrome is generally milder than that seen in cystinosis or tyrosinaemia, with acidosis and hypophosphataemia but minimal hypokalaemia [19]. The diagnosis is clinical, but with the isolation of the OCRL gene, mutation analysis is potentially feasible. There is no specific treatment for the disorder, but patients require specialized follow-up in order to manage the various ophthalmological and renal complications. In older patients (second to fourth decades), chronic glomerular failure develops.

Case 4

A 1-month-old baby girl is admitted with severe dehydration following a history of poor feeding and vomiting. She is febrile (38 °C), is estimated to be 15% dehydrated but has no other abnormalities on examination. Investigations are as follows:

Blood:
sodium	124 mmol/l
potassium	8.6 mmol/l
urea	7.0 mmol/l
creatinine	88 μmol/l
bicarbonate	15 mmol/l
calcium	2.58 mmol/l
phosphate	2.0 mmol/l

Urine:

sodium	60 mmol/l
potassium	3 mmol/l

This child presents in severe shock and requires urgent intravenous fluids (e.g. initially 10–20 ml/kg 0.9% saline over $\frac{1}{2}$–1 hour). Immediate management should also involve a septic screen and antibiotic administration, since overwhelming infection is by far the most common cause of such a presentation. There appear to be three other severe problems: hyperkalaemia, acidosis, and hyponatraemia. The plasma creatinine is approximately twice the normal value, suggesting renal impairment. Appropriate management of the electrolyte problems should include acute administration of calcium gluconate (as a cardioprotective manoeuvre in view of hyperkalaemia) and half correction of the acidosis with sodium bicarbonate. Four hours later, on repeating the biochemistry, there is an improvement in the bicarbonate and creatinine concentrations, but the hyperkalaemia and hyponatraemia persist.

Review of the urine biochemistry indicates an inappropriately high urine sodium in the context of severe hyponatraemia (and hypovolaemia). There is therefore clear evidence of tubular salt wasting. The differential diagnosis includes polyuric acute renal failure (ARF), congenital adrenal hyperplasia (CAH), and a renal tubulopathy. The degree of electrolyte imbalance is out of proportion to the elevation in creatinine for this to be due to ARF (although there is clearly some degree of impairment). A salt-wasting form of CAH is possible and appropriate biochemical investigations (e.g. 17-hydroxyprogesterone, urine steroid profile) should be undertaken. Plasma renin and aldosterone values should also be measured, and in this case are both very high. The 17-hydroxyprogesterone and steroid profile are normal and a trial of mineralocorticoid therapy has no appreciable effect. In summary, this child has hyper-reninaemia, hyperaldosteronism but severe salt-wasting and hyperkalaemia, evidence suggestive of tubular insensitivity to aldosterone, a disorder known as pseudohypoaldosteronism.

Pseudohypoaldosteronism type 1

Two forms of pseudohypoaldosteronism type 1 (PHA1) exist, a more severe, autosomal recessive type affecting several organ systems and persisting into adulthood, and an autosomal dominant form, involving only the kidney, which tends to improve with age [20]. The autosomal dominant form is due to mutations in the mineralocorticoid receptor gene (*MLR*) which prevents normal receptor function and hence causes salt wasting [21]. The autosomal recessive form of PHA1 is associated with mutations in the subunits of the epithelial sodium channel (ENaC) which the MLR regulates [22]. This channel, localized in the distal tubule, is the transporter for aldosterone-induced sodium reabsorption. Defects in the subunits of the channel prevent its function, so that sodium is inadequately reabsorbed and there is massive salt-wasting while, equally, potassium is inadequately excreted, causing hyperkalaemia. The logical treatment for PHA1 is therefore to give sodium chloride supplements, and this is effective although huge doses are commonly required (e.g. 50 mmol/kg/day). Adequate sodium replacement will restore circulating volume and lead to increased urinary excretion of potassium, thereby improving the biochemistry.

Case 5

An 8-month-old boy is brought to hospital having had a short generalized seizure. He has had a minor upper respiratory infection and has a history that 'he can't stop drinking'. He is noted to have a poor appetite, doesn't vomit but has infrequent and irregular bowel actions. He has a fever of 38 °C, his growth has tailed off in the past 2 months, although both length and weight remain above the 2nd centiles. His blood pressure is 90/55 and clinical examination is otherwise unremarkable. Investigations are as follows:

Blood:

sodium	118 mmol/l
potassium	4.0 mmol/l
urea	2.0 mmol/l
creatinine	45 μmol/l
bicarbonate	18 mmol/l
glucose	5.0 mmol/l

Urine:

sodium	59 mmol/l
potassium	12 mmol/l

An infant presenting with a 'febrile seizure' is a common general paediatric referral. Appropriate management for a child with febrile seizures was undertaken. What makes this case unusual is the profoundly low plasma sodium. Hyponatraemia is usually due to excessive salt losses (e.g. from the gut or kidney) or due to excess body water in relation to sodium (e.g. in acute renal failure). The high urine sodium level can be due to a number of disorders, including nephrotic syndrome, liver cirrhosis, cardiac failure or, in the context of hypervolaemia, may be secondary to renal failure, the syndrome of inappropriate secretion of ADH (SIADH) or 'psychogenic' polydipsia. In this case, there is no history of abnormal fluid losses and the normal plasma urea and creatinine concentrations are not consistent with acute renal failure. Clinical evaluation suggested a normal or elevated circulating volume.

In view of his seizure, he was given a slow infusion of hypertonic saline to partially correct his hyponatraemia towards a value of 125. Thereafter, fluid restriction led to an improvement in his plasma biochemistry. In reviewing the history, he had been receiving huge volumes (6–8 litres/day) of dilute juice for the last few months and was described as 'always thirsty'. Once stable and with normal plasma biochemistry, he underwent a water deprivation test. After a baseline weight and plasma biochemistry, fluids were withheld for 6–8 hours during which he was carefully observed on an investigation ward. Weight was recorded hourly and every urine sample sent for urine osmolality. After 6 hours his urine osmolality was 900 mOsm/kg, an essentially normal value for his age and one confirming that his renal concentrating capacity was intact. This problem is labelled as 'psychogenic polydipsia' in adults but in children the term 'habitual polydipsia' more accurately reflects the scenario in which they are offered large volumes of dilute juice. There are relatively few reports of this problem in the literature but these probably reflect only the most severe incidents and milder cases may be more prevalent. Such water intoxication and resultant hyponatraemia has also been recorded after swimming lessons, enemata, therapy with mist tents and has recently been recognized as a fatal form of child abuse [23].

Case 6

A 2-week-old boy, born at term after a normal pregnancy, is referred as an emergency with a history of poor feeding, fever, recurrent vomiting, and lethargy. On assessment, he is clinically dehydrated but no focus of infection is found. The results of preliminary investigations are as follows:

Blood:

sodium	148 mmol/l
potassium	4.0 mmol/l
chloride	112 mmol/l
urea	5.0 mmol/l
creatinine	75 μmol/l
bicarbonate	22 mmol/l

Urine:

sodium	8 mmol/l
potassium	40 mmol/l

These results show a raised plasma sodium, chloride, urea and creatinine, consistent with dehydration. Importantly, there is no disturbance of acid–base balance, despite the history of vomiting. In addition, plasma potassium is normal (as were the calcium, phosphate, and magnesium), which suggests that proximal and distal tubular functions are intact. The presentation and preliminary data are seen frequently in acutely ill children and the most important (and most common) cause is sepsis (urinary infection, meningitis, pneumonia, septicaemia, etc.). Appropriate broad-spectrum antibiotic treatment should be administered pending the results of cultures. At the same time, intravenous fluids (such as 0.9% saline or 0.45% saline with 2.5% glucose) should be given to restore circulating volume. In the majority of such children, this treatment would return the abnormal plasma levels towards normal. This child, however, became more irritable and plasma

sodium increased. He was noted to have very wet nappies and confirmed to be polyuric. Plasma and urine osmolalities were checked simultaneously and found to be 305 mosm/kg in plasma and 90 mosm/kg in urine. These data are highly suggestive of a defect in renal concentrating ability, which was confirmed by testing the osmolality of serial urines passed after intramuscular injection of DDAVP (a maximal value of 150 mosm/kg was obtained). This is proof that he has nephrogenic diabetes insipidus (NDI) and, given his age and sex, it is concluded that he has congenital X-linked NDI.

Nephrogenic diabetes insipidus

Nephrogenic diabetes insipidus (NDI) is a disorder in which the kidney fails to respond to arginine vasopressin, leading to defective urinary concentration. The most severe forms occur congenitally due to genetic defects in the AVP receptor or the associated water channels. Milder, secondary forms occur more commonly in children with renal damage or with some congenital renal abnormalities (e.g. nephrocalcinosis, dysplastic kidneys, cortical scarring), but this chapter will focus on congenital NDI. This is usually inherited in an X-linked manner and affected males typically present in the newborn period with poor feeding and growth, irritability, recurrent vomiting, and constipation [24]. The severe polyuria and polydipsia become evident within months. Older children can develop further problems, including poorer growth, delayed bladder control, learning and behavioural difficulties, and a flow uropathy (megaureter and megacystis) [25,26]. The biochemical abnormalities and assessment are detailed above. A renal ultrasound should also be requested to ensure there are two normally sized kidneys and to exclude nephrocalcinosis.

The treatment of NDI is a high water intake and a feed restricted in solute load (in particular by sodium restriction). Most babies are very irritable and have difficulties settling into a normal feeding regimen. Water should be offered after each milk feed. In addition, drug therapy with a combination of a diuretics (such as hydrochlorothiazide) and indomethacin, a prostaglandin synthetase inhibitor, is commenced [24]. These have the effect of reducing urine output, thus reducing slightly the excessive fluid intake. Clinically, the baby feeds better, settles well, and the biochemical abnormalities improve. Parents should be counselled that indomethacin can cause gastro-duodenal ulceration, so it should always be given with a feed and urgent medical attention sought if there is evidence of abdominal pain or bleeding. In practice, however, indomethacin is usually very well tolerated and significantly improves the child.

NDI occurs due to mutations in the gene encoding the arginine vasopressin receptor located in the collecting duct cells (V2R) [27,28]. When activated by binding of vasopressin, the V2R receptor, via a number of steps, causes an increase in cAMP which in turn, causes movement of intracellular vesicles containing aquaporin-2 (AQ-2) water channels, to the apical membrane, thereby increasing water permeability (see ref. 24 for a review). Female carriers of a V2R mutation in a CNDI family are generally asymptomatic. Rarely, NDI may occur in an autosomal recessive manner, in which case females are affected as often as males. In these families, affected individuals have heterozygous or homozygous mutations in the gene coding for the AQ-2 protein [29,30].

References

1. Mersin SS, Ramelli GP, Laux-End R, Bianchetti MG. Urinary chloride excretion distinguishes between renal and extrarenal metabolic alkalosis. Eur J Paediatr 1995; 154:979–982.
2. Rodriguez-Soriano J. Bartter and related syndromes: the puzzle is almost solved. Pediatr Nephrol 1998; 12:315–327.
3. Simon DB, Karet FE, Hamdam JM, Di Pietro A, Sanjad SA, Lifton RP. Bartter's syndrome, hypokalaemic alkalosis with hypercalciuria, is caused by mutations in the Na–K°2Cl cotransporter NKCC2. Nat Genet 1996; 13:183–188.
4. Simon DB, Karet FE, Rodriguez-Soriano J, Hamdan JH, DiPietro A, Trachtman H, Sanjad SA, Lifton RJ. Genetic heterogeneity of Bartter's syndrome revealed by mutations in the K⁺ channel, ROMK. Nat Genet 1996; 14:152–156.
5. Hebert SC. An ATP-regulated inwardly rectifying potassium channel from rat kidney. Kidney Int 1995; 48:1010–1016.
6. Simon DB, Bindra RS, Mansfield TA, Nelson-Williams C, Mendonca E, Stone R, Schurman S, Nayir A, Alpay H, Bakkaloglu A, Rodriguez-Soriano J, Morales JM, Sanjad SA, Taylor CM, Pilz D, Brem A, Trachtman H, Griswold W, Richard GA, John E, Lifton RJ. Mutations in the chloride channel ClC-Kb cause Bartter's syndrome type III. Nat Genet 1997; **17**:171–178.
7. Bettinelli A, Bianchetti MG, Girardin E, Caringella A, Cecconi M, Appiani AC, Pavanello L, Gastaldi R, Isimbaldi C, Lama G, Marchesoni C, Mateucci C, Patriarca P, Di Natale B, Stezu C, Vitucci P. Use of calcium excretion values to distinguish two forms of primary renal tubular hypokalaemia alkalosis: Bartter and Gitelman syndromes. J Pediatr 1992; 120:38–43.
8. Bettinelli A, Basilico E, Metta MG, Borella P, Jaeger P, Bianchetti MG. Magnesium supplementation in Gitelman syndrome. Pediatr Nephrol 1999; 13:311–314.
9. Simon DB, Nelson-Williams C, Bia MJ, Ellison D, Karet FE, Molina AM, Vaara I, Iwata F, Cushner HM, Koolen M, Gainza FJ, Gitelman HJ, Lifton RP. Gitelman's variant of Bartter's syndrome, inherited hypokalaemic alkalosis, is caused by mutations in the thiazide-sensitive NaCl cotransporter. Nature Genet 1996; 12:24–30.
10. Quamme GA. Renal magnesium handling: new perspectives in understanding old problems. Kidney Int 1997; 52:1180–1195.
11. Foreman J. Cystinosis and Fanconi syndromes. In Pediatric Nephrology, 4th edn, (eds Barratt TM, Avner ED, Harmon WE). Lippincott, Williams and Wilkins Baltimore 1999, Chapter 35, pp. 593–607.
12. Gahl, WA, Schneider, JA, Aula P. Lysosomal transport disorders. In The Metabolic and Molecular Bases of Inherited Disease, 7th edn, (eds Scriver CR, Beaudet AL, Sly WS, Valle D.). McGraw-Hill, New York, 1995, pp. 3763–3797.
13. Markello TC, Bernadini IM, Gahl WA. Improved renal function in children with cystinosis treated with cysteamine. N Engl J Med 1993; 328:1157–1162.
14. Town M, Jean G, Cherqui S, Attard M, Forestier L, Whitmore SA, Callen DF, Gribouval O, Broyer M, Bates GP, van't Hoff W, Antignac C. A novel gene encoding an integral membrane protein is mutated in nephropathic cystinosis. Nat Genet 1998; 18:319–324.
15. Forestier L, Jean G, Attard M, Cherqui S, Lewis C, van't Hoff W, Broyer M, Town M, Antignac C. Molecular characterisation of CTNS deletions in nephropathic cystinosis: development of a PCR-based detection assay. Am J Hum Genet 1999; 65:353–359.
16. Lindblad B, Lindstedt S, Steen G. On the enzymic defects in hereditary tyrosinemia. Proc Natl Acad Sci 1977; 74:4641–4645.
17. Lindstedt S, Holme E, Lock EA, Hjalmarson O, Strandvik B. Treatment of hereditary tyrosinaemia type I by inhibition of 4-hydroxyphenylpyruvate dioxygenase. Lancet 1992; 340:813–817.
18. Holme E, Lindstedt S. Tyrosinaemia type I and NTBC (2-(2-nitro-4-trifluoromethylbenzoyl)-1,3-cyclohexanedione). J Inherit Metab Dis 1998; 21:507–517.
19. Charnas L, Bernadini I, Rader D, Hoeg J, Gahl WA. Clinical and laboratory findings in the oculocerebrorenal syndrome of Lowe, with special reference to growth and renal function. N Engl J Med. 1991; 324:1318–1325.
20. Hanukoglu A. Type I pseudohypoaldosteronism includes two clinically and genetically distinct entities with either renal or mulitple target organ defects. J Clin Endocrin Metab 1991; 73:936–944.
21. Geller DS, Rodriguez Soriano J, Boado AV, Schifter S, Bayer M, Chang SS, Lifton RP. Mutations in the minerlacorticoid receptor gene cause autosomal dominant pseudohypoaldosteronism type 1. Nat Genet 1998; 19:279–281.

22. Chang SS, Grunder S, Hanukoglu A, Rosler A, Mathew PM, Hanukoglu I, Schild L, Lu Y, Schimkets RA, Nelson-Williams C, Rossier BC, Lifton RP. Mutations in subunits of the epithelial sodium channel cause salt wasting with hyperkalaemic acidosis, pseudohypoaldosteronism type 1. Nat Genet 1996; 12:248–253.

23. Arieff AI, Kronlund BA. Fatal child abuse by forced water intoxication. Pediatrics 1999; 103:1292–1295.

24. Knoers NVAM, Monnens LAH. Nephrogenic diabetes insipidus. In Pediatric Nephrology, 4th edn, (eds Barratt TM, Avner ED, Harmon WE). Lippincott, Williams and Wilkins, Baltimore 1999, Chapter 34, pp. 583–591.

25. Hoekstra JA, van Lieburg AF, Monnens LAH, Hulstijn-Dirkmatt GM, Knoers VV. Cognitive and psychometric functioning of patients with nephrogenic diabetes insipidus. Am J Med Genet 1996; 61:81–88.

26. van Lieburg AF, Knoers NVAM, Monnens LAH. Clinical presentation and long term follow up of thirty patients with nephrogenic diabetes insipidus. J Am Soc Nephrol 1999; 10:1958–1964.

27. van den Ouweland AM, Dreesen JC, Verdijk M, Knoers NV, Monnens LA, Rocchi M, van Oost BA. Mutations in the vasopressin type 2 receptor gene (AVPR2) associated with nephrogenic diabetes insipidus. Nat Genet 1992; 2:99–102.

28. Pan Y, Metzenberg A, Das S, Jing B, Gitschier J. Mutations in the V2 vasopressin receptor gene are associated with X-linked nephrogenic diabetes insipidus. Nat Genet 1992; 2:103–106.

29. Deen PM, Verdijk MA, Knoers NV, Wieringa B, Monnens LA, van Os CH, van Oost BA. Requirement of human renal channel aquaporin-2 for vasopressin-dependent concentration of urine. Science 1994; 264: 92–95.

30. van Lieburg AF, Verdiijk M, Knoers NVAM, van Essen AJ, Proesmans W, Mallman R, Monnens LAH, van Oost BA, van Os CH, Dee PMT. Patients with autosomal nephrogenic diabetes insipidus homozygous for mutations in the aquaporin-2 water-channel gene. Am J Hum Genet 1994; 55:648–652.

6

Imaging in paediatric nephrology

Helen Carty and Neville Wright

Introduction

Imaging has an important role in the investigation of urinary tract pathology and a large range of imaging modalities is available for this purpose. This chapter will discuss the advantages and disadvantages of these imaging procedures and the common pitfalls. The most important aspect of imaging is liaison with the clinical team involved in managing the child, be it the general practitioner, district general hospital, or tertiary referral centre. One of the most common problems encountered in radiological assessment is failure to have the appropriate clinical information and all the relevant imaging. This can lead to unnecessary investigation or incorrect diagnoses. Thus, it is important to emphasize that any imaging performed should not be reported or viewed in isolation from either the clinical information or from other investigations.

Diagnostic imaging

The available procedures can be divided into diagnostic imaging and interventional techniques. Imaging investigations provide information about anatomy and function to varying degrees. The information gained from the differing investigations is outlined in Table 6.1.

Table 6.1 Imaging techniques, anatomy, and function

Imaging technique	Anatomy	Function
Abdominal radiograph	+	−
Ultrasound	+ + +	−
Intravenous urography	+ + +	+ +
Scintigraphy	+	+ + + +
Renography	+	+ + + +
Computed tomography	+ + + +	+ +
Magnetic resonance	+ + + +	+

Abdominal radiography

Abdominal radiography is usually the starting point in the investigation of abdominal or loin pain. The radiograph should include the abdomen from the diaphragm to the symphysis pubis. Children with pain often have a gassy abdomen caused by crying. This, coupled with the paucity of perirenal fat in children, makes it more difficult to identify the renal outlines and ureteric stones in children than adults. The main value of the abdominal radiograph is as a general overview when the diagnosis is uncertain. The features to note are the presence of constipation or a mass, calcification, and renal, ureteric, or bladder calculi (Fig. 6.1). A careful search should be made for spinal or sacral anomalies (e.g. partial sacral agenesis) that might be associated

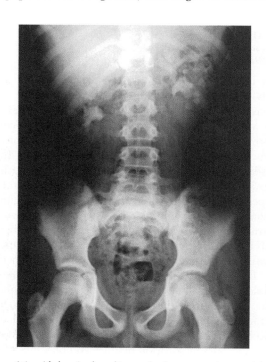

Fig. 6.1 Abdominal radiograph demonstrating multiple bilateral renal calculi.

Table 6.2 Indications for abdominal/kidneys, ureters, bladder (KUB) radiographs in nephrology

Suspected stone formation
Clinical history
Haematuria
Proteus urine infection
Mass lesion[a]
Suspected spinal anomalies[a]

[a] Not routine indications.

with neuropathic nephrological disease. It is important to note, however, that spina bifida occulta around the lumbo-sacral region is a common normal variant, which in itself does not require further investigation. Overall, the diagnostic yield of a straight abdominal radiograph in renal pathology is low, other than for the demonstration of stones and large mass lesions [1]. Occasionally, bowel wall thickening and ascites may be noted, for example in the haemolytic uraemic syndrome. The indications for a plain radiograph are summarized in Table 6.2. It should be noted that although radiographs are not generally required, the inevitable nature of tertiary referral work means that some children will ultimately have a plain X-ray taken when referred on for specialist advice.

Ultrasound (US)

General comments

An ultrasound examination of the renal tract and pelvis is an integral part of the investigation of suspected urinary tract pathology. The advantages of ultrasound include its ready availability, low cost, portability, and high sensitivity for the detection of structural renal abnormalities and renal stones. It is easily repeated, is painless, and has no radiation burden. The disadvantages are that it is operator dependent, may be technically difficult in a wriggling, crying child and abdominal gas may obscure visualization of ectopically placed kidneys. Five megahertz (MH$_z$) ultrasound probes are generally the most useful, although examination in neonates may benefit from higher frequency (7.5 MHz), and large adolescents from lower frequency (3.5 MHz) probes. The examination should be performed with a full bladder and there should be images of the kidneys and bladder to document pathology. Where relevant, pre- and post-micturition bladder volumes should be included. The examination in children who are not yet toilet trained should commence with the bladder, as

they are prone to micturate as soon as the abdomen is exposed. If the child is very fearful, the examination should start with the kidney area, with the child being cuddled by the parent until he or she gains confidence, the bladder being left to the last. It is important to get views of the bladder in order not to miss ureteroceles or distal ureteric dilatation. If bladder views are not achievable, then this should be recorded. Renal length and volume are useful for monitoring growth and can be compared with nomograms (see Chapter 28). The normal kidney (Fig. 6.2) is less echogenic than the liver, with the cortex being of a higher echogenicity than the medulla. The renal sinus echo is bright due to the presence of fat. There should be a single, central, contiguous renal sinus echo, with separation of the sinus echo suggesting that the kidney is duplex. The neonatal kidney may be more echobright than the liver, and has prominent hypoechoic papillae (Fig. 6.3). It should retain its normal shape and corticomedullary differentiation, although fetal lobulation may be present as a normal variant. The kidney reverts to normal echotexture at about 3 months. An end stage or dysplastic kidney is also echo bright, but loses the normal architecture and corticomedullary differentiation (Fig. 6.4). The indications for ultrasonography are summarised in Table 6.3 and discussed in detail below.

Infection and renal scarring

US appearances of acute pyelonephritis (Fig. 6.5) are a diffuse enlargement of the kidney, altered parenchymal

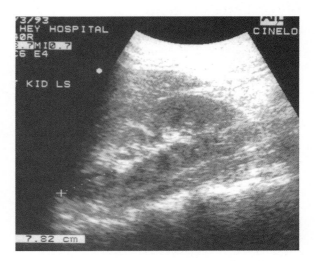

Fig. 6.2 Longitudinal ultrasound scan of the kidney showing normal echopattern and renal architecture.

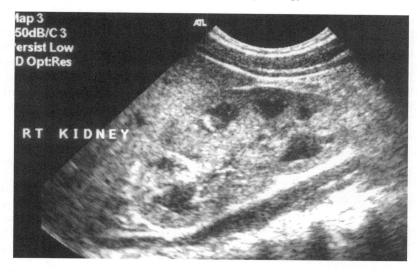

Fig. 6.3 Longtitudinal ultrasound scan of a normal neonatal kidney showing relatively echobright cortex with hypoechoic medullae. Contrast the echopattern of this kidney with that in Fig. 6.2.

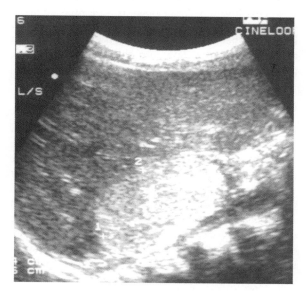

Fig. 6.4 Ultrasound showing renal dysplasia. The kidney is small and echobright with loss of the normal cortico-medullary differentiation.

Table 6.3 Indications for ultrasonography

Definite	Controversial
1. Acute pyelonephritis	1. Detection of renal scarring
2. Suspected hydronephrosis	2. Vesico-ureteric reflux
3. Suspected calculi ± nephrocalcinosis	
4. Renal cystic disease	
5. Renal mass	
6. Evaluation of the bladder	

echogenicity, loss of cortico-medullary differentiation, and dilatation of the pelvicalyceal system [2]. In the young child, renal enlargement can be up to 176% of normal [3,4]. This enlargement may result in a spurious reading as a baseline measurement for subsequent follow-up [5].

US is generally considered to be of low sensitivity for the detection of renal scarring (Fig. 6.6), with sensitivities often quoted around 37–39% [6,7], although careful detailed examinations with high-resolution equipment will improve this [8], as will colour flow and power Doppler imaging. Occasionally there is persistence of the inter-renicular septum in the upper pole of the kidney, a normal variant which may cause confusion, its appearance mimicking a scar.

Hydronephrosis

On US, hydronephrosis appears typically as dilated calyces of uniform size, distributed evenly around and communicating with a dilated central renal pelvis (Fig. 6.7). This is dissimilar to the disorganized cysts of varying sizes seen in a multicystic dysplasic kidney. Controversy exists concerning the measurement criteria to be used to define hydronephrosis. Most authors agree that a transverse renal pelvic

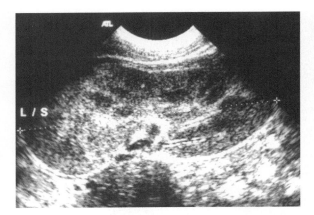

Fig. 6.5 Ultrasound of the kidney shows increased echogenicity and loss of cortico-medullary differentiation in the upper pole of this kidney, consistent with acute pyelonephritis in a child with confirmed urinary tract infection.

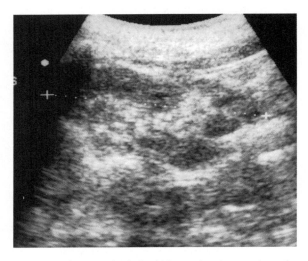

Fig. 6.6 Ultrasound of the kidney, showing an irregular contour with cortical thinning consistent with renal scarring.

diameter of greater than 10 mm is abnormal and, equally, most authors agree that a transverse pelvic diameter of less than 5 mm is normal. In the 5–10 mm range there is some disagreement (see further discussion in Chapters 12 and 14). The presence of calyceal dilatation, irrespective of pelvic diameter, should be viewed as abnormal.

A major pitfall in the use of ultrasound in children is 'over-reporting' of hydronephrosis, a prominent extrarenal pelvis being mistaken for hydronephrosis. The degree of pelvic dilatation can vary considerably with the state of hydration. Mild dilatation of the

renal pelvis is often exacerbated by an overfilled bladder. If doubt persists, a repeat renal scan with the bladder empty will often abolish or reduce the dilatation. It is important that measurement is standardized, with the maximum transverse diameter of the renal pelvis being measured at the hilar lip on a transverse image of the kidney (Fig. 6.8).

Vesico-ureteric reflux

The use of US to detect vesico-ureteric reflux (VUR) is controversial. A renal pelvis of 10 mm or less in transverse diameter has been considered a feature suggestive of VUR. One retrospective study of 455 children showed that the frequency of VUR was no different between dilated (≤10 mm) and non-dilated systems (≤2 mm) [9], and another showed no correlation between US and grade V reflux demonstrated by micturating cystourethography (MCUG) performed on the same day [10]. Conversely, Avni *et al.* [11] found features suggestive of VUR on US in 87% of neonates subsequently shown to have reflux. However, their selective population makes it difficult to extrapolate the data into the general paediatric population [12].

Calculi and nephrocalcinosis

US shows calculi and nephrocalcinosis as areas of increased echogenicity (brightness) with distal acoustic shadowing (Fig. 6.9), provided the calculus is large enough and the calcification dense enough. For stones over 5 mm, the overall sensitivity is 96% [13]. Calculi may be within the renal parenchyma, within the collecting system, ureter, bladder, or even the urethra. When obstructive, they may cause proximal dilatation of the urinary tract, but this is not always the case [14]. Ureteric stones may be missed and stones can move.

Renal cystic disease

US is excellent at demonstrating renal cystic abnormalities. Usually cysts appear as echo-free or hypoechoic, round lesions with distal acoustic enhancement (Fig. 6.10). Multiple, tiny cysts, such as those in autosomal recessive polycystic kidney disease, may appear echobright and cannot be discerned as individual cysts with US. The examination should assess renal size, symmetry, echogenicity, and cyst size, and whether there is unilateral or bilateral disease [15]. The examination

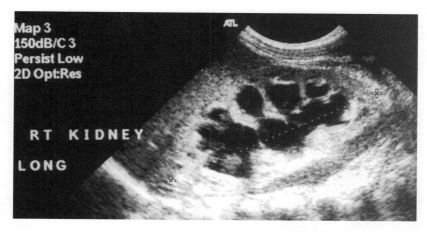

Fig. 6.7 Longitudinal ultrasound image of a neonatal kidney showing dilatation of the calyces and renal pelvis consistent with hydronephrosis.

TRANSVERSE IMAGE

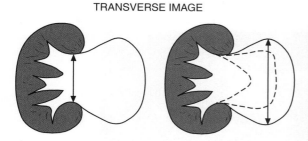

Fig. 6.8 Diagrammatic representation of (a) the appropriate site to measure the transverse renal pelvic diameter on ultrasound. The measurement should be obtained between the renal hilar lip. (b) The extrarenal pelvis should not be measured as it is prone to considerable variation, depending on the degree of hydration.

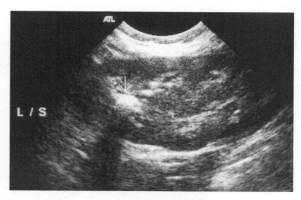

Fig. 6.9 Ultrasound showing typical appearances of renal calculi, with increased echogenicity and acoustic shadowing.

should also include a review of the liver and pancreas for cysts, hepatic fibrosis, and portal hypertension.

The renal mass

Ultrasound should be the first examination performed in the assessment of abdominal or pelvic mass lesions [16]. The examination should try to identify a number of features; the organ of origin of the mass, whether it is solid or cystic, the presence of calcium or fat, and the vascularity of the lesion. The presence of liver or nodal disease in tumours, normality of the contralateral kidney in renal tumours or nephroblastomatosis, and whether a tumour capsule is intact are also important aspects. Although ultrasound can suggest

the correct organ of origin of a tumour, further assessment by cross-sectional imaging will be required. Magnetic resonance imaging (MRI) is replacing many computed tomography (CT) examinations, especially in the pelvis, but CT remains the best method of demonstrating calcification. Most benign pelvic pathology can usually be identified with ultrasound, so that further cross-sectional imaging is not required.

The bladder

On ultrasound, the bladder wall thickness should not exceed 3 mm with normal distension, but a child with recurrent infection may not be able to maintain an adequate volume for assessment. In these circumstances subjective assessment is necessary. Echogenic

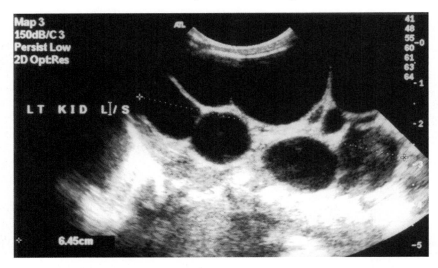

Fig. 6.10   Ultrasound showing multiple renal cysts of varying size and typical of multicystic renal dysplasia.

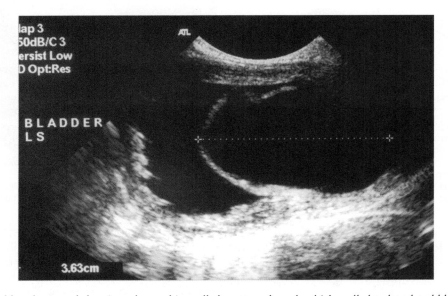

Fig. 6.11   Bladder ultrasound showing a large, thin-walled ureterocele and a thick-walled trabeculated bladder.

debris may be present within the bladder lumen with infection or chronic obstruction. The bladder should be examined for trabeculation, ureterocele (Fig. 6.11), and diverticulum formation. Careful assessment for ureteric dilatation is also essential. Occasionally persistent urachal remnants can be visualized, especially in the neonatal period, arising from the dome of the bladder. These often resolve without treatment [17].

Doppler, colour, and power imaging

Doppler studies of the extrarenal artery and vein and the intrarenal vessels are of value in some clinical situations—particularly in the assessment of transplanted kidneys, renal vein thrombosis, and in suspected renovascular hypertension. It must be emphasized that a normal Doppler study does not exclude renal artery stenosis as a cause for hypertension.

Small children are not able to hold their breath, so good-quality traces and measurement of resistive indices may be difficult. Altered colour flow signal has also been demonstrated in acute pyelonephritis (Fig. 6.12) [18].

A more recent development in ultrasound, power Doppler, enables renal cortical perfusion to be visible. Areas of altered perfusion will show as increased or decreased flow on the sonogram. Its use in small children is limited by the effect of movement. Decreased perfusion has been demonstrated in acute pyelonephritis [19].

Ultrasonic cystography

Attempts have been made to assess vesico-ureteric reflux using sonographic contrast agents. The technique used is similar to that of MCUG. The bladder is catheterized and filled with saline mixed with ultrasonic contrast medium. Ultrasound monitoring of the kidneys takes place during filling and micturition. If there is reflux to the kidneys, reflective echoes are obtained from the ultrasound contrast [20,21]. The technique, although radiation free, has not as yet found favour. It is time consuming, anatomical information is poor, and the urethra is not assessed. Grading according to conventional MCUG standards cannot be done and the technique obviously still requires catheterization and the child's co-operation.

Intravenous urography

Previously the cornerstone of the investigation of the renal tract, the role of intravenous urography has diminished with the advent of other imaging techniques. Its advantages include general availability and an excellent demonstration of anatomy. The disadvantages include a poor sensitivity in early scar detection, poor images with diminished renal function, an injection is required (always disliked by children), and a very small risk of allergic reaction to contrast media, although this is rare. Non-ionic, water-soluble contrast medium (1–2 ml/kg) should be administered intravenously. The examination should be tailored to answer the clinical question. A standard series of films should include a control film to include the symphysis pubis; a film taken within 3 min of the completion of the i.v. injection, in an attempt to see a nephrogram, if required; and a full-length film of the abdomen at 15 min (Fig. 6.13). This basic series can be altered and supplemented as required by delayed, prone, or oblique films. Excretion of contrast with blood clearance is rapid in children, so that even on a 3-minute film, a child with normal kidneys will show a pyelogram, and there is usually enough contrast still visible in the nephrographic phase to see a good renal outline (nephrogram). If there is hydronephrosis with a 'negative pyelogram' (i.e. renal pelvic dilatation is such that the calyces and collecting system are outlined by the contrast in the tubules), a prone film to show the point of

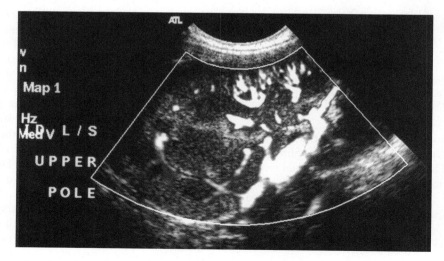

Fig. 6.12 Grey-scale colour flow ultrasound image of acute pyelonephritis, showing reduced vascularity in the area of acute infection in the upper pole.

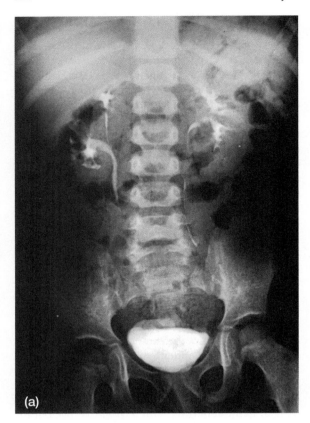

(a)

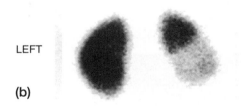

LEFT

(b)

Fig. 6.13 (a) Intravenous urogram shows a right-sided duplex system on the 15-minute film, with (b) dimercapto-succinic acid (DMSA) scan showing reduced uptake in the lower moiety.

obstruction should be delayed for at least 2 hours. For lesser degrees of obstruction, the film may be taken earlier. The appearances in autosomal recessive polycystic kidney disease are characteristic. Symmetrically enlarged kidneys with a streaky nephrogram and 'puddling' are considered diagnostic, although delayed films up to 24 hours may be required. Some authors have stated that an IVU is mandatory in suspected cases at 3–6 months of age [15]. The main indications for intravenous urography are summarized in Table 6.4.

Table 6.4 Indications for intravenous urography

1. The elucidation of anatomical lesions demonstrated by, but not interpretable by, other techniques, e.g. a malrotated kidney
2. The demonstration of point of obstruction by a ureteric stone [14] and occasionally assessment of pelvi-ureteric junction obstruction
3. The evaluation of trauma, if cross-sectional imaging and scintigraphy are not available [22]
4. To confirm scintigraphically suspected simple duplex systems as a cause of discrepancy in renal size
5. To confirm the diagnosis of autosomal recessive polycystic kidney disease [15]

Table 6.5 Indications for micturating cystourethrography

1. The demonstration and grading of vesico-ureteric reflux
2. The demonstration of urethral anatomy in suspected congenital malformation, e.g. posterior urethral valves
3. The investigation of terminal haematuria and trauma

Micturating cystourethrography

Micturating cystourethrography (MCUG) is an unpleasant examination for a child and their parents, even when carried out skilfully by experienced staff. The catheterization for those children who do not have a catheter *in situ* is ideally done in the radiology department. This minimizes the risk of the catheter falling out during transit, the use of unnecessary tape that can hurt on removal, or a balloon being inflated within the penis, causing added distress. The indications for MCUG are summarized in Table 6.5.

A sterile technique is used. All cleaning solutions should be warmed. Encouraging the parent to clean the perineum with the antiseptic may calm a fearful child and parent. Someone skilled in the procedure should do the catheterization and we usually use a size 5 or 6 feeding tube. Problems with catheterization are caused by labial adhesions, often not identified prior to the examination, and hypospadias. There should be an agreed policy in place about the management of these problems.

The examination should document the presence and degree of reflux (Fig. 6.14a), whether it occurs during filling or micturition, and the quality of ureteric peristalsis in very dilated ureters. Accurate description of the findings allows classification of the grade of reflux using the International Classification of Vesicoureteric

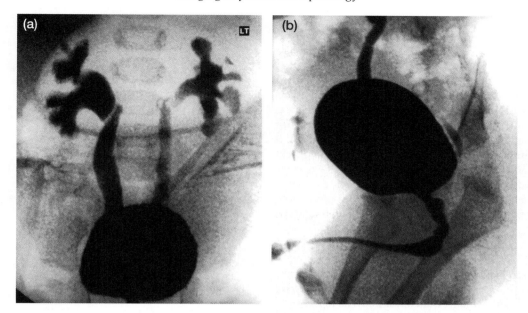

Fig. 6.14 Micturating cystourethrogram showing (a) bilateral vesico-ureteric reflux and (b) a normal male urethra.

Reflux [23,24] (see Chapter 11). Early filling films of the bladder should be obtained to identify ureteroceles, as these may be effaced when the bladder pressure rises, and may even evert [25]. There should also be oblique or true lateral views of the entire penis in boys—otherwise posterior urethral valves and the rare anterior urethral anomalies may be missed (Fig. 6.14b). Oblique views of the ureteric insertion into the bladder are indicated when there are low or ectopically inserted ureters. Cyclical voiding, that is multiple bladder fillings, may improve the sensitivity of cystography for the detection of VUR [26,27].

Controversy exists as to the preferred timing of MCUG in urinary tract infection. The demonstration of VUR is increased if the examination is done during an acute infection, but this carries a risk of increasing morbidity. Most advocate leaving the MCUG until 4–6 weeks after adequate treatment of an acute infective episode, maintaining the child on prophylaxis until the examination is done.

A policy about antibiotic cover for MCUG should be agreed by the paediatrician, urologist, and radiologist, and should be in place in each hospital. A suggested policy is given in Table 6.6.

The advantages of MCUG are excellent anatomical demonstration of VUR and ease of quantification, demonstration of urethral anatomy, reasonable sensitivity in showing reflux, and general availability.

Table 6.6 Antibiotic cover for MCUG

1. Full antibiotic cover for all neonates
2. Full antibiotic cover for all children in whom reflux is demonstrated, by either prescribing a therapeutic dose or increasing the prophylaxis to the therapeutic dose for a full course, reverting to prophylaxis after this
3. Maintain prophylaxis for those children already on it, in whom reflux is not demonstrated

The disadvantages include the unpleasantness and a moderately high radiation burden to the gonadal area. The latter can be reduced by removal of the antiscatter grid when screening, and the use of digital systems [28].

Direct and indirect radionuclide cystography

Direct cystography

Direct radionuclide cystography (DRC) is performed by catheterization of the bladder as for MCUG, following which the bladder is filled with sterile saline into which 25 MBq (megabecquerel) of technetium ($^{99}Tc^m$) pertechnetate is instilled. Filling of the bladder is performed with the child lying or sitting in front of a gamma-camera head. The examination is reviewed both as analogue images and with time/activity curves drawn over the kidneys. Reflux is seen on the former as activity in the ureters and kidneys and on the latter as a peak rise in the curve. The disadvantages of DRC include lack of anatomical detail, particularly of the posterior urethra, and inability to grade reflux in accordance with accepted classification. However, there is some evidence that it is more sensitive than MCUG for detecting reflux in children under 1 year of age [29]. If the examination is done as the primary screening technique and reflux is shown, then an MCUG may be required to delineate detail and to grade the reflux accurately. Advantages include continuous monitoring during filling and micturition and a low radiation dose.

Indirect voiding cystography

This examination is carried out following renography using technetium-labelled mercaptoacetyltriglycine (MAG3) thus avoiding catheterization. The renogram is carried out in the conventional way, following which the child is given fluid to drink. When the child desires to micturate, voiding takes place in the upright position in front of the gamma camera into an appropriate receptacle. Time–activity curves are created for the renal and bladder areas (Fig. 6.15). The examination is also recorded on images, usually using 1- and 5-second frames. The child must be co-operative and have bladder control for this technique to be successful. As it is combined with renography, information about divided renal function is obtained. The disadvantages are the requirement for co-operation, a low sensitivity in the detection of grade I reflux, variably reported sensitivity for grade II reflux, and the lack of anatomical information. It is generally used for the reassessment of children with known reflux, or as a screen in older children presenting with a urinary tract infection (UTI), who have a normal ultrasound examination and where the likelihood of significant reflux is low [30].

Renal cortical scintigraphy

Renal cortical scintigraphy uses a gamma-camera facility and is generally performed with technetium-99 m dimercaptosuccinic acid (DMSA). DMSA is a chelate extracted, but not excreted, by the renal tubules. This provides an image of functioning renal tubular tissue. The injected dose is based on a proportion of the adult dose of 80 MBq. DMSA scanning is currently accepted as the most sensitive technique for renal parenchymal imaging [31].

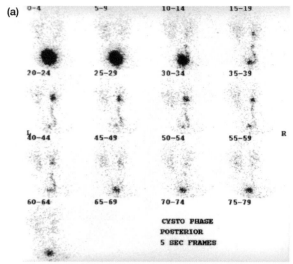

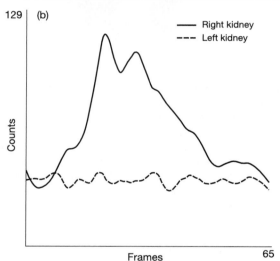

Fig. 6.15 Posterior analogue images (a) and time–activity curves (b) from an indirect cystogram showing right-sided vesico-ureteric reflux up into the renal pelvis.

Imaging is performed not less than 2 hours after intravenous injection of labelled DMSA, images in a co-operative child are taken in the posterior and both posterior oblique projections. Additional anterior images should be taken for any low-lying or ectopically placed kidneys. The relative uptakes of the kidneys are calculated. If there is an anteriorly placed kidney, the geometric mean is presented. The relative uptakes of normal kidneys should be about equal, in the range of 45–55%, although recently a study has suggested the left kidney can take up 57%

Table 6.7 Indications for DMSA scintigraphy

Demonstration and monitoring of renal scarring
Identifying ectopically placed kidneys
Demonstration of residual tissue after trauma
Identifying renal tissue in suspected renal aplasia

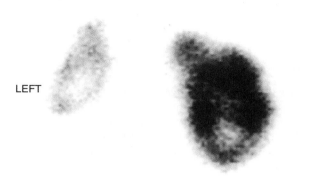

LEFT

Fig. 6.16 DMSA scan, showing bilateral renal scarring, left worse than right, in a child with proven *Proteus* infection.

and be normal [32]. DMSA uptake estimates the relative function of each of the kidneys and is not a measure of overall renal function. The indications for DMSA scintigraphy are shown in Table 6.7. The most frequent indication for DMSA scintigraphy is the demonstration of renal scarring in children with a history of urinary tract infection (Fig. 6.16). Other indications include the detection of ectopic renal tissue and assessing residual function following trauma. Its value in the assessment of tumours is limited, but neoplastic tissue or renal cysts will show as areas of reduced uptake (photopenia) on scintigraphy. The technique for the demonstration of ectopic tissue is to perform a standard posterior and anterior DMSA scan. If only one kidney is shown, both views should be repeated with the normally functioning kidney masked off. The ectopic renal tissue may lie anywhere from the pelvis to the renal bed.

Advantages of DMSA scintigraphy are its sensitivity in the detection of renal scars compared with urography or ultrasound, and its reproducibility. Sedation is not usually required as, if the child moves, the scan can be stopped and restarted. The disadvantage is that it is variably available, imparts a radiation burden, and has limited anatomical definition. DMSA scintigraphy is regarded as the gold standard in the detection of renal scars. It must always be viewed with other imaging studies and not reported

in isolation. If the DMSA scan is carried out in a nuclear medicine department, separate from the department of radiology, systems should be in place to ensure that all imaging is reviewed together.

DMSA single-photon emission tomography

With advances in gamma-camera technology, DMSA single-photon emission computed tomography (SPECT) has also been used to detect renal scars [33]. Rather than the planar images produced by standard studies, these images allow slices to be obtained through the kidneys in a fashion similar to CT. Current data suggest that the technique will improve the sensitivity of DMSA for detecting scars, although normal variants may produce increased false-positive rates [34].

Pitfalls of DMSA scintigraphy

Shallow, peripheral scars may be missed if oblique views are not done.

If the child is scanned during an acute episode of infection, photopenia in a kidney indicates acute pyelonephritis and is secondary to localized ischaemia and tubular dysfunction [35]. This may resolve without permanent scarring. The scan should be repeated a minimum of 6–8 weeks following treatment of the infection, if this is suspected. There is some evidence that resolution of changes can occur even later than 8 weeks after an acute infection. Some authors have suggested DMSA scans in the acute phase of infection are helpful in guiding management [31,36,37]. Others argue that a positive scan in the acute phase is immaterial, since all children with a febrile UTI are treated as if they have acute pyelonephritis [38], and the important long-term prognostic feature is the presence of renal scars [39,40].

An uncomplicated duplex kidney is usually larger than a single system [41]. This is reflected in the relative renal uptakes on DMSA scanning, the differential being greater than 10%. The 'small' kidney may be erroneously reported as growth failure. Ultrasound examination does not always show a split sinus echo in simple duplex systems. In these situations an IVU may clarify the situation.

Chronic pyelonephritis may occasionally result in smooth shrinking of a kidney without peripheral scarring. If the disease is symmetrical, the relative uptakes may be equal and the kidneys regarded as normal. In children with recurrent upper tract signs who have smooth kidneys on DMSA scintigraphy, an IVU is indicated to ensure that chronic pyelonephritis is not missed.

Dynamic renography

The main indication for dynamic renography is to confirm or exclude obstruction in a kidney shown to be hydronephrotic by ultrasound, IVU, or antenatal scanning. The examination is performed in a gamma-camera facility and involves i.v. injection of a radiopharmaceutical and often a diuretic. The radiopharmaceuticals in general use in children are technetium-labelled mercaptoacetyltriglycine (MAG3) [42] and diethylenetriaminepentacetic acid (DTPA).

Technique

Renography can be performed throughout childhood, including the neonatal period. The child should be normally hydrated. In order to identify obstruction more readily, it is standard practice to administer a diuretic intravenously. Ideally the diuretic is given 16 minutes after the isotope injection, but there is some variation in this. This practice is achievable in older children with an i.v. cannula *in situ*, but in young infants, the pragmatic approach, and this is the approach used by the authors, is to have the diuretic given immediately prior to the radiopharmaceutical injection as part of the same venepuncture. This avoids multiple injections, problems with difficult venous access, and the child being distressed by the sight of the needle. Some authors advocate injecting the diuretic between 7 and 15 minutes prior to the isotope injection, but for the same reasons stated above, this is not the authors' preference. With modern software programs, some compensation for movement can be made and satisfactory time–activity curves obtained. Sedation is occasionally necessary in a very distressed child. Posterior images of the kidneys and bladder are taken and time–activity curves over the renal areas are created. These show the progress of the radiopharmaceutical from renal artery to excretion. MAG3 is excreted by the tubules, 80% being extracted in the first pass, which gives an excellent signal to background ratio and thus good images. The effective renal plasma flow (ERPF) can be calculated for each kidney. This changes with age, being low in the neonate. The most valuable information from the renogram is the assessment of divided function and the curve shape.

DTPA is an alternative radiopharmaceutical to MAG3 and is excreted by glomerular filtration. If used for renography, individual kidney glomerular filtration rate (GFR) can be calculated, but because of a poorer blood/renal clearance than MAG3, the curves obtained with DTPA are flatter than those obtained with MAG3, making the latter easier to interpret.

Interpretation

The first summed image during renography shows the nephrographic phase of the examination before excretion takes place. It is sometimes possible to detect renal scarring on this image, which is a posterior view of the kidneys, and in some units this is substituted for DMSA scintigraphy, with which it correlates reasonably well. The limitations are a lower count rate than achievable by DMSA, rendering subtle scars difficult to see and inability to take oblique projections. For a full assessment of renal scarring, DMSA is the preferred technique.

Renographic curves can be described as obstructive, non-obstructive, and indeterminate. This is a contentious area, with some variability in reporting between centres. The clearly obstructive curve shows gradually increasing tracer activity within the renal pelvis. What defines a normal curve is less clear. In the authors' practice, if the curve falls beneath 50% of the peak activity within the time frame of the examination (32 min), the curve is considered normal and non-obstructive. If the curve plateaus out or fails to fall beneath the 50% cut-off, the curve is considered indeterminate. It cannot be overemphasized that correlation with other imaging modalities and clinical features is vital in this situation.

In poorly functioning kidneys the curve is flat and shows little or no response to diuretic. This does not indicate obstruction.

When interpreting renography, it is important that the analogue images are viewed as well as the curves and calculations. It may be easier to appreciate delayed renal perfusion on these images than on the time–activity curves. The configuration of the collecting system is easily appreciated on the images and it is possible to identify kidneys with a pelvi-ureteric junction (PUJ) configuration, or with hydroureters, on the images in the presence of normal curves, thus correlating the ultrasonic findings of hydronephrosis with normal function (Fig. 6.17). It is possible

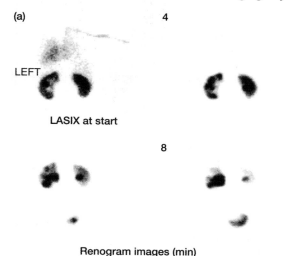

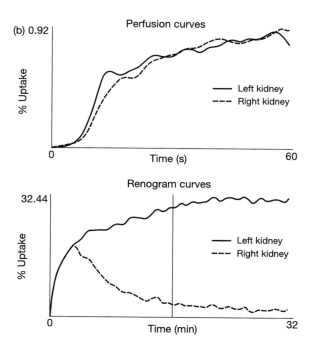

Fig. 6.17 MAG3 isotope renogram, with (a) posterior analogue images and (b) time–activity curves, showing a left pelvi-ureteric junction obstruction.

to have an obstructive curve with normal renal function. If a rise in the count rate is noted late in the acquisition on the time–activity curve, this may indicate vesico-ureteric reflux to the kidney.

Pitfalls

A pitfall of interpretation occurs in young children's scans if a diuretic is given at injection and calculations of divided renal function are based on the uptake at 3 min. By 3 min, excretion has already commenced on the non-obstructed side and causes a fall in count rate in the normal kidney. It may thus appear to have less function than the abnormal dilated side. The uptake at 1 min is a more reliable estimate of function in this situation.

In a poorly functioning kidney the renal curve may be very flat and obstruction cannot be assessed in such a kidney.

Estimates of divided renal function based on renography are unreliable in ectopically placed kidneys due to differing count rates from the kidney distant from the camera face. Time–activity curves are reliable and obstruction can be confirmed or excluded, subject to the usual limitations of renography. Relative renal function estimates will need to be done with DMSA scintigraphy.

A further pitfall of renography is that a very full bladder may cause hold-up of tracer in the upper tracts, resulting in delayed excretion, giving an 'obstructive' curve. An image taken following bladder emptying will show good and rapid wash-out and should be done in these patients.

Captopril renography

Children with hypertension may have normal renal scintigraphy and renography despite the presence of renal artery stenosis—most commonly due to fibromuscular hyperplasia. Captopril-enhanced scintigraphy and renography may help to demonstrate the secondary effects of renal artery stenosis by impairing the autoregulation mechanism. The standard renogram may be normal but when repeated with captopril, an angiotensin converting enzyme inhibitor, the effect of dilatation of the efferent arterioles and decrease in the transcapillary pressure gradient in the glomerulus leads to a significant but reversible fall in renal function. Different tracers demonstrate this in slightly different ways. In DTPA renography this shows as decreased tracer in the affected kidney at 5 min, with a delayed time to peak activity when compared with the baseline renogram. The normal kidney is unaltered by captopril. With MAG3, there is prolonged cortical retention of tracer as there is uptake in the renal tubular cells due to preservation

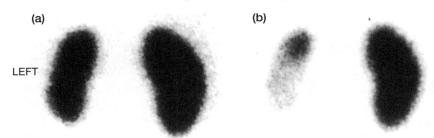

Fig. 6.18 Captopril scintigraphy. (a) A control DMSA shows a small left kidney and normal right kidney. (b) Following captopril, there is significantly reduced activity on the subsequent scan in the lower pole of the left kidney. There was renal artery stenosis of the lower pole vessel supplying this area.

of some reduced blood flow, even though GFR is reduced. The cortical activity is prolonged because there is reduced urine production. DMSA shows reduced relative function on the affected side. One pitfall of the technique is the presence of multiple renal arteries, which may show asymmetrical decrease in function in the affected kidney (Fig. 6.18).

Captopril renography is only positive for renal artery stenosis when the vessel lumen is sufficiently narrow. However, marked reduction in luminal calibre may not produce a positive result, because the renin–angiotensin mechanism is no longer effective. Medication with ACE inhibitors must be withdrawn for 48 hours prior to the test.

Computed tomography

Indications

Computed tomography (CT) is a cross-sectional imaging technique that gives excellent anatomical information based on the attenuation of tissue by a fine X-ray beam generated by the scanner. The indications for CT in the investigation of children's urinary tracts are shown in Table 6.8.

Children presenting with an *abdominal* or *pelvic mass* will usually have had an ultrasound examination prior to CT, so the organ of origin is usually known. The role of cross-sectional imaging is to further characterize the lesion, to assess its local extent and operability, and, in the case of malignant lesions, to stage the tumour [16] (Fig. 6.19). The choice of CT or MRI depends on the suspected nature of the lesion. In relation to renal tumours, MRI and CT are equally sensitive in both diagnosis and staging. CT has the added advantage that the lungs can be assessed for metastatic spread at the same examination. Renal tumours

Table 6.8 Indications for computed tomography

1. Abdominal or pelvic mass
2. Renal infection or abscess
3. Pyonephrosis
4. Suspected calculi or nephrocalcinosis
5. Trauma
6. Biopsy

rarely invade the spinal canal but, if suspected clinically, then MRI is indicated.

Pelvic tumours in children arise from the urinary tract (e.g. rhabdomyosarcoma), the female reproductive organs (e.g. ovarian teratomas, rarely uterine or vaginal tumours), or in the pre-sacral area—the most frequent here being a sacrococcygeal teratoma, presacral neuroblastoma, or pre-sacral PNET (primitive neuro-ectodermal tumour), and more rarely anterior sacral meningoceles. Pseudotumours, which may appear as a pelvic mass, are pelvic abscesses almost invariably due to a ruptured appendix and hydrocolpos or hydrometrocolpos. These latter two have a characteristic ultrasound appearance and CT is not indicated. In appendix abscess, CT is helpful in delineating its extent and suitability for percutaneous drainage. For most pelvic tumour assessment, MRI is the cross-sectional imaging technique of choice.

Renal stones and *nephrocalcinosis* are usually identified easily by ultrasound. However, in some children, such as those with a scoliosis, evaluation may be difficult. In these circumstances, a non-contrast-enhanced CT of the kidneys can be very helpful in resolving the issues.

Contrast-enhanced CT will demonstrate areas of *acute pyelonephritis* as areas of underperfusion, but whether the technique is practical in the paediatric setting, when DMSA scanning is relatively easy to

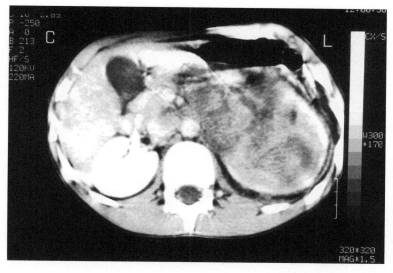

Fig. 6.19 Transverse, post-intravenous contrast, computed tomography scan of the upper abdomen, showing a large left-sided Wilms' tumour with para-aortic lymphadenopathy. There is a normal right kidney.

perform and readily available, is debatable. Lavocat *et al.* [43] compared US, DMSA, and CT in acute pyelonephritis, and concluded that DMSA is more sensitive. However, CT has the advantage of better anatomical resolution and detection of perinephric disease and thus may be helpful in difficult cases [44].

Children with a *renal abscess* or *pyonephrosis* present with fever, loin pain, and a mass. Both are easily identified by ultrasound but contrast-enhanced CT is helpful in mapping the lesion and assessing suitability for percutaneous drainage if this is not clear from the ultrasound examination. *Xantho-granulomatous pyelonephritis* usually presents as a mass lesion and is often mistakenly thought to be a neoplasm. However, it contains calculi and fatty densities easily demonstrated by CT [45].

With *trauma* the CT is exquisitely sensitive in detecting renal contusion, lacerations, perirenal collections, and renal pedicle avulsion. The examination should also include the pelvis, looking for bladder rupture and intra- or extraperitoneal leakage of urine. Complications of renal trauma, e.g. urinoma or infection of a perirenal collection, may also be assessed by CT as required, though monitoring of the kidney after the initial CT is by ultrasound.

Technique

CT of the kidneys is undertaken as part of an abdominal CT examination. Oral contrast is not generally required, but intravenous contrast medium should be administered, with images obtained both pre- and post-injection, except in trauma, when post-contrast images alone are adequate. Contiguous slices should be obtained, preferably with breath holding but this may obviously be difficult in the young child. With the more recent advances in CT technology, spiral (helical) CT may obviate the need for sedation and breath holding in view of the rapid acquisition time of the images. Slice thickness is generally in the order of 7–10 mm.

CT technique modification

For calcification CT scans used to identify calcification must be performed without i.v. contrast medium (Fig. 6.20) in the first instance, as the contrast will obscure the calcification.

For mass lesions The paucity of intra-abdominal fat in children may make it difficult to distinguish lymph nodes from bowel loops and to identify the margins of a lesion. Therefore, abdominal CT should ideally be done with prior administration of oral contrast, but if the child is too sick to co-operate and will not drink the contrast, a satisfactory examination is achievable in most instances without it. Oral contrast is not required in children with suspected appendix abscess. Images should be obtained pre- and post-injection of i.v. contrast medium, the former to identify calcification and fat. CT of the chest should also be performed, where appropriate, if pulmonary metastases may be present.

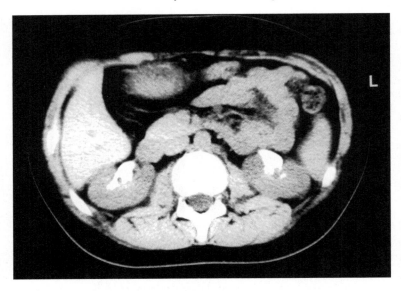

Fig. 6.20 Non-enhanced computed tomography scan of the kidneys, showing bilateral renal calculi.

Disadvantages and pitfalls

The major disadvantage of CT is the considerable radiation burden imparted by the scan. It has been estimated that a single abdominal CT in an adult has a radiation dose equivalent to 500 chest radiographs [46]. Most modern CT scanners allow variation in scan technique to reduce this significantly. It is important that both the clinician and radiologist are aware of the clinical problem to be solved, so the examination can be tailored to minimize the radiation dose.

One pitfall of CT occurs in right-sided renal mass lesions. Due to the partial volume effect, renal masses may appear to infiltrate the liver on CT. Movement of the organs relative to each other is better assessed by ultrasound.

If i.v. contrast is administered without obtaining images pre-injection, calculi and nephrocalcinosis may be masked by contrast in the renal parenchyma and collecting system.

Magnetic resonance imaging

Indications and technique

Magnetic resonance imaging (MRI) currently has a relatively limited role in nephrology. Its main input is in the assessment of renal masses and pelvic pathology, especially gynaecological disease, but it also has a developing a role in evaluating renal vessels, particularly renal artery stenosis, and in defining the extent of central venous thrombosis related to long-term central-line placement. The advantages of magnetic resonance imaging include multiplanar images; easy detection of bony metastatic disease; excellent soft-tissue contrast, giving clearly defined interfaces between pathological and normal tissue; and no radiation burden.

The disadvantages are the cost of the equipment and that the length of time required to obtain images leads to a greater need for sedation.

Obtaining good MR images in the child's abdomen, especially in children under 4 years, is technically challenging. This is due to the increased respiratory rate in the young child and the greater diaphragmatic excursion and abdominal movement during normal respiration compared with adults. Scanning times are relatively long and children's attention spans are limited. Consideration should be given to referring children to a MRI unit with a large paediatric workload for imaging, rather than attempting to do it on an occasional basis.

In general terms, images are divided into T_1-weighted images, which demonstrate anatomy, and T_2-weighted images, which highlight pathology due to altered water content (Fig. 6.21). Further delineation of pathology can be achieved with fat-suppression techniques and contrast enhancement with gadolinium.

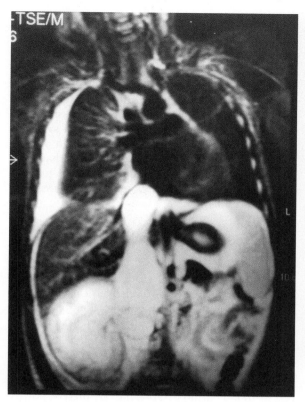

Fig. 6.21 Coronal T$_2$-weighted magnetic resonance scan of the abdomen, showing a large Wilms' tumour with extension of tumour into the inferior vena cava.

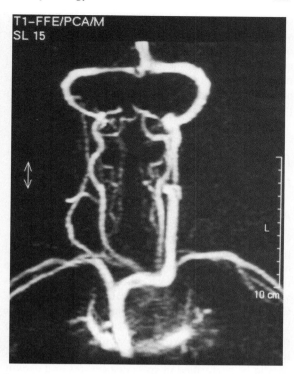

Fig. 6.22 Magnetic resonance venography, showing occlusion of the right internal jugular vein with prominence of the right external jugular. There are normal subclavian, left internal jugular, and brachiocephalic veins.

All masses should be imaged in the transverse plane and supplemented by coronal and sagittal projections as appropriate. Pelvic tumours should have sagittal and transverse views, the coronal plane being less useful. Abdominal and retroperitoneal tumours should be imaged in transverse and coronal planes. Images taken before and after contrast medium are essential for tumour evaluation. It is especially important to scrutinize the contralateral kidney when there is a renal-based mass such as a Wilms' tumour, to identify synchronous lesions or areas of nephroblastomatosis. Nephroblastomatosis shows as relatively avascular tissue on post-contrast MR images [47].

Metastatic deposits in the lungs are not demonstrated as well as on CT. Large calcific deposits can be identified as a signal void, but fine calcification, which is often diagnostically important, is easily overlooked with MRI and is best demonstrated by CT.

Magnetic resonance angiography and venography

MR angiography and venography are useful non-invasive methods for demonstrating abnormal vasculature. MR angiography has been used to demonstrate renal artery stenosis, and is more sensitive closer to the renal artery ostium. However, large studies have not been performed in children, most work being based on adults. Time-of-flight, phase contrast, and contrast-enhanced MR angiography techniques are all in use [48]. MR venography has an increasing role in identifying complications of intravenous central lines (Fig. 6.22) and can be used to assess the renal veins.

Magnetic resonance urography

MR urography is a recently described technique which generally involves the use of heavily T$_2$-weighted sequences to generate images that have similar appearances to an IVU [49]. These images can be obtained without an i.v. injection, although contrast-enhanced MR urography is also feasible. The clinical use of such a technique is currently limited, but reports have demonstrated its use in hydronephrosis [50] and its use will undoubtedly increase [51].

Invasive and interventional techniques

Angiography

Conventional contrast angiography is an invasive procedure that is rarely required in the assessment of nephrological problems in children. Its main role is in the demonstration of a vasculitis and in the diagnosis and treatment of renal artery stenosis (Fig. 6.23). Occasionally arteriovenous malformations of the kidney may present with haematuria and these may require delineation with angiography, possibly leading to therapeutic embolization. These procedures should be performed in specialist centres and usually the angiogram and therapeutic intervention is the last of a long series of diagnostic tests performed on the child.

Venography

Conventional venography is still occasionally required for demonstration of the central venous system, particularly with children in whom there are problems with long-term catheter placement. These studies are gradually being replaced by MR venography, which gives a non-invasive method of venous assessment.

Inferior vena cava (IVC) and renal vein sampling for renin levels is occasionally indicated in a small number of children when it is thought that their hypertension may be due to increased renin production by the diseased kidney, and that nephrectomy may be indicated.

Antegrade pyelography and the Whitaker test

Percutaneous puncture of the renal collecting system under ultrasound control is a relatively easy procedure in a dilated system. The main indication for an antegrade pyelogram is to demonstrate complex anatomy, especially in duplex kidneys with an ectopically placed ureteric opening, and to identify the level of obstruction, i.e. at the renal pelvis or distally at the vesico-ureteric junction (VUJ) if there is doubt. It is also the best method of demonstrating the rare ureteric polyps, most of which are found by serendipity.

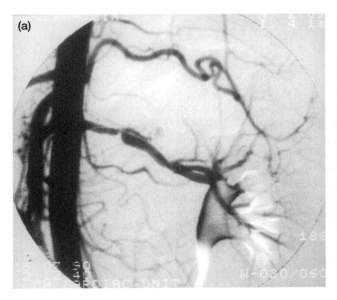
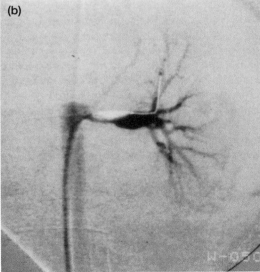

Fig. 6.23 Renal angiograms showing: (a) left renal artery stenosis in a 3-year-old child; (b) balloon dilatation of a stenosis in another 3-year-old with neurofibromatosis type I. (Courtesy Drs DA Gould and LJ Abernethy.)

Technique

The procedure is generally carried out under general anaesthetic. Antibiotic prophylaxis is given to cover the procedure. With the child prone, the kidney is identified by ultrasound and a 22G needle is inserted into the collecting system. For antegrade pyelography without pressure measurement, contrast medium is hand injected. Passage of contrast through the system into the bladder is monitored with fluoroscopy.

If pressure measurements are required (the Whitaker test) to distinguish dilatation from obstruction in children with equivocal renograms, a second needle can be inserted and attached to a pressure monitor. The kidney is then perfused through one needle with concurrent monitoring of renal pelvic and vesical pressures. A pressure differential between renal pelvis and bladder of 22 mm of water or greater indicates obstruction. Below 15 is normal and figures in between are indeterminate, the results being reviewed with the clinical and other imaging information.

Complications of antegrade pyelography and Whitaker tests are few. Haematuria is the most frequent and is due to inadvertent puncture of a renal vessel when attempting to enter a calyx. This is seldom severe and settles spontaneously in 24 hours. Extravasation of contrast in the perirenal area may occur if the needle becomes dislodged during injection. This does not require drainage but antibiotic cover should be continued.

Percutaneous drainage of the kidney or abdominal collection

Insertion of a renal drainage catheter percutaneously is now a preferred option to surgical nephrostomy. Indications include relief of acute obstruction, drainage of a pyonephrosis or renal abscess, and occasionally drainage of post-traumatic or post-transplant urinomas or lymphoceles. Sometimes a trial of drainage in a poorly functioning obstructed system is performed to see if renal function improves with relief of obstruction. French gauge 5 or 6 catheters are used to drain non-infected systems. Abscesses and pyonephrosis may require larger systems, depending on the viscosity of the pus. Antibiotic prophylaxis is required for the procedure and must be therapeutically continued in infected systems. Clotting studies should be performed before the procedure and any deficit corrected. Prior to removal of the drainage tube a nephrostomy study should be performed to establish the site of any obstruction and to ensure ureteric peristalsis in large dilated ureters, and to confirm free flow of contrast into the bladder.

Renal biopsy

The histological diagnosis and staging of nephropathy may necessitate percutaneous renal biopsy. Dependent on the co-operation of the child, it is done either under local or general anaesthetic usually using ultrasound guidance. Prior to biopsy, a full blood count and clotting studies should be done, together with blood grouping and saving of the serum, so that cross-matching may be performed if required. Routine cross-matching is not necessary. Contraindications to renal biopsy are given in Table 6.9. Most are relative rather than absolute contraindications and when clinical circumstances necessitate they may be overridden. The most common exception is the transplanted kidney, even though this is a single kidney; repeated biopsy is indicated if there are problems with graft dysfunction. Indications for renal biopsy are discussed in the relevant chapters.

Biopsy specimens are obtained using a minimum of a 16G needle. Automated devices have been shown to produce fewer complications than a manually operated biopsy needle. The specimen should be checked immediately to ensure that adequate glomeruli have been obtained, and usually at least two core biopsies are obtained. Specimens should be obtained from either upper or lower pole of the kidney to avoid the major vessels centrally, but obviously the lower pole is usually most amenable to biopsy. Complications of renal biopsy are given in Table 6.10 [52].

Image-guided percutaneous biopsy of a mass is also an alternative to open biopsy. The decision as to the best method of biopsy in an individual case is made by clinical discussion and depends on the

Table 6.9 Contraindications to renal biopsy [52]

Uncontrolled bleeding diathesis (absolute
  contraindication)
Uncontrolled hypertension
Severe and uncorrected anaemia
Single kidney
Large and/or multiple cysts
Gross hydronephrosis
Acute pyelonephritis/perinephric abscess
Obesity
Uncooperative patient

Table 6.10 Complications of renal biopsy [52]

Perirenal haematoma	2–3%
Frank haematuria	2%
Blood transfusion	1%
Arteriovenous fistula	1%

Table 6.11 Dosimetry

Technique	Chest X-ray equivalents	Typical effective dose
Abdominal X-ray	50	1.0 mSv
IVU	125	2.5 mSv
DMSA scan	50	1.0 mSv
Computed tomography of the abdomen/pelvis	500	10 mSv
Ultrasound	0	0
Magnetic resonance	0	0

IVU, intravenous urogram; DMSA, dimercaptosuccinic acid.

suspected nature of the mass, its location and vascularity. Biopsy material must be taken from viable tumour. Adequate tissue must be obtained for histopathology and for molecular genetic and cytokine studies. For these reasons there is a trend away from percutaneous tumour biopsy back to operative surgical biopsy, be it by excision during mini laparatomy or laparoscopy. If the biopsy is to be performed surgically and without image guidance, then prior imaging should be reviewed to identify the most appropriate biopsy site.

Dosimetry

It is important when investigating a child with a radiological technique that some consideration is given to the radiation burden that may be placed upon the child. Ultrasound and MR are particularly advantageous as they do not involve the use of any ionizing radiation, but the other imaging techniques used impart a radiation dose to the child. One study has compared the radiation doses of DMSA scans and IVU, and concluded that in a child with suspected renal scarring from urinary tract infection, DMSA is the preferred technique [53]. Table 6.11 gives an overview of the doses of radiation and chest X-ray equivalents related to some of the tests [46].

Transplant imaging

Most renal transplant imaging is based around ultrasound assessment, occasionally supplemented by isotope renography and, rarely, angiographic and antegrade studies. Departments dealing with transplant patients will need to become familiar with the normal post-transplant ultrasound appearances. Many departments perform a base-line ultrasound immediately following renal transplantation and this may need to be done as a portable study. Assessment includes evaluation of the renal echo pattern and kidney size, Doppler and colour flow assessment of renal vessels, including calculation of the resistive indices, and careful assessment for the presence of perinephric fluid collections and dilatation of the collecting system. Occasionally isotope renography is required in the acute phase to distinguish acute tubular necrosis from vascular occlusion. Long-term complications of stricture formation at vessel anastamosis sites and the site of ureteric implantation may require more invasive studies such as angiography and antegrade renal puncture, possibly leading to therapeutic balloon dilatation. These latter procedures would require specialist input at tertiary referral centres.

References

1. Kenney IJ, Arthur RJ, Sweeney LE *et al.* (1991) Initial investigation of childhood urinary tract infection: does the plain abdominal x-ray still have a role? Br J Radiol 64:1007–1009.
2. MacKenzie JR, Fowler K, Hollman AS *et al.* (1994) The value of US in the child with an acute urinary tract infection. Br J Urol 74:240–244.
3. Dinkel E, Orth S, Dittrich M, Schulte-Wisermann H (1986) Renal sonography in the differentiation of upper from lower urinary tract infection. Am J Roentgenol 146:755–780.
4. Johansson B, Troell S, Berg U (1988) Renal parenchymal volume during and after acute pyelonephritis measured by ultrasonography. Arch Dis Child 63:1309–1314.
5. Pickworth FE, Carlin JB, Ditchfield MR *et al.* (1995) Sonographic measurement of renal enlargement in children with acute pyelonephritis and time needed for resolution: implications for renal growth assessment. Am J Roentgenol 165:405–408.
6. Tasker AD, Lindsell DRM, Moncrieff M (1993) Can US reliably detect renal scarring in children with urinary tract infection. Clin Radiol 47:177–179.
7. Bjorgvisson E, Madj M, Eggli KD (1991) Diagnosis of acute pyelonephritis in children: comparison of sonography and 99 m Tc-DMSA scintigraphy. Am J Roentgenol 157:539–543.

8. Barry BP, Hall N, Broderick NJ *et al.* (1998) Improved ultrasound detection of renal scarring. Clin Radiol 53:747–751.

9. Davey MS, Zerin JM, Reilly C, Ambrosius WT (1997) Mild renal pelvic dilatation is not predictive of vesicoureteral reflux in children. Pediatr Radiol 27:908–911.

10. Blane HH, Di Pietro MA, Zerin JM *et al.* (1993) Renal sonography is not a reliable screening examination for vesicoureteric reflux. J Urol 150:752–755.

11. Avni EF, Ayadi K, Rypens F *et al.* (1997) Can careful US examination of the urinary tract exclude vesicoureteric reflux in the neonate? Br J Radiol 70:977–982.

12. Postlethwaite RJ, Wilson B (1997) Ultrasonography vs Cystourethrography to exclude vesicoureteric reflux in babies. Lancet 350:1567–1568.

13. Middleton WD, Dodds WJ, Lawson TL, Foley WD (1988) Renal calculi: sensitivity for detection with US. Radiology 167:239–244.

14. Webb JAW (1990) Ultrasonography in the diagnosis of renal obstruction. BMJ 301:944–946.

15. De Bruyn R, Gordon I (2000) Imaging in cystic renal disease. Arch Dis Child 83:401–407.

16. Carty H. Wilms' tumour and associated neoplasms of the kidney. In Husband JES, Reznek RH (eds) *Imaging in Oncology.* Oxford: Isis Medical Media, 1998; 671–689.

17. Zieger B, Sokol B, Rohrschneider WK *et al.* (1998) Sonomorphology and involution of the normal urachus in asymptomatic newborns. Pediatr Radiol 28:156–161.

18. Eggli KD, Eggli D (1992) Color Doppler sonography in pyelonephritis. Pediatr Radiol 22:422–425.

19. Dacher J-N, Pfister C, Monroc M *et al.* (1996) Power doppler sonographic pattern of acute pyelonephritis in children: Comparison with CT. Am J Roentgenol 166:1451–1455.

20. Darge K, Troeger J, Rohrschneider W *et al.* (1997) Contrast sonography for the detection of vesicoureteric reflux in children. Abstracts of 34th Congress of ESPR, p. 72.

21. Bosio M (1998) Cystosonography with echocontrast: a new imaging modality to detect vesicoureteric reflux in children. Pediatr Radiol 28:250–255.

22. Mayor B, Gudinchet F, Wicky S, Reinberg O, Schnyder P (1995) Imaging evaluation of blunt renal trauma in children: diagnostic accuracy of intravenous pyelography and ultrasonography. Pediatr Radiol 25:214–218.

23. International Reflux Committee (1981) Medical versus surgical treatment of primary vesicoureteric reflux. Pediatrics 67:392–400.

24. Lebowitz RL, Olbing H, Parkkulaien KV, Smellie JM, Tammuren-Mobius TE (1985) International system of radiographic grading of VUR. Pediatr Radiol 15:105–109.

25. Bellah RD, Long FR, Canning DA (1995) Ureterocele eversion with vesicoureteric reflux in duplex kidneys: Findings at voiding cystourethrography. Am J Roentgenol 165:409–413.

26. Jequier S, Jequier J-C (1989) Reliability of voiding cystourethrography to detect reflux. Am J Roentgenol 157:807–810.

27. Ditchfield MR, de Campo JF, Nolan TM *et al.* (1994) Risk factors in the development of early renal cortical defects in children with urinary tract infection. Am J Roentgenol 162:1393–1397.

28. Bazopoulos EV, Prassopoulos PK, Damilakis JE *et al.* (1998) A comparison between digital fluoroscopic hard copies and 105-mm spot films in evaluating vesicoureteric reflux in children. Pediatr Radiol 28:162–166.

29. McLaren CJ, Simpson ET (2001) Direct comparison of radiology and nuclear medicine cystograms in young infants with vesico-ureteric reflux. BJU International 87:93–97.

30. Bissett III GS, Strife JL, Dunbar JS. (1987) Urography and voiding cystourethrography: findings in girls with urinary tract infection. Am J Roentgenol 148:479–482.

31. MacKenzie JR (1996) A review of renal scarring in children. Nucl Med Commun 17:176–190.

32. Pusuwan P, Reyes L, Gordon I (1999) Normal appearances of technetium-99 m dimercaptosuccinic acid in children on planar imaging. Eur J Nucl Med 26:483–488.

33. Groshar D, Moskovitz B, Gorenberg M *et al.* (1994) Quantitative SPECT of technetium-99 m-DMSA uptake in the kidneys of normal children and in kidneys with vesicoureteric reflux: detection of unilateral kidney disease. J Nucl Med 35:445–449.

34. Rossleigh MA (1994) The interrenicular septum: a normal anatomical variant seen on DMSA SPECT. Clin Nucl Med 19:953–955.

35. Majd M, Rushton HG (1992) Renal cortical scintigraphy in the diagnosis of acute pyelonephritis. Semin Nuc Med 22:98–111.

36. Jakobsson B, Berg U, Svensson L (1994) Renal scarring after acute pyelonephritis. Arch Dis Child 70:111–115.

37. Rushton HG (1997) The evaluation of acute pyelonephritis and renal scarring with technitium 99 m-dimercaptosuccinic acid renal scintigraphy: evolving concepts and future directions. Pediatr Nephrol 11:108–120.

38. Seigle R, Nash M (1995) Is there a role for renal scintigraphy in the routine initial evaluation of a child with urinary tract infection? Pediatr Radiol 25:S52–S53.

39. Goonasekara CDA, Shah V, Wade AM, Barrat TM, Dillon MJ (1996) 15-year follow-up of renin and blood pressure in reflux nephropathy. Lancet 347:640–643.

40. Jacobson SH, Eklof O, Eriksson CG *et al.* (1989) Development of hypertension and uraemia after pyelonephritis in childhood. BMJ 299:703–706.

41. Privett JTJ, Jeans WD, Roylance J (1976) The incidence and importance of renal duplication. Clin Radiol 27:521–530.

42. Pickworth FE, Vivian GC, Franklin K, Brown EF (1992). 99 Tcm-mercapto acetyl triglycine in paediatric renal tract disease. Br J Radiol 65(769):21–29.

43. Lavocat MP, Granjon D, Allard D, Gay C, Freycon MT, Dubois F (1997) Imaging of pyelonephritis. Pediatr Radiol 27:159–165.

44. Dacher J-N, Boillot B, Eurin D *et al.* (1993) Rational Use of CT in acute pyelonephritis: Findings and relationships with reflux. Pediatr Radiol 23:281–285.

45. Cousins C, Somers J, Broderick N *et al.* (1994) Xanthogranulomatous pyelonephritis in childhood: ultrasound and CT diagnosis. Pediatr Radiol 24:210–212.

46. Royal College of Radiologists (1998) Making the best use of a Department of Clinical Radiology, 4th edition. The Royal College of Radiologists, London.

47. Gylys-Morin V, Hoffer FA, Kozakewich H *et al.* (1993) Wilms' tumor and nephroblastomatosis: Imaging characterization at Gd-enhanced MRI. Radiology 188:517–521.

48. Borrello JA (1997) Renal MR angiography. Magn Reson Imaging Clin N Am 5:83–93.

49. Hussain S, O'Malley M, Jara H, Sadeghi-Nejad H, Yucel EK (1997) MR Urography. Magn Reson Imaging Clin N Am 5:95–106.

50. Sigmund G, Stoever B, Zimmerhackl LB *et al.* (1991) MR urography in the diagnosis of upper urinary tract abnormalities in children. Pediatr Radiol 21: 416–420.

51. Borthne A, Pierre-Jerome C, Nordshus T, Reiseter T (2000) MR urography in children: current status and future development. Eur Radiol 10:503–511.

52. Boulton-Jones M (2000) Renal biopsy. In Johnson RJ, Feehally J (eds), Comprehensive Clinical Nephrology. Mosby pp. 7·1–6.

53. Smith T, Gordon I, Kelly JP (1998) Comparison of radiation dose from intravenous urography and 99 Tcm DMSA scintigraphy in children. Br J Radiol 71:314–319.

7

How and when to measure blood pressure

Graham C. Smith and Carol Inward

Introduction

There are two questions to address when managing blood pressure problems:

1. Is the value obtained from the blood pressure measurement an accurate representation of the child's systemic blood pressure?

2. Is the measured blood pressure considered potentially harmful to the child's health?

Hypertension is undoubtedly a risk factor for ischaemic heart disease and cerebrovascular accidents in adults and contributes to the deterioration in renal function in patients with renal impairment. Patients with severe hypertension clearly need active treatment, but the benefits of the treatment of mild hypertension are less clear. Nevertheless, the detection of hypertension in children has its benefits if it can help target health education to initiate preventative measures at an early age.

The need for accurate measurement of blood pressure and clear guidelines as to what levels of blood pressure require active management are therefore an important part of this process. This chapter aims to help readers decide how best to measure blood pressure and to interpret the results obtained.

How to measure blood pressure

As with any biological variable, when deciding whether a measurement is normal or abnormal, the result obtained must be compared with data from the 'normal' population, collected by the same method, under identical conditions. This is particularly important with respect to blood pressure, which varies significantly depending upon the physiological conditions under which it is measured and for which there is no distinct cut-off between normal and abnormal.

Standardization of blood pressure measurement in children was first attempted in a report commissioned by the National Heart, Lung and Blood Institute in 1977 and revisions were carried out in the Report of the Second Task Force on Blood Pressure Control in Children, published in 1987 [1]. The most recent update was published in 1996 [2]. This latter report recognizes a number of changes which have occurred over the past couple of decades with respect to the diagnosis and management of hypertension in children, particularly in relation to the recognition of the origins of essential hypertension in childhood.

The mercury sphygmomanometer

The use of a mercury sphygmomanometer, with the cuff around the upper right arm and a stethoscope placed over the brachial artery pulse, remains the gold standard for measurement of blood pressure. The mercury column should be vertical and positioned so as to be easily and correctly read. It is important to select the correct cuff size. The earliest recommendation was to use the largest cuff that allowed access to the antecubital fossa with a stethoscope. However, accumulating evidence suggests that as well as blood pressure being overestimated if the cuff is too small, it may be underestimated if the cuff is too large [3]. The most recent recommendation is that the cuff must be of an adequate size and the cuff bladder width (not the cloth covering) should be approximately 40% of the arm circumference midway between the olecranon and the acromion. The cuff bladder length will usually be 80–100% of the circumference of the arm [2].

In order to minimize anxiety-induced elevation of blood pressure, so-called 'white-coat' hypertension, readings should be taken in as relaxed an environment as possible. The Task Force studies stipulated that measurements should be taken after 3 to 5 minutes of rest in the seated position with the antecubital fossa supported (held beneath the elbow) at heart level, defined by the midsternum. If the arm is below heart level, then systolic and diastolic pressures can be over-estimated by up to 10 mmHg and the opposite is true if the arm is elevated. If the arm is not supported, then the muscle contraction required to keep the arm elevated can also raise heart rate and blood pressure. Diastolic blood pressure may be increased by up to 10% if the arm is extended and unsupported. Posture will also affect blood pressure, with a tendency for it to increase from the lying to the sitting or standing position.

The blood pressure cuff should be inflated rapidly to a pressure approximately 20 mmHg greater than that needed to occlude the brachial pulse as detected by palpation. It is then recommended that the cuff is deflated at about 2–3 mmHg/s whilst listening over the brachial artery with the bell of the stethoscope. Systolic blood pressure is taken as the point when the 'tapping' Korotkoff sounds (K1) are first heard. It is important to palpate the brachial pulse as the cuff is inflated, as in some instances the K1 sounds disappear as pressure is reduced and then reappear at a lower level—the auscultatory gap. If inflation pressure is then judged on the basis of auscultation, the systolic pressure may be underestimated. The systolic pressure has been an easily defined point, in contrast to the controversy over the definition of diastolic pressure in children. The fourth Korotkoff sound (K4) is the point at which there is a distinct abrupt muffling of sounds, which become soft and blowing in quality. The fifth Korotkoff sound (K5) is the point at which all sounds disappear completely. It is recognized that there may be a significant difference between K4 and K5. Sinaiko *et al.*, in a study of 19 274 children aged between 10 and 15 years, found that in 20% the K4–K5 difference was 5–10 mmHg, in 11% it was 11–20 mmHg and in 3% it was greater than 21 mmHg [4]. In younger children it is also possible to hear Korotkoff sounds down to 0 mmHg, although when this occurs it is felt that diastolic hypertension is excluded. Because of these difficulties with assessing K5, the Second Task Force Report used K4 for children up to 13 years of age and K5 in older children. This approach has been modified in the most recent update [2] and K5 has now been recommended in all age groups. However, there is an ongoing debate, with some evidence that K4 is a more reliable measure of diastolic blood pressure in childhood and a better predictor of the development of hypertension

in adult life than K5 [5]. In order to ensure that measurement of blood pressure in an individual patient is consistent, it may be sensible to record all the relevant information e.g. BP: 120/75/ 69 mmHg, right arm, sitting with 9 cm cuff.

The mercury sphygmomanometer is a simple tool but must be in good order if reliable results are to be obtained. The rubber tubing should be in good condition as leaks make controlled deflation of the cuff difficult. There should be at least 70 cm of tubing between the cuff and manometer and 30 cm between the pump and cuff [6]. Connections must be airtight and the control valve should also function correctly, as leaks will again hamper control of pressure release.

A problem with the mercury sphygmomanometer is the toxicity of mercury. Staff who use and service them should be aware of this risk and be familiar with the guidelines for handling mercury and dealing with spillages [7]. These concerns have led a number of European countries to ban their use from hospitals, although the superior reliability of the mercury sphygmomanometer over its alternatives has led to its retention in the United Kingdom and Ireland.

Key points: The mercury sphygmomanometer

- Is the gold standard device for measuring blood pressure.

- Must be in good working order if reliable results are to be obtained.

- The cuff must be of an adequate size:
  – the cuff bladder width (not the cloth covering) should be approximately 40% of the arm circumference midway between the olecranon and the acromion;
  – the cuff bladder should cover 80–100% of the circumference of the arm.

Blood pressure centiles

The Task Force data were obtained from 61 206 children in North America. These data were collected using the mercury sphygmomanometer and this measurement technique must be used when comparing readings against them. Similar cross-sectional data have been obtained from a population of 28 043

Table 7.1 BP levels for the 90th and 95th percentiles of BP for girls aged 1 to 17 years by percentiles of height. Reproduced with permission from Pediatrics, Vol 98, pages 649–658, Table 3, Copyright 1996.

Age (yr)	BP percentile	SBP by percentile of height (mmHg)							DBP by percentile of height (mmHg)						
		5%	10%	25%	50%	75%	90%	95%	5%	10%	25%	50%	75%	90%	95%
1	90th	97	98	99	100	102	103	104	53	53	53	54	55	56	56
	95th	101	102	103	104	105	107	107	57	57	57	58	59	60	60
2	90th	99	99	100	102	103	104	105	57	57	58	58	59	60	61
	95th	102	103	104	105	107	108	109	61	61	62	62	63	64	65
3	90th	100	100	102	103	104	105	108	61	61	61	62	63	63	64
	95th	104	104	105	107	108	109	110	65	65	65	66	67	67	68
4	90th	101	102	103	104	106	107	108	63	63	64	65	65	66	67
	95th	105	106	107	108	109	111	111	67	67	68	69	69	70	71
5	90th	103	103	104	106	107	108	109	65	66	66	67	68	68	69
	95th	107	107	108	110	111	112	113	69	70	70	71	72	72	73
6	90th	104	105	106	107	109	110	111	67	67	68	69	69	70	71
	95th	108	109	110	111	112	114	114	71	71	72	73	73	74	75
7	90th	106	107	108	109	110	112	112	69	69	69	70	71	72	72
	95th	110	110	112	113	114	115	116	73	73	73	74	75	76	76
8	90th	108	109	110	111	112	113	114	70	70	71	71	72	73	74
	95th	112	112	113	115	116	117	118	74	74	75	75	76	77	78
9	90th	110	110	112	113	114	115	116	71	72	72	73	74	74	75
	95th	114	114	115	117	118	119	120	75	76	76	77	78	78	79
10	90th	112	112	114	115	116	117	118	73	73	73	74	75	76	76
	95th	116	116	117	119	120	121	122	77	77	77	78	79	80	80
11	90th	114	114	116	117	118	119	120	74	74	75	75	76	77	77
	95th	118	118	119	121	122	123	124	78	78	79	79	80	81	81
12	90th	116	116	118	119	120	121	122	75	75	76	76	77	78	78
	95th	120	120	121	123	124	125	126	79	79	80	80	81	82	82
13	90th	116	118	119	121	122	123	124	76	76	77	78	78	79	80
	95th	121	122	123	125	126	127	128	80	80	81	82	82	83	84
14	90th	119	120	121	122	124	125	126	77	77	78	79	79	80	81
	95th	123	124	125	126	128	129	130	81	81	82	83	83	84	85
15	90th	121	121	122	124	125	126	127	78	78	79	79	80	81	82
	95th	124	125	126	128	129	130	131	82	82	83	83	84	85	85
16	90th	122	122	123	125	126	127	128	79	79	79	80	81	82	82
	95th	125	126	127	128	130	131	132	83	83	83	84	85	86	86
17	90th	122	123	124	125	126	128	128	79	79	79	80	81	82	82
	95th	126	126	127	129	130	131	132	83	83	83	84	85	86	86

European children aged 4–19 years [8]. K5 was used as the measure of diastolic blood pressure in both of these reports. Data from these two studies are shown in Tables 7.1 and 7.2 and Fig. 7.1. It is recognized that body size is an important determinant of blood pressure in childhood and adolescence. The physical size of the child must therefore also be taken into account when assessing blood pressure, and both the North American and European studies include height-specific centiles. While weight also has an influence on blood pressure, the association between obesity and hypertension is thought to be causal, with obesity contributing to higher blood pressure and increased risk of cardiovascular disease.

One problem with the updated Task Force data is that with the change to using K5 for estimation of diastolic blood pressure in younger children, some of the data from the Second Task Force Report had to be discarded where no K5 reading was available, leaving only 561 measurements in 371 children under 4 years of age. There was also no update of the reference values for children under 1 year of age (Fig. 7.2).

Another recognized variable which influences blood pressure is ethnicity. The most recent Task Force report [2] contains data from a heterogeneous, although predominantly White, population (White 56%, African-American 29%, Hispanic 9%, Asian 3%, Native American 1%, Other 3%). There are

Table 7.2 Levels for the 90th and 95th percentiles of BP for boys aged 1 to 17 years by percentiles of height. Reproduced with permission from Pediatrics, Vol 98, pages 649–658, Table 2, Copyright 1996.

Age (yr)	BP percentile	SBP by percentile of height (mmHg)							DBP by percentile of height (mmHg)						
		5%	10%	25%	50%	75%	90%	95%	5%	10%	25%	50%	75%	90%	95%
1	90th	94	95	97	98	100	102	102	50	51	52	53	54	54	55
	95th	98	99	101	102	104	106	106	55	55	56	57	58	59	59
2	90th	98	99	100	102	104	105	106	55	55	56	57	58	59	59
	95th	101	102	104	106	108	109	110	59	59	60	61	62	63	63
3	90th	100	101	103	105	107	108	109	59	59	60	61	62	63	63
	95th	104	105	107	109	111	112	113	63	63	64	65	66	67	67
4	90th	102	103	105	107	109	110	111	62	62	63	64	65	66	66
	95th	106	107	109	111	113	114	115	66	67	67	68	69	70	71
5	90th	104	105	106	108	110	112	112	65	65	66	67	68	69	69
	95th	108	109	110	112	114	115	116	69	70	70	71	72	73	74
6	90th	105	106	108	110	111	113	114	67	68	69	70	70	71	72
	95th	109	110	112	114	115	117	117	72	72	73	74	75	76	76
7	90th	106	107	109	111	113	114	115	69	70	71	72	72	73	74
	95th	110	111	113	115	116	118	119	74	74	75	76	77	78	78
8	90th	107	108	110	112	114	115	116	71	71	72	73	74	75	75
	95th	111	112	114	116	118	119	120	75	76	76	77	78	79	80
9	90th	109	110	112	113	115	117	117	72	73	73	74	75	76	77
	95th	113	114	116	117	119	121	121	76	77	78	79	80	80	81
10	90th	110	112	113	115	117	118	119	73	74	74	75	76	77	78
	95th	114	115	117	119	121	122	123	77	78	79	80	80	81	82
11	90th	112	113	115	117	119	120	121	74	74	75	76	77	78	78
	95th	116	117	119	121	123	124	125	78	79	79	80	81	82	83
12	90th	115	116	117	119	121	123	123	75	75	76	77	78	78	79
	95th	119	120	121	123	125	126	127	79	79	80	81	82	83	83
13	90th	117	118	120	122	124	125	126	75	76	76	77	78	79	80
	95th	121	122	124	126	128	129	130	79	80	81	82	83	83	84
14	90th	120	121	123	125	126	128	128	76	76	77	78	79	80	80
	95th	124	125	127	128	130	132	132	80	81	81	82	83	84	85
15	90th	123	124	125	127	129	131	131	77	77	78	79	80	81	81
	95th	127	128	129	131	133	134	135	81	82	83	83	84	85	86
16	90th	125	126	126	130	132	133	134	79	79	80	81	82	82	83
	95th	129	130	132	134	136	137	138	83	83	84	85	86	87	87
17	90th	128	129	131	133	134	136	136	81	81	82	83	84	85	85
	95th	132	133	135	136	138	140	140	85	85	86	87	88	89	89

data to suggest that both African- and Asian-American children have higher blood pressures than White children. The European study by de Man [8] does not give any information about ethnicity. Ideally, the normal data used should be from the same population as the patient, and a case could be made in the United Kingdom for using normal values from the Brompton study [9], which obtained longitudinal rather than cross-sectional data from children from birth to 10 years of age.

Blood pressure should be recorded at least twice on each occasion, and the average of systolic and diastolic readings used as a measure of blood pressure. One criticism of the Task Force Report is that while it stresses the need to take multiple blood pressure readings before judging blood pressure, the nomograms are based on the first blood pressure readings in each of the subjects. Readings above the 95th centile are considered abnormal and those below the 90th centile as normal. Measurements between the 90th and 95th centile are deemed as high-normal and warranting further observation.

White-coat hypertension

It is also important that hypertension should only be diagnosed if measurements are consistently raised on at least three separate occasions. One reason for this

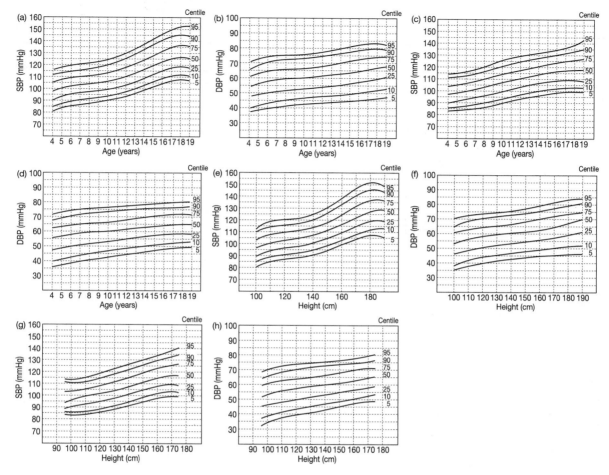

Fig. 7.1 (a) Age-specific percentiles of systolic blood pressure (SBP) in boys. (b) Age-specific percentiles of diastolic blood pressure (DBP) in boys. (c) Age-specific percentiles of systolic blood pressure (SBP) in girls. (d) Age-specific percentiles of diastolic blood pressure (DBP) in girls. (e) Height-specific percentiles of systolic blood pressure (SBP) in boys. (f) Height-specific percentiles of diastolic blood pressure (DBP) in boys. (g) Height-specific percentiles of systolic blood pressure (SBP) in girls. (h) Height-specific percentiles of diastolic blood pressure (DBP) in boys. Reproduced from de Man S *et al*. Blood pressure in childhood: pooled findings of six European studies. J Hypertens 1991; 9:109–114 with permission from Lippincott Williams and Wilkins.

is the phenomenon of 'white-coat' hypertension [10]. The strict definition of this is a persistent rise in blood pressure when in a medical setting, which is not attenuated with time or repeated blood pressure measurements. However, the definition has been used more loosely to describe patients whose blood pressure may come down with repeated measurements. It should not be underestimated, and the few studies which have investigated this phenomenon in children have reported a prevalence ranging from 44 to 88%, depending on the choice of threshold values of normality.

Systolic versus diastolic hypertension

The need to ensure that K5 is used as the measure of diastolic blood pressure when making comparisons with the normal data quoted, has already been made. However, the arguments over the measurement of diastolic pressure may, in practice, be of little consequence as there has been a move, particularly in adult practice, from an emphasis on diastolic blood pressure to a recognition that the systolic blood pressure may be of greater clinical importance. The previous preoccupation with diastolic blood pressure arose from the observation that systolic blood pressure rises

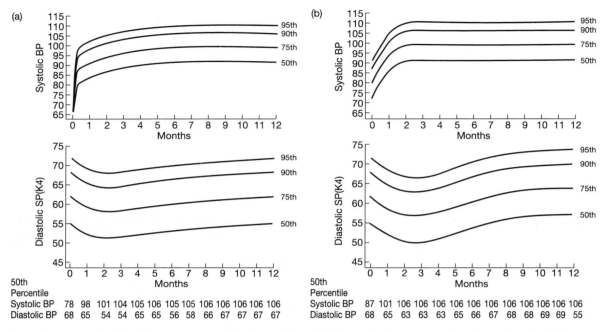

Fig. 7.2   Age-specific blood pressure percentiles in (a) girls and (b) boys, birth to 12 months of age: Korotkoff phase IV (K4) used for diastolic blood pressure. Reproduced with permission from Pediatrics, Vol 79, pages 1–25. Figure 1 and 2, Copyright 1987 [1].

with age whereas diastolic blood pressure does not. Recruitment into adult studies of hypertension therefore tended to be based on the detection of a diastolic blood pressure greater than 90 mmHg, regardless of systolic blood pressure. Data from adult studies now indicate that systolic hypertension is far more common than diastolic hypertension, and that elevated systolic blood pressure, independent of diastolic blood pressure, shows a linear relationship with coronary heart disease death rates, at every level of diastolic blood pressure [11]. Two intervention studies have also demonstrated the clinical importance of systolic hypertension [12,13].

Systolic blood pressure is therefore becoming the major criterion for the diagnosis and management of hypertension in adults. While increased stiffness of large arteries secondary to atherosclerotic disease, the postulated cause of systolic hypertension in many adults, is rare in childhood, there is increasing evidence that systolic hypertension may also be important in paediatric practice, and this has recently been reviewed by Sorof [14]. While studies of hypertension in adults can use objective outcomes such as stroke, congestive heart failure, and myocardial infarction, such events in the paediatric population

are fortunately rare. In its place left ventricular wall thickness has been used as a surrogate marker of hypertensive injury. Two large studies have looked at the effects of hypertension in children: the Bogalusa Heart Study and the Muscatine Study. Burke *et al.*, in one of the Bogalusa study reports [15], demonstrated that left ventricular wall thickness and the ratio of left ventricular wall thickness to chamber size correlated with systolic rather than diastolic blood pressure. They showed that even in children with normal blood pressure, left ventricular wall thickness increased in proportion to systolic blood pressure. The Muscatine study also demonstrated a strong positive linear relationship between left ventricular mass and age, height, weight, and both systolic and diastolic blood pressures, with each exerting an independent influence [16]. Amongst these variables, only weight and blood pressure are modifiable and therefore risk factors for cardiovascular disease.

A further study by Daniels *et al.* [17] found that age, weight, height, fat mass, lean body mass, sexual maturation, systolic blood pressure, and diastolic blood pressure were each univariate correlates of left ventricular mass. However, when multivariate analysis was carried out, only fat mass, lean body mass, and systolic blood pressure were statistically significant independent factors affecting left ventricular mass.

Similar studies have been carried out in children with a family history of hypertension and, again, an independent correlation between left ventricular mass index and systolic blood pressure, but not diastolic pressure, was identified [18]. A stronger relationship between systolic rather than diastolic blood pressure and left ventricular morphology has also been demonstrated in hypertensive children [19,20].

Key points: Measurement of blood pressure

- Ensure that staff measuring blood pressure are adequately trained.

- Ensure equipment is in proper working order.

- Do not rely on a single blood pressure measurement for the diagnosis of hypertension.

- Assess blood pressure against normal values comparable for height/age, sex, and measurement technique.

- Be aware of the phenomenon of 'white-coat' hypertension in children.

- Systolic blood pressure is becoming the major criterion for the diagnosis of hypertension in adults and there is evidence to support its use in children.

How accurate is blood pressure measurement?

An important aspect of making any measurement is to try and ensure its accuracy. Errors will occur as a result of failures of the equipment and the user. Observer errors have been classified into three categories [21]:

Systematic errors. These will be recurring faults caused by lack of concentration and inappropriate recognition of the auditory cues, leading to inaccurate interpretation of the Korotkoff sounds. This may lead to the diastolic pressure being recorded wrongly. These problems lead to inter- and intra-observer errors.

Terminal digit preference. On occasions the observer may round the last digit of the pressure measurement to a number of their choosing, usually one ending in a zero or five.

Observer prejudice and bias. This refers to problems arising from the observer recording a result which fits with the preconceived notion of what the result should be, rather than what it actually is. An example of this may be where a 95th centile limit has been ascribed to the subject and, in an attempt to avoid diagnosing hypertension, a result below this value is recorded.

In order to try and reduce these errors it is important to ensure that staff responsible for measuring blood pressure are adequately trained. Some of these problems have been countered by the increased use of automated devices for measuring blood pressure, but the gold standard for measurement of blood pressure remains the mercury sphygmomanometer. Various training aids are available, including videos and CD-ROMs [22].

Alternatives to the mercury sphygmomanometer: the anaeroid sphygmomanometer and automated devices

Anaeroid sphygmomanometer

Because of concerns with the safety of mercury, in many settings, e.g. home use, the mercury sphygmomanometer has been replaced by the anaeroid manometer. Pressure is measured by means of a bellows and lever system. The machinery is more complex and jolts suffered during its routine use can lead to inaccuracies in the readings given. A mean difference, when compared with a mercury sphygmomanometer, of 3 mmHg is considered satisfactory, but in one study, 58% of anaeroid sphygmomanometers were shown to produce errors of more than 4 mmHg and a third had errors greater than 7 mmHg [23]. Therefore, if anaeroid equipment is used it must be serviced regularly.

Automated blood pressure measurement

One of the difficulties with measuring blood pressure in children, particularly small children and infants, is that the Korotkoff sounds are difficult to hear. An alternative to the stethoscope is a Doppler ultrasound probe that can be used to measure systolic blood pressure, as the point when pulsation is first heard. However, this method has been largely superceded by automated devices which, in many units, have also replaced sphygmomanometers for the routine measurement of blood pressure. Most of these machines rely on oscillometric technology which detects initial (systolic blood pressure) and maximal (mean arterial pressure) arterial vibrations. These measurements are then used to calculate diastolic pressure by means of proprietary formulae. The advantage of these machines is their ease of use, particularly in small children, and the ability to obtain repeated measurements, important in intensive care settings. However, drawbacks include requirements for frequent calibration and the lack of established reference standards. Earlier oscillometric devices had a tendency to overestimate blood pressure when compared to mercury sphygmomanometry, but newer models produce much closer estimations of blood pressure. It must, however, be appreciated that the nomograms available for assessment of blood pressure are obtained using a mercury sphygmomanometer and ideally similar nomograms should be produced for each of the automated devices available. The problem is that as soon as the normal data become available it is likely that the equipment will have been superceded by further technological advances.

A refinement on the instruments described above is the Dinamap® monitor. This machine is also based on the oscillometric principle but measures diastolic pressure directly, as the point at which there is a sudden decrease in oscillation of the vessel wall. A study comparing the Dinamap® monitor with blood pressure obtained either via a radial artery line or auscultation using a mercury sphygmomanometer, on a paediatric intensive care unit, showed an excellent correlation between the Dinamap® and the radial artery pressure. This was superior to that between the auscultatory method and the radial artery line [24]. While the blood pressures recorded from a radial artery line are not necessarily error free, the conclusion was that the lack of observer variation when using the Dinamap® outweighed inaccuracies of the machine when compared with the traditional auscultatory method.

An alternative to the oscillometric monitors are those based on auscultation. These devices 'listen' for Kortokoff sounds with either single or dual microphones sited over the brachial artery. There can be problems with error readings as a result of noise interference and these machines are not generally used in the paediatric setting.

Key points: Automated devices for measuring blood pressure

- Are easy to use, particularly in small children.

- Early devices had a tendency to overestimate blood pressure.

- Devices which measure blood pressure using an oscillometric technique are the most accurate.

- It must be appreciated that the available normal data have been generated using the mercury sphygmomanometer.

Measurement of blood pressure in neonates

Accurate monitoring of physiological parameters is an important aspect of neonatal care. Blood pressure is one such variable, although hypotension rather than hypertension is generally the main concern. The relationship between blood pressure and blood flow and the complications of cerebral ischaemia and intraventricular haemorrhage is a complex one and the correct response to hypotension is a difficult clinical issue [25]. Nevertheless, unless there is arterial access allowing direct blood pressure measurement, the only reliable non-invasive method of measuring blood pressure is with an oscillometric device such as a Dinamap® [26].

Home blood pressure monitoring

One way of trying to counter the problem of 'white-coat' hypertension is to facilitate the measuring of blood pressure at home. This should give a better measure of the child's true blood pressure and involves the parents in the child's care. Home blood pressure measurement is particularly useful in patients with known hypertension to help in management. Parents can be taught how to measure blood pressure by the auscultatory method using an aneroid sphygmomanometer or given an automated measuring device. The problems with measuring blood pressure in small children may make it impractical in this patient group and there are concerns, raised by adult studies, over the reliability of reporting of results. Again, improved automated devices with storage capabilities may be helpful.

Ambulatory blood pressure monitoring

This technology has been taken one step further with the development of ambulatory blood pressure monitoring (ABPM). The technique is attractive in that the measurements are free from human bias, they are obtained during the night-time as well as during the day, it can be used even in small children, with the availability of suitable-sized cuffs, and measurements are obtained during normal activities. The devices are reasonably light-weight and well tolerated by paediatric patients as young as 6 months of age [27].

The equipment should have passed through a validation process laid down by the American Association for the Advancement of Medical Instrumentation (AAMI) or the British Hypertension Society (BHS). Validation by the AAMI is voluntary, although the Food and Drug Administration look for new devices to meet the minimum requirements of these guidelines. As a part of this, the equipment must meet certain performance standards at varying humidities, altitudes, and temperatures. Comparison is made with standard auscultation techniques or with intra-arterial standards. There is no specific assessment of use with children, but validation for lower ranges of blood pressure down to systolic pressure less than 100 mmHg and diastolic pressures less than 60 mmHg takes place, as well as for small arm circumferences less than 25 cm. BHS validation also includes standards for observer training before those for equipment validation and interdevice reliability, but does not require inclusion of individuals with lower blood pressure or smaller arm sizes.

Adult studies suggest that these ambulatory monitors are generally accurate. Compared to intra-arterial blood pressure, they tend to underestimate systolic blood pressure by approximately 6 mmHg and overestimate diastolic pressure by about 6 mmHg [28]. Comparison with mercury sphygmomanometers showed that both auscultatory and oscillometric devices underestimated systolic blood pressure by less than 3 mmHg and oscillometric devices underestimated diastolic blood pressure by less than 2 mmHg [29]. Comparison with mercury sphygmomanometers has been made in children and again confirmed their accuracy [30]. This study of 10- and 11-year-olds found systolic pressures to be slightly higher

Table 7.3 Practical issues in ambulatory blood pressure monitoring

Instruct the patient adequately about the aims of the study
Use the non-dominant arm
Instruct the patient in the use of the patient-activated button
Use the real bedtime to calculate daytime and night-time mean values. If these are not known, use a standard timeframe leaving out the transitional hours, e.g. 'day' = 08.00 to 20.00 hours and 'night' = 00.00 to 06.00 hours
Tell patients to avoid water and not to remove monitor
Tell patients to avoid intense exercise during the study
Instruct patients to hold arm motionless during actual readings
Avoid placing the cuff too low on elbow
Ensure that the monitor is within ±5 mmHg of the mercury sphygmomanometer before and at the end of the study
Give the patient a contact person for any problems during the study
Instruct the patient to call if he or she develops any pain or discoloration of the skin distal to the cuff

(4–6 mmHg) as measured by the ambulatory monitors, whereas diastolic pressures were equivalent. The same study showed the results to be reproducible and the system well tolerated by the children.

Some practical aspects with regard to the use of ambulatory blood pressure monitors are given in Table 7.3 [31]. Diaries should be provided for the patient or parent to record activities, medication, and sleep periods. During the daytime blood pressure is measured every 15–20 minutes and overnight the frequency of measurements is every 30 minutes in order to minimize any disturbance to sleep. At the end of the study period the data collected is downloaded on to a computer and the following measurements obtained:

- individual systolic, diastolic, and mean blood pressures and pulse;

- 24-hour mean blood pressure values;

- mean daytime (awake) and night-time (sleep) systolic and diastolic blood pressures;

- blood pressure load (see below).

As with one-off (casual) blood pressure measurements, there is a need for nomograms with which to compare data obtained from an individual patient with normal values for the population from which the subject comes. It is essential that ambulatory blood pressure readings are not compared with normal data from casual blood pressure measurement. ABPM in children is still in its infancy, but some normal data exist and results from one such study are shown in Figs 7.3 and 7.4 and Table 7.4 [32]. In this study, ABPM was carried out on 1141 healthy German children aged between 5 and 21 years and the nomograms were plotted for height. The participants were recruited in schools on a voluntary basis and tested on a regular school day. Two oscillometric

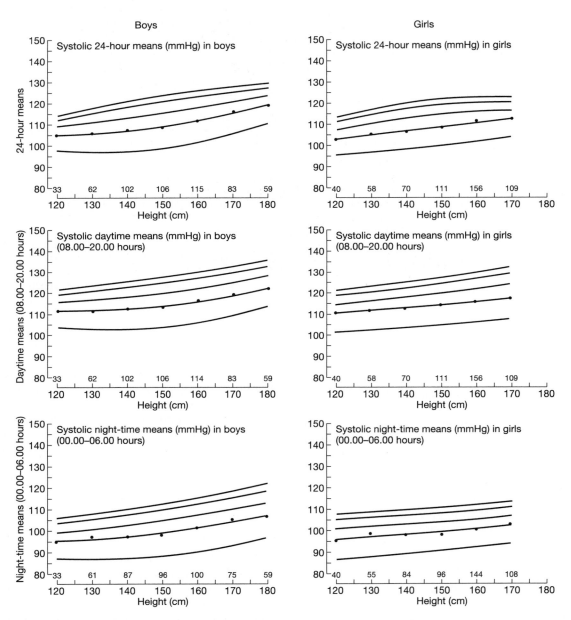

Fig. 7.3 Systolic ambulatory blood pressure in boys (left) and girls (right), related to height: 24-hour (top), daytime (middle), and night-time (bottom) means. The points show the raw median values for each height group. The lines represent the fitting polynomials for the 10th, 50th, 75th, 90th, and 95th percentiles. The smaller numbers on the *x*-axis indicate the number of subjects for each height group. Reproduced from [32] with permission from Mosby Inc.

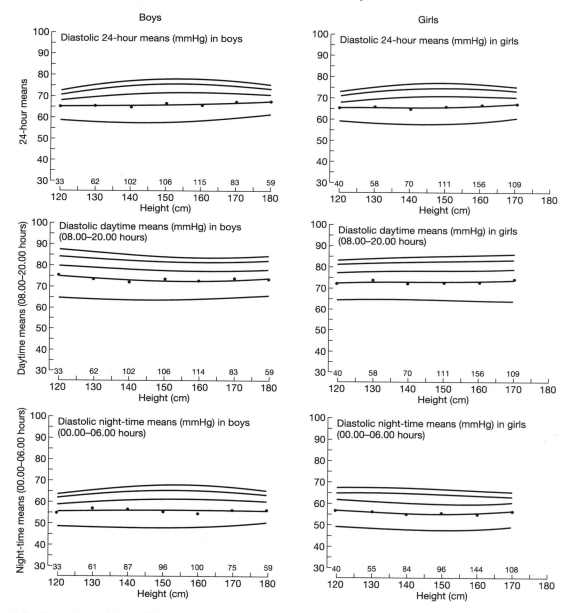

Fig. 7.4 Diastolic ambulatory blood pressure in boys (left) and girls (right), related to height: 24-hour (top), daytime (middle), and night-time (bottom) means. The points show the raw median values for each height group. The lines represent the fitting polynomials for the 10th, 50th, 75th, 90th, and 95th percentiles. The smaller numbers on the *x*-axis indicate the number of subjects for each height group. Reproduced from [32] with permission from Mosby Inc.

devices were used in the study (Spacelabs 90207® and Meditech®) and the results from each were found to be comparable. Daytime means were calculated for data collected between 08.00 hours and 20.00 hours and in order to ensure that night-time measurements were collected during periods of sleep, these data points were collected between 00.00 and 06.00 hours. In comparison with reference values for casual blood pressure measurement [2,8], mean systolic daytime blood pressure rose only slightly with increasing height. For boys this was 112–124 mmHg and in girls from 111 to 120 mmHg, while there was

Table 7.4　Oscillometric mean ambulatory blood pressure values in healthy children: summary for clinical use. Reproduced from [32] with permission from Mosby Inc.

Height (n) (cm)	Percentile for 24-hour period		Daytime percentile*		Night-time percentile[†]	
	50th	95th	50th	95th	50th	95th
Boys						
120 (33)	105/65	113/72	112/73	123/85	95/55	104/63
130 (62)	105/65	117/75	113/73	125/85	96/55	107/65
140 (102)	107/65	121/77	114/73	127/85	97/55	110/67
150 (108)	109/66	124/78	115/73	129/85	99/56	113/67
160 (115)	112/66	126/78	118/73	132/85	102/56	116/67
170 (83)	115/67	128/77	121/73	135/85	104/56	119/67
180 (69)	120/67	130/77	124/73	137/85	107/56	122/67
Girls						
120 (40)	103/65	113/73	111/72	120/84	96/55	107/66
130 (58)	105/66	117/75	112/72	124/84	97/55	109/66
140 (70)	108/66	120/76	114/72	127/84	98/55	111/66
150 (111)	110/66	122/76	115/73	129/84	99/55	112/66
160 (156)	111/66	124/76	116/73	131/84	100/55	113/66
170 (109)	112/66	124/76	118/74	131/84	101/55	113/66
180 (25)	113/66	124/76	120/74	131/84	103/55	114/66

* Daytime: 08.00–20.00 hours.
[†] Night-time: 00.00–06.00 hours.

no significant change in diastolic daytime blood pressure. Smaller children were found to have both systolic and diastolic mean ambulatory blood pressures significantly above levels found in the studies of casual blood pressure [2,8], although this finding was less pronounced in older children. An explanation suggested for this difference was that the younger children were more physically active. When using these data, as with casual blood pressure measurements, the 95th centile is considered the upper limit of normal.

The individual readings may also be shown graphically. Normal results are characterized by a fall in blood pressure (and pulse) when sleeping compared to when awake (Fig. 7.5). This is known as dipping, and can be quantified:

$$\frac{\text{Mean daytime BP} - \text{Mean night-time BP}}{\text{Mean daytime BP}} \times 100\%$$

In the study of healthy German children [32], the nocturnal fall in blood pressure was normally distributed and averaged $13\% \pm 6\%$ (mean $\pm$ SD) for systolic and $23\% \pm 9\%$ for diastolic blood pressure. The dipping of systolic and diastolic blood pressure was closely correlated ($r = 0.69$; $P < 0.0001$). For the sake of analysing test results, normality has been defined as a nocturnal fall of more than 10%. Dipping may be absent or even inverted in patients with secondary hypertension ('non-dippers') with high nocturnal blood pressure (Fig. 7.6). In contrast, most patients with essential hypertension retain a nocturnal fall in blood pressure.

A final means of analysing the data is to calculate the 'blood pressure load'. This is the percentage of blood pressure measurements above a predetermined threshold. In adults, blood pressure load appears to be a better measure of the haemodynamic stress that is placed on end organs susceptible to hypertensive injury [33]. The night-time and daytime results should be analysed separately and a reasonable threshold is the 95th centile value for the respective time period. An arbitrary limit of 30% of readings exceeding the threshold has been suggested. The software should be able to calculate this percentage and, while it will default to adult values, values specific for the subject being studied should be entered. Sometimes it is easier to do this when the device is being programmed prior to data collection and the limits should therefore be specified on the request form. Nevertheless, it should be appreciated that the data can be re-analysed if criteria need to be changed.

It is important that trained staff are available to back up the use of these devices [34]. This may be a doctor, a technician, or a nurse who is able to spend an adequate amount of time with the child and their parents to fit the device and explain the procedure. A variety of monitors are available on the market and many have accessories, in particular cuffs, suitable

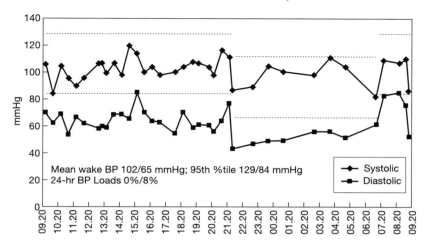

Fig. 7.5 Normal ambulatory blood pressure pattern in a normal 11-year-old girl. The graph shows the systolic and diastolic blood pressure tracing for the 24-hour monitoring period. Blood pressure in mmHg is shown on the vertical axis and time of day is shown on the horizontal axis. The solid horizontal lines within the graph show the age- and size-adjusted 95th percentile for both wake and sleep periods. Reproduced from Sorof JM *et al.* Ambulatory blood pressure monitoring in the paediatric patient. J Pediatr 2000; 136:578–586 with permission from Mosby Inc.

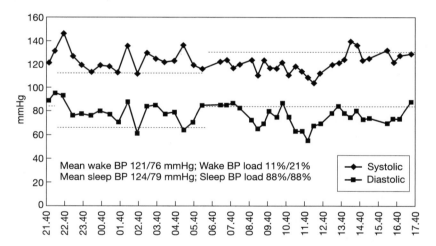

Fig. 7.6 Non-dipping ambulatory blood pressure monitoring trace in a 12-year-old girl after renal transplantation. The mean sleep blood pressure is higher than the mean awake blood pressure. Sleep blood pressure loads are elevated, but awake blood pressure loads are normal. Reproduced from Sorof JM *et al.* Ambulatory blood pressure monitoring in the paediatric patient. J Pediatr 2000; 136:578–586 with permission from Mosby Inc.

for paediatric use. Other considerations are whether the machine is validated by the BHS or AAMI, the cost of machine and software, suitability of the software, cost of consumables (batteries, etc.), after sales support, and complexity. The use of oscillometric devices appears logical, as the available normal data were generated using these and the majority of successful paediatric experience has been with them.

Use of ABPM is growing and will be further stimulated as more normal data become available to help in interpreting the results. Certain patients may particularly benefit from ABPM:

- Children with white coat hypertension: the phenomenon of 'white-coat' hypertension has already been discussed. Use of ABPM may help avoid unnecessary investigation and treatment.

- Children with borderline hypertension: with the increased recognition that hypertensive children become hypertensive adults, the use of ABPM will hopefully help ensure that children who end up being treated are correctly assigned as being hypertensive.

- Nocturnal hypertension: ABPM is the only non-invasive method of assessing blood pressure during sleep. The importance of nocturnal hypertension is unclear, but nocturnal blood pressure has been shown to be independently related to end organ damage in adults, over and above the risk associated with daytime measurements [35].

- Children known to be at significant risk of hypertension: children with end stage renal failure and renal transplants, polycystic kidney disease, insulin-dependent diabetes mellitus, etc.

- Children with resistant hypertension: children who have been placed on antihypertensive medication but remain hypertensive when they come to clinic may be exhibiting a white-coat phenomenon and this may be demonstrated by ABPM.

- To help adjust antihypertensive therapy: investigations continue to examine how ABPM may help in guiding drug treatment in adult patients. One recent study has demonstrated that when ABPM was used, the amount of antihypertensive medication prescribed was significantly reduced [36]. ABPM allows a better assessment of response to treatment, removing white-coat effects and showing the effects of treatment over a whole 24-hour period.

Key points: Ambulatory blood pressure monitoring

- The measurement of ambulatory blood pressure requires the availability of staff who are appropriately trained and experienced in the use of the relevant devices.

- The use of ambulatory blood pressure monitoring reduces the potential for the misdiagnosis of hypertension due to the white-coat effect.

- Most successful experience has been with oscillometric devices. These are also the devices with which the majority of the normal data were obtained.

- Appropriate normal data should be used: ambulatory blood pressure readings should not be compared with normal data from casual blood pressure measurement.

- Mean blood pressure values can be obtained for the entire 24-hour period and separate values for daytime (awake) and night-time (sleep) periods.

- Normal children show a nocturnal fall in blood pressure known as 'dipping'.

- Blood pressure 'load' determines the percentage of values above a predetermined threshold, and may be a better measure of haemodynamic stress placed on end organs.

When should blood pressure be measured in children?

The second part of the question posed in the title of this chapter is when to measure blood pressure. Blood pressure levels within the population are normally distributed, with no clear cut-off between normal and abnormal. The size of the problem is therefore dependent on the value deemed to be abnormal. If we take the 95th centile as the upper acceptable limit, then we would expect at least 5% of the population to be hypertensive, as the population studies have excluded children with known problems. In practice the numbers are closer to 1–2%, probably reflecting the circumstances under which the 'normal' data are collected. Nevertheless, while it

is clear that treating severe hypertension and hypertension in children with underlying problems, such as renal disease, is beneficial, the management of children with mild hypertension, who will often not have an identifiable cause, i.e. with essential hypertension, is less clear. At present there are no longitudinal studies on the outcome of children with mild to moderate hypertension. However, the evidence suggests that the level of blood pressure is maintained into adult life, and children with elevated blood pressure should continue to be monitored, if not treated.

As a relatively simple non-invasive measurement, it is not unreasonable to expect blood pressure to be measured alongside height and weight in the general paediatric outpatient setting as well as in children admitted to hospital, for whatever reason, particularly with the availability of automated measuring devices. In clinics dealing with children at increased risk of hypertension, such as a renal clinic, routine measurement of blood pressure is mandatory. There is certainly a trend now for antihypertensive therapy to be used more aggressively in patients with renal disease, aiming at a target blood pressure in the lower half of the normal range. Adult studies have shown diabetic nephropathy to progress more rapidly when the blood pressure is maintained in the upper rather than the lower normal range [37].

At present, population screening in the paediatric age group is not recommended, although the potential benefits of monitoring blood pressure, alongside promotion of appropriate nutrition and exercise and discouragement of smoking, in the fight against cardiovascular disease, are an important public health issue [2].

Key points: When to measure blood pressure

- Blood pressure measurement should be a routine part of the assessment of a child attending hospital, at least on the first visit.

- Children at risk of developing hypertension, e.g. with known renal disease, must have their blood pressure checked routinely.

- At present, population screening in the paediatric age group is not recommended.

References

1. National Heart, Lung, and Blood Institute. Report of the Second Task Force of Blood Pressure Control in Children—1987. *Pediatrics* 1987; 79:1–25.
2. National High Blood Pressure Education Program Working Group on Hypertension Control in Children and Adolescents. Update on the 1987 Task Force Report on High Blood Pressure in Children and Adolescents: A Working Group Report from the National High Blood Pressure Education Program. *Pediatrics* 1996; 98:649–658.
3. Gómez-Marín O, Prineas RJ, Råstam L. Cuff bladder width and blood pressure measurement in children and adolescents. *J Hypertens* 1992; 10:1235–1241.
4. Sinaiko AR, Gomez-Marin O, Prineas RJ. Diastolic fourth and fifth phase blood pressure in 10–15-year-old children. The Children and Adolescent Blood Pressure Program. *Am J Epidemiol* 1990; 132:647–655.
5. Elkasabany AM, Urbina EM, Daniels SR, Berenson GS. Prediction of adult hypertension by K4 and K5 diastolic blood pressure in children: The Bogalusa Heart Study. *J Pediatr* 1998; 132:687–692.
6. Beevers G, Lip GYH, O'Brien E. Blood pressure measurement Part 2—Conventional sphygmomanometry: technique of auscultatory blood pressure measurement. *BMJ* 2001; 322:1043–1047.
7. European Standard EN 1060–2 (British Standard BSSEN 1060–2:1996) *Specification for non-invasive sphygmomanometers. Part 2. Supplementary requirements for mechanical sphygmomanometers.* 1995. European Commission for Standardisation, Brussels.
8. de Man SA, André J-L, Bachmann H, Grobee DE, Ibsen KK, Laaser U, Lippert P, Hofman A. Blood pressure in childhood: pooled findings of six European studies. *J Hypertens* 1991; 19:109–114.
9. de Swiet M, Fayers P, Shinebourne EA. Blood pressure in first 10 years of life: the Brompton study. *BMJ* 1992; 304:23–26.
10. Sorof JM. White coat hypertension in children. *Blood Pressure Monitoring* 2000; 5:197–202.
11. Neaton JD, Blackburn H, Jacobs D, Kuller L, Lee DJ, Sherwin R, Shih J, Stamler J, Wentworth D. Serum cholesterol level and mortality findings for men screened in the Multiple Risk Factor Intervention Trial. Multiple Risk Factor Intervention Trial Research Group. *Arch Intern Med* 1992; 152:1490–1500.
12. SHEP Cooperative Research Group. Prevention of stroke by antihypertensive drug treatment in older persons with isolated systolic hypertension. Final results of the Systolic Hypertension in the Elderly Program (SHEP). *JAMA* 1991; 265:3255–3264.
13. Staessen JA, Thijs L, Fagard R, O'Brien ET, Clement D, Leeuw PW de, Mancia G, Nachev C, Palatini P, Parati G, Tuomilehto J, Webster J. Predicting cardiovascular risk using conventional vs ambulatory blood pressure in older patients with systolic hypertension. Systolic Hypertension in Europe Trial Investigators. *JAMA* 1999; 282:539–546.
14. Sorof JM. Systolic hypertension in children: benign or beware? *Pediatr Nephrol* 2001; 16:517–525.
15. Burke GL, Arcilla RA, Culpepper WS, Webber LS, Chiang YK, Berensen GS. Blood pressure and echocardiographic measures in children: the Bogalusa Heart Study. *Circulation* 1987; 75:106–114.
16. Malcomn DD, Burns TL, Mahoney LT, Lauer RM. Factors affecting left ventricular mass in childhood: the Muscatine Study. *Pediatrics* 1993; 92:703–709.
17. Daniels SR, Kimball TR, Morrison JA, Khoury P, Witt S, Meyer RA. Effect of lean body mass, fat mass, blood pressure, and sexual maturation on left ventricular mass in children and adolescents. Statistical, biological, and clinical significance. *Circulation* 1995; 92:3249–3254.
18. Treiber FA, McCaffrey F, Pflieger K, Raunnikar RA, Strong WB, Davis H. Determinants of left ventricular mass in normotensive children. *Am J Hypertens* 1993; 6:505–513.
19. Daniels SR, Meyer RA, Loggie JM. Determinants of cardiac involvement in children and adolescents with essential hypertension. *Circulation* 1990; 82:1243–1248.

20. Sorof JM, Mielke TR, Portman RJ. Ambulatory blood pressure monitoring data are correlated with LV mass index and predictive of LV hypertrophy in children with hypertension (abstract). *Am J Hypertens* 2000; 13:39A.

21. Rose G. Standardisation of observers in blood pressure measurement. *Lancet* 1965; 1: 673–674.

22. The British Hypertension Society. Blood pressure measurement CD ROM. London: BMJ Books, 1998.

23. Burke MJ, Towers HM, O'Malley K, Fitzgerald D, O'Brien E. Sphygmomanometers in hospitals and family practice: problems and recommendations. *BMJ* 1982; 285:469–471.

24. Park MK, Menard SM. Accuracy of blood pressure measurement by the Dinamap monitor in infants and children. *Pediatrics* 1987; 79:907–914.

25. Engle WD. Blood pressure in the very low birth weight neonate. *Early Human Development* 2001; 62:97–130.

26. Nuntnarumit P, Yang W, Bada-Ellzey HS. Blood pressure measurements in the newborn. *Clin Perinatol* 1999; 26:981–996.

27. Gellermann J, Kraft S, Ehrich JHH. Twenty-four-hour ambulatory blood pressure monitoring in young children. *Pediatric Nephrol* 1997; 11:707–710.

28. Graettinger WF, Lipson JL, Cheung DG, Weber MA. Validation of portable noninvasive blood pressure monitoring devices: comparisons with intra-arterial and sphygmomanometer measurements. *Am Heart J* 1988; 116:1155–1160.

29. Santucci S, Cates EM, James GD, Schussel YR, Steiner D, Pickering TG. A comparison of two ambulatory blood pressure monitors, the Del Mar Avionics Pressurometer IV and the Spacelabs 90202. *Am J Hypertens* 1989; 2:797–799.

30. Portman RJ, Yetman RJ, West MS. Efficacy of 24-hour ambulatory blood pressure monitoring in children. *J Pediatr* 1991; 118:842–849.

31. Mansoor GA, White WB. Ambulatory blood pressure monitoring is a useful clinical tool in nephrology. *Am J Kid Dis* 1997; 30:591–605.

32. Soergel M, Kirschstein M, Busch C, Danne T, Gellerman J, Holl R, Krull F, Reichert H, Reusz G, Rascher W. Oscillometric twenty-four-hour ambulatory blood pressure values in healthy children and adolescents: A multicenter trial including 1141 subjects. *J Pediatr* 1997; 130:178–184.

33. White WB. Hypertensive target organ damage involvement and 24-hour ambulatory blood pressure measurement. In: Waeber B, O'Brien E, O'Mallet K, Brunner H, eds. Ambulatory blood pressure monitoring. New York: Raven, 1994, 47–60.

34. O'Brien E, Beevers G, Lip GYH. Blood pressure measurement. Part III—Automated sphygmomanometry: ambulatory blood pressure measurement. *BMJ* 2001; 322:1110–1114.

35. Verdecchia P, Schillaci G, Guerrieri M, Gatteschi C, Benemio G, Boldrini F, Porcellati C. Circadian blood pressure changes and left ventricular hypertrophy in essential hypertension. *Circulation* 1990; 81:528–536.

36. Staessen JA, Byttebier G, Buntinx F, Celis H, O'Brien E, Fagard R for the Ambulatory Blood Pressure Monitoring and Treatment Investigators. Antihypertensive treatment based on conventional blood or ambulatory blood pressure measurement. A randomised controlled trial. *JAMA* 1997; 278:1065–1072.

37. Dillon JJ. The quantitative relationship between treated blood pressure and progression of diabetic renal disease. *Am J Kidney Dis* 1993; 22:798–802.

8 | The child with hypertension

Chulananda D.A. Goonasekera and Michael J. Dillon

Introduction

Severe untreated hypertension in childhood carries a high risk of morbidity and mortality [1]. In the majority of cases it is secondary to an underlying cause and often remediable [2,3]. The benefits of recognizing mild to moderate degrees of hypertension are not so clear-cut, but are now considered of importance since individuals predisposed to adult essential hypertension might be detected this way [4,5].

The prevalence of hypertension in children in general is assumed to be 1–3% [6], but this is partly a reflection of its arbitrary definition (i.e. blood pressure above 95th centile) laid down by the task forces [7,8]. The prevalence of severe hypertension is perhaps much lower, at around 0.1% [6,9]. The group of children affected by severe hypertension is often dealt with by paediatric nephrologists, since in more than two-thirds of cases the problem is either of renal origin or renal impairment may occur as a consequence of ongoing untreated hypertension causing renal vascular damage.

Inevitably, the diagnosis of hypertension has to depend on an arbitrary cut-off figure, since we tend to consider only the absolute level of blood pressure for this process. Blood pressure variability (such as circadian rhythm, emotional influence, activity versus rest, etc.), geographical variations [10], and physiological increase in blood pressure with age [7] makes diagnosing hypertension difficult using a simple cut-off point. Overt and covert errors of measurement further complicate interpretation [11]. Therefore, the diagnosis of hypertension by measurement of blood pressure alone should not necessarily lead to initiation of therapy, but should alert the physicians to look for more evidence in support of a rise in blood pressure being pathological, with benefits of treatment outweighing the risks of no therapy.

The thrust of this chapter is not so much to delve into the controversies of hypertension definition or errors of measurement, but to introduce an acceptable outline of management when a child is labelled hypertensive utilizing prevailing methods of blood pressure measurement, for example, office blood pressure, home blood pressure, or ambulatory blood pressure. We recommend, however, that the same and validated method of blood pressure measurement [12] should be used for re-assessment during follow-up and also in assessing response to therapy. This would allow assessment of progress in relative terms rather than utilizing absolute levels of blood pressure. For example, a child treated for hypertension based on office blood pressure measurement using mercury sphygmomanometry had his antihypertensive therapy altered to normalize the blood pressure measurements, but was subsequently unable to stand up without fainting due to covert postural hypotension that was not obvious by routine blood pressure measurement. This illustrates the importance of interpretation of blood pressure in relative terms rather than in absolute terms.

What to do if blood pressure is found to be elevated

Ensure that it is truly elevated

If a child's blood pressure (BP) is diagnosed to be high, it is first necessary to ensure that his or her blood pressure is truly elevated. This can be achieved by following a simple step by step approach as described below.

1. Repeat the blood pressure measurements to demonstrate a persistent rise. The time span over which this should be undertaken should be determined by clinical circumstances, i.e. a child in an emergency situation may need his BP checking several times within a few minutes whereas a borderline

rise demonstrated during a routine school examination may be re-checked several months later. In certain situations, such as a phaeochromocytoma, the rise in BP could be intermittent (approximately 12% of cases), but this scenario is relatively uncommon [13].

2. Carefully exclude errors in measurement. This can be achieved by following the recommendations of the task forces [8,14]. Use of inappropriate cuff sizes [15], incorrect use of the mercury sphygmomanometer with poor auscultation technique [16,17], or use of an unvalidated instrument are some of the common mistakes that may be rectified [11,18].

3. Use a consistent setting and method. Use of the same method of blood pressure measurement and the setting is important to avoid confusion at follow-up, i.e. a distinction between office, home, or ambulatory blood pressure should be maintained when assessing progress at follow-up [11].

4. Correct interpretation. Preferably, the measured blood pressure should be interpreted using an appropriate nomogram, i.e. a nomogram that has been developed utilizing the same methodology that was used to measure blood pressure in the subject. Variations related to geography, age, sex, weight, or height should also be accounted for by the use of appropriate nomograms [11].

Exclude reactive increases in blood pressure

It is also important that reactive increases in blood pressure are excluded [19]. If the reactive increase is due to emotion, time of the day, or any other temporary cause, such as pain, then management should be directed to the aetiology of raised blood pressure and not so much the blood pressure itself. In certain situations, the increase in blood pressure may reflect an increase in sympathetic tone, for example, in hypovolaemia [20] and heart failure [19]. The correction of hypovolaemia or treatment of heart failure is then the treatment of choice. In another situation an increase in blood pressure may be a protective mechanism, as in cerebrovascular disease with critically impaired cerebral perfusion. Inadvertent reduction in blood pressure in these states may precipitate cerebral infarcts. Thus, one should be certain that the rise in blood pressure is not a natural protective phenomenon or an epiphenomenon before embarking on treatment. In the presence of raised intracranial pressure (ICP),

blood pressure may be raised as a reflex phenomenon to maintain adequate cerebral perfusion. This situation should not be confused with hypertensive encephalopathy, where the ICP pressure may also be raised. Treatment of high blood pressure in the former situation would be detrimental unless combined with specific measures to reduce raised ICP concomitantly, whereas in the latter, gentle reduction of blood pressure over 2–3 days would suffice to ameliorate the effects of 'malignant' hypertension.

A careful history and clinical examination, especially looking for clinical features of raised intracranial pressure, hypovolaemia, and anxiety, is the key to the diagnosis of reactive increase in blood pressure. In the event of borderline hypertension or a doubtful interpretation, the child should be labelled hypertensive and followed up until proven otherwise.

Recognize transient increases in blood pressure

There are other conditions associated with short-lived increases in blood pressure that may rarely go on to develop sustained hypertension [21]. Within this group, acute renal disease (nephritis) predominates. Less commonly, Guillain–Barré syndrome, lead poisoning, hypercalcaemia, familial dysautonomia, and drug therapy (steroids) or overdose, excess administration of blood, plasma, or saline, may be associated with a rise in blood pressure. These subjects may carry the risk of developing hypertension-associated complications, hence appropriate antihypertensive therapy should be instituted until the subject has recovered sufficiently to remain normotensive without drugs. Concomitant treatment of the primary disease is also important to reduce mortality and morbidity that may not be related directly to hypertension (e.g. lupus nephritis).

Key points: What to do if BP is found to be elevated

- Ensure that the blood pressure is truly elevated.

- Exclude reactive increases in blood pressure.

- Consider conditions that cause short-lived increases in BP.

How to approach management of a truly hypertensive child

Can we classify hypertensive children at presentation?

Many of the children with severe hypertension may have evidence of existing target organ damage (e.g. cardiomegaly, retinopathy, renal impairment, and encephalopathy) at presentation. If this is found, there is no doubt as to the necessity for antihypertensive treatment. In a few others, blood pressure may be extremely high at diagnosis without evidence of target organ damage. In this group, onset of target organ damage or complications in the short term should be anticipated. In a third group, where blood pressure is elevated to mild to moderate levels, treatment may be considered after a period of follow-up. As the aim of treatment of high blood pressure is prevention of complications and target organ damage, hypertension in children may best be classified by the duration of time before these consequences are anticipated (a new concept). This concept transpires from the clinical observation that there is a poor correlation between the level of blood pressure *per se* and the onset of complications.

With the current evidence two broad categories of hypertensive children may be recognized:

Category 1. Increased BP with anticipated onset of complications in the short term (this includes subjects

who already have established complications or target organ damage at presentation or may do so in the near future if untreated, and are usually children with secondary hypertension).

Category 2. Increased BP with anticipated onset of complications in the long term (this includes children with high BP who would develop complications late in life as adults; mainly essential hypertension, with no evidence of target organ damage at presentation).

There is no clear dividing line between the two categories, but features mentioned in Table 8.1 are useful in distinguishing them. This classification will be most useful in determining timing, forms of antihypertensive treatment, and the degree of investigation. Category 1 patients should certainly be commenced on antihypertensive therapy earlier rather than later, whereas those in Category 2 may be observed until a definitive diagnosis is established or the diagnosis is ascertained on regular follow-up.

Key points: Approach to the truly hypertensive child

- Search for target organ damage.
- Consider how high the BP is and how likely complications are.

Table 8.1 Clinical features that may be useful in distinguishing the two clinical groups of subjects who will develop complications of hypertension within the short-term or long-term

	Category 1: Hypertension associated with the onset of complications in the short term (days, months, or years)	Category 2: Hypertension associated with the onset of complications in the long term (years to decades)
Complications	Usually seen at presentation or during childhood	Usually occur late in life as adults
Age	Usually younger children	Usually post-pubertal children
Symptoms	Commonly symptomatic (irritability, behavioural changes, failure to thrive, facial palsy, headache, seizures, etc.)	Often asymptomatic
Aetiology	Usually secondary with identifiable cause	Usually cause cannot be identified
Target organ damage (heart, brain, kidney, eyes)	Commonly found at diagnosis	May not be evident at presentation
Level of blood pressure	Usually clearly elevated (except in the presence of established complications such as heart failure)	Borderline or mild to moderate

The following case histories illustrate the above.

Case 1

A 5-year-old boy presenting with facial palsy was diagnosed to be hypertensive with a blood pressure of 156/110 mmHg. Further investigation revealed that this child had an enlarged heart and mild proteinuria. A diagnosis of hypertension needing urgent therapy was made and he was treated with a calcium-channel blocker and a beta-blocker. Further investigation revealed bilateral renovascular disease. This scenario falls into Category 1 since, if untreated, he was likely to develop complications of hypertension within the short term.

Case 2

A 13-year-old post-pubertal obese asymptomatic girl was diagnosed to have a blood pressure of 140/90 mmHg at school examination. The fundi, heart, and urine examination were normal. She was seen regularly by her general practitioner and, despite regular exercise and a low-salt diet, no improvement in her blood pressure could be detected. This scenario would fit into Category 2, where benefits of immediate pharmacological treatment are controversial.

Antihypertensive measures

Aims

The true aim of treatment of high blood pressure is to reduce the cardiovascular risk to what it might be in normal circumstances. This cannot be achieved only by normalizing blood pressure by pharmacological and other means, although this plays a part [13]. In childhood practice, it is unusual to focus on other factors that increase cardiovascular risk, for example lipid disorders, passive smoking, and dietary habits, etc., but these are important [13]. In addition, adequate blood pressure control aids the recovery from some of the damage that has already occurred as a consequence of high blood pressure.

In general, control of blood pressure should not be achieved precipitously, particularly in the presence of encephalopathy and in accelerated or malignant hypertension. In these situations the reduction of BP should be carefully controlled and slow [22].

Emergency therapy

A few clinical situations need emergency treatment of hypertension. These include encephalopathy presenting with convulsions and altered level of consciousness due to raised blood pressure, and arteriopathy (malignant hypertension) following severe hypertension with rapidly deteriorating renal function, fundal changes, and evidence of cardiac and respiratory decompensation [23]. These patients should have antihypertensive therapy established immediately, preferably in an intensive care environment, in addition to cranial imaging to confirm diagnosis [24]. The blood pressure should be reduced extremely slowly, without instituting precipitous falls, and allowing preservation of target organ function [25]. In general, the slow reduction in BP should be planned, aiming to reduce the BP by one-third of the total desired reduction within the first 12–24 hours. The BP should be monitored continuously during the process, and this should be achieved by the use of intravenous infusions of sodium nitroprusside or labetalol titrated against the response. The supportive care of vital functions, i.e. cardiac and respiratory support to maintain adequate tissue perfusion as well as oxygenation and nutrition, should continue through this acute period. Thereafter, investigations to identify the precise aetiology of the hypertension may be commenced. Specific treatment of the aetiology, such as angioplasty, may be delayed until the patient has recovered from the effects of high blood pressure and has stabilized. Hence the aim in such emergency situations is to carefully achieve control of blood pressure over a few days rather than hours.

Choice of pharmacological antihypertensive agent

When a pharmacological agent is necessary to achieve adequate control of blood pressure in childhood hypertension, the following factors should be taken into account in determining which drug or drugs to use.

1. Is the hypertensive child hyper-, hypo-, or normovolaemic? Calcium antagonists and diuretics are useful agents for blood pressure control in salt overloaded and hypervolaemic hypertensives [23]. Vasodilators are useful in hypovolaemic hypertensives, but concomitant adequate fluid replenishment may be necessary to maintain tissue perfusion and avoid precipitous falls in blood pressure. The latter group includes severe hypertensives with phaeochromocytoma and children in whom hypertension is due to extremely high levels of renin, as in renovascular disease. In very high renin states, the increased peripheral resistance and pressure natriuresis may contribute to hypovolaemia. In cases with only one kidney affected, the 'pressure natriuresis' by the normal kidney may even produce a salt-depleted hypovolaemic state at presentation. Such patients may need salt replenishment concomitantly with the introduction of antihypertensives.

2. Is the subject in heart failure? Some children may be in heart failure at presentation. If cardiac function is severely compromised, the presenting blood pressure may be recorded as normal or low and the hypertensive state only becomes evident with effective treatment of heart failure. In these cases beta-blockers should initially be avoided and inotrophic support may be required. Once heart failure is controlled, however, beta-blockers may be of use in the treatment of these children.

3. Is there renal impairment? It is good practice to avoid the use of angiotensin converting enzyme (ACE) inhibitors until renovascular disease had been excluded. The use of ACE inhibitors in this situation may initiate renal hypoperfusion, leading to permanent kidney damage and even loss of the affected kidney. In specialized hands, however, ACE inhibitors may be used judiciously in cases with small-vessel renovascular disease.

4. Is there a possibility of compromised cerebovascular blood flow? The reduction of blood pressure should not jeopardize cerebral blood flow, and this is a special concern in children with hypertensive encephalopathy or cerebrovascular disease. The same principles may apply in renovascular disease, where reduction in BP may jeopardize renal blood flow. Caution, therefore, is indicated when blood pressure reduction is taking place.

Therapeutic approach

The therapeutic approach in childhood hypertension is mainly pharmacological. Surgery may be useful in a selected number of cases. Dietary measures may have a role in some cases, especially in adolescence.

- Pharmacological therapy is indicated as an urgent measure in hypertensives belonging to Category 1, in whom complications are anticipated within the short term if BP remains untreated, or in patients who already have established complications.

- Dietary measures (weight reduction [26] and reduced salt intake) and lifestyle adjustment (regular exercise) can be of value in all cases of hypertension. This may be tried, at least initially, as the sole method of therapy in Category 2 children, in whom complications are not anticipated within the short term even when untreated.

> ## Key points: General hypotensive measures
>
> - The aim of treatment is to reduce cardiovascular risk to normal.
>
> - In hypertensive emergencies, reduction of BP should be carefully controlled and slow.
>
> - In choosing an antihypertensive agent consider:
>   – is the child hyper-, hypo-, or normovolaemic?
>   – is the child in heart failure?
>   – is there a possibility of compromised cerebrovascular blood flow?
>
> - The therapeutic approach in children:
>   – is mainly pharmacological;
>   – surgery may be useful in selected cases;
>   – dietary measures have a role in some cases, particularly in adolescence.

Basic investigation

There are many sophisticated investigations that are undertaken in hypertensive children. It is, however, noteworthy that a thorough clinical examination and simple ward tests are the most useful in deciding on the most appropriate method of emergency treatment. For example, four-limb examination of blood pressures and radio-femoral delay will help diagnose a coarctation that is surgically remediable.

The purpose of investigation

The investigation of a hypertensive child has as its aim clarification of three areas:

1. Is there any target organ damage and what is its extent?

2. Are there any established complications?

3. What is the aetiology?

The following investigations should be performed as routine in all Category 1 childhood hypertensives and would be expected to give a basic assessment of aetiology, current status in terms of target organ damage, and established complications. These investigations include a full blood count, plasma urea and electrolytes, calcium, creatinine, renin, aldosterone and catecholamines, a renal ultrasound examination, a renal isotope study [dimercaptosuccinic acid (DMSA), diethylenetriaminepentacetic acid (DTPA), or mercaptoacetyltriglycine (MAG3) scans before and after ACE inhibitor priming [27], a chest X-ray, an electrocardiogram (ECG), an echocardiogram, urine for steroid profile, urine for vanillylmandelic acid (VMA) [28], and preferably a plasma lipid profile. A careful fundoscopy by an ophthalmologist could also be considered as a relevant investigation, as the general paediatrician may not be geared to interpret subtle changes of the retinal

vasculature that may occur as a result of long-standing hypertension.

Advanced investigation (mainly in search of aetiology)

These advanced investigations are best carried out in specialized centres and are mainly a quest for aetiology (for example, Liddle syndrome). They are valuable in planning specific long-term therapy and counselling. An algorithm for management of a newly diagnosed hypertensive child and relevant investigations are illustrated in Fig. 8.1 and Table 8.2, respectively.

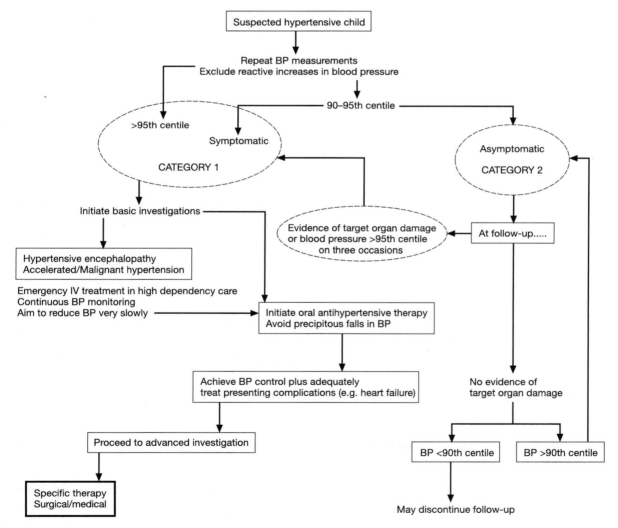

Fig. 8.1 An algorithm for the management of a newly diagnosed hypertensive child.

Table 8.2 Relevant specialized investigations based on clinical features at presentation

Investigation	Purpose	Clinical features that would justify the investigation
Doppler ultrasound and magnetic resonance/spiral CT scan angiography	Exclude main vessel renovascular disease	Severe hypertension, abdominal bruit, neurological abnormalities in an older child
Renal vein renin study	Identify disproportionate renin levels between kidneys or within segments of the same kidney (may have therapeutic implications)	Very young child, raised peripheral renin, hypokalaemia, evidence of renal dysfunction, asymmetric kidney sizes, abdominal bruit
Renal angiography	The 'gold standard' for the diagnosis of renovascular disease	Very young children, severe hypertension, hyponatraemia, evidence of vasculitis, abdominal bruits
Glomerular filtration rate/creatinine clearance	Base line assessment of renal function to monitor progress	Raised plasma creatinine
Cerebral isotope scan	Identify abnormalities in cerebral perfusion	Suspected renovascular disease, neurological complications such as convulsions, nerve palsies, cranial bruits
Metaiodobenzylguanidine (MIBG) scan using ^{131}I or ^{123}I label [29], venous catecholamine sampling [30]	Identify and localize tumours with MIBG uptake	Suspected phaeochromocytoma, raised vanillylmandelic acid (VMA) in urine, raised plasma catecholamine
Somatostatin receptor imaging (SRI) by ^{111}In octreotide scan [31]	Supplement MIBG scan findings and especially to localize metastatic phaeochromocytomas	
Genetic studies for Liddle syndrome, apparent mineralcorticoid excess, glucocorticoid remediable hypertension, von Hippel–Lindau syndrome, multiple endocrine neoplasias and neurofibromatosis	Molecular recognition of syndromes that need special drug therapy and family counselling	Strong family history, hypokalaemia, low renin, dysmorphism, café-au-lait spots
Cerebral angiography	'Gold standard' for the recognition of cerebrovascular disease	Abnormal cerebral isotope scan, MRI/CT scan, cerebral bruit

---

Key points: Investigation of hypertension

- The aims of investigation are:
  - to assess the presence and severity of target organ damage;
  - to identify any complications;
  - to establish aetiology.
- Advanced investigations should be performed in specialized centres.

Choosing a specific therapy based on aetiology

Surgical measures

Some causes of hypertension in children are surgically remediable, for example, renal artery stenosisx [32,33],

coarctation of aorta [34], and phaeochromocytoma. Renal angiography is the gold standard for the diagnosis of renovascular disease as other measures (such as spiral CT, magnetic resonance imaging) may not have sufficient sensitivity to pick up small-vessel disease that is common in children. Renal vein renin sampling may be useful in lateralization of renin production. This may assist in deciding which kidney to operate on first, or in identifying segmental areas of relevance in the kidney that may need surgical removal. Negative investigations should not preclude a surgical approach if indicated otherwise; for example, a contracted scarred kidney with an undoubtedly normal contralateral one. Metaiodobenzylguanidine (MIBG) scanning is useful in obtaining information in relation to the location of chromaffin-staining tumours such as phaeochromocytomas and paragangliomas.

Coarctation of the thoracic or abdominal aorta may present with hypertension. Radio-femoral pulse delay and blood pressure differences between upper and lower limbs clinically support this diagnosis. Although surgical correction of the mechanical obstruction may relieve the problem of hypertension in the majority, in some patients this may not improve. This is because the coarctation may not be an isolated lesion but a feature of diffuse vessel disease that may jeopardize renal perfusion (mid-aortic syndrome) [35].

Pharmacological agents in specific situations

We have previously discussed the choice of antihypertensive agents in general. However, there are specific circumstances where certain agents are specifically beneficial. For example, angiotensin converting enzyme inhibitors or angiotensin receptor blockers are definitely useful in raised renin states. This is applicable in general but may not be appropriate in the presence of severe main renal artery stenosis. In Liddle syndrome, where there is a sodium-channel mutation [36], triamterene is indicated. In glucocorticoid remediable aldosteronism, in which the formation of a chimeric gene between 11β-hydroxylase and aldosterone synthase results in 'ectopic' synthesis of aldosterone under the control of adrenocorticotrophic hormone (ACTH) [37], dexamethasone is required to achieve adequate control of blood pressure by suppressing the feedback loop. In apparent mineralocorticoid excess (AME), in which there is inadequate conversion of cortisol to cortisone in mineralocorticoid target tissues due to an inactivating mutation in the type 2 isoform of 11β-hydroxysteroid dehydrogenase [38,39], spironolactone and triamterene have roles. In phaeochromocytoma there is a place for nifedipine, phenoxybenzamine, propranolol, labetalol, and prazosin, etc. More recently newer drugs such as amlodipine (a calcium-channel blocker) [40] and esmolol (a beta-blocker) [41] have been used in the treatment of childhood hypertension. A guide for the starting and maintenance dosages of antihypertensive agents is given in Table 8.3.

Lifestyle adjustments

Non-pharmacological measures are often useful in post-pubertal children with essential hypertension, in other words children belonging to Category 2. A low-salt diet makes particular sense in this regard, regular exercise is known to reduce blood pressure, and reducing weight is beneficial in the obese.

Key points: Choosing a specific therapy

- Surgery may be useful in coarctation, renal artery stensosis, phaeochromocytoma.

- Lateralization of renin production may be helpful in guiding surgery.

- MIBG scanning localizes some tumours.

- See text for specific pharmacological agents in specific situations.

- Category 2 patients are usually managed with non-pharmacological measures.

Control of blood pressure: what target?

The 'target' blood pressure in antihypertensive therapy should be the level at which the progressive deterioration in vital functions has come to a halt, with the beginning of repair of the damage that has already occurred due to hypertension. The target blood pressure should not aggravate vital function impairment by reducing perfusion, for example in cerebrovascular disease or renovascular disease.

To avoid difficulties in interpretation (against height, weight, or age) and errors between devices (e.g. mercury versus Dinamap®), it is best to use the same method of BP measurement during follow-up that was used to diagnose the increase in BP; i.e. if originally ambulatory blood pressure monitoring (ABPM) was used to diagnose hypertension, then ABPM should also be used subsequently to assess response to treatment (see previous chapter for further discussion).

Long-term management and counselling

Inevitably, children with hypertension need long-term follow-up and appropriate referral to adult physicians late in adolescence, as the management in many cases is life-long. The purpose of follow-up is mainly twofold, as shown below.

Table 8.3 A list of commonly used antihypertensive drugs in children

Drug	Route	Normal starting dose	Normal dose range	Divided doses/day
Amiloride[a]	Oral	0.1 mg/kg/dose	0.4 mg/kg/day; 20 mg/day (maximum)	1–2
Atenolol	Oral	1 mg/kg/dose	1–2 mg/kg/day	1
Captopril	Oral	0.05 mg/kg/dose	0.5–3 mg/kg/day	3
Clonidine	i.v.	0.002 mg/kg/dose	0.002–0.006 mg/kg/day	2
	Oral	0.005 mg/kg	0.01–0.08 mg/kg/day	2
Diazoxide[a]	i.v.	0.5–1 mg/kg	1–10 mg/kg/day	By rapid infusion
Enalapril	Oral	0.2 mg/kg	0.2–1 mg/kg/day (max. 40 mg/day)	1
Esmolol	i.v.	50 µg/kg/min	100–300 µg/kg/min	Infusion only
Frusemide	i.v.	0.5 mg/kg/dose	0.5–4 mg/kg/day	1–4
	Oral	0.5 mg/kg/dose	1–4 mg/kg/day	1–4
Hydralazine	i.v. stat followed by infusion	0.1 mg/kg/dose stat (max.10 mg)	Infusion 10–50 µg/kg/h	As an infusion
	Oral	0.2 mg/kg/dose	1–8 mg/kg/day	3–4
Hydrochlorothiazide	Oral	1 mg/kg/dose	1–4 mg/kg/day	2
Labetalol	i.v.	0.5 mg/kg/h	1–3 mg/kg/h	Infusion only
Metolazone	Oral	0.1 mg/kg/dose	0.1–3 mg/kg/day	1
Minoxidil	Oral	0.1 mg/kg/dose	1–2 mg/kg/day	2
Nifedepine	Oral/ sublingual	0.25 mg/kg/dose (capsular contents drawn by syringe to make correct dose)	1–2 mg/kg/day	4
	Slow release tablets	0.5 mg/kg/dose	1–2 mg/kg/day	2–3 (used in older children)
Phenoxybenzamine[a]	Oral	0.2 mg/kg/dose	1–4 mg/kg/day	2
	i.v.	0.5 mg/kg over 1 h (stat dose)	1–2 mg/kg/day	2–4 (need intensive care facilities)
Phentolamine[a]	i.v.	0.1–0.2 mg/kg/dose	Titrated to response	Infusion only (used for control of hypertensive episodes during phaeochromocytoma surgery)
Prazosin	Oral	0.005 mg/kg/dose; max. 0.25 mg	0.05–0.4 mg/kg/day	4
Propranolol	Oral	1 mg/kg/dose	1–10 mg/kg/day	3
Sodium nitroprusside[a]	i.v.	0.5 µg/kg/min	0.5–8.0 µg/kg/min	Infusion only (protect from light and monitor blood cyanide levels)
Spironolactone	Oral	0.5 mg/kg/dose	1–3 mg/kg/day	2
Triamterene[a]	Oral	1 mg/kg/dose	1–6 mg/kg/day	1–3

[a] Drugs used under special circumstances for specific indications.

At regular follow-up

1. Look for target organ damage in eyes, heart, and renal function as a measure of assessing adequacy of blood pressure control, and adjust treatment accordingly. This is often necessary as the requirement for antihypertensive therapy changes frequently in children. With advancing age the formulations that are used also need changing (for example liquid to tablets, etc.), and adjustments are needed for weight gain. In some children the antihypertensive requirements do not increase with weight gain and this is a reflection of improvement in antihypertensive requirements. Rarely, in some patients the need for antihypertensive treatment wears off completely.

2. Look for emergence of previously unsuspected aetiologies or syndromes. In some cases new diagnoses, such as neurofibromatosis, emerge with time. Some

Summary points

Several points need to be remembered in treating a hypertensive child:

- Hypertension may present with bizarre features such as facial palsy, pulmonary oedema, irritability, and unexplained vomiting, especially in young children.

- Some hypertensive children may have a normal blood pressure if they are in heart failure at presentation.

- Reduce blood pressure slowly: precipitous falls are hazardous.

- Not all hypertensives have salt and water overload or hypervolaemia, and many are salt and water depleted at presentation.

- Controlling blood pressure is important even if the aetiology is not established.

- The target for controlling blood pressure should be tailored individually.

- Follow-up is crucial. New diagnoses may emerge with time.

- The treatment of children with established acute complications of hypertension and advanced investigations are best carried out in specialized centres.

patients previously labelled as essential hypertensives go on to develop features of other syndromes. Therefore, a full clinical examination at each visit is essential in these children who are on regular antihypertensive therapy. Some may develop side-effects of antihypertensive treatment, which would need dealing with on their merits at follow-up visits.

At counselling

1. Explain why control of BP is important, the risks involved and recurrence of risk in family.

2. Educate patient and parents about: lifestyle, complications, exercise, diet, relevance of body weight, etc.

It is important to give a complete picture of the condition to the patient (if old enough) or to parents, since compliance with medication is a problem, particularly during adolescence. Adequate compliance can only be achieved by explanation of the problem. The ways and means of minimizing the cardiovascular risk should also be explained and the family may be interested to know the recurrence risk for siblings and offspring. Thus, appropriate referral to geneticists for counselling may be indicated, for example in Liddle syndrome and AME.

References

1. Still JL, Cottom D. Severe hypertension in childhood. *Arch Dis Child* 1967; 42: 34–39.
2. Ingelfinger JR, Dillon MJ. Evaluation of secondary hypertension. In: Holliday MA, Barratt TM, Avner ED, eds. Pediatric Nephrology, 3rd edn. Baltimore: Williams & Wilkins, 1994: 1146–1164.
3. Gruskin AB, Dabbagh S, Fleischmann LE. Mechanisms of hypertension in childhood diseases. In: Holliday MA, Barratt TM, Avner ED, eds. Pediatric Nephrology, 3rd edn. Baltimore: Williams & Wilkins, 1994: 1096–1115.
4. Gillman MW, Ellison RC. Childhood prevention of essential hypertension. *Pediatr Clin N Am* 1993; 40: 179–194.
5. Lauer RM, Clarke WR, Mahoney LT, Witt J. Childhood predictors for high adult blood pressure. *Pediatr Clin N Am* 1993; 40: 23–40.
6. Leumann EP. Blood pressure and hypertension in childhood and adolescence. *Ergeb Inn Med Kinderheilk* 1979; 43: 109–183.
7. Blumenthal S, Epps RP, Heavenrich R, *et al.* Report of the task force on blood pressure control in children. *Pediatrics* 1977; 59: I–II,797–820.
8. National Heart, Lung and Blood Institute, Bethesda, Maryland. Report of the second task force on blood pressure control in children. *Pediatrics* 1987; 79: 1–25.
9. Rames LK, Clarke WR, Conner WE, Reiter MA, Lauer RM. Normal blood pressures and the evaluation of sustained blood pressure elevation in children. The Muscatine Study. *Pediatrics* 1978; 61: 245–251.
10. Menghetti E, Virdis R, Strambi M, *et al.* Blood pressure in childhood and adolescence: the Italian normal standards. Study Group on Hypertension of the Italian Society of Pediatrics. *J Hypertens* 1999; 17: 1363–1372.
11. Goonasekera CDA, Dillon MJ. Measurement and interpretation of blood pressure. *Arch Dis Child* 2000; 82: 261–265.
12. Reid JL. Validation of blood pressure measuring systems [editorial]. *J Hypertens* 1993; 11: i–ii.
13. Swinford RD, Ingelfinger JR. Evaluation of hypertension in childhood diseases. In: Barratt TM, Avner ED,

Harmon WE, eds. Pediatric Nephrology, 4th edn. Baltimore: Williams & Wilkins, 1999: 1007–1030.

14. O'Brien E, Coats A, Owens P, *et al.* Use and interpretation of ambulatory blood pressure monitoring: recommendations of the British Hypertension Society. *BMJ* 2001; 320: 1128–1134.

15. Arafat M, Mattoo TK. Measurement of blood pressure in children: recommendations and perceptions on cuff selection. *Pediatrics* 1999; 104: e30.

16. Elkasabany AM, Urbina EM, Daniels SR, Berenson GS. Prediction of adult hypertension by K4 and K5 diastolic blood pressure in children: the Bogalusa Heart Study. *J Pediatr* 1998; 132: 687–692.

17. Beevers G, Lip GYH, O'Brien E. Blood pressure measurement Part 2—Conventional sphygmomanometry: technique of auscultatory blood pressure measurement. *BMJ* 2001; 322: 1043–1047.

18. Beevers G, Lip GYH, O'Brien E. Blood pressure measurement Part 1–Sphygmomanometry: factors common to all techniques. *BMJ* 2001; 322: 981–985.

19. Kaplan NM. Management of hypertensive emergencies. *Lancet* 1994; 344: 1335–1338.

20. Houtman PN, Shah V, Barratt TM, Dillon MJ. Reduction of hypertension in hypovolaemia. *Lancet* 1990; 336: 1454.

21. Dillon MJ. Hypertension. In: Clinical Paediatric Nephrology, 2nd edn. Oxford: Butterworth Heinemann, 1995: 175–195.

22. Deal JE, Barratt TM, Dillon MJ. Management of hypertensive emergencies. *Arch Dis Child* 1992; 67: 1089–1092.

23. Sinaiko AR. Treatment of hypertension in children. *Pediatr Nephrol* 1994; 8: 603–609.

24. Cooney MJ, Bradley WG, Symko SC, Patel ST, Groncy PK. Hypertensive encephalopathy: complications in children treated for myeloproliferative disorders—report of three cases. *Radiology* 2000; 214: 711–716.

25. Adelman RD, Coppo R, Dillon MJ. The emergency management of severe hypertension. *Pediatr Nephrol* 2000; 14: 422–427.

26. Dustan HP. Mechanisms of hypertension associated with obesity. *Ann Int Med* 1983; 98: 860–864.

27. Chandar JJ, Sfakianakis GN, Zilleruelo GE, *et al.* ACE inhibition scintigraphy in the management of hypertension in children. *Pediatr Nephrol* 1999; 13: 493–500.

28. Bravo EL, Tarazi RC, Gifford RW, Stewart BH. Circulating and urinary catecholamines in pheochromocytoma. *N Eng J Med* 1979; 301: 682–686.

29. Leung A, Shapiro B, Hattner R, *et al.* Specificity of radioiodinated MIBG for neural crest tumors in childhood. *J Nucl Med* 1997; 38: 1352–1357.

30. Mather CM. Paediatric blood pressure and anaesthesia. *Anaesthesia* 1991; 46: 381–382.

31. van der Harst E, de Herder WW, Bruining HA, *et al.* [I(123)I] metaiodobenzylguanidine and [(111)In] octreotide uptake in benign and malignant pheochromocytomas. *J Clin Endocrinol Metab* 2001; 86: 685–693.

32. Hiner LB, Falkner B. Renovascular hypertension in children. *Pediatr Clin N Am* 1993; 40: 123–140.

33. Chalmers RT, Dhadwal A, Deal JE, Sever PS, Wolfe JH. The surgical management of renovascular hypertension in children and young adults. *Eur J Vasc Endovasc Surg* 2000; 19: 400–405.

34. Rocchini AP. Cardiovascular causes of systemic hypertension. *Pediatr Clin N Am* 1993; 40: 141–147.

35. Leandro J, Balfe JW, Smallhorn JF, Benson L. Coarctation of the aorta and hypertension. *Child Nephrol Urol* 1992; 12: 124–127.

36. Shimkets RA, Warnock DG, Bositis CM, *et al.* Liddle's syndrome: heritable human hypertension caused by mutations in the beta subunit of the epithelial sodium channel. *Cell* 1994; 79: 407–414.

37. Lifton RP, Dluhy RG, Powers M, *et al.* A chimeric 11 beta hydroxylase/aldosterone synthase gene causes glucocorticoid-remediable aldosteronism and human hypertension. *Nature* 1992; 355: 262–265.

38. Wilson RC, Krozowski ZS, Li K, *et al.* A mutation in the HSD 11 beta 2 gene in a family with apparent mineralocorticoid excess. *J Clin Endocrinol Metab* 1995; 80: 2263–2268.

39. Mune T, Rogerson FM, Nikkila H, Agarwal AK, White PC. Human hypertension caused by mutations in the kidney isozyme of 11 beta-hydroxysteroid dehydrogenase. *Nat Genet* 1995; 10: 394–399.

40. Pfammatter JP, Clericetti-Affolter C, Truttmann AC, Busch K, Laux-End R, Bianchetti MG. Amlodipine once-daily in systemic hypertension. *Eur J Pediatr* 1998; 157: 618–621.

41. Wiest DB, Garner SS, Uber WE, Sade RM. Esmolol for the management of paediatric hypertension after cardiac operations. *J Thorac Cardiovasc Surg* 1998; 115: 890–897.

9 | Disorders of micturition

Jonathan Evans and Manoj Shenoy

Introduction

Wetting is the most common urinary tract disorder in children. In most children, there is no underlying organic pathology and the long-term prognosis is excellent in that the majority will eventually become dry even without treatment. Despite these reassuring facts, children with wetting problems can be amongst the most challenging for doctors. This is probably because the problem is poorly understood, there is no readily identifiable 'medical pathology', and because treatment is usually time consuming and arduous. There is a great demand for treatment because wetting is an unpleasant symptom that can cause a great deal of stress and anxiety in the family and at times frustration for the child and parents. There may also be other coexisting problems such as urinary tract infection, constipation, soiling, and behavioural or emotional difficulties. One author described the characteristics of the ideal doctor treating wetting, as somebody with the anatomic and physiological expertise of a urologist, the patience of a paediatrician or nurse practitioner, and the insight of a psychologist!

This chapter focuses on the child with functional incontinence and enuresis, the other urological disorders and the neurogenic bladder are dealt with in other chapters. The terminology used in the chapter is summarized in Table 9.1. Central to management is a good understanding of the normal development of continence, an understanding of the functional disturbances of bladder and urine production that lead to wetting, and an ability to recognize the many different patterns of wetting that demand differing therapeutic approaches. For most children, a detailed history and physical examination supported by very limited investigations are all that are needed to make a diagnosis and select appropriate treatment. Only rarely are complex investigations necessary.

Table 9.1 Terminology

Term	Definition
Urinary incontinence	The involuntary loss of urine
Enuresis	A normal void occurring at a socially unacceptable time or place
Nocturnal enuresis (NE)	Voiding in bed while asleep
Monosymptomatic nocturnal enuresis	NE without any other bladder symptoms
Primary nocturnal enuresis	NE in a child who has never been reliably dry
Onset nocturnal enuresis	NE in a child who was previously dry for 6 months or more after the age of 5 years
Urge syndrome and urge incontinence	The frequent attacks of imperative urge to void that may be accompanied by incontinence
Dysfunctional voiding	Functional disturbances of voiding due to overactivity of the pelvic floor during micturition (recognized by variable urinary stream, prolonged voiding and incomplete bladder emptying)
Diurnal enuresis	Voiding in the day at a socially unacceptable time or place

Embryology and anatomy

The urinary bladder develops from the vesical part of the urogenital sinus. The trigone, however, is derived from the caudal ends of the mesonephric ducts. The endoderm of the vesical part of the urogenital sinus forms the epithelium of the bladder and the other layers of the wall develop from the adjacent splanchnic mesenchyme [1].

The bladder is made of an interlacing network of smooth muscle fibres; the detrusor muscle, with a lining of transitional epithelium [2]. The trigone has a superficial layer of muscle that is histologically different from the rest of the bladder musculature.

The bladder receives its motor innervation from the pelvic splanchnic nerves (S2, S3, S4). Onuf's nucleus is a series of neurons clustered in the midventral spinal grey matter at S2 and S3 and supplies the innervation to the external urethral sphincter, the anal sphincter, and most pelvic floor muscles. The sympathetic fibres are derived from the L1 and L2 segments of the spinal cord and come via the superior hypogastric and pelvic plexuses. The pudendal reflex pathways at the spinal level are modulated by supraspinal influences [3,4]; the brainstem, specifically the neurons of the pontine-mesencephalic grey matter, are the origins of control over the bladder motor neurons. The Barrington's nucleus is a group of neurons in the anterior pontine area and it is here that facilitatory impulses to the bladder are believed to originate. The pontine micturition centre (PMC) receives input from the cerebellum, basal ganglia, thalamus, hypothalamus, and the cerebral cortex. The PMC projects to the sacral intermediolateral column and to the sacral intermediomedial column or the dorsal grey commissure (DGC) [5]. The excitatory PMC projection to the bladder motor neurons causes an increase in bladder pressure and the excitatory PMC projection to the GABA-ergic interneurons in the DGC causes relaxation of the external urethral sphincter. The processing of the sensory input from the bladder to the brainstem is more complex than previously recognized and is relayed in part by the periaqueductal grey matter.

Another group of neurons in the pons is involved in the storage of urine during continence; they are located more ventrally and laterally than the PMC. This is known as the pontine storage centre (PSC) or the L-region, and projects to the motor neurones of the urethral sphincter in the nucleus of Onuf. Stimulation of the PSC results in strong excitation of the pelvic floor musculature and an increase in the urethral pressure.

The cerebellum receives sensory input from the bladder and pelvic floor muscles. Its efferents maintain the tone and co-ordination of the pelvic floor striated muscles and also co-ordinate the relaxation of the pelvic floor with detrusor contraction. The basal ganglia are believed to have an inhibitory role on the pontine micturition centre. The superomedial portion of the frontal lobes and the genu of the corpus callosum are responsible for the lower urinary tract control. Cortical stimulation has an inhibitory influence on the pontine micturition centre.

Normal emptying results from contraction of the detrusor muscle and reciprocal relaxation of the external sphincter (innervated by the perineal branch of the pudendal nerve, S2, S3, S4) and pelvic floor.

Physiology of micturition

The lower urinary tract has two important functions, namely storage of urine and emptying at a suitable time. The bladder is a very compliant organ and accommodates an increase in volume without a significant increase in pressure until a critical point is reached. This is due largely to the viscoelastic properties of the bladder wall. Once a critical intravesical pressure is reached, the autonomic and somatic nervous systems are activated. Somatic fibres, through the pudendal nerve, activate the striated sphincter. Additionally, a spinal sympathetic reflex is evoked and its efferent fibres are carried via the hypogastric nerve. This leads to inhibition of detrusor contractility, activation of bladder base and urethra and inhibition of transmission through the ganglia.

The process of micturition involves a sensation of fullness perceived by the frontal lobes of the cerebral cortex. These signals are transmitted by myelinated afferents, passing superiorly via the dorsal columns of the spinal cord, to the cortex. If the social circumstances are appropriate, signals are sent down to the pontine micturition centre, from where they are conveyed down the cord to the intermediolateral zones of the grey matter at the S2, S3 segments, where the Onuf's nucleus is present. This nucleus contains the motor efferents that initiate detrusor contraction.

The supraspinal stimulation of the parasympathetic neurons initiates detrusor contraction and also triggers the inhibition of the sympathetic nervous system and the pudendal nerve reflex. A bladder contraction then occurs together with a relaxation of the bladder outlet with dilatation of the urethra, leading to a funnelled configuration with a low resistance to flow.

Normal developmental milestones of urinary control

The development of control of the external sphincter and voluntary initiation of the detrusor contraction by centres in the midbrain and cerebral cortex determines the degree of neuromuscular maturation. The different patterns of voiding dysfunction are seen if one area of maturation lags behind the other. By 3 years of age most children have some conscious control over micturition and achieve daytime control, but enuresis and accidents during daytime can occur. At approximately 4 years of age, the bladder volume is adequate and central control, which needs an intact brainstem, is complete in most children, with most nights being dry.

Key points: Milestones of urinary control

- Newborn: reflex voiding about 20 times per day.

- >6 months: frequency of void decreases and volume increases.

- 1–2 years: child recognizes sensation of bladder fullness.

- 3 years: some conscious control over micturition; achieve daytime control; accidents do occur.

- 4 years: bladder volume adequate; central control; mostly dry nights.

Psychological factors

It has long been recognized that there is an association between wetting in the absence of an organic disorder and psychological disorders. However, the nature of this relationship is far from clear, as it is difficult to ascertain whether any association is causal and, indeed, whether wetting is causing psychological disorders or vice versa [6]. Some of the more important issues are shown in Table 9.2.

The impact of wetting varies greatly between children and is likely to be determined by factors such as age, parental attitude and response, peer influences, and the child's own personality. There are harrowing anecdotes of how distressing enuresis can be; yet for other children there is little if any distress [9]. Nocturnal enuresis and daytime wetting are often said to adversely affect self-esteem, a view that is supported in a number of studies, usually in selected children attending specialist clinics. Low self-esteem is most prevalent amongst those who have had repeated unsuccessful attempts at treatment [10].

Table 9.2 Psychological factors and wetting problems

Stressful life events such as parental separation may predate enuresis. Such events are also known to cause emotional and behavioural problems [7]

Children with daytime wetting are more likely to have emotional or behavioural problems than those with NE [8]

Children with voiding dysfunction and voiding postponement have a high incidence of psychological disorder [8]

Children with NE tend to have significantly higher scores on behavioural checklists than controls; however, most still have scores that are in the normal range [8]

NE, nocturnal enuresis.

In contrast, when a community-based population of children with enuresis is studied, only a small and clinically insignificant difference in self-esteem is found. Interestingly, and most encouraging for the practitioner, successful treatment does improve self-esteem but even those who do not become dry demonstrate significant improvements [11].

Assessment

The general approach to assessment is applicable to any type of wetting and is based on a careful history of wetting and voiding, physical examination, and patient/parental recording of information about bladder function. Typically, children are unable to communicate a subtle voiding problem to the parents or physicians. Consequently significant disorders may go undetected for some time.

A history suggestive of subtle CNS disorder, such as a traumatic birth, neonatal anoxia, convulsive disorder, and head or back trauma, may explain many voiding abnormalities despite the absence of apparent neurological disease.

History

All children require a full medical history. Particular emphasis should be placed on the features highlighted in Table 9.3.

Clinical examination

In additional to a standard medical examination, specific points to note are set out in Table 9.4.

Table 9.3 Features to assess in the history of a child with wetting

The frequency and circumstances of daytime wetting:
  Is it with or without urge?
  Before or after micturition?
  Associated with exertion/Valsalva manoevres or with laughter?
  Is wetting constant and unremitting or variable, with some periods of dryness?
The frequency and pattern of bedwetting
The severity of wetting—is it dampness or a full void?
The voiding history should include:
  the frequency and urgency of micturition
  indicators of deferring/suppressing micturition
  the nature of micturition (stream, duration, completeness, and posture)
  ability to initiate voiding at will
  volume of urine passed
The fluid intake should be documented and the amount, type, and the times of drinks recorded
An assessment of behavioural and psychosocial disturbances is essential as these undoubtedly affect bladder function
A psychosocial history to assess the family dynamics and school performance is important
During the clinic consultation a note should be made of the parent–child interaction
It is important to assess the impact of the wetting on both the child and parents, and also to explore the reactions of child and parent to the wetting
If wetting is of secondary onset, an attempt to identify any psychosocial or physical precipitants should be made
Urinary tract infections and the presence of constipation or soiling
Any management prior to the clinic visit, medical and/or surgical, should be noted

Table 9.4 Specific points in the examination of a child with wetting

Perineal sensation, lumbosacral reflexes (bulbocavernosus reflex, anal reflex and tone, standing on toes), asymmetry of buttocks, legs or feet, and gait abnormalities. Signs of occult spinal dysraphism (hairy patch, naevus, sinus, haemangioma, and lipoma over the back) should be looked for
Measurement of blood pressure
Abdominal examination should detect bladder distention or a loaded colon
The ability to express urine by suprapubic pressure should be noted
Presence of skin excoriation over the genitalia, a sign of incontinence, should be recorded
Anatomical abnormalities, namely meatal stenosis, hypospadias, labial and anal anomalies, should be documented
Palpate spine, particularly the sacrum

Parent/child record

A baseline frequency volume chart gives a record of the episodes of wetting and number of voidings in the day and night. If need be, voided volumes may also be documented to estimate functional bladder capacity. Additional items such as fluid intake and bowel actions can also be charted. Remember that these charts are time consuming and intrusive and few people will continue to record all these items for more than a few days.

Investigations

These are summarized in Table 9.5. The purpose of investigations should be to detect important urinary tract pathology and to provide information that will influence management. It is easier to justify the frequent use of simple, harmless, non-invasive investigations than it is to justify the use of investigations that involve venepuncture, catheterization, or the use of ionizing radiation.

The need for investigations will therefore vary, depending on the clinical problem. All children require urinalysis and urine culture but other tests are not always necessary. For a child with straightforward monosymptomatic NE, no other investigation is needed. The same is probably true for a child with classical urge incontinence, although some people choose to undertake renal tract ultrasound. Urinary tract infections are often present in children with voiding dysfunction or detrusor instability and will need investigating appropriately (Chapters 10 and 11). For the child with wetting without urge, or unresponsive to initial attempts at treatment, some further investigation is needed.

Plain abdominal radiographs, which are widely used, are, in our experience, of negligible value, as calculi are uncommon and almost invariably detected on ultrasound, while minor lumbo-sacral anomalies are so common in the normal population that their detection is of little value. The decision to perform detailed urodynamics should be taken on an individual patient basis. In a child with a normal appearance to the bladder and upper urinary tract, in whom non-invasive bladder assessment using ultrasound has documented normal bladder filling and emptying and normal urine flow rates, urodynamic investigation is highly unlikely to reveal useful information.

One circumstance where detailed investigations are often undertaken is in the child who fails to respond to treatment. There is certainly some justification for a more thorough evaluation, but clinicians should be

Table 9.5 Investigation of a child with wetting

Investigation	Indication
Urinalysis (blood, protein, glucose, nitrite, leucocytes)	Screen for urinary tract anomalies and renal disease and UTI in any child with wetting
Ultrasound of renal tract	Screen for urinary tract anomalies in a child with UTI or persistent daytime wetting
Ultrasound of the bladder pre- and post-micturition	Assess bladder emptying in a child with daytime wetting
Urine flow measurement	Evaluate voiding in a child with post-void residual or suspected voiding dysfunction
Urine concentrating capacity	Child in whom polyuria/polydipsia are present
Urodynamics	Detailed evaluation of bladder and urethral function in children with wetting unresponsive to conventional where non-invasive investigations indicate the therapy, or possibility of neuropathic bladder or urethral obstruction
Serum creatinine	Child with polyuria or documented urinary tract disease
Plain X-ray of the abdomen	Screen for spinal anomalies and renal calculi
Overnight urine volume	Bedwetting child with suspected polyuria

UTI, urinary tract infection.

aware that the most common reason for treatment failure is non-adherence to the treatment regime or the presence of substantial psychological or social problems, and urological investigations will not help alleviate these problems!

Daytime wetting

Daytime wetting may occur as a result of a number of different disorders and characterization of the wetting is dependent on the clinical and investigation findings. The most common functional disturbances are shown in Table 9.6 and are subsequently described in detail. Clinical features suggestive of neuropathic bladder are discussed further in Chapter 10 (see Tables 10.1 and 10.2).

Incidence

The prevalence of daytime wetting decreases with age. In a recent longitudinal study of British schoolchildren, 12.5% of 11-year-olds (7% of boys, 16% of girls) and 3% of 15–16-year-olds (5% of girls, 1% of boys) reported occasional daytime wetting [12]. The most common provoking factor was laughter. Approximately half of those wet at 15 years of age had been dry at 11 years. It is likely that a much smaller number of children have regular wetting of sufficient severity to seek treatment. In this study and others, urgency of micturition was the most common urinary symptom.

Table 9.6 Common patterns of daytime wetting

Detrusor overactivity leading to urge incontinence
Dysfunctional voiding
Giggle micturition
True diurnal enuresis

Urge syndrome and urge incontinence

In urge syndrome, the imperative urge to void is caused by overactive detrusor contractions early in the filling phase, countered by voluntary pelvic floor contraction and hold-manoeuvres such as squatting which aim to externally compress the urethra [13,14]. The attacks start towards the latter part of the morning, and increase in frequency and severity over the course of the day with peaks in the afternoon. Some children have a nocturnal component and have loss of urine at night. The bladder capacity is usually small for the child's age, causing an increase in frequency. However, micturition is essentially normal, with complete relaxation of the pelvic floor.

The urge to void is very sudden and the escape of urine can only be countered by the hold manoeuvres. The method of external compression varies from one child to the other; a common one is an asymmetrical squat, first described by Vincent [15] as the 'curtsey sign' wherein the child squats on one foot, with the heel of the foot on the perineum. This is usually sustained until the urge to void has passed. Unfortunately, most children do not succeed completely and this results in a small volume of urine loss, which is involuntary and incomplete. Kondo *et al.* [16], in their experience with over 200 children, described different types of holding postures in children with unstable bladders; younger children used straightforward holding postures, while older children adopted more sophisticated and less recognizable positions. Every child usually possesses two or three holding postures and selects one, depending on the circumstances. It is probably useful for the clinician to suspect an unstable bladder in a child who demonstrates any of these postures.

The urge syndrome is very infrequently seen in boys. The prevalence in girls aged 4–12 years is about 1–3/1000 [13]. The onset of symptoms is usually described as being around the age of 4–5 years, and starts to decrease around puberty and is low in adolescence.

> ## Key points: Characteristics of urge syndrome
>
> - Frequent attacks of imperative urge to void.
> - Attacks increase in frequency during the day, peaking in the afternoon.
> - Hold manoeuvres such as squatting or Vincent's 'curtsey sign' [15].
> - Some children have a nocturnal component.
> - Very infrequently seen in boys.

Consequences of the urge syndrome

Urinary tract infections usually occur in conjunction with the syndrome and may contribute to the persistence and severity of symptoms.

Children with the urge syndrome also have a higher prevalence of *vesico-ureteric reflux* and *reflux nephropathy* [17,18].

The secondary effects on inappropriate postponement of defecation lead to *constipation* and *faecal soiling*. The association of chronic constipation with urinary tract infections is well known and it should be treated aggressively in children with the urge syndrome.

Children with long-standing urge syndrome develop *secondary behavioural problems*. At times these are significant enough for a child to be labelled as having primary behavioural problems with 'psychogenic enuresis' [19]. However, a careful enquiry shows that the behaviour is usually secondary to acceptance and understanding of the incontinence by peers and parents [20].

> ## Key points: Consequences of the urge syndrome
>
> - Urinary tract infection.
> - Vesico-ureteric reflux [17,18].
> - Constipation.
> - Behavioural problems.

Urodynamic findings

The urge to void coincides with unstable detrusor contractions early in the filling phase and these are accompanied by forceful contraction of all pelvic floor muscles, as shown on electromyography [21–23]. The urge to void grows stronger with the amplitude of the detrusor contraction, and the bladder pressure will rise to a very high level.

Management

Bladder retraining. Bladder retraining forms the mainstay of treatment for children with the urge syndrome. The training consists of three components: education, scheduled voiding, and positive reinforcement. The children have to learn to recognize the early sensations of urge and to suppress these by central inhibition rather than by 'holding manoeuvres'. They are also taught to void with a completely relaxed pelvic floor. Biofeedback using electronic or mechanical instruments to provide information to patients about the status of the pelvic floor may also be used.

Anticholinergic medications. Anticholinergic medications are a useful adjunct to bladder retraining, reducing the detrusor overactivity, leading to an increased threshold for the development of unstable detrusor contractions and an increased functional bladder capacity. It should be stressed, however, that medication is not a substitute for bladder retraining and a routine of regular, relaxed voiding.

Oxybutynin is the most widely used, and widely studied, of the anticholinergic medications. Its activity is attributable to its anticholinergic effect, inhibiting the parasympathetic innervation of the detrusor muscle. In addition, it has a direct antispasmodic action on smooth muscle that further inhibits bladder contractions. It also has local anaesthetic properties. Oxybutynin is absorbed rapidly from the gastrointestinal tract and reaches maximum plasma concentrations in less than 1 hour. Maximum effect is seen within 3–4 hours, with some effect still evident at 10 hours. The usual starting dose for children over 5 years is 2.5 mg 2–3 times daily, the last dose given before bed. This dosage can be doubled if not beneficial at the lower dose. Adverse effects such as dry mouth, constipation, blurred vision, nausea, abdominal pain, and facial flushing are common and were reported in 17% of children in one study [24]. As a result of these adverse effects, newer anticholinergic drugs such as tolterodine are now being studied in children. It is also possible that the use of a slow-release (once daily) preparation of oxybutynin will be better tolerated.

Antibiotic prophylaxis. Antibiotic prophylaxis has a definite place in the treatment regime for children with recurrent symptomatic urinary tract infections, but benefits are not proven in children with asymptomatic infection in whom the eradication of UTI does not usually result in improvement of the incontinence.

It is disappointing to find that there are few rigorous, published trials of treatment interventions. In one uncontrolled, long-term follow-up study, Curran *et al.* [25] concluded that incontinence due to idiopathic detrusor instability is amenable to medical management, with 87% of their patients achieving complete resolution or significant improvement in symptoms, although treatment was often needed for several years.

Key points: Management of the urge syndrome

- Bladder retraining:
  - education;
  - scheduled voiding;
  - positive reinforcement.

- Anticholinergic medication.

- Antibiotic prophylaxis.

Dysfunctional voiding

This is probably an abnormal, learned voiding behaviour, often evolving from attempts to suppress impending or active bladder contractions by inappropriately contracting the pelvic floor muscles, thereby tightening the urinary sphincter complex [14,26]. There are several patterns.

Staccato voiding is a peculiar rhythmic voiding pattern caused by bursts of pelvic floor activity during micturition, resulting in peaks in bladder pressure coinciding with interruptions in flow. The pelvic floor contraction is triggered by a flow rate above a certain threshold; once the contraction has reduced the flow rate the pelvic floor relaxes and the flow rate regains the threshold. The flow duration is prolonged and the bladder emptying tends to be incomplete.

Fractionated voiding occurs in several small fractions with incomplete bladder emptying. It is caused by hypoactivity of the detrusor with unsustained detrusor contractions. Abdominal pressure is often exerted to speed the voiding. Increase in abdominal pressure triggers reflex activity of the pelvic floor muscles, resulting in a highly irregular flow rate. The bladder capacity is large for the child's age and the voiding frequency tends to be low and the wetting is a form of overflow incontinence.

Lazy bladder syndrome is the result of long-term dysfunctional voiding. Detrusor contractions are absent secondary to detrusor decompensation and abdominal pressure is the driving force for voiding. The end result is large residual volume of urine and recurrent urinary tract infections.

Key points: Patterns of dysfunctional voiding

- Staccato voiding.

- Fractionated voiding.

- Lazy bladder syndrome.

A variety of unusual urodynamic patterns have been described, but the common denominator is failure to co-ordinate detrusor and sphincter activity. Allen and Bright [22] postulated that these patterns represent persistence of the transitional phase in the development of micturition control, whereby the child learns to prevent wetting by forceful contraction of the external urethral sphincter. They also noted what appeared to be a high incidence of internal stress within the families of many of the children, and suspected that emotional tensions had a major part in the problem.

Vereecken and Proesmans [27] noted urethral instability in 8 of the 15 girls studied with dysfunctional voiding, and highlighted another possible mechanism. They concluded that dysfunctional voiding was not an anomaly of voiding only, but detrusor and pelvic floor structure behaviour throughout bladder filling was often affected as well. Instability of the detrusor was present frequently, but instability of the urethra may also be present.

Farhat et al. [28] developed a dysfunctional voiding symptom score (DVSS), wherein 10 voiding dysfunction parameters were assigned scores of 0–3 according to prevalence, and possible total scores ranging from 0 to 30. This scoring system, in their study, appeared to provide an objective and numerical grading of voiding behaviours of children.

Dysfunctional voiding can disrupt laminar flow of urine through the urethra and lead to 'milk back' of urine from the meatus to the bladder and UTI [29,30]. Infections can increase bladder instability and lead to incontinence. The pelvic floor dysfunction can cause incomplete emptying of the bowel as well, causing constipation and soiling.

Management

Maintenance of a *frequency voiding chart*, which should be the responsibility of the child and not the parent. Girls should be taught to void while sitting on the toilet with their feet resting on the floor and thighs spread, back held straight and tilted slightly forward to provide maximal relaxation of the pelvic floor. This *posture* has been shown to provide maximal relaxation of the pelvic floor [31]. Investigations include uroflowmetry, ultrasonography, and urodynamics.

De Paepe et al. [32] showed that a training programme of *pelvic floor relaxation biofeedback* was effective in treating recurrent UTIs in 83% of girls with urodynamically proven dysfunctional voiding. Porena et al. [33] used voiding biofeedback therapy consisting of pelvic floor electromyography during uroflowmetry and achieved perineal synergy and symptom resolution in patients with detrusor–sphincter dyssynergia. Interactive computer games have also been used for pelvic floor retraining [26]. It must be

appreciated that whatever the technique used for biofeedback, it is important to associate the relaxation and tightening of the voluntary muscles with visual or acoustic signals. Biofeedback appears to reinforce a physiological mechanism that was not completely developed and usually leads to a good outcome.

Simple behavioural therapy without biofeedback techniques is also an effective first-line management strategy for children with daytime wetting, as shown by Weiner et al. [34] Their programme included timed voiding, modification of fluid intake, positive reinforcement techniques, and pelvic floor (Kegel) exercises to promote strengthening and relaxation. The Kegel exercises were used in a previous study [35] and consisted of tightening the pelvic muscles and holding the contraction for 5–10 seconds, followed by a rest period of 5 seconds. Proper use of the exercises was demonstrated with the 'start and stop' technique. Children were instructed to void, starting and then stopping the urinary stream two or three times by means of pelvic contractions. Approximately 74% of patients showed improvement in symptoms during the first year following therapy, and almost 60% of children demonstrated long-term improvement in daytime wetting and a similar proportion documented reduction in urinary tract infections.

Key points: Management of dysfunctional voiding

- Frequency of voiding chart.
- Correct posture for micturition.
- Simple behavioural therapy.
- Biofeedback training.

Giggle incontinence

Wetting associated with laughter, is so common as to be considered normal, provided it is infrequent in occurrence. Laughter may also trigger wetting in children with detrusor instability and in children with voiding dysfunction, particularly the 'lazy bladder syndrome' where laughter, by increasing intraabdominal pressure, may result in stress incontinence. These children will have other urinary symptoms and laughter usually results in a small amount of incontinence. Although it may be a very common condition, the incidence may be underreported because the individuals affected often change their social life to avoid embarrassment. In a study by Glahn [36], of the 99 student nurses questioned, nearly a quarter had experienced 'giggle incontinence' at some time, and in 10% it had persisted beyond the age of 20 years.

True giggle incontinence refers to involuntary complete bladder emptying induced by giggling or laughing. Full-scale micturition is triggered by laughter and it cannot be stopped, until the bladder is empty. It has been suggested to occur only with certain types of laughter, namely giggle or suppressed, on the one hand, and excited wild laughter, on the other.

MacKeith [37] first coined the term 'giggle micturition' to separate this condition from other causes of incontinence induced by laughter. Although it can occur in both sexes, it is more common in females. It typically starts before the onset of puberty, is most common during school age and tends to improve or disappear with increasing age. However, it may persist into adult life [38]. There may be a family history of a similar or related disorder.

The exact pathophysiology of giggle incontinence is not known. Neurological examination, EEG studies and urodynamics have not shown any obvious abnormalities; there are no reports in the literature where urodynamics were obtained during uncontrolled laughter. It is possible that it may be caused by a CNS disorder. Rogers *et al.* [39] reported two cases of giggle incontinence; one patient was shown to have a convulsive disorder together with giggle incontinence and anticonvulsant therapy prevented the incontinence; the second patient had a cystometrogram performed while she was laughing. This demonstrated bladder tetany with off-scale ($>100\,cm\,H_2O$) high pressure, in contrast to lower transient increases associated with 'stress manoeuvres'. This second patient also had a sensation of numbness in the suprapubic area and both upper thighs for a few seconds before the onset of laughter and incontinence.

Management of this distressing condition is difficult. To curb one's sense of humour and maintain a straight face may not always be practical. Brocklebank and Meadow [40] reported cure in two patients treated. It was not clear, however, how much of the success was due to the general sympathetic and confidence-building measures used, advice about posture (one patient wet himself only if he laughed vigorously while standing, but remained dry if he laughed sitting; he was advised to sit down if he started to laugh), or to the drug propantheline.

Sher and Reinberg [41] used methylphenidate to treat seven patients with giggle incontinence, and reported continence in all during treatment with 1–5 years of follow-up. There is an association of laughter-induced generalized or localized muscular hypotonia in cataplexy and possibly in giggle incontinence, which led them to consider a common pathophysiological basis for the two conditions. The positive clinical outcome in their patients suggested that giggle incontinence was a centrally mediated, and likely hereditary, disorder, which may be related to a receptor-mediated imbalance of cholinergic and monoaminergic systems.

Self-administration of a harmless, painless electric shock to the back of one hand, at the moment when micturition was induced by laughter, led to inhibition of the voiding reflex, and later replacing the electric shock by an imaginary shock was used to treat children with enuresis risoria [42]. Wetting was diminished by about 80% and, although none of the children became totally dry, all children benefited from the programme, by a reduction of the wetting incidents and emotionally, by gaining more self-confidence and self-esteem.

Diurnal enuresis

This is seen more commonly in boys who delay emptying their bladder until it becomes too late. Urgency is therefore uncommon and when they are wet it is often a complete bladder emptying. Voiding is infrequent but otherwise normal. In these children, with essentially normal bladder function, psychological disorders are common. Management involves behaviour modification and encouragement of a timelier pattern of voiding.

Pollakiuria: extraordinary daytime urinary frequency

Pollakiuria [43–45] (*pollakis*: Greek, often) is a benign, self-limiting condition, characterized by urination as often as every 5–20 minutes and occurs during the waking hours only. It is seen most commonly in pre-school children who have been toilet trained and is not associated with incontinence. Although more than 80% of children in one series presented in the cold weather, others have not found any particular relationship between the season and the occurrence of symptoms.

The exact aetiology of this condition remains unknown. Some kind of anxiety-producing situations, such as fear of death and other stresses, have been noted in some patients, although the causal relationship is difficult to prove.

Typically, patients present with sudden onset of daytime frequency and there is no associated dysuria; symptoms of nocturia or nocturnal frequency are usually absent. Physical examination and urinalysis are essentially normal. The condition is self-limited and usually lasts for 1–4 weeks. Invasive investigations are not warranted, but an ultrasound to rule out upper-tract pathology may be justified in some patients.

Treatment with anticholinergics or antibiotics have not been shown to have any benefit; reassurance of the parent and child is all that is necessary. If a precipitating factor is uncovered at the clinic visit or subsequently, a sympathetic discussion may help alleviate anxiety. Whether this actually contributes to resolution of symptoms remains a matter of debate.

In conclusion, pollakiuria is an easily recognizable condition, which can be managed without expensive invasive investigations, reassuring the family of the benign nature of the condition and awaiting spontaneous resolution.

Urofacial (Ochoa) syndrome

This is a rare autosomal recessive disorder characterized by abnormal facial expression and urinary abnormalities [46–48]. The gene has been mapped on chromosome 10q23–q24. The children have enuresis and urinary tract infection in association with 'inversion' of facial expression when laughing, so that they appear to be crying when they smile. Urodynamic studies show features of mild neuropathic bladder and urinary tract damage. Some of the affected children also have constipation. This facial expression is so characteristic that it is possible to identify most, if not all, of the patients with an underlying neuropathic bladder

and start treatment before damage to the urinary tract occurs. The treatment is essentially the same as that described above for the different types of voiding dysfunction, namely a combination of bladder retraining, anticholinergics, and prophylactic antibiotics.

Nocturnal enuresis

Bedwetting refers to children who wet when asleep; this is usually at night but can also occur during daytime naps. By far the most common cause of bedwetting is nocturnal enuresis (NE). Other rare causes of bedwetting are shown in Table 9.7.

In the past, NE was essentially a diagnosis of exclusion, being defined as regular bedwetting in a child over 5 years, in the absence of neurological disease or structural abnormalities of the urinary tract. The current International Children's Continence Society definition (see Table 9.1) is a more precise definition of NE that takes into account our current understanding of the different causes of bedwetting [14]. This definition, by emphasizing that the wetting is a normal voiding while asleep in a child with a normal bladder, allows the clinician to make a positive diagnosis and avoids the pitfall of including children with other conditions, such as detrusor overactivity or dysfunctional voiding. Unfortunately, at the time of writing there is no definition that has been uniformly adopted. One reason for this may be that the ICCS definition is less easy to use for epidemiological studies.

Epidemiology

Bedwetting is a common problem with a high prevalence reported in the international literature. The widely quoted prevalence in the United Kingdom and important epidemiological data are shown in Table 9.8. Other countries report a similar prevalence.

Table 9.7 Conditions that cause bedwetting

Diagnosis	Clinical indicators
Urinary tract infection	Other urinary tract symptoms, secondary onset wetting
Neuropathic bladder	Constant severe daytime wetting, soiling, lumbosacral dimple or naevus, abnormal gait, abnormal perianal or lower-limb neurology, palpable bladder
Posterior urethral valves	Poor urinary stream, daytime wetting, palpable bladder
Ectopic ureter	A constant dribble of urine between voidings
Detrusor instability	Daytime symptoms of urinary frequency, urgency, and urge incontinence usually with a minor degree of wetness and worse in the afternoons
Chronic renal disease	Chronic ill health, hypertension, palpable kidneys or bladder, anaemia, polydipsia
Diabetes mellitus	Recent illness with weight loss, thirst, and polydipsia

Table 9.8 Epidemiology of nocturnal enuresis

Prevalence [49]
  15–20% of 5-year-olds
  5% of 10-year-olds
  1–2% of 15-year-olds
Boys are affected more frequently than girls
Between the ages of 5 and 18 years 15% of enuretics
  become dry each year *without treatment*
25% have daytime wetting in addition to bedwetting
Onset wetting accounts for 20% of cases of bedwetting
<3% of children referred to an enuresis clinic have an
  identifiable 'organic' disorder [50]

Aetiology/trigger factors

Many factors have been shown to be associated with the presence of enuresis. It has long been recognized that there is a *genetic predisposition* to NE. As many as 75% of affected children will have an affected first-degree relative, there is a greater concordance for the presence of NE in monozygotic compared to dizygotic twins, and linkage analysis of several families with enuresis indicates an 'enuresis gene' on chromosome 13q [51–53]. Early life events are also important, with growth retardation *in utero* and the absence of breast-feeding increasing the incidence of NE [54]. Social factors also play a part, with low social class, paternal unemployment, and 'stressful life events', particularly between 2 and 3 years, also predisposing to NE.

Most children become dry at night by 5 years of age. This appears to be the age at which bladder capacity first exceeds nocturnal urine production and hence in most instances the children are able to hold their urine all night without the need to wake up [55]. In children with NE a number of *physiological abnormalities* have been identified that explain their predisposition to wetting.

In contrast to normal individuals, children and young adults with enuresis may have *relative nocturnal polyuria*, in that they produce a greater amount of urine than their bladder capacity overnight and lack the nocturnal reduction in urine production. This polyuria is associated with a loss of the normal nocturnal increase in vasopressin secretion [56,57]. Furthermore, the nocturnal urine output has been shown to be greater on nights that the child is wet than on a dry night. This pattern is usually present in those with monosymptomatic NE. In children with voiding dysfunction, nocturnal polyuria has also been reported, but is associated with increased sodium and water losses at night, suggesting a different cause [58].

Children with NE have been shown to wet when their bladder reaches close to its functional capacity and the wetting episode is a normal co-ordinated micturition [59]. Although their bladders appear normal, as a group they tend to have *smaller functional bladder capacities*, and on urodynamic testing it may be easier to provoke *unstable detrusor contractions*. For children with daytime symptoms, and in some children with resistant enuresis, overt detrusor instability may be demonstrated [60].

Parents will often state that their bedwetting child is a 'deep sleeper' and difficult to wake, and it is evident that few bedwetting children wake when they wet at night. However, non-enuretic children are rarely required to wake at night, and achieve dryness not by waking to void, but by lasting until morning. Furthermore, fluid challenging non-enuretic children may provoke enuretic episodes. Overnight EEG studies have shown that wetting episodes occur in all stages of sleep and are not associated with the deepest levels of sleep [61]. Shortly before the voiding, children demonstrate a variable degree of arousal associated with increased pelvic floor muscle activity, but fail to fully awaken or to inhibit the micturition reflex. In comparison to age-matched non-enuretic children, bedwetting children are less likely to wake to a noise stimulus [62]. It thus appears that although sleep is essentially normal, *poor arousability* in a child whose bladder has become full is a contributing factor.

Key points: Aetiological/trigger factors in nocturnal enuresis

- Genetic factors [51–53].

- Early life events [54]:
  – growth retardation *in utero*;
  – absence of breast-feeding.

- Social factors:
  – low social class;
  – paternal unemployment;
  – 'stressful life events'.

- Physiological factors:
  – nocturnal polyuria;
  – small functional bladder capacity;
  – detrusor instability;
  – poor arousability.

Management strategies

A great variety of treatments have been used over the years on children with bedwetting. Few, however, have been shown to actually work! Nocturnal enuresis is a condition where most children get dry over time without any intervention, and with this background and the 'placebo effect' of being assessed, monitored, and given a treatment by a sympathetic clinician, means that almost any treatment is likely to result in some improvement.

Recently, there have been several high-quality systematic reviews of interventions, focusing on information from randomized, controlled trials. These reviews thus form the basis from which the true value of many interventions can be assessed [63–66].

There are a number of *simple behavioural interventions* for which good-quality evidence of effectiveness is lacking, but which are at worst harmless and at best appear to improve effectiveness of treatment in the eyes of a large body of professionals. *Star Charts*, rewarding dry nights or helpful behaviour may be beneficial and appear to help motivation if used properly. *Retention control training* is aimed at enhancing bladder capacity, but there is no evidence that it is helpful. There is no evidence that *fluid restriction* is helpful, but it seems sensible to avoid excessive fluid intake before bedtime. *Increasing daytime fluids* may encourage the development of a good bladder capacity and reduce the likelihood of excessive fluid intake in the evening. There is no good evidence it is helpful but it is a 'healthy living' measure. *Lifting* may help achieve dry nights but there is little evidence that it works on its own. It is best combined with waking, in order to avoid training the child to void in their sleep! *Waking*, as for lifting, may be helpful as part of a 'dry bed training regime'. *Treatment of constipation* demonstrated benefit in one uncontrolled trial in children with voiding dysfunction.

There are only two *drugs* with good evidence of effectiveness in NE: desmopressin and imipramine.

Desmopressin (DDAVP®; 1-deamino-8-D-arginine vasopressin) is a synthetic analogue of human arginine vasopressin (AVP) and acts by binding to V2 receptors in the renal tubules and collecting system, leading to an increase in water permeability and thus water reabsorption, leading to smaller volumes of more concentrated urine being produced. DDAVP® is available as a nasal spray or in tablet form. Both formulations have been compared in a double-blind crossover trial and shown to be equally effective. Although only about 10% of a nasal dose is absorbed,

it is absorbed quickly and reaches maximum plasma concentration about 40–55 minutes after dosage. Its half-life is 4–6 hours, with the duration of action of around 10–12 hours. AVP is degraded principally by the liver, kidney, brain, and within plasma, and DDAVP® is probably eliminated in a similar way.

Desmopressin is most effective in children with monosymptomatic NE and particularly if there is nocturnal polyuria and lower nocturnal AVP levels. Other good prognostic factors include: those with less severe enuresis, those with large functional bladder capacities, and those with primary, rather than secondary enuresis. Unfavourable social and psychological factors are associated with treatment failure, as is the presence of daytime wetting.

Overall, desmopressin improves the wetting in about 65–80%, typically by 1–2 dry nights per week, but only 46% will be completely dry. Patients treated with desmopressin are 4.6 times more likely to achieve 14 consecutive dry nights compared with placebo [63,65]. When treatment is stopped, relapse is likely, as the placebo-controlled trials show that DDAVP®-treated patients had no lasting benefit. Those who do not respond may have a different pathophysiology to their bedwetting, such as detrusor instability. DDAVP® has been compared directly with alarm treatment (see below). There is a faster initial response (in the first 3 weeks) with DDAVP®, but a much higher relapse rate when drug treatment is withdrawn [67].

The starting dose for the nasal spray is 20 µg at night (0.2 mg for the tablets). This starting dose is used irrespective of the age of the child. The dose can be doubled if there is a poor response to the lower dose. DDAVP® can be prescribed initially for 3 months to assess response. It can be used for much longer periods if successful. Clearly, though, intervals off the treatment are needed from time to time to see if the child has become dry. It is well tolerated with few side-effects. There are a small number of case reports of hyponatraemic convulsions and cerebral oedema, and so patients should be advised to avoid excessive fluid intake in the evening or overnight. Mild asymptomatic hyponatraemia may develop in 1–10% of patients on DDAVP® for primary enuresis [68].

Imipramine is the best studied of the tricyclic antidepressants. The mode of action is not clear as the drug has anticholinergic effects and seems to have central effects on sleep level and perception, making arousal from sleep with a full bladder more possible. In addition, imipramine has an antidiuretic effect. Imipramine is rapidly and completely absorbed orally and has an active metabolite, desmethylimipramine. The mean half-life is about 18 hours but there is significant inter-patient variation.

In the short term, patients treated with imipramine and other tricyclic antidepressants are five times more likely to achieve 14 consecutive dry nights compared to placebo, a similar degree of improvement as that seen with desmopressin. Overall, about 60% improve but only 40% become dry. As with DDAVP®, there is a high relapse rate off treatment [63,66]. Overall, there is no significant difference in effectiveness in the trials of imipramine and the trials of DDAVP®, but there have been no large-scale trials comparing the two drugs directly.

The dose of imipramine is age/weight determined and should not exceed 2.5 mg/kg. It should be taken as a single dose at bedtime. It is often most effective taken 2–3 hours before bedtime, particularly if wetting occurs in the first few hours of sleep. The maximum period of treatment should not exceed 3 months (including slow withdrawal).

Imipramine has many common side-effects; these include anticholinergic effects such as dry mouth, constipation, visual disturbance, and urinary retention. Central side-effects, such as nausea, tremor, confusion, insomnia, agitation, or sedation, are also reported, as well as disturbance in cognitive function. However, the major concern with this group of drugs is accidental poisoning. Tricyclics are clearly cardiotoxic and potentially lethal in overdose, but there is little hard evidence of danger at therapeutic doses used in enuresis. Because it is hepatically metabolized and highly protein bound, there are many drugs that interact with imipramine.

Because of the adverse effects, most practitioners are reluctant to prescribe imipramine as a first-line treatment for NE.

Oxybutynin is the most widely used of the anticholinergic drugs. The only controlled trial to date failed to demonstrate a positive effect above placebo in monosymptomatic nocturnal enuresis [24]. It may, however, have a role in bedwetting when there are significant daytime symptoms suggesting bladder instability, and in children with monosymptomatic NE unresponsive to other treatment. In one study, patients with diurnal voiding disturbances and bedwetting had a 71% 'success rate' with DDAVP® and oxybutynin combined [69].

Enuresis alarm based treatments

The enuresis alarm is an alarm that is triggered when urine comes in contact with a sensor. The alarm is a conditioning device, using a noise to link the stimulus of a full bladder beginning to void with the desired behaviour of inhibiting micturition and waking (classical conditioning). Rewards for using the alarm may enhance its effectiveness (operant conditioning) and in a few children the unpleasantness of treatment may also contribute to its effectiveness (aversive conditioning). Physiologically, the alarm results in waking, contraction of the pelvic floor, and inhibition of the micturition reflex. Over a period of weeks and months children become dry; in most instances this occurs not by learning to wake, but by holding on until the morning.

Enuresis alarms have consistently been shown to be the most effective treatment in terms of 'cure'. Typically 60–70% of children with NE will become dry and at least two-thirds of these will remain dry after treatment [63,64]. There is, however, a high drop-out rate from treatment, reflecting its arduous, protracted, and demanding nature. Alarm treatment is therefore usually combined with star charts, rewards, and frequent contact with a supportive professional. Thus, alarm therapy is not suitable for all children. Over the past 40 years there have been many changes in the design and technology of alarms, but there is no evidence that this has improved success rates of treatment.

A combination of the alarm and desmopressin, where the desmopressin is used for the first 6 weeks only, has been shown to improve the overall success rate compared to the alarm alone. The benefits are greatest in children with severe enuresis, who do least well with the alarm alone [70].

Dry bed training refers to a multidimensional training programme that combines an enuresis alarm with waking regimes, positive practice routines, and cleanliness training. The main advantage over an enuresis alarm is a more rapid achievement of dryness. A number of modified versions of the regime also exist and it is recognized that the enuresis alarm is the single most important component of the regime. Overall there is probably no greater success rate than using the alarm on its own [64].

Other treatments

Acupuncture, chiropractic, hypnotherapy, and homeopathy have all been used for the treatment of enuresis. None of these treatments have been evaluated rigorously and it is thus difficult to comment on their effectiveness.

Table 9.9 Management strategy for nocturnal enuresis

Under 5 years	Explanation, reassurance and simple advice
5–7 years	Star charts and rewards, consider enuresis alarm/desmopressin if the impact of wetting is sufficient
Over 7 years	For monosymptomatic NE the choice lies between alarm and a trial of desmopressin. The alarm is most likely to effect a cure. If there are symptoms of detrusor instability, consider treatment of daytime wetting first or desmopressin combined with oxybutynin. If an alarm is being used, consider combining with desmopressin if adverse prognostic factors are present.

A management strategy for nocturnal enuresis

Explanation and information are an essential component of management. The precise treatment will differ between patients because the nature, severity, impact of wetting, and attitudes towards treatment, will vary. Nevertheless, in most instances the strategy shown in Table 9.9 is appropriate.

Key points: Management of nocturnal enuresis

- There are a number of simple behavioural interventions, for which good-quality evidence of effectiveness is lacking; nevertheless a large number of professionals feel that they are effective.

- Desmopressin and imipramine are the only drugs with good evidence of effectiveness in NE.

- Enuresis alarms have been shown consistently to be the most effective treatments in terms of 'cure'. Typically 60–70% of children with NE will become dry and at least two-thirds of these will remain dry after treatment.

- A combination of alarm and desmopressin increases the overall success rate.

- Dry bed training achieves dryness more rapidly, but overall the success is no greater than with the alarm on its own.

- Unfavourable social and psychological factors and daytime wetting are associated with treatment failure.

References

1. Moore KL, Persaud TVN (eds) Before we are born. Essentials of Embryology and Birth Defects, 5th Edition, W.B.Saunders Company, Philadelphia, 1998.
2. McMinn RMH (ed.) Last's Anatomy Regional and Applied, 9th Edition, Churchill Livingstone, Edinburgh, 1994.
3. Bhatia NN, Bradley WE. Neuroanatomy and physiology: innervation of the urinary tract. In Raz S (ed.): Female Urology, WB Saunders, Philadelphia, 1983, pp. 12–32.
4. de Groat WC. Anatomy and physiology of the lower urinary tract. Urol Clin North Am 1993; 20, 3: 383–401.
5. Blok BFM, Holstege G. The central control of micturition and continence: implications for urology. BJU International 1999; 83, Suppl. 2: 1–6.
6. Butler RJ. Nocturnal Enuresis: The Child's Experience, Butterworth-Heinmann, Oxford, 1994.
7. Jarvelin MR, Vikevainin-Teronen L, Moilanen I, Huttunen NP. Life changes and protective capacities in enuretic and non-enuretic children. J Child Psychol. Psychiatry 1990; 31: 763–774.
8. Von Gontard A, Lehmkuhl K, Mauer-Mucke, Rassouli R. Association of child psychiatric diagnoses with different forms of enuresis/incontinence. International Children's Continence Society Monograph Series No 1 1995: 55–59.
9. Anonymous. My enuresis. Arch Dis Child 1987; 62: 866–868.
10. Paesbrugge S, Theunis M, Van Hoecke E, Raes A, Hoebeke P, Vande Walle J. Self image and performance in children with nocturnal enuresis. Proceedings of the The International Children's Continence Society, 1999 Abs 35.
11. Moffatt MEK, Kato C, Pless IB. Improvements in self concept after treatment of nocturnal enuresis: a randomised controlled trial. J Pediatr 1987; 110: 647–652.
12. Swithinbank LV, Brookes ST, Shepherd AM, Abrams P. The natural history of urinary symptoms during adolescence. BJU 1998; 81, Suppl. 3: 90–93.
13. Van Gool JD, De Jonge GA. Urge syndrome and urge incontinence. Arch Dis Child 1989; 64: 1629–1634.
14. Norgaard JP, Van Gool JD, Hjalmas K, Djurhuus, Hellstrom AL. Standardization and definitions in lower urinary tract dysfunction in children. BJU 1998; 81, Suppl. 3: 1–16.
15. Vincent SA. Postural control of urinary incontinence: the curtsey sign. Lancet, 1966; ii: 631–632.
16. Kondo A, Kato K, Takita T, Otani T. Holding postures characteristic of unstable bladder. J Urol 1985, 134: 702–704.
17. Taylor CM, Corkery JJ, White RHR. Micturition symptoms and unstable bladder activity in girls with primary vesicoureteric reflux. Br J Urol 1982, 54: 494–498.
18. Koff SA, Lapides J, Piazza DH. Association of urinary tract infection and reflux with uninhibited bladder contractions and voluntary sphincter obstruction. J Urol 1979, 122: 373–376.

19. Hinman F Jr. Nonneurogenic neurogenic bladder (the Hinman syndrome)—15 years later. J Urol 1986; 136: 769–777.

20. Millard RJ, Oldenburg BF. The symptomatic, urodynamic and psychodynamic results of bladder re-education programs. J Urol 1983, 130: 715–719.

21. Van Gool JD, Tanagho EA. External sphincter activity and recurrent urinary tract infection in girls. Urology 1977; 10: 34–53.

22. Allen TD, Bright TL. Urodynamic patterns in children with dysfunctional voiding problems. J Urol 1978; 119: 247–249.

23. Borzyskowski M, Mundy AR. Videourodynamic assessment of diurnal urinary incontinence. Arch Dis Child 1987; 62: 128–131.

24. Lovering JS, Tallett SE, McKendry JB. Oxybutynin efficacy in the treatment of primary enuresis. Pediatrics 1988; 82: 104–106.

25. Curran MJ, Kaefer M, Peters C, Logigian E, Bauer SB. The overactive bladder in childhood: Long-term result with conservative management. J Urol 2000; 163: 574–577.

26. McKenna PH, Herndon CD, Connery S et al. Pelvic floor muscle retraining for pediatric voiding dysfunction using interactive computer games. J Urol 1999; 162: 1056.

27. Vereecken RL, Proesmans RL. Urethral instability as an important element of dysfunctional voiding. J Urol 2000; 163: 585–588.

28. Farhat W, Bagli DJ, Capolicchio G, O'Reilly S, Merguerian PA, Khoury A, McLorie GA. The dysfunctional voiding scoring system: Quantitative standardization of dysfunctional voiding symptoms in children. J Urol 2000, 164: 1011–1015.

29. Tanagho EA, Miller EA, Lyon RP. Spastic striated external sphincter and urinary tract infections in girls. Br J Urol 1971; 43: 69–82.

30. Van Gool JD, Tanagho EA. External sphincter activity and recurrent urinary tract infection in girls. Urology 1977; 10: 384–387.

31. Wennegren HM, Oberg BE, Sandstedt P. The importance of leg support for relaxation of the pelvic-floor muscles. Scand J Urol Nephrol 1991, 25: 205–13.

32. De Paepe H, Hoebeke P, Renson C, Van Laecke E, Raes A, Van Hoecke E, Van Daele J, Vande Walle J. Pelvic-floor therapy in girls with recurrent urinary tract infections and dysfunctional voiding. Br J Urol 1998; 81, Suppl. 3: 109–113.

33. Porena M, Costantini E, Rociola W, Mearini E. Biofeedback successfully cures detrusor–sphincter dyssynergia in paediatric patients. J Urol 2000; 163: 1927–1931.

34. Weiner JS, Scales MT, Hampton J, King LR, Surwit R, Edwards CL. Long-term efficacy of simple behavioral therapy for daytime wetting in children. J Urol 2000; 164: 786–790.

35. Schneider MS, King LR, Surwit RS. Kegel exercises and childhood incontinence: a new role for an old treatment. J Pediatr 1994; 124: 91–92.

36. Glahn BE. Giggle incontinence (enuresis risoria). A study and an aetiological hypothesis. Br J Urol 1979; 51: 363–366.

37. MacKeith RC. Micturition induced by giggling. Guy's Hospital Reports, 1964; 113: 250–260.

38. Giggle incontinence. Lancet 1982; 1, 1(8279): 1000–1001.

39. Rogers MP, Gittes RF, Dawson DM, Reich P. Giggle incontinence. JAMA 1982 Mar 12; 247(10): 1446–1448.

40. Brocklebank JT, Meadow SR. Cure of giggle micturition. Arch Dis Child. 1981 March; 56(3): 232–234.

41. Sher PK, Reinberg Y. Successful treatment of giggle incontinence with methylphenidate. J Urol 1996; 156: 656–658.

42. Elzinga-Plomp A, Boemers TML, Messer AP, Vijverberg, DeJong TPVM, Van Gool JD. Treatment of enuresis risoria in children by self-administered electric and imaginary shock. Br J Urol 1995; 76: 775–778.

43. Asnes PS, Mones AL. Pollakiuria. Pediatrics 1973; 52: 615–617.

44. Bass LW. Pollakiuria, extraordinary daytime urinary frequency: Experience in a pediatric practice. Pediatrics 1991; 87: 735–737.

45. Walker J, Rickwood AMK. Daytime urinary frequency in children. BMJ 1988; 297: 455.

46. Ochoa B, Gorlin RJ. Urofacial (ochoa) syndrome. Am J Med Genet 1987; 27(3): 661–667.

47. Wang CY, Hawkins-Lee B, Ochoa B, Walker RD, She JX. Homozygosity and linkage-disequilibrium mapping of the urofacial (Ochoa) syndrome gene to a 1-cM interval on chromosome 10q23–q24. Am J Med Genet 1997; 60(6): 1461–1467.

48. Ochoa B. The urofacial (Ochoa) syndrome revisited. J Urol 1992, 148: 580–583.

49. Blackwell C, Dobson P, eds. A guide to enuresis. Enuresis Resource and Information Centre, Bristol, 1995.

50. Forsythe WI, Redmond A. Enuresis and spontaneous cure rate. Arch Dis Child 1974; 49: 259–263.

51. Bakwin H. Enuresis in twins. Am J Dis Child 1971; 121: 222–225.

52. Bakwin H. The genetics of enuresis. Clin Dev Med 1973; 48/49: 73–77.

53. Eiberg H, Berendt I, Mohr J. Assignment of dominant inherited nocturnal enuresis (ENUR1) to chromosome 13q. Nat Genet 1995; 10: 354–356.

54. Jarvelin MR. Developmental history and neurological findings in enuretic children. Dev Med Child Neurol 1989; 31: 728–736.

55. Vande Walle J, Hoebeke P, Van Laecke E, Castillo D, Milicic D, Maraina C, Hussein C, Raes A. Persistent enuresis caused by polyuria is a maturation defect of the nycthemeral rhythm of diuresis. Br J Urol 1998; 81, Suppl. 3: 40–45.

56. Norgaard JP, Pedersen EB, Djurhuus JC. Diurnal antidiuretic hormone levels in enuretics. J Urol 1985; 134: 1029–1031.

57. Rittig S, Knudsen UB, Norgaard JP, Pedersen EB, Djurhuus JC. Abnormal diurnal rhythm of plasma vasopressin and urine output in patients with enuresis. Am J Physiol 1989; 256: 664–671.

58. Vande Walle J, Thijs J, Dehoorne J, Raes A, Van Laecke E, Hoebeke P. Nocturnal polyuria associated to bladder dysfunction is rather related to an abnormal

nycthermeral rhythm of renal function and salt handling than to a vasopressin related concentration disorder. Proceedings of the The International Children's
Continence Society, 1999; Abs. 15.

59. Noorgard JP, Hansen JH, Willdschiotz G. Cysto-
metries in children with nocturnal enuresis. J Urol
1989; 141: 1156–1159.

60. Medel R, Ruarte AC, Castera R, Podesta ML.
Primary enuresis: a urodynamic evaluation. Br J Urol
1998; 81, Suppl. 3: 50–52.

61. Hunsballe JM, Rittig S, Djurhuus JC. Sleep and
arousal in adolescents and adults with nocturnal
enuresis. Scan J Urol Nephrol 1995; 173, Suppl.
59–61.

62. Wolfish NM. Sleeping patterns and their effects on the
etiology and treatment of nocturnal enuresis. Can
Enuresis J 1996; 5: 5–7.

63. Houts AC, Berman JS, Abramson H. Effectiveness of
psychological and pharmaceutical treatments for nocturnal enuresis. J Consult Clin Psychol 1994; 62:
737–745.

64. Lister-Sharpe D, O'Meara S, Bradley M, Sheldon TA.
A Systematic review of the effectiveness of interven-
tions for managing childhood nocturnal enuresis,
CRD Report 11. University of York, NHS Centre for
Reviews and Disseminations 1977.

65. Glazener CMA, Evans JHC. Desmopressin for nocturnal enuresis in children (Cochrane Review). The
Cochrane Library, Issue 2. Update Software, Oxford,
2000.

66. Glazener CMA, Evans JHC. Tricyclic and related
drugs for nocturnal enuresis in children (Cochrane
Review). The Cochrane Library, Issue 2. Update
Software, Oxford, 2000.

67. Wille S. Comparison of desmopressin and enuresis
alarm for nocturnal enuresis. Arch Dis Child 1986;
69: 30–33.

68. Robson W, Norgaard J, Leung A. Hyponatraemia in
patients with nocturnal enuresis treated with desmopressin. Eur J Pediatr 1996; 155: 959–62.

69. Caione P, Arena F, Biraghi M, Cigna RM, Chendi D,
Chiozza ML, De Lisa A, De Grazia E, Fano M,
Formica P, Garofalo S, Gramenzi R, von Heland M,
Lanza P, Lanza T, Maffei S, Manieri C, Merlini E,
Miano L, Nappo S, Pagliarulo A, Paolini Paoletti F,
Pau AC, Porru D, Artibani W *et al.* Nocturnal enure-
sis and daytime wetting: a multicentric trial with
oxybutinin and desmopressin. Eur Urol 1997; 31:
459–463.

70. Bradbury MG, Meadow SR. Combined treatment
with enuresis alarm and desmopressin for nocturnal
enuresis. Acta Paediatr 1995; 84: 1014–1018.

Neuropathic bladder: identification, investigation, and management

Malgorzata Borzyskowski

Introduction

There are many causes of incontinence in childhood, including neuropathic bladder. Thus, when assessing a child with wetting it is important to consider this possibility. The causes of a neuropathic bladder are numerous and include open and closed spina bifida, sacral agenesis, spinal cord tumour and trauma, transverse myelitis, and autonomic neuropathy. In a small group in whom a cause is not found, the bladder behaves as though there is a neurological problem with all the same risks to the kidneys (occult neuropathic bladder).

Children with neuropathic bladder may have many other problems which need to be addressed when planning management. This has to take into account the child's deformities, orthopaedic, manipulative and intellectual problems, and motivation. However, a significant number will have only a minor neurological deficit or none at all, so that the neuropathic bladder is their major handicap. This in itself can lead to delayed diagnosis and psychological problems in the child, who appears physically normal.

The management has changed greatly in the past 25 years and has been influenced by the advent of video-urodynamic studies (VUDs) to assess bladder and urethral function, which in turn has led to a greater understanding of the pathophysiology and natural history of this condition. The introduction of clean intermittent catheterization (CIC) by Lapides *et al.* in 1972 [1], availability of various pharmacological agents, reconstructive bladder surgery, and the artificial urinary sphincter (AUS) have all played their part in the improved management and have resulted in preservation of renal function, improved continence, and enhanced quality of life. It also means that management can be tailored to each child's needs and factors that are dangerous to the kidneys can be identified early.

Despite the introduction of antenatal screening and the recognition of the role of preconception folic acid in the prevention of neural tube defects, spina bifida, open and closed, remains the most common cause of the neuropathic bladder in childhood. We are still seeing a significant number of children born each year with spina bifida, particularly with closed lesions, where the diagnosis is often not made antenatally and may not be made until the child presents with urinary tract infections, voiding difficulties, or incontinence, by which time there may be renal damage.

Clinical assessment

Children who are referred to a specialist service because of incontinence can usually be divided into three categories:

1. The child who presents mainly with incontinence, in whom it is important to exclude a neuropathic bladder. This group will include those in whom closed spina bifida and sacral agenesis have not previously been diagnosed, and the child with the so-called occult neuropathic bladder in whom the bladder behaves as though there were a neurological abnormality, although none can be detected. However, the vast majority of the children in this group are neurologically normal and do not have a neuropathic bladder, although it is obviously important to ensure that they do not have a structural abnormality such as an ectopic ureter. It is also important to remember that the child who has developmental delay will not achieve continence until the appropriate developmental stage is reached.

2. The child who has an overt spinal problem such as spina bifida, spinal cord tumour, or trauma.

3. The child who is at risk of bladder problems, for example the child with anorectal anomaly, cerebral palsy, or transverse myelitis.

It is therefore crucial that in any child presenting with incontinence, a thorough history and examination are undertaken.

History and examination

A careful and thorough history will pay dividends and should focus on factors related to acquisition of continence and micturition (see p. 165). It is important to exclude congenital abnormalities of the urinary tract, such as ectopic ureter (which will be suggested by constant daytime wetting), and developmental abnormalities. Family history and social factors are also obviously important. Enquiry should be made about factors associated with a neuropathic bladder (Table 10.1). The specific features that should be addressed in the examination are summarized in Chapter 9 (p. 166).

Worrying features in the clinical assessment that might lead one to suspect a neuropathic bladder are shown in Table 10.2. Any child with these features requires further assessment and investigation to exclude a neuropathic bladder. In the first instance this should include pre- and post-micturition renal and bladder ultrasonography, assessment of bladder

Table 10.1   Associations of neuropathic bladder

Family history of any type of spina bifida
Maternal pre-gestational insulin-dependent diabetes
  (associated with sacral agenesis)
Maternal anticonvulsant therapy in pregnancy
Talipes equinovarus

Table 10.2   Clinical features suggestive of a neuropathic bladder

Poor or impaired urinary stream
Straining to pass urine
Impaired/lack of bladder sensation
Small urine volumes
Continual dribbling
Infrequent micturition
Impaired bladder emptying
Recurrent urinary tract infections
Abnormality of the spine
Abnormality of the lower limbs
Associated constipation

and urethral function by means of a VUD, postero anterior and lateral X-rays of the lumbo-sacral spine, or, if the facility is available, a magnetic resonance imaging (MRI) scan of the whole spine to exclude a spinal cord abnormality.

If an abnormality is found on the MRI scan, the child needs referral to a neurologist or a neurosurgeon and the bladder and kidneys need to be investigated and managed in the same way as in those children with an obvious neuropathic bladder, as discussed later.

Key points: Clinical assessment

- Remember the possibility of a neuropathic bladder when assessing a child with wetting.

- Spina bifida, open and closed, remains the most common cause of neuropathic bladder.

- In the clinical assessment include enquiry about:
  – factors associated with spina bifida (Table 10.1);
  – clinical features suggestive of neuropathic bladder (Table 10.2).

The child with an overt spinal problem

Any child with an obvious spinal problem requires assessment of renal, bladder, and urethral function when first seen, in order to assess baseline function and identify those most at risk for renal damage.

Assessment of renal status

The preservation of renal function is the most important aim when planning management and a significant number of children already have damaged kidneys when first seen, particularly when the diagnosis has been delayed. Baseline investigations are detailed in Table 10.3.

It should be noted that in children who have abnormal lower limbs and reduced muscle bulk, the serum creatinine might consequently be misleadingly normal when there is significant renal impairment. Glomerular filtration rate (GFR) is, therefore, the only reliable way to assess and follow long-term renal function in children who have abnormal muscle bulk. Either inulin or

Table 10.3 Baseline renal assessment of the child with an overt spinal problem

Creatinine, urea, and electrolytes
Glomerular filtration rate
Renal and bladder ultrasonography
DMSA scan
MAG3 or DTPA renogram (only if there are concerns about uretero-vesical obstruction)

DMSA, dimercaptosuccinic acid; MAG3, mercaptoacetyltriglycine; DTPA, diethylenetriaminepentaacetic acid.

$[^{51}Cr]$EDTA clearance methods can be used, as they are not dependent on urine collection. GFR calculated in ml/min uncorrected for surface area can be used for serial measurements in patients in whom it is not possible to assess the surface area accurately.

Renal and bladder ultrasonography has made a great difference to the management of these children. It can be carried out frequently in worrying situations and enables problems, such as poor bladder emptying and ureteric and pelvicalyceal dilatation secondary to high bladder pressures and poor emptying, to be detected early.

Dimercaptosuccinic acid (DMSA) scanning of the kidneys excludes renal scarring and assesses differential renal function. Diethylenetriaminepentaacetic acid (DTPA) or mercaptoacetyltriglycine (MAG3) renography is required if there are concerns about uretero-vesical obstruction. It should be noted that these tests are not useful in excluding vesico-ureteric reflux (VUR) in those children not able to void voluntarily.

Assessment of bladder and urethral function

It is difficult to predict the type of bladder dysfunction from the clinical assessment alone; the best way of doing this is by carrying out a VUD which consists of a filling and voiding cystometrogram combined with a micturating cystourethrogram (MCU). The two are displayed simultaneously on a television screen and recorded on videotape for playback at a later date. Thus, events occurring in the bladder and urethra can be correlated with pressure changes and vice versa. VUD requires the insertion of a bladder catheter, urethrally or suprapubically, and a rectal pressure probe for measurement of intra-abdominal pressure. A MCU on its own provides only static films and thus is not applicable to the dynamic nature of the problem. However, if VUD is not available, a MCU will provide useful information about the appearance of the bladder and urethra, the presence or absence of VUR, and bladder emptying.

The child cannot be sedated for the investigation as this affects detrusor activity. However, it is very important that the child and his or her carers are well prepared for the test and know what to expect. We have found handouts to take home and time spent with a dedicated nurse explaining the procedure to be very helpful. It should be stressed that these examinations should only be performed in specialist centres on a dedicated paediatric list and by personnel who are able to interpret the results. We prefer the urethral route for catheterization, although some workers prefer the suprapubic route. The latter involves a general anaesthetic and usually an overnight stay in hospital.

Some clinicians prefer to combine cystometry with electromyography to assess sphincter dysfunction. However, this does not give information on VUR and bladder emptying and a formal MCU will then need to be performed separately to obtain this information. Natural-fill cystometry also has advocates. However, it is very time-consuming and does not exclude the need for catheterization or a MCU in order to obtain all the required information.

The indications for a VUD in children with incontinence are shown in Table 10.4.

Key points: Assessment of the child with an overt spinal problem

- Any child with an overt spinal problem needs assessment of renal and bladder/urethral function.

- Preservation of renal function is the most important aim.

- Initial assessment includes:
  – assessment of renal function (Table 10.3);
  – assessment of bladder and urethral function by VUD Table 10.4.

- It is very important that the child and carers are well prepared for the VUD.

VUD abnormalities in the neuropathic bladder

The information provided by VUD is set out in Table 10.5.

Table 10.4 Indications for video-urodynamic studies in children with incontinence

A neuropathic bladder
Proven urinary tract infections
Previous investigations suggestive of VUR
Impaired bladder emptying
Impaired urinary stream
No response to conventional treatment, e.g. no response
 to anticholinergics in a child with a history strongly
 suggestive of detrusor instability

Table 10.5 Information obtained from a video-urodynamic study

Bladder outline, shape, and capacity
The detrusor pressure at rest, during filling and voiding
 or leakage
Bladder sensation
State of the bladder neck and distal urethral sphincter at
 rest, during filling and in response to a detrusor
 contraction
Degree of bladder emptying
Presence or absence of VUR
Voiding or leak pressure
Urine flow rate

VUR, vesico-ureteric reflex.

In the normal situation (Fig. 10.1) the bladder fills with a minimal rise in pressure until bladder capacity is reached. Urine is held in the bladder by the bladder neck and distal urethral sphincter mechanism. Voiding is voluntarily initiated (at an appropriate time) by contraction of the detrusor muscle, which opens the bladder neck. The distal sphincter relaxes and voiding empties the bladder. This is followed by closure of the bladder neck and contraction of the distal sphincter. Normal bladder capacity data are shown in Chapter 28, but in the child up to 12 years can be calculated using the formula: 30 ml/year of life, plus an extra 50 ml [2].

Classification of the bladder dysfunction based on the type and level of neurological deficit in children with congenital spinal cord abnormalities is difficult, and is made even more complex because the spinal cord lesions are often incomplete, and sensory and motor deficits may be patchy. It is very difficult to predict the bladder and urethral abnormalities from the neurological examination, and individuals with low lesions and minor or absent neurological deficits often have the type of bladder dysfunction which poses the greatest threat to the kidneys.

The current approach is based on the VUD findings and takes into account the overall ability of the

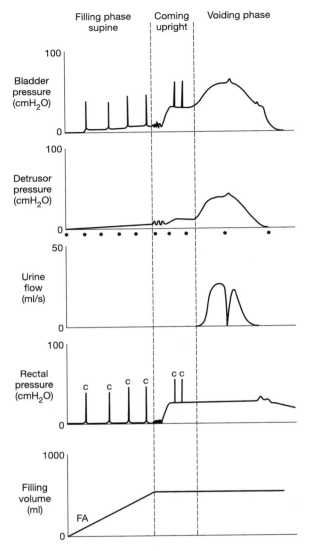

Fig. 10.1 Detrusor pressure during filling and voiding in the normal patient.

bladder to hold and void urine. Three types of dysfunction are recognized [3].

1. *Contractile dysfunction*: in this type of bladder, the bladder wall compliance is normal but all patients have hyperreflexic contractions, with a competent bladder neck in 50% and detrusor sphincter dyssynergia (DSD) in most. DSD describes the picture seen when the bladder contracts and, instead of relaxing, the distal urethral sphincter also contracts. This can lead to very high intravesical pressures. In the majority

there is incontinence with reduced bladder capacity and incomplete emptying. If VUR is present, then the risk of renal damage is high, particularly in the presence of an infection (Fig. 10.2).

2. *Intermediate*: during filling, the bladder pressure slowly rises due to reduced bladder wall compliance, thus constantly exposing the kidneys to raised pressure. The hyperreflexic contractions are rather ineffectual and in the majority the bladder neck is incompetent and there is a static or fixed distal sphincter, which is therefore both obstructive and incompetent, and

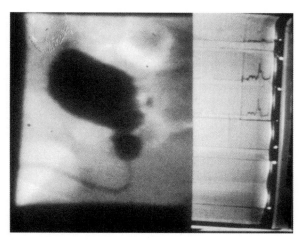

Fig. 10.2 The appearance in contractile dysfunction with detrusor sphincter dyssynergia in response to high-pressure contraction. Note the bladder diverticula.

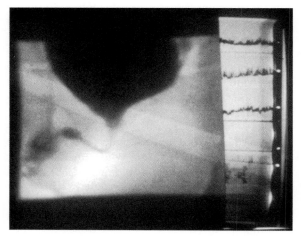

Fig. 10.3 Slowly rising baseline pressure during filling and the open bladder neck with incomplete relaxation of the distal sphincter.

leakage occurs at a critical pressure. This is the most common type and most dangerous to the kidneys, with a picture of incontinence, reduced capacity, raised pressure, and residual urine (Fig. 10.3).

3. *Acontractile*: the bladder fills with little or no evidence of detrusor activity. However, incontinence occurs at critical volumes because of sphincter weakness and, again, because the distal sphincter is fixed there is both incontinence and impaired emptying. This is the safest bladder because of the low intravesical pressure, and incompetent sphincters allow leakage. However, if an obstruction to outflow such as an artificial urinary sphincter (AUS) is implanted to prevent leakage, then this type of bladder can also develop hyperreflexia and reduced compliance.

VUDs are carried out to identify those most at risk of renal damage and the above classification helps to do this, as well as predicting the treatment modalities which are most likely to improve continence. VUDs have also highlighted the importance of the role of the urethra in the pathogenesis of this dysfunction. In 1982, Mundy *et al.* [4] reviewed 402 studies in 207 children with congenital cord lesions, with ages ranging from 1 month to 16 years. The bladder behaviour was classified as above and the findings were of almost universal urethral dysfunction. In the 73 children with contractile dysfunction, the bladder neck was incompetent in 50% and DSD was present in 95%. In the 82 children with intermediate and 52 with acontractile dysfunction, the bladder neck was incompetent at normal bladder volumes and the distal sphincter was both incompetent and obstructive, due to its fixed or static nature, resulting in leakage and incomplete emptying. Bladder-neck obstruction did not occur in any of these children and it is now recognized that in patients with spina bifida the obstruction occurs at the distal sphincter, which is either dyssynergic in the contractile group or fixed/static in the other two groups. It is important to know this when planning management in children who present with dilated upper tracts secondary to obstruction. Thus the term 'neuropathic vesico-urethral dysfunction' more accurately describes this abnormality.

It is now recognized that anything that raises intravesical pressure is potentially dangerous to the kidneys and the importance of DSD, reduced bladder compliance, and hyperreflexia, particularly in the presence of VUR and an infection, are well known.

Timing of VUD

There has been considerable debate about the timing and predictive value of VUDs, particularly in babies with spina bifida. Bauer *et al.* in 1984 [5] described the findings in 36 newborn infants with myelodysplasia of whom 18 had DSD and 13 later developed hydroureteronephrosis. This only happened in 2 of 9 without reflux and 1 of 9 with no sphincter activity. All 16 who developed hydronephrosis improved after decompression with a vesicostomy or clean intermittent catheterization (CIC). The authors felt that those with DSD were at great risk and needed close monitoring and that CIC should be started early. These findings have been confirmed by other workers and all have stressed the importance of regular monitoring even in those with less dangerous bladders, as bladder behaviour may change with time. In 1991, Galloway *et al.* [6] described an objective score based on urodynamic findings in myelodysplasia which could be used to predict upper tract deterioration. The parameters used were VUR, bladder wall compliance, hyperreflexia, leak pressure, and activity of the distal sphincter during detrusor contractions. Each was given a score of 0–2 with a maximum score of 10, i.e. the most threatening to the kidneys. This can be used as a guide to time intervention, and any child with a score of 5 or more is considered to be at risk. However, the authors stress that it is important to monitor all children regularly as problems can occur even in those at least risk.

We now recognize that the first 5 years of life and the teenage/adolescent years are the most dangerous to the kidneys. It is often found that children who have been well managed deteriorate when they reach puberty, with a worsening of bladder compliance, DSD, and hyperreflexia, all of which combine to put the kidneys at risk and continence deteriorates. In addition, in these children renal scarring can occur at any age in the presence of reflux, high pressure, and infection.

It is our practice in babies born with open spina bifida to perform VUDs as soon as it is feasible, after the back is closed and hydrocephalus dealt with. In those in whom the diagnosis is made later, or in whom a neuropathic bladder is suspected, VUDs should form part of the initial assessment. It is difficult to predict the type of dysfunction that occurs in those with minor neurological signs and deficits, where the voiding history may appear normal but urodynamics can reveal a high urodynamic score and the kidneys may be damaged at presentation.

Key points: VUD assessment of overt spinal problems

- The severity of vesico-urethral dysfunction cannot be predicted from the clinical assessment.

- VUD identifies three patterns of bladder dysfunction:
  – contractile;
  – intermediate;
  – acontractile.

- Urethral dysfunction is commonly present and must also be assessed.

- Anything that raises intravesical pressure is potentially deleterious to the kidneys.

- VUD should be performed as soon as the back is closed in babies with open spina bifida and at presentation in other children.

Management

The aims are to preserve renal function and improve continence. It is important to take into account any other problems the child might have, and the child and carers need to understand the problem and the reasons for the management strategies proposed. This often requires a great deal of time and explanation to ensure success. We have found it helpful, in difficult situations, for our specialist nurse to visit the family at home and discuss further the issues that have been raised during the hospital consultation.

The best way of preserving renal function is by keeping the bladder empty, at low pressure, and free of infection. Factors dangerous to the kidneys that need to be taken into account when planning management are:

1. Raised intravesical pressure due to hyperreflexia (which can be reduced with anticholinergic agents), DSD (can be overcome by CIC), a fixed distal sphincter (can be overcome by CIC), and reduced bladder wall compliance (which may respond to anticholinergics, although surgery is often required).

2. VUR, which is managed by keeping the bladder empty by CIC, reducing intravesical pressure

with the use of anticholinergics, and prophylactic antibiotics. However, surgery may be required eventually if there is evidence of deteriorating renal function.

3. Urinary tract infections (UTI).

In order to achieve continence, the requirements are:

- a means of emptying the bladder, which is usually by CIC;

- a reasonable bladder capacity, which may be improved medically by anticholinergics or, if that fails, surgically;

- competent urinary sphincters, which may respond to ephedrine or require surgery (AUS).

Management can be divided into non-surgical and surgical means.

Key points: Management of neuropathic bladder

- The aims are to preserve renal function and improve continence.

- To preserve renal function:
  – keep bladder empty;
  – keep bladder pressure low;
  – control urinary tract infections.

- To improve continence the following are needed:
  – a means of emptying the bladder, usually CIC;
  – reasonable bladder capacity;
  – competent urinary sphincters.

Non-surgical management of neuropathic bladder

Bladder expression (the Credé manoeuvre) has been used extensively and is often the first recommended management. However, it should not be used until DSD and VUR have been excluded. An acontractile bladder with incompetent sphincters responds best to this management, but there is often associated leakage. It is rarely indicated in children and is disliked by them as a means of management.

Bladder straining can work well in those with low-pressure bladders and incompetent sphincters with reasonable abdominal muscles. The child must be able to understand what to do and in my experience this method is used infrequently in this age group.

Clean intermittent catheterization (CIC) has made a tremendous difference to the management of these problems, with an improvement in continence, reduction of renal problems and infections. However, it is purely a means of emptying the bladder at regular intervals and may not be suitable for all children. The indications for CIC are:

- a poorly emptying bladder;

- detrusor sphincter dyssynergia;

- evidence of back pressure on the kidneys.

In those children who are found to have a bladder dangerous to the kidneys, this form of management should be started early in order to protect the kidneys, even though, in the infant, continence is not an issue. CIC is often combined with anticholinergic medication, which reduces hyperreflexia and intravesical pressure and indirectly increases bladder emptying, thus improving continence.

In our experience, wherever possible the parents and child prefer to be taught at home, and a specialist nurse often needs to make several visits to prepare all involved before the technique is instituted. Children learn to self-catheterize (SCIC) at around 6 years of age, although this will be dependent on the child's intelligence, motivation, manipulative skills, and skeletal deformities. However, even children with significant problems can learn to self-catheterize successfully, as has been shown by Robinson *et al.* [7]

Drugs. Anticholinergic agents, such as oxybutynin, propantheline, and the newer drug, tolterodine (Table 10.6), reduce intravesical pressure, resulting in improved continence and bladder capacity. The kidneys are thus exposed to lower intravesical pressures and this may also reduce reflux.

These drugs are very effective and we have found children suffer fewer side-effects than adults. However, they do need to be used with caution as they can adversely affect bladder emptying, which is obviously not an issue when CIC is being used, but is in those not catheterizing. Bladder emptying is easily

Table 10.6 Drugs useful in the management of the neuropathic bladder

Drug	Type	Dose
Propantheline	Anticholinergic	1 month to 12 years: 1 mg/kg/day in 3 doses >12 years: 15 mg 8-hourly
Oxybutynin	Anticholinergic	<5 years: 0.1 mg/kg/day in 3 doses increasing to 0.1 mg/kg 3 times a day >5 years: 2.5 mg twice daily, increasing to 5 mg 3 times a day
Tolterodene	Anticholinergic	Licensed for use >12 years only: 0.5 mg twice daily, increasing to 2 mg twice daily
Ephedrine	Alpha-adrenergic	1 month to 12 years: 2.5 mg/kg/day in 3 doses >12 years: 30 mg 8-hourly

monitored by ultrasonography and portable machines are now available, which means that bladder emptying can be assessed easily in the outpatient clinic or in the child's home.

Alpha-adrenergic agents, such as ephedrine (Table 10.6), are used to increase the tone in the bladder neck region. However, in the author's experience they are not effective if there is significant stress incontinence, and it is important to ensure bladder emptying.

A large number of children with neuropathic vesico-urethral dysfunction will ultimately be managed by a combination of CIC to empty the bladder and anticholinergics to reduce leakage. In addition, some will also require alpha-adrenergics. However, it is sensible to introduce these measures sequentially and ensure that CIC is established before adding anticholinergics in a child with poor bladder emptying. Alpha-adrenergics should only be added when the above combination has failed and there is stress incontinence.

Prophylactic *antibiotics* should be prescribed for all children who have VUR and those who suffer recurrent symptomatic infections. It is important to check the bladder emptying technique and to exclude stones in the latter group. CIC in itself is not an indication for prophylaxis.

Children who develop symptomatic UTIs require treatment. However, there are some children on CIC, or who have an indwelling catheter and do not have VUR,

---

Key points: Non-surgical management of neuropathic bladder

- Bladder expression should not be used until DSD and VUR have been excluded.

- Bladder straining requires the patient's understanding, so is little used in children.

- CIC is purely a means of emptying the bladder.

- CIC is not suitable for all children.

- Indications for CIC include:
  - a poorly emptying bladder;
  - detrusor sphincter dyssynergia;
  - evidence of back pressure on the kidneys.

- Many children are best managed with a combination of CIC, anticholinergics, and sometimes alpha-adrenergics.

- Antibiotics should be given:
  - to treat symptomatic infections;
  - prophylactically in the presence of VUR or recurrent symptomatic infections.

---

in whom organisms are frequently cultured in the urine but who are well. It is generally felt that these do not require treatment, as often this leads to the emergence of resistant strains. However, each case needs careful evaluation. Circumcision should be considered in boys on CIC, particularly if there are recurrent infections.

Bladder neck obstruction is extremely rare in these children, thus there is no indication for alpha-blockers. There is currently no cholinergic agent available which significantly improves bladder emptying in these children.

Continuous catheterization may be indicated in the child who presents with gross hydronephrosis, in order to decompress the upper tracts, before further management is instituted. We have experience of some children, who have presented with severe renal impairment, who have been managed with an indwelling catheter for many years, and this has preserved enough renal function to delay renal transplantation, or even allowed them to go through the pubertal growth spurt without further significant impairment. It may be the only means of managing a severely handicapped wheelchair-bound girl where other methods are not feasible. There are a few children who for various reasons will not contemplate CIC, but who do require drainage in order to protect the kidneys and choose to have an indwelling catheter (urethral or suprapubic).

There is now a whole range of *appliances* available to improve the management of incontinence. These include penile appliances for boys, though very few boys use them as it is notoriously difficult to get a good fit. In addition, a wide variety of pads, nappies, pants with inbuilt pads, and bedding products are now available to improve the quality of life of these patients. Many different types of catheters are available for use in CIC, so that each individual child's needs can be met.

Surgical management

The indications for surgical intervention are:

- failure of conservative methods to prevent upper tract dilatation and progressive renal damage;

- failure of conservative methods to produce an acceptable level of continence;

- a combination of the above.

Timing of intervention is entirely dependent on the problem. If the kidneys are at risk, then there is no choice but to intervene. However, if surgery is being done for incontinence alone, then it is really up to the child. It is important that the child has a clear understanding of what is involved, in what is major surgery, and should include the fact that SCIC will almost certainly be required after surgery even if the child is not catheterizing prior to surgery. Indeed, most surgeons would not undertake the procedure unless the child is able to catheterize and willing to do so.

The small, hyperreflexic, poorly compliant bladder is the type of bladder which often leads to deterioration of function and problems with continence. It also produces obstruction to urinary flow. This may be compounded by the presence of reflux, particularly if the child suffers from symptomatic urinary tract infections. If reconstructive bladder surgery is performed to preserve renal function, it will also improve continence.

Vesicostomy may be indicated in babies to protect the kidneys and decompress the upper tract if an indwelling catheter or CIC are not feasible. This allows the urine to drain directly into the nappy from the bladder and reduces the intravesical pressure and keeps the bladder empty. This is only a temporary measure and ultimately CIC will be required to empty the bladder when the vesicostomy closes. Reconstructive surgery may also be necessary.

Bladder reconstruction has been a major advance in protecting the kidneys and improving continence by increasing the capacity of the bladder and reducing intravesical pressure. This is usually at the expense of bladder emptying.

Bowel is used to augment the bladder in the so-called clam cystoplasty, whereas a substitution cystoplasty describes the situation whereby virtually the whole of the bladder is removed and substituted with bowel. The latter is more likely if the bladder is small, thick-walled and poorly compliant. The decision on which procedure is required will depend on the characteristics of the bladder and may not be made until the surgery itself. Nearly all parts of the bowel have been used, although a clam ileocystoplasty remains the most common procedure [8].

Currently this is the best option available to protect the kidneys and improve continence when non-surgical means have failed. However, careful selection is required as the procedure is not without problems, which include mucus production, stone formation, infection, perforation, metabolic problems (particularly if renal function is compromised), and the possibility of malignancy [9]. Perforation of the bladder is a surgical emergency which is life threatening, and often occurs when there is infection secondary to poor bladder emptying, therefore the importance of regular and complete emptying cannot be overstressed. It is clear that continued meticulous lifelong follow-up and monitoring are required.

Sphincter weakness incontinence can be improved in mild cases by alpha-adrenergic drugs, as already discussed. In addition the removal of residual urine will also help if ephedrine alone fails. A reduction in intravesical pressure by drugs or surgery, i.e. cystoplasty, also improves the situation. However, if despite these measures the child still has significant stress incontinence, some form of *bladder neck suspension procedure* may help.

In those in whom there is a severe degree of sphincter weakness (usually in the absence of a significant degree of obstruction) the implantation of an *artificial urinary sphincter* may be required. Many of these children will have already undergone bladder reconstruction, although the two procedures can be combined.

In those children with large, atonic bladders who have stress incontinence, bladder behaviour may change after the insertion of an AUS, and thus careful monitoring is required to detect these changes early, before hydronephrosis develops secondary to raised intravesical pressure. The majority will need to continue to empty their bladder by SCIC.

The AUS is a mechanical device and thus any of the components may fail or erode. However, the most serious complication is infection, which necessitates removal of the whole device. It is preferable, but not mandatory, to defer this procedure until after puberty, although many have been implanted successfully in younger children.

The Mitrofanoff procedure (continent urinary diversion) can be created in those who are not able to catheterize per urethra. This may be because of skeletal deformities, manipulative problems, or visuospatial problems. Urethral catheterization may be tolerated poorly because of pain if urethral sensation is preserved. This can be overcome, however it may be another indication for the Mitrofanoff procedure. The appendix is reimplanted into the bladder wall to produce a continent, catheterizable abdominal channel [10]. In children without an appendix, other tubular structures can be used and continence rates of 94% are reported [11]. Selection of patients and site of the stoma are important and need to take into account the child's body habitus. This procedure has undoubtedly given independence to some children and adolescents who have not been able to self-catheterize per urethra.

Urinary diversion is now rarely performed, as there are much better methods available to achieve continence. However, in the very occasional child, when all else fails, it can be very successful.

Vesico-ureteric reflux can be a very difficult problem and is most troublesome in those with high-pressure, thick-walled bladders, in whom reimplantation often leads to obstruction at the vesico-ureteric junction and thus hydronephrosis. It is important to make the bladder safe by keeping it at low pressure, empty, and free of infection. If a combination of CIC, anticholinergics, and prophylactic antibiotics fail to prevent problems, then the next step is usually to perform a bladder augmentation, at which time the ureters can be reimplanted into the bowel segment, or the surgeon may decide not to reimplant if it is thought that a reduction in detrusor pressure

secondary to the augmentation procedure is sufficient to alleviate the situation.

Key points: Surgical management of neuropathic bladder

- Indications for surgical intervention are:
  - failure of conservative measures to prevent upper tract dilatation, and progressive renal damage;
  - failure of conservative measures to produce acceptable continence;
  - a combination of the above.

- Bladder reconstruction should only be undertaken if the children or carers are willing and able to catheterize.

- Bladder reconstruction is the best option to protect the kidneys when non-surgical measures have failed.

- Bladder perforation is a life-threatening complication of bladder reconstruction, and so meticulous life-long follow-up is necessary.

- The Mitrofanoff procedure can be utilized in those children who cannot catheterize urethrally.

Case 1

This girl, now aged $3\frac{1}{2}$, was referred at the age of 12 days as she was noted to have a sacral mass at birth with reduced movement of the right leg. MRI showed a large complex lipomeningocele with tethering. Neurosurgical opinion had been sought and, because of the complexity of the lipomeningocele, it was decided not to operate but to monitor closely. Urodynamics at the age of 2 months showed a slightly increased bladder capacity with hyperreflexia to 16 cm of water and a bladder that emptied completely. She was therefore monitored quite closely and was noted on ultrasonography to show poor bladder emptying, and she subsequently developed a urinary tract infection. She was therefore commenced on CIC and prophylactic antibiotics. Urodynamics were repeated at the age of 1 and she demonstrated left grade III reflux with a large, poorly emptying bladder, and consequently oxybutynin was added to her management regime to reduce the intravesical pressure. Antibiotics controlled her infections and at the age of $3\frac{1}{2}$ she has a normal DMSA and renal function. She is being catheterized four times a day and is dry by day and damp at night, and will require close monitoring. This case demonstrates that in these children the bladder behaviour may change and significant reflux can develop.

It is important that these children are fully investigated when first seen. The timing and nature of further investigations is dependent on each individual, their renal function, and response to management. They need to be seen at least every 6 months, with a minimum of an annual renal ultrasound. However, infants are seen much more frequently, often with monthly ultrasonography if their upper tracts are felt to be at risk. We recommend a repeat VUD at the end of the first year of life or 6 months after any surgical procedure to the spine and spinal cord. Further urodynamics are indicated if management is not controlling the situation, i.e. the child is wet, suffering recurrent infections, or there is evidence of upper tract deterioration, and when surgical intervention is being planned. As already stated, the first 5 years and adolescence are particularly difficult times and most children should have a full assessment of renal function (to include ultrasound, GFR, and DMSA) every year to 18 months during these critical periods.

None of this is straightforward, and the management of these difficult problems requires a multiprofessional team approach, with the paediatrician/paediatric neurologist, nephrologist, paediatric urologist, and nurse all working together, and preferably seeing the patients together. It is clear that these investigations should be performed in specialized centres where there is a great deal of expertise in the assessment and interpretation of the results of investigations, and that the surgery is performed by experienced paediatric urologists. The specialist nurse has a major role to play in the management of these children undergoing this complex surgery, both in the pre-and post-operative assessment and in management.

Closed spina bifida

Closed spina bifida describes a skin-covered congenital cord fusion defect and consists of a heterogeneous group of developmental anomalies, which include meningocele, lipomeningocele, primary tethered cord, diastematomyelia, intradural lipoma, and dermoid cyst. It may be manifest at birth by a skin lesion such as a deep sacral pit, lipoma, hairy tuft, or naevus overlying the spine, or a limb deformity secondary to a neurological abnormality. The abnormalities result in distortion of the developing neural tissue, with subsequent damage of the spinal cord and/or nerve roots.

Although often diagnosed at birth, this is not always the case and the lesion may not be recognized until the child presents with the onset of urinary incontinence or failure to achieve continence, recurrent urinary tract infections, soiling, or orthopaedic problems in later childhood. Often there is no clinical neurological abnormality or only a minor deficit. It is now recognized that these children do have neuropathic vesico-urethral dysfunction which can lead to renal damage [12]. This condition should not be confused with simple failure of fusion of the neural arches of L5 and S1 found in a proportion of the normal population, which is not associated with spinal cord pathology.

It is crucial that these patients are identified early and that bladder, urethral, and renal function are assessed. This was highlighted by Johnston and Borzyskowski (1998) [13], who reported clinical and VUD findings in a group of 51 patients with closed spina bifida at the time they first presented to a specialist paediatric neuro-urology clinic. The mean age at referral was 3.3 years (range 6 months to 10 years). Only 12 presented with neurological problems, whereas 25 presented with urinary tract disturbance. Thirty-three had a normal neurological examination or only minor objective signs. At presentation 21 had normal renal tract ultrasonography, whereas only two had normal VUDs. DMSA scanning showed that 12 children had already developed renal scars (eight unilateral and four bilateral), all of whom had had at least one UTI.

Management of the bladder was based on the VUD findings and 30 of the children required CIC. Anticholinergic agents and antibiotics were used as indicated, and only six had remained dry without medical treatment. Five children had a cystoplasty, and four, ureteric reimplantation. Twenty-two had neurosurgical intervention because of neurological or neuro-urological deterioration.

The authors concluded that neither the history of voiding habits nor the neurological examination were reliable indicators of bladder dysfunction and subsequent renal damage, and this was consistent with the findings of other workers (Mevorach *et al.* [14]; Dator *et al.* [15]). Therefore all patients with known or suspected closed spina bifida should have VUD assessment and assessment of renal function if the urodynamics are abnormal. Follow-up and reassessment should be as discussed for children with open spina bifida, as the bladder behaves in exactly the same way and may indeed be more dangerous to the kidneys.

Key points: Closed spina bifida

- Closed spina bifida describes a skin-covered congenital cord fusion defect and consists of a heterogeneous group of developmental anomalies.

- This condition should not be confused with simple failure of fusion of the neural arches of L5 and S1 found in the normal population.

- Often not diagnosed at birth.

- May not be recognized until the child presents with urinary incontinence, recurrent urinary tract infections, soiling, or orthopaedic problems.

- It is crucial that these patients are identified early and bladder, urethral, and renal function are assessed.

- Management depends on VUD findings.

Case 2

This 2-year-old boy presented at the age of 6 months with a urinary tract infection and urinary retention. At the referring hospital he was catheterized and was found to have 240 ml of urine in his bladder. The catheter was removed on two occasions but on each occasion he developed recurrent retention. Cystoscopy at the referring hospital showed a mildly trabeculated bladder and on admission he was noted to have a sacral pit with an overlying tuft of hair. He was transferred for further management with an indwelling catheter *in situ*. VUD showed contractions during filling to 117 cm of water. There was no evidence of reflux. He had detrusor sphincter dyssynergia and impaired bladder emptying. MRI scan showed him to have a cord that ended at L1. It was rather blunted, split at the lower end with thickening of the filum terminale and tethering. He was also noted to have a deficiency of the sacrum. His spinal cord was surgically untethered at the age of 10 months and he has been managed on CIC, prophylactic antibiotics, and oxybutynin. Repeat urodynamics 6 months after his spinal cord untethering were unchanged. He has a normal DMSA scan, normal renal function, and has had no further infections. His development is proceeding normally and he is walking normally.

Case 3

This 15-year-old girl was referred at the age of $13\frac{1}{2}$ years. At birth she had been noted to have abnormalities of her fingers and toes which had required surgery. She was also noted to have a pea-sized lump at the base of her spine and this was removed at the age of 4 years. She gave a history of never being dry at night, with daytime frequency, urgency, and

recurrent urinary tract infections. DMSA scan at the age of 10 showed the left kidney to contribute 45% of the total function and there was a suggestion of a scar. An ultrasound had shown incomplete bladder emptying. A MAG3 renogram was performed and was normal with no vesico-ureteric reflux. She was reinvestigated at the age of 13 years because of recurrent infections, frequency, urgency and night-time wetting, and a DMSA scan at that time showed no uptake in the right kidney. Ultrasound showed gross hydronephrosis on the right and a bladder volume of 410 ml with a post-micturition residue of 264 ml. At referral she was noted to have wasting of the left calf and rudimentary toes of both feet, with increased tone bilaterally in the legs and absent ankle jerks. An MRI scan at the referring hospital had shown a sacral lipomyelomeningocele. VUD showed a large trabeculated bladder, holding 680 ml of urine with multiple diverticulae, with hyperreflexia to 53 cm of water and compliance reduced to 20 cm of water, gross reflux on the right, and a residue of 380 ml. She was immediately commenced on CIC, prophylactic antibiotics, and oxybutynin to try and regain some of the function in the right kidney. Her GFR at that time was 73 ml/min/1.73 m². However, 18 months later there was no recovery of function in the right kidney and she started having recurrent infections and is awaiting a right nephroureterectomy. She was referred for a neurosurgical opinion; however, it was decided that intervention, which would be technically difficult at this time, was not required unless she showed a neurological deterioration. This case demonstrates the importance of excluding a neuropathic bladder at birth or early in life in anyone who has any abnormality noted at the base of the spine.

Neuropathic bowel

Children with neuropathic bladder very commonly have associated bowel problems, with constipation and soiling, which must be addressed, as there is little point in performing complex surgery to achieve urinary continence if soiling continues to be a problem. Soiling is socially much less acceptable than urinary incontinence and it is often much more difficult to achieve bowel continence for these children. It is often those with only a minor neurological deficit who are most difficult to treat.

Early intervention and training is important. Attention needs to be paid to the diet and the establishment of a regular routine (particularly after meals). Some children will require laxatives, whereas in others regular manual evacuation will achieve faecal continence without soiling inbetween times. The same result can be obtained by the regular use of suppositories or enemas of various types.

There are some children in whom it is very difficult to achieve a satisfactory regime, or the child does not wish to, or is unable to, perform manual evacuations or enemas and wishes to be independent of others. In this situation surgical intervention may be required to provide a catheterizable colonic stoma, the so-called ACE procedure (antegrade colonic enema) [16]. It may take several weeks for the bowel to adjust to these regular antegrade washouts; however, the results are encouraging. The ACE stoma can be performed at the same time as reconstructive bladder surgery, with or without a Mitrofanoff procedure.

Key points: Management of neuropathic bowel

- Bowel problems are commonly associated with neuropathic bladder.

- There is little point in performing complex surgery to achieve urinary continence if soiling continues to be a problem.

- Early intervention and training are important.

- The ACE procedure should be considered in children in whom it is difficult to achieve a satisfactory regime

---

Conditions that may be associated with a neuropathic bladder

Sacral agenesis

This is a rare disorder and any defect of the sacrum which involves more than one sacral vertebra can cause a neuropathic bladder, with a defect between S2 and S4 being most likely to lead to bladder dysfunction. It is not possible to predict the type of abnormality from the neurological dysfunction.

Key features include constipation and urological symptoms of persistent diurnal wetting, difficulty voiding, and recurrent UTIs. Physical examination may reveal flattening of the buttocks, loss of the gluteal cleft, widely spaced buttock dimples, or a palpable sacral defect. These children may have a widely based flat-footed gait or pes cavus, and previous history may reveal orthopaedic abnormalities, particularly equinovarus abnormalities. Neurological examination may be completely normal. Delayed diagnosis increases the risk of renal impairment.

The association with maternal pre-gestational insulin-dependent diabetes mellitus (IDDM) is well recognized, with 1% of infants born to IDDM mothers having sacral agenesis and 12–16% of infants with sacral agenesis having a mother with IDDM [17]. In 1999 Wilmshurst *et al.* [18] reviewed children referred to a paediatric neuro-urology service over a 20-year period in whom a diagnosis of sacral agenesis had been made. Twenty-two of these children were studied retrospectively, 10 presented after a year of age and the oldest was diagnosed at 12 years of age. Most had persistent dribbling of urine associated with frequency, urgency, recurrent urinary tract infections (19), and constipation. In 12 there was a history of maternal pre-gestational IDDM; 20 had abnormal neurology in the lower limbs and VUDs were abnormal in all, with VUR in 11, renal scarring in seven, and renal impairment in three at presentation. CIC was recommended in 20 of the children and bladder or bowel surgery had been performed in seven. Twenty of the 22 children had undergone operative procedures, and 10 of these procedures, which included rectal biopsy to exclude Hirschsprung's disease, orthopaedic surgery on the feet, manual evacuation of the faeces under anaesthetic, and an ACE procedure were carried out prior to the diagnosis of sacral agenesis being made. Over a third of these children had required psychological support over the years.

The authors state that it is very important for paediatricians to have a high level of suspicion of sacral agenesis in children presenting with persistent wetting and constipation, particularly if there is a history of maternal IDDM, spinal skin defects, or lower-limb abnormalities. All should have a VUD at the time of diagnosis. Early diagnosis enables early intervention to avoid renal damage, improved continence and quality of life. These children who are found to have a neuropathic bladder should obviously be managed in the same way as those with open and closed spina bifida.

Key points: Sacral agenesis

- Sacral agenesis should be suspected in children with persisting wetting, constipation, spinal skin defects, or lower-limb abnormalities.

- Maternal IDDM is an important association (see Table 10.1).

- It is not possible to predict the type of vesicourethral dysfunction from the neurological dysfunction.

- All should have VUD at diagnosis.

- Management depends on the findings on VUD.

Case 4

This girl is now $16\frac{1}{2}$ years old and was referred to us at the age of 4 years. The diagnosis of sacral agenesis had been made at 15 months. At referral her parents complained that she had constant dribbling of urine, her urine was infected, and she had minor foot abnormalities. VUD revealed a small hyperreflexic bladder with an incompetent bladder neck and detrusor sphincter dyssynergia. She leaked only with contractions and had poor emptying. She was started on CIC and propantheline at the age of $4\frac{1}{2}$ years. At this time she did not have reflux and had normal renal function. At the age of 10 years she was still wet despite regular self-catheterization and regular anticholinergics. There were no symptomatic urinary tract infections and her parents were not keen for her to be on prophylactic antibiotics. VUD at the age of 10 years showed grade III right-sided reflux with contractions to over 100 cm of water. She had reduced compliance of 35 cm of water and again detrusor sphincter dyssynergia with poor emptying and a capacity of only 100 ml. A DMSA scan carried out at the same time showed a possible scar on the right kidney. She underwent a clam cystoplasty with a possibility of having an artificial sphincter at a later date. However, at the age of 16 she is dry, self-catheterizes three to four times a day, wakes at night once to empty her bladder, and is very occasionally wet in the morning. She has a GFR of 93 ml/min/1.73 m^2 and no significant change on her DMSA scan. She has, however, had psychological problems and this is particularly related to the fact that she appears absolutely normal but has had to deal with this very significant bladder problem and at times has felt very isolated.

Cerebral palsy

It has been increasingly recognized that children with cerebral palsy have an increased incidence of bladder problems [19] which are not attributable to reduced ability, manipulative skills, cognitive impairment, or communication problems. However, there are little published data. In 1993, Reid and Borzyskowski reviewed the management of 27 patients with cerebral palsy referred to a paediatric neuro-urology service over a 10-year period [20]. Symptoms included urinary incontinence, urgency, and frequency, with failure to respond to the usual forms of management. Mean age of referral was 9.9 years (range 3–20 years). VUDs were abnormal in 85%, with hyperreflexia and reduced bladder capacity being the most common finding (20 out of 23). Five children had DSD, 13 had a UTI, reflux neuropathy was present in two at referral, and a further patient was shown to have VUR. The children were treated with anticholinergics, CIC, or a combination of the two as indicated, and two underwent surgery. No treatment was indicated in five. All but one of those treated improved.

This study showed a high incidence of VUD abnormalities and the mean age of referral was nearly 10 years. Thus it is clearly important to think about the possibility of a bladder problem in any child with cerebral palsy who would be expected to be dry, particularly if there is a history of urinary tract infection.

Key points: Bladder dysfunction in children with cerebral palsy

- Children with cerebral palsy have an increased incidence of bladder problems.

- It is important to consider this possibility in children with cerebral palsy who would be expected to be dry, particularly if there is a history of urinary tract infection.

Anorectal anomalies

These occur in approximately 1 in 5000 live births [21] and are part of the spectrum of congenital abnormalities in which the anus fails to open on to the perineum. This can vary from minor anomalies where the anus terminates close to the perineal skin to major cloacal abnormalities seen in girls where the rectum, vagina, and urethra fail to develop, and drain via a single abnormal channel on to the perineum.

Approximately 25% of patients with anorectal anomalies have lower urinary tract dysfunction which is poorly understood [22]. However, a significant number have associated sacral anomalies and an abnormality of the spinal cord. Thus these children may well have neuropathic vesico-urethral dysfunction.

It is important to be aware of this association. These children should all have an MRI of the whole spinal cord and VUD to exclude problems. They may present in urinary retention, with a urinary tract infection or with wetting, at which time renal damage may already be present.

Key points: Anorectal anomalies and bladder dysfunction

- 25% of children with anorectal anomalies have lower urinary tract dysfunction.

- All these children should have:
  – MRI of the whole spine;
  – VUD.

Acute transverse myelitis

Acute transverse myelitis (ATM) is a clinical syndrome with acute flaccid paraparesis with segmental sensory dysfunction without evidence of cord compression, which may result from a variety of mechanisms. Bladder dysfunction is common and may be the presenting symptom [23]. The natural history of urinary tract abnormalities has not been described in children in the past. However, we have reviewed 10 children with ages ranging from 8 months to 16 years with this diagnosis [24]. All had VUDs, which showed a combination of detrusor hyperreflexia and DSD in most. These children have been followed for a mean of 3 years (6 months to 10 years) and all had residual bladder dysfunction. Only four were asymptomatic on *no* treatment. There was no relationship between the severity of residual motor symptoms and long-term urinary tract dysfunction. Of the seven children who had recovered sufficiently to achieve independent community ambulation, five were incontinent and one of the other two required CIC to achieve continence. Urinary tract dysfunction may persist in these children even if they make a full motor recovery.

Key points: Acute transverse myelitis and bladder dysfunction

- Bladder dysfunction is common and may be the presenting symptom.

- There is no relationship between the severity of the residual motor symptoms and long-term urinary tract dysfunction.

- Urinary tract dysfunction may persist even if there is complete motor recovery.

The occult neuropathic bladder (occult neurological bladder, non-neurogenic neurogenic bladder, pseudoneurogenic bladder, Hinman syndrome)

This describes a situation seen in children who are neurologically normal (with normal spinal cord imaging) who present with diurnal incontinence, incomplete bladder emptying, and urinary tract infections, and in whom VUDs may reveal high pressure detrusor contractions with DSD and poor emptying, with or without VUR. These changes can be severe and progressive and lead to renal impairment.

Hinman and Baumann in 1973 [25] reported the condition in a series of 14 boys with urinary incontinence, recurrent UTIs, urinary tract structural changes, and often encopresis. They described them as having timid, shy, and anxious 'failure personalities'. As well as short-term treatment with anticholinergics and correction of constipation, they achieved a good response with re-education, suggestion therapy, and hypnosis. These authors felt the underlying problem was an acquired functional incoordination between the detrusor and external urethral sphincter rather than a subclinical neurological lesion. This was supported 4 years later by Allen [26] who described 21 children with similar problems. However, Mix [27] reviewed the arguments between an organic or psychogenic origin of the syndrome and noted that not all authors found a high incidence of psychological and family disturbance.

Koff *et al.* [28] studied 53 neurologically normal children with similar symptoms. They were found to have bladder sphincter incoordination, characterized by voluntary contractions of the distal urinary sphincter, in an attempt to maintain continence during involuntary uninhibited detrusor contractions. This incoordination produced high intravesical pressures with VUR in 50%. They postulated that this may represent a delay in maturation of control, or regression to the infant pattern of bladder control.

Case 5

This girl is now 13 years old, and was referred at the age of $9\frac{1}{2}$ years with a history of wetting, constipation, and recurrent urinary tract infections, when a VUD had shown mild bladder instability with high voiding pressures and incomplete emptying. She had not been able to tolerate oxybutynin and propantheline. An MRI had shown an entirely normal spinal cord. When she was seen her bladder contained 230 ml of urine with a post-micturition residue of 170 ml. The problem here was that she was known to have detrusor instability but obviously anticholinergics would make the bladder emptying worse, and she was therefore started on SCIC. She was also noted to have psychological problems and was referred to our psychologist. The current situation is that she catheterizes at least three times a day, but is not very happy to catheterize in school and does suffer breakthrough infections. Her renal function is entirely normal and she only wets when she has a urinary tract infection. There has been no improvement in her bladder emptying over the years and she will need to self-catheterize for the foreseeable future.

These children can present at all ages and, in some, if a careful history is taken, there is evidence that the child required infrequent nappy changes, being dry for many hours at a time and, in some, potty training has never been achieved. In others, there is a deterioration of continence or a history of urinary tract infections and infrequent voiding. There may be evidence of behaviour disturbance due to a disruptive family background or a significant life event. For example, two sisters were referred with severe bladder and upper tract changes and impaired renal function 5 years after the death of their mother in childbirth. It is also important to remember that wetting may lead to psychological problems in the child and family, and must be taken into account when planning management.

It is clear that these children require a detailed assessment of bladder, urethral, and renal function. It is important to exclude a neurological problem, which includes an MRI investigation of the whole spinal cord and spine, in those with poorly emptying bladders and involuntary DSD.

These bladders have to be managed in exactly the same way as a true neuropathic bladder, with CIC, anticholinergics, antibiotics, and surgery as indicated, to prevent renal damage and improve continence. Psychological intervention should also be offered where appropriate, whether the psychological problems are a primary cause of the bladder dysfunction or as a result of the impact of the bladder problem. A great deal of support is required for these children and their families.

Key points: Occult neuropathic bladder

- These children can present at all ages.

- A history of infrequent micturition, failure to achieve potty training, or subsequent deterioration in continence may be elicited.

- There may be evidence of behaviour disturbance due to disruptive family background or a significant life event.

- The wetting may lead to psychological problems in the child and/or family.

- These bladders should be managed in the same way as overt neuropathic bladders.

- Psychological intervention should be offered where appropriate.

Miscellaneous

There are other groups of children with bladder problems, whose lives can be improved greatly by careful assessment and management, e.g. those with spinal cord tumours. We have recently become aware that boys with Duchenne muscular dystrophy often have bladder problems (74% of 88 males when specifically asked). It seems that continence is achieved in the normal way and then lost when the boys are still mobile. VUDs were carried out in nine boys and showed that eight had detrusor hyperreflexia and one had DSD and hyperreflexia following spinal fusion. The reasons for hyperreflexia are unclear; however, the quality of life of these boys has been improved significantly with appropriate management (MacLeod *et al.*, personal communication).

Specialist nurse

The role of the specialist nurse (Table 10.7) cannot be overemphasized and, indeed, the neuropathic bladder service cannot function adequately without a dedicated nurse as a member of the team who plays a crucial role in overall management.

Table 10.7 The role of the specialist nurse in the management of the child with a neuropathic bladder

Part of the initial assessment team
Advice on available aids
Teaching CIC or SCIC
Liaison with local services and schools
Discussing and planning treatment options with child and family, both in hospital and at home
Performing bladder function assessments
Involvement in preoperative and postoperative care and follow-up after discharge from hospital

The role of the general paediatrician

The general paediatrician is often the first person to see and assess the child. Some of the investigations can be performed locally, but more detailed assessment, particularly VUDs, should be performed in specialist centres, where decisions regarding management, non-surgical and surgical, are made. However, these specialist centres may be a considerable distance from the child's home and it is important that the child is known to the local team, as these children often have very complex problems and require a great deal of input.

Conclusions

It is clear that there are many causes of neuropathic vesico-urethral dysfunction in children. These problems are complex and lifelong. Thus there must be a full initial multidisciplinary specialist assessment and regular reassessment and lifelong follow-up by a specialist team.

References

1. Lapides J, Diokno AC, Silber SJ, Lowe BS. Clean intermittent self-catheterisation in the treatment of urinary tract disease. *J Urol* 1972, 107, 458–461.
2. Rickwood AMK. Investigations. In: Borzyskowski M, Mundy AR (Eds) *Neuropathic Bladder in Childhood. Clinics in Developmental Paediatrics No 111.* London, MacKeith Press, 1990, 12–13.
3. Rickwood AMK, Thomas DG, Philip NM, Spicer RD. Assessment of congenital neuropathic bladder by combined urodynamic and radiological studies. *Br J Urol* 1982, 54, 512–518.
4. Mundy AR, Shah PJR, Borzyskowski M, Saxton HM. Sphincter behaviour in myelomeningocele. *Br J Urol* 1982, 54, 645–649.
5. Bauer SB, Hallett M, Khoshbin S. Predictive value of urodynamic evaluation in newborns with myelodysplasia. *JAMA* 1984, 252, 650–652.
6. Galloway NTM, Mekras JA, Helms M, Webster GD. An objective score to predict upper tract deterioration in myelodysplasia. *J Urol* 1991, 145, 535–537.
7. Robinson RO, Cockram M, Strode M. Severe handicap in spina bifida: no bar to intermittent self-catheterisation. *Arch Dis Child* 1985, 60, 760–762.
8. Woodhouse RC. Reconstruction of the lower urinary tract for neurogenic bladder: lessons from the adolescent age group. *Br J Urol* 1992, 69: 589–593.
9. Mundy AR, Nurse DE. Calcium balance, growth and skeletal mineralization in patients with cystoplasties. *Br J Urol* 1992, 69, 257–259.
10. Mitrofanoff P. Cystostomie continente trans-appendiculaire dans le traitement des vessies neurologiques. *Chir Paediatr* 1980, 21, 297–305.
11. Woodhouse CRJ, Gordon EM. The Mitrofanoff principle for urethral failure. *Br J Urol* 1994, 73, 55–60.
12. Borzyskowski M, Neville BGR. Neuropathic bladder and spinal dysraphism. *Arch Dis Child* 1981, 56, 176–180.
13. Johnston L, Borzyskowski M. Bladder dysfunction and neurological disability at presentation in closed spina bifida. *Arch Dis Child* 1998, 79, 33–38.
14. Mevorach RA, Bogaert GA, Baskin LS, Lazzaretti CC, Edwards MSB, Kogan BA. Lower urinary tract function in ambulatory children with spina bifida. *Br J Urol* 1996, 77, 593–596.
15. Dator DP, Hatchett L, Dyro FM, Shefron JM, Bauer SB. Urodynamic dysfunction in walking myelodysplastic children. *J Urol* 1992, 148, 362–365.
16. Malone PS, Ransley PG, Kiely EM. Preliminary report: the antegrade continence enema. *Lancet* 1990, 336, 1217–1218.
17. Guzman L, Bauer SB, Hallett M, Khoshbin S, Colodny AH, Retik AB. Evaluation and management of children with sacral agenesis. *Urology* 1983, XXII, 506–510.
18. Wilmshurst JM, Kelly R, Borzyskowski M. Presentation and outcome of sacral agenesis: 20 years' experience. *Dev Med Child Neurol* 1999, 41, 806–812.
19. McNeal DM, Hawtrey CE, Wolraich ML, Mapel JR. Symptomatic neurogenic bladder in a cerebral palsied population. *Dev Med Child Neurol* 1983, 25, 612–616.
20. Reid CJD, Borzyskowski M. Lower urinary tract dysfunction in cerebral palsy. *Arch Dis Child* 1993, 68, 739–742.
21. Rowe MI, *et al. Essentials of Paediatric Surgery*, 1st edn. St Louis, Missouri, Mosby, 1995, 596–609.
22. Boemers T, Beck F, de Jong T, Bax K. Urologic problems in anorectal malformations. Part 1 urodynamic findings and significance of sacral anomalies. *J Pediatr Surg* 1996, 31(3), 407–410.
23. Knebusch M, Strassburg HM, Reiners K. Acute transverse myelitis in childhood: nine cases and review of the literature. *Dev Med Child Neurol* 1998, 40, 631–639.
24. Ganesan V, Borzyskowski M. Characteristics and course of urinary tract dysfunction after acute transverse myelitis in childhood. *Dev Med Child Neurol* 2001, 43, 473–475.
25. Hinman F, Baumann FW. Vesical and ureteral damage from voiding dysfunction in boys without neurologic or obstructive disease. *J Urol* 1973, 109, 727–732.
26. Allen TD. The non-neurogenic neurogenic bladder. *J Urol* 1977, 117, 232–238.
27. Mix LW. Occult neuropathic bladder. *Urology* 1977, 10, 1–9.
28. Koff SA, Lapides J, Piazza DH. Association of urinary tract infection and reflux with uninhibited bladder contractions and voluntary sphincter obstruction. *J Urol* 1979, 122, 373–377.

11 | The child with urinary tract infection

Heather Lambert and Malcolm Coulthard

Background

Urinary tract infection (UTI) in childhood is a significant and common problem encountered by primary, secondary, and tertiary healthcare professionals. UTI is an important cause of acute illness; it may be a marker of an underlying urinary tract abnormality, and may be associated with scarring which can cause significant long-term morbidity, particularly hypertension and renal impairment.

The true incidence of UTI is uncertain, but is reported in Sweden as 2.2% in boys and 2.1% in girls cumulative incidence by age 2 years [1]. Cumulative referral rates in northern England are similar, rising to 2.8% of boys and 8.2% of girls by the age of 7 years and 3.6% and 11.3% respectively by the age of 16 years [2]. It is generally accepted that the true rates are higher than those reported in earlier epidemiological studies from the 1970s and 1980s [3–6]. It is not known whether this represents a true rise in incidence or difference in rates of ascertainment. Some underdiagnosis is likely as there is evidence from Scandinavia that, even when strict diagnostic criteria are applied, rates vary between regions and are higher from centres with special interest [1].

UTI may be recurrent; about a third of girls having a further UTI within a year. The recurrence rate in boys is much lower. It causes considerable distress, anxiety, and inconvenience to children and their families. In some cases, UTI is associated with long-term problems, including hypertension and renal failure. Renal scarring is probably the most important aetiological factor in the development of hypertension in children and young adults. The terms renal scarring (renal damage associated with UTI) and reflux nephropathy (renal disease associated with vesicoureteric reflux) are ill-defined and often used interchangeably. Scarring, once present, is irreversible and, if severe, may lead to chronic renal failure (CRF). This usually presents many years later. In some cases it presents after several decades, and is often called chronic pyelonephritis. The incidence of chronic and end stage renal failure in childhood caused by reflux nephropathy varies worldwide. In Sweden there appears to be a falling incidence of end stage renal failure (ESRF) secondary to reflux nephropathy. It has been suggested that this may be due in part to increased awareness of UTI [1,7].

Large numbers of children with UTI are seen in the community by general practitioners, but there is frequently delay in treatment and not all are referred for further investigation [8]. There are considerable problems in the diagnosis of UTI, especially in younger patients, including lack of awareness, non-specific symptoms, and difficulties collecting and analysing specimens. There is evidence that many cases are misdiagnosed in the community and it is our experience that diagnosis and referral of cases increase when there is targeted information and education. Accurate diagnosis is fundamental in directing subsequent management and investigation.

For such a common problem it is perhaps surprising that there is no established consensus on investigation and management in childhood. However, given the paucity of knowledge of some of the basic pathophysiology, and lack of evidence comparing long-term outcomes with different management and intervention strategies, inconsistencies are to be expected.

Management and investigation of children with UTI consumes considerable healthcare resources in the United Kingdom and the rest of the world. It is important to optimize diagnostic and management strategies. The aim should be to:

(1) recognize the child at risk of UTI;

(2) diagnose early and definitively;

(3) treat acute UTI promptly;

(4) refer appropriately for evaluation after UTI;

(5) identify underlying renal tract abnormalities by appropriate investigation;

(6) identify those who have, or are at risk of, renal damage;

(7) prevent further renal damage;

(8) organize appropriate long-term follow-up for those who need it;

(9) avoid over-investigation and unnecessary follow-up.

Key points: General points

Urinary tract infection:

- affects many children;

- may be difficult to diagnose;

- may cause acute illness and symptoms;

- is frequently over- or underdiagnosed;

- may have long-term sequelae: hypertension, renal scarring, renal failure.

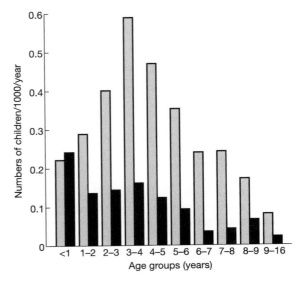

Fig. 11.1 Incidence of UTI. Number of children in Newcastle per 1000 total population referred with a diagnosis of UTI per years. Black bars, boys; grey bars, girls.

Clinical features

Classical symptoms of lower UTI (dysuria, frequency, and incontinence) and upper UTI (fever, systemic upset, loin pain, and renal tenderness) are frequently not seen in paediatric practice. Attempts to distinguish between upper and lower urinary tract infection on clinical grounds are unreliable and clinical history is not closely related to findings on imaging. Boys and girls are equally affected in infancy but after that the ratio of girls to boys progressively rises [1]. After puberty the incidence of UTI is low in both sexes, but rises in females who are sexually active (Figure 11.1).

The young child

In general terms, the younger the child the more diverse and less specific are the symptoms and signs. There may be a history of smelly urine or of crying on passing urine. Dysuria, urgency, frequency, or hesitancy may occur even in young children, but these are easier to identify in older children who are out of nappies and who are more articulate. Children may have an altered pattern of micturition, so a child who has recently stopped wearing nappies may start wetting again or night-time wetting may recur. Non-specific manifestations, such as poor feeding, vomiting, irritability, abdominal pain, failure to thrive, lethargy, and restlessness, should always lead to a suspicion of UTI, but there are no data that assess the sensitivity, specificity, or predictive value of these symptoms. Fever is frequently, but not always, present and UTI should be suspected in any young child with unexplained fever. There is evidence that UTI is found in around 5% of under 2-year-olds with unexplained fever [9,10].

The older child

Older children may have more typical signs and symptoms localizing to the urinary tract, including dysuria, frequency, urgency, hesitation, and enuresis. Some may have loin pain, but absence of loin pain does not exclude upper urinary tract involvement. Generalized symptoms are common, including fever, lethargy, anorexia, abdominal pain, nausea, and vomiting.

Not all children with dysuria have a urinary tract infection. Febrile or mildly dehydrated children may complain of pain, stinging, or discomfort on passing concentrated, or what they term 'strong', urine. Some other causes of dysuria are listed in Table 11.1.

Table 11.1   Causes of frequency/dysuria in pre-adolescent girls

Local irritants
  Bubble bath
  Shampoo
  Detergents
  Fabric softeners
  Tight-fitting garments
  Vulvovaginitis
  Chemicals in food, drink, medication
  Hypercalciuria
Highly concentrated urine
  Dehydration
UTI

Recurrent UTI

About one-third of girls will have a further UTI within a year and some go on to have repeated infections. Recurrent infections may be associated with an underlying urinary tract abnormality or renal scarring [11], but, in practice, a significant number of girls with non-scarred and non-refluxing urinary tracts have recurrent symptomatic UTI. This may cause considerable distress, anxiety, and frustration to the child and family. It is unusual for boys to have repeated infections in the absence of a urinary tract abnormality [11]. UTI may be associated with dysfunctional voiding and bladder instability [12] (see Chapter 15). There has long been evidence that UTI is more common in children with constipation [13,14]. There is reported evidence of post-micturition residue and upper tract dilatation in constipated children which improves with treatment [15]. A history of constipation should be sought, and may be suspected on abdominal palpation. In children with recurrent UTI, constipation should be treated aggressively and the rationale discussed with the family. UTI may be more frequent in girls suffering sexual abuse and this diagnosis should not be overlooked during assessment. Teenage girls may be sexually active and this may be a contributing factor in a recent onset of recurrent UTI.

Assessment

It is important to take a full clinical history from any child with a UTI, and to perform appropriate examination. Details should be sought of antenatal and perinatal history, drinking and voiding patterns, bowel habits, and family history of urinary infection, vesico-ureteric reflux (VUR), renal disease or hypertension. Examination should include measurement of blood pressure, abdominal palpation for masses (bladder, kidney), inspection of external genitalia and lower back, assessment of lower limb sensation and reflexes, and examination of the urine. When UTI is recurrent, it is particularly important that bladder and bowel habits are evaluated.

There has been much written about the distinction between upper and lower urinary tract infection. Indicators such as temperature, C-reactive protein, and loin pain have been used. However, although there is some evidence that those with classical clinical pyelonephritis may have an increased risk of scarring, there is no convincing evidence that any particular clinical pattern is associated with an 'uncomplicated or lower' UTI. Renal scarring may occur in association with few or no symptoms.

After the first year of life there is a marked sex difference in incidence of UTI, with girls being far more susceptible. This is usually explained by the difference in urethral length; the short female urethra providing easy access to the bladder for bacteria. While urine provides a good culture medium for bacteria, the bladder normally provides some resistance to infection. Repeated voiding and complete emptying of the bladder helps remove bacteria. Increasing fluid intake is often helpful in encouraging regular voiding, if the child and family understand the rationale. The bladder epithelium may also have some antibacterial activity. Incomplete emptying of the bladder may have an important role to play in recurrent UTI. Infection may affect normal ureteric peristalsis. Children with VUR, bladder outlet obstruction, constipation, neuropathic bladder, and dysfunctional voiding may have significant residual urine in the bladder, reducing the ability to decrease bacterial colonization by simple washout.

Key points: Clinical features of UTI

- Evaluation of any sick child must include examination of urine.

- Every young child with unexplained fever should have their urine examined.

- Clinical features of UTI are often non-specific.

- Boys seldom get recurrent UTI in the absence of urinary tract abnormalities.

Urine collection and testing

It is easy to under- or overdiagnose UTI in children if the urine is not examined. Underdiagnosis is especially common among infants presenting only with non-specific symptoms [16,17], and overdiagnosis is frequent among girls with vulvitis, and among children with febrile illness and anorexia who complain of dysuria (because of highly concentrated urine). The diagnosis must be correct if children at risk of scarring are to be appropriately treated and investigated, while those without UTI are to be spared unnecessary antibiotics, tests, and radiation.

Unfortunately, it is common for some children to receive an antibiotic for a presumed UTI without a urine sample being either collected or tested [8,18]. After such 'blind' treatment, the diagnosis remains uncertain, and it can only be an educated guess whether any individual should have imaging investigations. Often, urine is not collected because doctors imagine that uncontaminated samples are difficult to obtain (especially from the very young), or difficult to transport to the laboratory quickly enough. These practical problems are addressed later.

Urine collection

General

The ideal urine collection method would have zero contamination, be quick and easy for parents to undertake with a child of any age, be cheap, and would use little special equipment. Sadly, no such technique exists. Instead, there is a range of methods, and the best choice for a particular child will depend on the clinical setting and the child's age. Every method produces some contaminated samples, and opinions as to which is best differ between individual doctors, units, and families (Table 11.2). Unfortunately, infants who

Table 11.2 Specificity of urine cultures compared with suprapubic aspiration

Catheter sample of urine [9]
  Any growth 83–89%
  >1000 cfu/ml 95%
Clean catch urine 95% [19]
Bag specimen of urine 14–84% [10]

There are reasons to question the gold-standard status of SPA collections (page 201). We argue that bacterial quantification by phase contrast microscopy allows contaminated samples to be identified immediately, virtually eliminating this as a clinical problem (page 204).

are at the highest risk of scarring are also the most challenging to collect urine from. Many parents asked to collect a specimen at home are given no guidance on how to do this [8].

Older children

In older children urine can be voided directly into a sterile universal collection bottle after gently washing the genitalia with cotton wool and water. Disposable plastic funnels make this easier in girls. Collecting the mid-stream urine is ideal because the initial flow is likely to have washed off contaminating bacteria, but cleanly caught complete samples have relatively little contamination [20]. The glans should be washed in boys whose foreskin retracts easily. In girls, bacterial contamination may occur from the labia, or from urine flowing into the vagina before being collected. If this happens, most girls can produce a urethral stream by voiding into a bath while sitting on the side with their legs and labia parted.

Toddlers

Some potty-trained toddlers refuse to void into a sterile bottle, but will use a carefully cleaned potty. Potties cannot be adequately sterilized with bleach, household antiseptic, or boiling water, whereas simply washing them up in hot water and detergent reliably removes the bacteria with the biofilm [21]. Some clinics find it convenient to place a sterile dish in the potty.

Infants

Clean catch. Good association has been shown between the results of urine culture by clean-catch method (CCU) and suprapubic aspiration of urine [19]. CCU has also been shown to be superior to pad specimens and bag specimens for culture of the urine [20]. There are, however, practical problems with this method of urine collection, particularly in the home setting. Parents' views of doing this at home are mainly negative [22]. They consider it time consuming, messy, and difficult. In practice, collection failures are frequent. Gentle suprapubic tapping [23] has not been confirmed to induce immediate voiding.

Urine collection pads. Urine can be extracted from collection pads, which are modified sanitary towels without antiseptics or absorbent gel, placed inside the nappy (Ontex UK Ltd, Corby NN17 4JN, UK) [24].

The urine has only brief skin contact. It can be aspirated using a syringe without a needle, or squeezed from a minimally wetted pad by placing some fibres within a syringe barrel. Parents like them, though some find the urine extraction fiddly [22]. They are cheap. Some white cells are retained by the pad, but it is argued below that this is unimportant. Bacterial contamination rates using pads are similar to those seen using bags [22,23]. In practice, it is sensible to have a sterile bottle available when the nappy is removed, to put the pad in place, so a clean catch can be collected if the baby happens to void at once.

Sterile adhesive bags. These can be stuck to the skin around the genitalia. The inevitable contact time between the urine and genitalia is reduced in bags designed to drain the urine into an inner bag. Most parents are upset by the redness and discomfort on removing the bag, and many find decanting the urine difficult [22]. Their cost deters many general practitioners from using them [8].

Suprapubic aspiration. Urine may be obtained safely by suprapubic aspiration (SPA) with a syringe and needle. This is relatively easier in infants than older children because their bladders extend into the abdomen even when they are only partially full [25,26]. It is made easier by locating the bladder with ultrasound [26]. Studies clearly show that SPA urine samples have much less contamination than voided ones [25,27,28].

SPA is often referred to as being the 'gold standard'. It is widely assumed that *any* concentration of bacteria grown from an SPA urine *always* indicates a certain UTI (which implies that they have 100% sensitivity and specificity). However, this has not been rigorously assessed. Indeed, there is suggestive evidence that this is not so. Very low colony counts, presumably due to contaminating organisms, have been recorded in 16% of SPA samples [25]. Also, cases have been reported where paired urines were positive when collected by SPA, but negative when voided into a bag [19,29]. These authors state that the voided urines were falsely negative, and do not suggest how this could happen, or discuss the possibility that the SPA results could have been falsely positive. If they were false positives, the rates would be between 11% [35] and 29% [29]. To clarify this, it would be necessary to design a study in which the SPA was repeated in uncertain cases. Since blood cultured after clean venepuncture may contain contaminating

bacteria, it is implausible that urine collected by bladder puncture cannot; suprapubic skin is no less likely to be colonized than the arm. Also, if the needle was advanced too far, it might enter the bowel transiently during the process of bladder aspiration [30].

SPA is undoubtedly of value in ill infants who require immediate antibiotics, if voiding cannot be induced by suprapubic pressure. It has no role in the home or in general practice, where most infants are screened for a UTI. Its value for collecting urine in hospital in non-emergency cases is debatable. The main disadvantage of using non-invasive collection methods is the greater risk of obtaining contaminated samples, something which largely disappears if fresh urine can be screened by phase-contrast microscopy, and repeat samples collected if necessary.

Urethral catheterization

Bladder taps may not yield specimens, success rates varying between 23 and 90%; 100% success rates have been achieved with ultrasonographic guidance [10]. Because of these problems with SPA, practitioners often use transurethral catheterization to obtain urine specimens for culture. This may be justifiable in a child who is unable or too ill to co-operate.

> ## Key points: Obtaining a urine sample
>
> - Collect urine before starting treatment.
> - Pad, bag, and clean catch all result in contamination of some urines.
> - Potties can be used for clean catches if they are washed thoroughly.
> - SPA has a much lower contamination rate (but not zero).
> - Catheterization is preferred to SPA by some clinicians.

Minimizing post-collection bacterial growth

It is important to minimize the overgrowth of contaminating organisms during storage and transfer to the laboratory. Storage and transport difficulties may be why general practitioners are less likely to culture a urine sample from a child presenting during an evening or weekend [8].

Dipslides. These provide a method of culturing fresh urine, which can be used at any time or location. Thus the problem of post-collection overgrowth of bacteria is minimized. They, therefore, have great potential in culture of urine where there is a delay before the urine reaches the laboratory. Dipslides consist of a sterile bottle with a miniature culture plate attached to the inside of the lid. The manufacturers suggest inoculating the agar by briefly immersing the culture plate in a 20 ml sample bottle of urine. They have been used successfully for schoolgirls [31], but a report of their use for a wide age range of children reported that agar often became detached [32]. These may have been shaken vigorously to try to coat the agar with a small sample. An effective alternative for small urine samples is to 'plate out' urine on to the agar using a sterile swab. In a research study where parents were given a demonstration, augmented by written instructions, they found it easy to do [22].

Once wetted, the dipslide can be posted to the laboratory for incubation, or kept at 37 °C in the primary-care department. Dipslides with few or no colonies after 24 hours at 37 °C can be discarded [33]. Ones with significant growth require laboratory subculture for sensitivity testing.

Refrigeration. Refrigeration to 4 °C is another very effective way of miminizing post-collection contamination. It provides highly effective storage for 72 hours [47], but is not always convenient. Always placing urine in a fridge at 4 °C when there is any delay in getting the sample to the laboratory has a dramatic impact on the number of false-positive results.

Boric acid preservation of urines. Collection bottles containing boric acid are widely used, but may produce false-negative results [32,34]. They are designed to be completely filled with urine to produce bacteriostatic concentrations of boric acid, so small paediatric samples may result in bactericidal levels. Smaller borate bottles are available.

Urine testing

Theoretical considerations

When considering criteria for the diagnosis of UTI there are a number of factors that need to be taken into account (Table 11.3).

There are the competing considerations of false-negative and false-positive diagnoses. A false-negative diagnosis will leave patients at risk of serious complications. A false-positive diagnosis will lead to unnecessary, invasive, and expensive investigations. Kass' seminal paper [35] that introduced quantitative urine culture recognized this dilemma. He recognized that the cut-off of 10^5/ml colony forming units (cfu) of one bacterial species on culture was, to some extent, arbitrary and was 1000 times lower than the concentration seen in most UTI [35]. A lower cut-off point increases the sensitivity of the test but reduces the specificity, with the converse for a higher cut-off point. There is no doubt that this figure has been adhered to too rigidly and that most have not had the sophisticated understanding of this that the original paper assumed.

Sensitivity and specificity are constant criteria that can be applied to any diagnostic test irrespective of the characteristics of the population on which the test is used. However, the clinical importance of the test result is determined not only by the sensitivity and specificity of the test but also by the prevalence of the condition in the population being studied. This is illustrated in the matrix for an almost ideal test with a sensitivity and specificity of 90% (Table 11.4) [36]. The dramatic effect of the prevalence on the significance of the test is immediately obvious.

The prevalence of UTI among febrile infants between 2 and 24 months of age has been shown in a number of studies to be ~5% [9,10]. There is very little information about the prevalence of UTI in children with other symptoms or signs or at other ages;

Table 11.3 Some considerations in assessing diagnostic tests for UTI

Sensitivity and specificity of the test
Variability and quality control
Assumed prevalence of UTI in the population being tested
Post-collection bacterial growth
Gold standard
Practicalities and timing of results

Table 11.4 Positive predictive value of a test with sensitivity and specificity of 90% in populations with different prevalence of disease [36]

Prevalence	Positive predictive value
50%	90%
10%	50%
2%	16%

See comments about phase-contrast microscopy in Table 11.2

but, particularly in infants, the prevalence in most other clinical situations is not likely to be higher than for febrile children. Thus in clinical situations, the incidence of UTI is low and the positive predictive value of the results correspondingly low. Furthermore, most of the tests used in the diagnosis of UTI have sensitivities and specificities of well below 90%.

Another consequence of these considerations is that tests will have different significance in different clinical settings where the 'prevalence' of UTIs differs. A test which performs well in a hospitalized population might give quite different results in a primary-care setting.

Pre- and post-test probability predicted from the likelihood ratio nomogram is another, more convenient, way of estimating the significance of a test result [37].

Finally, because young children with UTI may be acutely unwell, and are at risk of rapid scarring, an instant near-patient test that is reliable and convenient would be a major advantage. Urine culture cannot provide this. This would allow immediate treatment with the 'best guess' antibiotic, adjusted later according to the bacterial sensitivities. Although helpful, none of the near-patient tests are ideal. Without an immediate certain diagnosis, the options are to delay treatment pending the culture results (increasing the risk of scarring), or start treatment on clinical suspicion, and stop if the culture is negative (risking overusing antibiotics). The younger the child, the stronger the argument for immediate treatment, guided by a near-patient diagnostic test.

Diagnostic tests for UTI

Bacterial culture

The diagnostic criteria for bacteriuria suggested by Kass [35], and some of the problems with this, have been discussed above. The cut-off concentration of 10^5/ml is also very convenient for practical laboratory reasons. One wire-loop of urine containing bacteria at 10^5/ml produces confluent colonies on a Petri dish; to count higher numbers requires predilution. Thus, bacterial numbers below 10^5/ml can be quantified, but all higher concentrations are reported as greater than 10^5/ml.

Kass reported that using his criteria, 4% of asymptomatic men and 6% of asymptomatic women in outpatients were diagnosed as having UTI [19]. We have found similar rates of 8% in infants [22] and 6.6% in children [38]. Others have reported growing more

than 10^5 coliforms/ml in bag or clean catch samples from preterm [25] and term neonates [25,39], infants [39,40], and older children [40] who did not have urine infections (confirmed by sterile SPAs). Guidelines suggest that all infants with an unexplained fever above 38.5 °C should have a urine cultured [9,17]. This means that a child with three febrile illnesses would have a 1 in 5 chance of being falsely labelled as having a UTI.

Standard laboratory urine culture takes up to 24 hours. If positive, the organism is identified and subcultured with antibiotic-impregnated discs to determine its sensitivity and to guide treatment. Culture has an inherent delay. Four or five days may easily elapse between a general practitioner seeing a child and receiving the laboratory report. This is a major disadvantage. Occasionally, a UTI may be caused by anaerobic organisms which produce a false-negative result by standard culture.

Urinary white blood cells

Many children with UTI have an increased number of urinary white blood cells (WBCs), and this is commonly regarded as an important diagnostic feature. However, the evidence does not support this. This is partly because the laboratory WBC count may be artificially low, and partly because children can have UTI without increased WBCs, and increased WBCs without a UTI.

Urinary WBCs survive intact for variable periods of time, perhaps related to factors such as urinary pH [41]. Some are very short lived, and fall to a low number or disappear by the time the urine reaches the laboratory [38]. Additionally, the number of urine WBCs varies widely between children with UTI, even when freshly voided urine is examined microscopically. Rarely, a young child with an overwhelming infection may be unable to maintain a urinary WBC response [42]. Similarly, children being treated with immunosuppressant drugs may be unable to produce a pyuria. On the other hand, girls may have moderately high WBC count from the vagina, and children with a pyrexia from any cause tend to have increased urinary WBC numbers [43], perhaps because of an increase in the mobility and number of circulating white cells in the blood.

None of these factors suggests that the urine WBC count is reliable in distinguishing a child with a UTI from one without [9,10,17]. The slight reduction in WBC numbers in urine samples collected by pad [24] is, therefore, unimportant.

Leucocyte esterase (LE) test

A urine stick test is available to detect excess WBCs, but this does not make their presence or absence any easier to interpret. This is not the common view. In our experience, many doctors are less likely to accept the bacteriological diagnosis of a UTI if the laboratory does not report an excess of white cells.

Nitrite stick tests

Most bacteria that cause UTI produce nitrite as a result of their metabolism, which can be detected using a urine stick test. The nitrite test has a high specificity (90–100%) but the sensitivity is only 53% (range 15–82%) [10], because it sometimes take hours for the bacteria to produce detectable quantities of nitrite [44], and children with UTIs tend to void much more frequently than this. The nitrite test may, therefore, be useful for ruling in UTI when it is positive, but it has little value in ruling out UTI [10]. Samples that test negative should therefore still be cultured or examined microscopically. In practice, some doctors interpret them as if they can reliably exclude a UTI, and only culture ones that test positive [8]. Reviews supporting this use inappropriate statistical tests [45]. The negative predictive value of a test depends not only on its sensitivity, but also on the population frequency of the condition being tested. For example, a totally flawed test, with a sensitivity of 0%, would have a negative predictive value of 99.9% if the condition for which it was introduced had a prevalence of only 1 in 1000. For nitrite sticks, where the sensitivity is only about 50%, the negative predictive value will be very low if it is tested on a population with a high chance of having a UTI, such as in a clinic for children who perform self-catheterization. By contrast, it will be very high (and may therefore be recommended as a useful test [45]) if nitrite sticks were used to screen children where the prevalence of UTI is relatively low. However, it must be remembered that in both situations half the children with UTI will have the diagnosis missed.

Phase-contrast microscopy

Bacteria are readily identified in urine by Gram staining, but this is time consuming, and unsuitable for routine urine screening [35]. Unstained bacteria are difficult to see using standard light microscopy. However, phase-contrast makes it very easy [38].

Bacteria are clearly defined as black organisms against a light background in uncentrifuged fresh urine (Fig. 11.2). Therefore, phase-contrast microscopy can provide a fast, reliable, efficient, and economic near-patient UTI diagnostic service.

Urine microscopy is a simple and satisfying skill to learn (Table 11.5). Most samples are likely to be uninfected. Focusing on the counting grid, no bacteria will be seen. If no bacteria are seen, the urine is sterile and can be discarded. Infected urine typically has tens, hundreds, or thousands of identical rods per high power field, equivalent to bacterial counts of between 10^6 and 10^9/ml (all reported as $>10^5$/ml on culture). Antibiotics can be commenced immediately, but culture and sensitivity testing is also needed to guide treatment. Occasionally UTIs are caused by *Streptococcus faecalis* which is easily recognized as chains of cocci. These must not be confused with phosphate crystals which are a similar size, but are seen individually or in clumps, and not chains. If a UTI is diagnosed by phase-contrast, but the culture is negative, consider whether the urine was a small volume in a boric acid bottle, or whether the child has an anaerobic UTI.

A few urine samples will give uncertain results, either because just one or two bacteria are seen, both rods and streptococci are present, or there is amorphous debris, cotton strands etc. Because this result is available at once, an immediate careful second sample can be collected. Rarely, this confirms a UTI. Occasionally, children on antibiotic prophylaxis have unusually small numbers of bacteria. This can be due to partial antibiotic resistance, identified microscopically if bacilli are seen in chains with swellings at their junctional walls. The majority of repeat specimens are completely clear, indicating that the first sample was contaminated. They can therefore be discarded. It is interesting that if these first samples are cultured, some would be recognized as contaminated, and others would grow more than 10^5/ml coliforms. These are false-positive UTIs which cannot be distinguished from genuine cases except by urine microscopy. In our experience 6.6% of sterile paediatric urine samples give a false-positive result by culture [38].

Phase-contrast is also better than standard microscopy for examining cells in the urine. White cells can be seen in detail. Red cell morphology is clear, and can differentiate glomerular from lower tract bleeding. The content of casts is clearly visible. Many older girls have vaginal epithelial cells in the

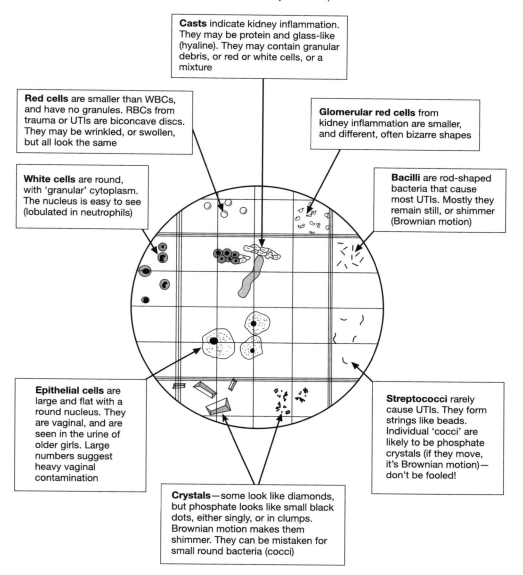

Casts indicate kidney inflammation. They may be protein and glass-like (hyaline). They may contain granular debris, or red or white cells, or a mixture

Red cells are smaller than WBCs, and have no granules. RBCs from trauma or UTIs are biconcave discs. They may be wrinkled, or swollen, but all look the same

Glomerular red cells from kidney inflammation are smaller, and different, often bizarre shapes

White cells are round, with 'granular' cytoplasm. The nucleus is easy to see (lobulated in neutrophils)

Bacilli are rod-shaped bacteria that cause most UTIs. Mostly they remain still, or shimmer (Brownian motion)

Epithelial cells are large and flat with a round nucleus. They are vaginal, and are seen in the urine of older girls. Large numbers suggest heavy vaginal contamination

Streptococci rarely cause UTIs. They form strings like beads. Individual 'cocci' are likely to be phosphate crystals (if they move, it's Brownian motion)—don't be fooled!

Crystals—some look like diamonds, but phosphate looks like small black dots, either singly, or in clumps. Brownian motion makes them shimmer. They can be mistaken for small round bacteria (cocci)

Fig. 11.2 Phase-contrast microscopy of urine.

urine and occasionally long rods which are anaerobic vaginal lactobacilli. Children with metabolic stones may have identifiable crystals. Phosphate crystals are common in normal concentrated urines.

In our paediatric department, phase-contrast microscopy has saved considerable sums of money. This is because sterile urine samples (the majority) are not cultured, and the running costs are negligible. Many nurses and all junior doctors are trained to examine urines. Each examination is recorded on an adhesive result label and stuck in the case notes. Most staff find it very satisfying to be able to give an instant diagnosis to a worried parent.

Causative organisms

Escherichia coli are cultured from about 85% of urines from boys and girls with a first UTI [46,47].

Table 11.5 Phase-contrast microscopy: practicalities

Our experience is that ease, convenience and accuracy of use of the phase-contrast microscope is aided by:

- keeping microscopes in clinical areas (e.g. outpatients, ward, day-unit), dedicated for urine microscopy only
- having a binocular eyepiece (with a second teaching head)
- having only one objective (to give a total magnification of ×400) and removing the other objectives (so the microscope is left 'in focus')
- using a glass slide counting chamber with two recessed areas 0.1 mm deep, each with a grid etched on a lightly mirrored surface, together with a coverslip to create two chambers 0.1 mm deep
- using a urine dipstrip to test for blood, protein, etc., then touching its wet tip on the edge of one of the chambers so urine is drawn in by capillary action
- using the grid to aid focusing; there is nothing to focus on with a negative urine on a plain slide
- inspecting five grid squares (0.02 μl, or about five high-power fields)
- frequent practice and by having an experienced person available to review puzzling findings via a teaching eyepiece

It has long been thought that the bacteria originate from the patient's own bowel, and this has now been confirmed definitively by genetic 'fingerprinting' techniques [48]. The other responsible organisms include *Klebsiella* and *Proteus*, as well as *Streptococcus faecalis* and a variety of other species. Children with abnormal urinary tracts are much more likely to have UTI due to less virulent organisms such as *Pseudomonas* or *Staphylococcus aureus*. These bacteria often contribute to the flora which may cause contamination from the genitalia and skin.

Children with *Proteus* UTI are at particular risk of developing stones within the urinary tract. This occurs because the bacteria produce ammonia by metabolizing urea. This increases the urinary pH, which tends to make calcium and magnesium phosphate salts precipitate. This may occur particularly in the mucus and cellular debris caused by the inflammatory process, and create a thick sludge that takes up the shape of the drainage tract. Further chemical precipitation may make it more solid. In the pelvicalyceal system these become stag-horn calculi, and in the ureter they become shaped like a date stone.

Key points: Summary of urine collection and testing

- Accurate diagnosis of UTI is vital to appropriate subsequent management.
- Antibiotic treatment should be started as soon as a suitable sample has been collected.
- Urine can be collected in any setting by pad, bag, or by clean catch into a bottle or washed potty.
- All urine collecting methods may fail or result in contamination.
- All methods result in some (up to 8%) false positives (e.g. pure growth $> 10^5$/ml coliforms).
- Phase-contrast microscopy is easy to learn, and quick to perform.
- Microscopy can immediately identify and prevent false positives.
- Positive nitrite stick tests diagnose UTI, but negative ones do not exclude UTI.
- Urine white cell counts do not help make the diagnosis of UTI.
- Urine samples that cannot be transported to the laboratory quickly should be refrigerated, or inoculated onto a dipslide.
- Boric acid bottles should be avoided for small samples, as underfilled bottles may produce false-negative results.
- Hospital paediatric departments could help general practitioners by offering a urinary collection and diagnostic service for children, especially the youngest, where the diagnosis of UTI is not clear.

Treatment

The aim of treatment is to eliminate the acute infection and reduce or prevent renal damage. There is evidence in animal models of scarring of susceptible kidneys occurring if infection lasts more than a few days before treatment [49,50]. For obvious reasons there are no good prospective studies in children, but retrospective studies suggest that delayed treatment increases the risk of renal scarring [51–53].

If UTI is suspected, 'best guess' antibiotics should be started while awaiting results of the urine culture. This is particularly important in younger children. Sensitivities should be available within 48–72 hours and antibiotics can be changed if indicated. It is important that procedures are implemented for obtaining reports on urine cultures quickly and that, for patients at home, information is conveyed rapidly to parents. Cephalexin, trimethoprim, or nitrofurantoin are frequently used, but discussion with the local microbiologist should help guide general advice about resistance patterns in community-acquired infection in the local paediatric population. Recent antibiotic use by the patient should also be taken into account when prescribing. It is common practice to encourage increased intake of fluids when treating UTI.

Children, particularly infants, who are clinically dehydrated, toxic, or unlikely to retain oral fluids, should be referred to hospital for parenteral antibiotics initially. Fever should settle within 48 hours in the majority of infants treated with parenteral antibiotics. Prolonged fever alone has not been shown to be associated with complications [54]. However, if the clinical condition does not improve within this time, a repeat urine specimen should be obtained and further urgent investigation should be considered, for example renal tract ultrasound to look for dilatation related to obstruction. Normally there should be an aim for discharge on appropriate oral antibiotics once the child is improving and sensitivities are known. There is no clear evidence about the ideal length of therapy to eradicate acute infection in children. In adults, studies suggest improved efficacy of a 3-day treatment versus a one-dose treatment. In children longer courses of antibiotics (7–10 days) achieve better results than short courses (one dose or up to 3 days) [9,10]. These studies support the common practice of using a longer rather than shorter course in children because of the risk of long-term sequelae if infection is not eradicated. Because of the association between recurrent UTI and scarring [4], after the acute course of antibiotics a urine specimen should be checked and a prophylactic dose of a suitable antibiotic should be continued until investigations are completed and assessed [9,17].

In children with a normal urinary tract, but recurrent UTI, there is evidence that a long course of antibiotics (6 months) is associated with not only a reduced frequency of UTI while the antibiotics are being taken, but also for the subsequent 2 years [55]. Rotation of prophylactic antibiotics is sometimes advocated. Cranberry juice has been used for many years for prevention of UTI, but the few small studies that exist are currently inconclusive as to the effectiveness of cranberry products [56]. Clinical experience suggests simple measures like increasing fluid intake, regular voiding, and avoiding perineal irritants may be helpful in the prevention of recurrent UTI in some girls.

There is an association between recurrent UTI and both constipation and dysfunctional voiding. Active treatment of constipation may reduce recurrent UTI in patients with normal urinary tracts. In one study of children with constipation, 46% had problems with day or night wetting and a third of girls had UTI. In children who had no anatomical urinary tract abnormalities, with successful treatment of constipation there was no recurrence of UTI and wetting improved [57]. Post-micturition residue and upper tract dilatation have been found to be increased in children with constipation, and improved after treatment [15]. UTI may be associated with dysfunctional voiding and bladder instability [12], and it is important that bladder and bowel habits are evaluated, especially when UTI is recurrent. There is, however, little evidence regarding efficacy of interventions such as bladder training, behaviour modification, or anticholinergic drugs in affected individuals. Clinical experience suggests that these approaches warrant further study.

The treatment of children known to have vesicoureteric reflux is addressed later.

Children with complex urinary tract problems, who require interventions such as intermittent catheterization, frequently have both asymptomatic bacteriuria and symptomatic UTI. These children should all be managed in conjunction with a specialist centre, and decisions on management and treatment will vary depending on the individual circumstances and underlying problems (see Chapters 9 and 10).

There is no evidence of benefit from treatment of asymptomatic bacteriuria in girls with normal urinary tracts. They do not therefore require routine screening of urine when well. However, the patient in whom it is discovered by chance presents a dilemma. Scarring may be found in patients with asymptomatic bacteriuria and progression can occur in a minority of those with scarring. Thus such patients should be evaluated to establish whether or not renal damage is present.

Circumcision

The risk of UTI in uncircumcized boys under the age of 1 year is reported to be increased between 3 and 15 times compared to those who are circumcised [58,59]. However, that increased risk, when countered against the risks of circumcision, is not considered sufficient to recommend it as a routine preventative measure [60,61] (this is further discussed in Chapter 12).

Key points: Treatment of UTI

- Treatment goal is prevention of renal injury and symptoms associated with UTI.

- Start 'best guess' antibiotic as soon as urine obtained.

- Change antibiotic if indicated by culture result.

- If clinical condition does not improve after 48 hours, repeat urine culture and consider urgent investigations to exclude urological problems.

- Treatment antibiotics should be given for 7–10 days.

- Prophylactic antibiotics should be given to children under 4 years of age until investigations are complete.

- Clinical experience suggests a benefit from increasing fluid intake and treatment of constipation.

Investigation

There is considerable controversy about the appropriate investigation of the child with UTI, and no perfect solution. Some understanding of the pathophysiology and an appreciation of some of the unanswered questions are essential in developing a pragmatic approach to investigation of UTI. Investigation will need to be tailored to the individual patient in many cases, and developments in techniques and new uses of current techniques will change current investigation schemes. The general aims of investigation are summarized in Table 11.6.

Renal scarring

Risk factors for development of renal scarring include young age, delay in antibiotic treatment of

Table 11.6   Aims of investigations in UTI

To identify those:
   with an underlying renal tract abnormality or
      predisposition to UTI, e.g.
         -structural abnormality of urinary tract
         -urinary tract obstruction
         -vesico-ureteric reflux
         -abnormal bladder emptying
   who have already sustained damage to their kidneys
   who are likely to sustain damage to their kidneys

UTI [50], recurrent infections [11,62], vesico-ureteric reflux [63], and obstruction of the urinary tract.

Timing of scarring

The timing of scarring is often not clear. Young children appear to be at most risk of scarring [64]. In one study children with normal investigations after UTI were re-investigated by repeat [^{99}Tc^m]dimercapto-succinic acid (DMSA) scan 2–11 years later. Very few first scars were found in children who were older than 3 years at the time of their original DMSA, and none in those who were older than 4 years [65]. The reasons for this are not clear. It is possible that children 'grow out' of their tendency to scar, or simply that if a child is going to get a UTI leading to scarring they are likely to have already done so by the time they reach the age of 4 years. However, the frequency of renal scars in children presenting with their first *documented* UTI does not appear to be related to age [2,66]. The apparent paradox may be explained by scarring having occurred when a child had an earlier undiagnosed UTI. There is now evidence from pig models that kidneys remain susceptible to scarring at any age [67]. Other factors such as failure of diagnosis or delay in initiating treatment may explain the apparent age relationship between UTI and scarring seen in man [68].

Vesico-ureteric reflux

Vesico-ureteric reflux (VUR) is a major risk factor for progressive renal damage associated with UTI. VUR is the retrograde flow of urine from the bladder into the upper urinary tract. It is usually congenital but may occasionally be acquired, for example after surgery. Because of the difficulties and ethics of studies, the true incidence of VUR in the normal population at various ages is not known, but is in the order of 1% in infants [68,69] and is increased in certain risk groups. VUR is found in up to one-third of children investigated after symptomatic UTI and in up to 50% of infants with UTI [69]. Babies with antenatal identification of renal pelvis dilatation have an increased risk of VUR. The figures depend on the population investigated postnatally but are in the region of 10–40% [70,71]. VUR is found in association with congenital abnormalities of the urinary tract, such as ureteric duplication, contralateral multicystic dysplastic kidney or renal agenesis. There is evidence of a 20- to 50-fold increased risk of VUR in children with a family history of VUR [69,72]. There is good evidence that VUR is a genetic disorder [73]. Different modes of inheritance have been proposed, including dominant and polygenic inheritance [73].

Grading of vesico-ureteric reflux

Grades of severity of VUR are recognized, designated grades I to V by the International Reflux Study Committee in 1981 and still generally accepted worldwide (Fig. 11.3) [74].

VUR is not an 'all or none' phenomenon. It is well described as being intermittent and variable in grade at different times during an examination [75]. VUR in both humans and animals can be influenced by variations in urine flow [76,77], which may be related to changes in ureteric peristalsis. Despite that, grading of VUR remains important because higher grades of reflux are associated with increased chance of renal scarring [63,78], of reflux-associated dysplasia, and with less chance of spontaneous resolution [79].

Abnormal urodynamic patterns associated with vesico-ureteric reflux

There is an association between abnormal urodynamic variables and a diagnosis of VUR in infants, especially boys [80]. Urodynamic dysfunction, bladder instability, or high intravesical pressures are commonly found in infants with high-grade VUR [81,84] (see also Chapters 9 and 10). Urodynamics in normal infants are not easily studied for comparison, and the relationship of abnormal urodynamic patterns to the pathogenesis or resolution of VUR is not known. In the growing pig, sterile VUR has been shown not to affect renal growth or uptake of DMSA, even in the presence of raised voiding pressures and abnormal bladder function [85]. Bladder dysfunction may predispose to infection.

Relationship of vesico-ureteric reflux, renal scarring, and reflux nephropathy

Details of these relationships are far from clear, despite the recognition of an association between VUR and scarring since the 1960s. VUR is thought to predispose to renal damage by facilitating passage of bacteria from the bladder to the upper urinary tract. An immunological and inflammatory reaction is caused by renal infection, leading to renal injury and scarring. Extensive renal scarring causes reduced renal function, reduced renal growth, renal failure, hypertension, and increased incidence of pregnancy-related hypertension. While these sequelae may occur in childhood they frequently do not arise until many years or decades later.

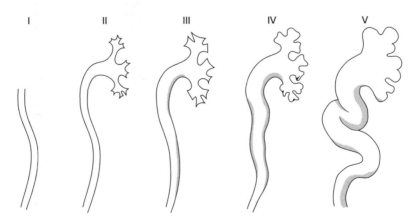

Fig. 11.3 Grading of vesico-ureteric reflux: I, into ureter only; II, into ureter, pelvis, and calyces with no dilatation; III, with mild to moderate dilatation, slight or no blunting of fornices; IV, with moderate dilatation of ureter and/or renal pelvis and/or tortuosity of ureter, obliteration of sharp angle of fornices; V, gross dilatation and tortuosity, no papillary impression visible in calyces [74].

Our understanding of the mechanism of focal scarring has been greatly advanced by the piglet model developed by Ransley and Risdon. In their studies they found that neither VUR alone (with sterile urine), nor lower UTI alone (with no VUR) led to scarring [50,86]. However scars, developed in some segments of kidneys when there was VUR and UTI, leaving the adjacent segments unaffected. They found that the scarred and unscarred segments had different-shaped papillae. The scarred segments had compound papillae that were flat or concave in shape whereas the unscarred segments had simple, cone-shaped papillae (Fig. 11.4). Compound papillae with open, gaping orifices allow intrarenal reflux, whereas simple papillae with slit-like orifices do not [87].

Post-mortem examination of kidneys from young children who died of a non-renal cause reveals similar variation in papillary form, likely to have led to intrarenal reflux in about two-thirds [88]. This figure is higher than can be demonstrated radiologically in children with VUR [89,90]. A number of factors may interfere with demonstration of intrarenal reflux, including timing of films, back flow of urine, or details obscured by bowel shadows. It is thus suggested that intrarenal reflux may be present more often than can be demonstrated [88]. There is good evidence in humans that the reflux of infected urine into the kidney in the presence of compound papillae can cause acute pyelonephritis and subsequent renal

parenchymal scarring [89]. The presence of both types of papillae in one kidney explains why scarring is segmental and why adjacent areas can remain pristine [87]. It is possible that the development of a scar can distort the intrarenal architecture to such an extent that adjacent papillae may develop intrarenal reflux, leading to extension of scarring with subsequent infections. The absence of refluxing papillae may explain why some kidneys with a refluxing ureter do not scar, even in the presence of infection.

Some babies born with VUR have associated dysplastic or hypoplastic renal malformations or *in utero* damage; all of which may impair renal function [91,92]. These abnormalities are usually associated with severe grades of VUR, and sometimes with obstruction. It is not clear whether severe VUR is simply associated with renal abnormalities or whether there is a causal link. There is some evidence from work with fetal lambs suggesting that fetal sterile reflux may impair GFR as well as concentrating ability [93]. Work with piglets has shown an association between sterile VUR and impaired concentrating ability [94]. Thus renal abnormalities may be found on imaging, associated with VUR *in utero* but in the absence of any history of UTI. Confusingly, these abnormalities may often also be referred to as scars. Therefore when a child being investigated following a UTI is found to have abnormalities on DMSA scan it may be difficult to distinguish whether this is scarring caused by UTI or a congenital renal abnormality, or both. Progressive renal impairment from dysplasia is probably not preventable and presumably results from lack of normal growth potential of abnormal renal tissue. Development of new or additional renal scarring secondary to UTI may be preventable, and it is to this end that investigation and management strategies should be aimed.

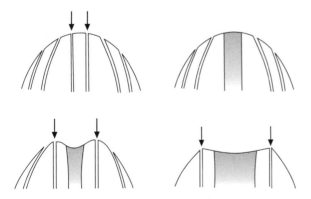

Fig. 11.4 Intrarenal reflux: a diagram illustrating the suggested mechanism whereby some apparently non-refluxing papillae with ducts opening at the very tip of the papilla might be transformed into a refluxing papilla under the influence of high pressure vesico-ureteric reflux. The arrows indicate ducts allowing intrarenal reflux and the stippled areas represent the subsequent scar formation. (Reproduced from [86] with permission from BMJ Publishing Group.)

The child with scarring but no vesico-ureteric reflux

While it is clear that VUR is a major risk factor for development of renal scarring, many children are found to have a scarred kidney but no evidence of VUR [95]. A number of theories have been proposed to explain this:

- The child had VUR but has now grown out of it.

- The child has VUR but the test failed to detect it.

- The diagnosis is wrong, they don't have scarring but have some other abnormality, e.g. dysplasia or hypoplasia.

- Infection can ascend in the absence of demonstrable VUR.

- The scar was not caused by ascending infection but by some other mechanism, e.g. blood-borne infection or local toxin release.

The first of these theories may be the correct explanation in many cases when scarring is discovered at initial investigation but the timing of the development of scarring is not known. However, there are sufficient anomalies, for example when there is evidence of acute involvement of the kidney in the absence of VUR [95], to require an open mind to be kept about the whole nature of the relationship of VUR and scarring.

Who to investigate

Young children and infants warrant intensive investigation because a UTI is more likely to be a marker of underlying urinary tract abnormality like severe VUR or obstruction. In addition, because of the non-specific symptoms in this age group, there is more likely to be a delay in treatment and diagnosis of UTI. Younger children appear to be at higher risk of sustaining renal damage associated with UTI. Older children warrant investigation after their first documented UTI because the detection of scarring does not appear to be related to age [2,71,96]. Despite clear and generally accepted guidance from the Royal College of Physicians [17] that all children should be referred for some form of investigation after a first UTI, there is evidence that this does not always happen [8]. While most very young children are referred after a first UTI, the referral rate declines for older children, particularly for girls [8].

An intensive investigation programme, for example of abdominal X ray, DMSA scan, renal ultrasound, and micturating cystourethrogram (MCU) for all children with a UTI would identify those with renal damage and risk factors like VUR or urethral abnormalities. However, UTI is so common that many children with no urinary tract abnormalities would be subjected to invasive investigations without benefit. Therefore, ideally one would like to be able to identify children who are at high risk of renal damage and thus of long-term sequelae, and only investigate them.

Much has been written about trying to identify those with *upper* versus *lower* urinary tract infection. However, clinical features are non-specific and there is conflicting evidence on the association of parameters such as C-reactive protein with scarring [96,97].

There is an association, which is widely accepted, between renal scarring and VUR. The more severe the VUR, the more likely the chance of finding scarring. However, the converse is not true. Renal scarring is found in kidneys drained by a ureter not found to be refluxing. The evaluation and investigation of VUR and its relationship to scarring is problematic. There are anomalies that are difficult to explain. There may be renal involvement on early DMSA (done at the time of infection) that does not go on to leave a permanent scar. However, when permanent scars do form, they do so at the same site as the acute involvement. We do not fully understand what factors are involved in resolution of acute renal involvement as opposed to progression to permanent scarring. There may be renal involvement on acute DMSA but no evidence of VUR. This is one of many unresolved questions. What we currently understand about the relationship of VUR, UTI, and scarring should be regarded as the beginning of the story not the end. However, both research and clinical evaluation and management are hampered by the nature of the techniques available to study it and by the intermittent, fluctuant nature of VUR itself.

Key points: Investigation of UTI

- All children should have some investigation after a first proven UTI.

- Unnecessary investigations should be avoided.

- First scars rarely occur after the age of 4 years.

- VUR is found in up to 30% of children with UTI.

- There is a 20- to 50-fold increased risk for VUR if there is a family history of VUR.

- Relationships between VUR, renal scarring, and reflux nephropathy are not clear.

- Young children and infants warrant intensive investigation.

Techniques commonly used for investigating UTI in childhood

Ultrasonography

Pros:

- No ionizing radiation.

- Widely available.

- Good for detecting differences in density, therefore detects structural abnormality, i.e. dilated kidneys and ureters, and cysts in kidneys.

- Capable of detecting parenchymal abnormality, including scars, if there is a good operator and equipment, and sufficient time with a co-operative subject (e.g. in a research centre).

- Colour flow imaging may be useful in detection of VUR (controversial)

Cons:

- Very operator-dependent.

- Often misses scars.

- Difficult if patient uncooperative.

- Cannot readily be reviewed retrospectively from still pictures.

DMSA study

Pros:

- Good at detecting scars.

- Provides differential renal function (although this is tubular function, it corresponds well with glomerular filtration rate).

- Original data can be reviewed for second opinions/ reporting of difficult studies/comparison with previous or later studies.

- Can be standardized.

Cons:

- Radiation dose.

- Intravenous injection.

- Timing is important—DMSA during or soon after acute infection may show areas of reduced uptake, which may not be permanent scars.

- Sometimes difficult to interpret, especially in babies.

MCU *direct contrast study*

Pros:

- Shows detail of anatomy, including bladder, urethra, and ureters. Demonstrates timing and grade of vesico-ureteric reflux.

- May demonstrate intrarenal reflux.

Cons:

- Requires insertion of bladder catheter.

- Radiation dose to gonads.

- May miss intermittent vesico-ureteric reflux.

MCU *direct radio-isotope study*

Pros:

- Can do prolonged imaging.

- May detect intermittent VUR.

- Lower radiation dose than contrast MCU.

Cons:

- Requires insertion of bladder catheter.

- Anatomy not defined.

- Grading of reflux not possible.

- Dilatation of ureters not easily seen.

- Reflux into ureter but not up to kidney may be missed.

- Radiation dose.

Indirect radio-isotope study

Pros:

- No bladder catheter required.

- Lower radiation dose than contrast MCU.

Cons:

- Substantial false negative rate.

- No anatomical information provided.

- Requires co-operation, so difficult in young children

- Unable to assess filling-phase reflux which occurs in some patients without micturition reflux.

- Intravenous injection.

- Radiation dose.

Contrast-enhanced ultrasonography

Pros:

- No ionizing radiation.

Cons:

- Requires bladder catheter.

- Requires co-operative and suitable patient.

- Requires experienced operator.

Abdominal radiography

Pros:

- Identification of spinal defects.

- Localization of stones—useful in selective cases (e.g. *Proteus* infection) or where there is a suggestive history.

Cons:

- Radiation dose.

Intravenous urography

Pros:

- Can be useful for distinguishing anatomy when unclear from DMSA and US, e.g. demonstration of a scar in a duplex or horseshoe kidney.

Cons:

- Radiation dose of multiple X-rays.

- Scars only demonstrated after a number of months or years.

- Misses scars on anterior and posterior surfaces of kidney.

- Small anaphylaxis risk.

- Risk of acute tubular necrosis if patient prepared by withholding fluids, but poor pictures if patient not prepared.

- Injection of contrast is unpleasant (metallic taste, flushing, etc.).

General comments on investigations

It should be remembered that anatomical variants may yield misleading results which are difficult to interpret and may require comparison of more than one investigation. For example, horseshoe kidney may not be detected on ultrasound but is clearly seen on DMSA; a duplex kidney on DMSA may simply be reflected by an abnormal split function on DMSA but the anatomy will be often be clarified on US. Occasionally, additional investigations such as intravenous urography (IVU) or magnetic resonance imaging (MRI) may be useful to aid diagnosis. Whereas IVU was previously a common investigation, it should not now be used routinely for investigation after a UTI, but may be useful in specific cases, usually after discussion with a specialist unit.

In general, technological advances are leading to improved imaging and resolution, as well as reductions in radiation doses. With centralization of tertiary specialists and the need for 'second opinions' and shared care with general paediatricians, transfer of results and images between centres is frequently required. Increasingly, this can be done electronically. It should be remembered that images are susceptible to change by alteration of settings and use of different equipment. Interpretation of DMSA scans done in different centres with unfamiliar formats is sometimes difficult. In that situation it is often necessary to return to the raw data of the test. Ease of review of investigations varies. For example, the image obtained during a DMSA scan reflects the full examination, whereas ultrasound is reported in real time and mostly the pictures obtained only reflect 'highlights' of the examination.

Some common questions about imaging in urinary tract infection

It is important that clinicians acknowledge that there is no single test that answers all the essential questions in a child who has had a UTI. In addition, one needs to be aware of the limitations of any combination of tests in order to interpret them intelligently.

Uncertainty about the accuracy of the diagnostic test used also needs to be taken into account when deciding on investigation of the individual patient.

The effects of this are illustrated in Table 11.7. The number of 'unnecessary' investigations might be 6.5 times those required if good diagnostic approaches are used [10]. This example takes no account of post-collection factors which might further reduce the accuracy of the diagnosis. We stress the value of phase–contrast microscopy of the urine which should virtually eliminate unnecessary investigations.

Detection of scars by DMSA scan or ultrasound

There are several comparisons of DMSA scan and US for detecting scars which report a widely varying degree of concurrence [98]. US is extremely operator dependent. The overall view, for which there is much evidence, is that there is good agreement for widespread and diffuse scarring but that US misses focal scars [99,100]. However, under research conditions, in experienced hands with the best equipment and sufficient time and with a co-operative subject, US can detect scars as well as a DMSA scan [101]. The challenge is to recreate these conditions in the routine clinical setting if US is to be considered instead of DMSA for routine detection of scars. Currently, most units would be advised to rely on DMSA scans for scar detection.

Detection of reflux

There is no perfect test for detection of VUR. The contrast MCU is often described as the gold standard, but it has limitations. It only shows whether VUR exists over a very short period of time; it is unphysiological because of the presence of a catheter; and the

child is unlikely to be relaxed. The use of general anaesthetic or sedatives for insertion of the catheter is controversial, but is likely to make the test less physiological unless the effect of drugs used has worn off. Since VUR is known to be a fluctuant and intermittent phenomenon, repeat filling of the bladder is often advocated. Contrast MCUG is the only study to give good anatomical detail (Fig. 11.5) and should be the investigation of choice in young babies, especially males, to exclude urethral abnormalities. It is the only technique providing information on the grade of VUR. This is an important consideration since the risk of renal scarring, and probability of resolution of VUR, can be predicted from the grade at the outset [79]. Thus the grade may alter subsequent management.

Direct radionuclide cystography has the major advantage of being able to scan the child over a longer period of time with less radiation than a contrast MCU. It may therefore detect intermittent VUR more often but may miss lower grades of VUR [102]. These studies require bladder catheterization and the child to micturate on demand in a strange environment without privacy, which may cause considerable problems. Attempts to quantify VUR detected on nuclear cystography have shown it not to predict

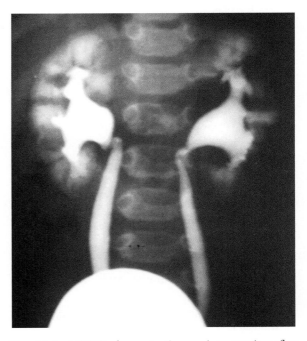

Fig. 11.5 MCUG demonstrating vesico-ureteric reflux and intrarenal reflux.

Table 11.7 Number of investigations performed in a cohort of infants with prevalence of UTI of 5% with different investigation strategies [10]

Strategy	Missed UTI	Investigations performed
Catheter or SPA urine sample	0	5 000
Bag urine culture	0	33 500
LE or nitrite	580	13 050

SPA, suprapubic aspiration; LE, leucocyte esterase. See comments about phase–contrast microscopy in Table 11.2

outcome [103]. The arguments for using indirect radionuclide cystography are compelling because of the major advantage of not requiring bladder catheterization. However, it has a number of drawbacks and is generally considered less reliable. The test is unable to assess filling-phase reflux, which occurs in some patients without micturition reflux. Studies showing high sensitivity and specificity have been done on highly selected patients [104]. and other units have found difficulty reproducing these results when applied to the general population of patients with UTI. It has been shown to have a high false-negative rate [105]. It is therefore considered useful if VUR is demonstrated but does not reliably exclude it. Modifications of technique and careful selection of patients may improve reliability.

Contrast-enhanced ultrasonography is a new technique, which still requires bladder catheterization for introduction of sonicated albumin or saline but avoids a radiation dose. Controversial results have been reported using colour flow Doppler to detect VUR. Neither of these ultrasound techniques has been fully evaluated.

Suggested investigation scheme

This is summarized in Table 11.8.

Table 11.8 Suggested simplified investigation scheme following UTI

Aged 0–1 year
   Ultrasound (US)
   DMSA
   MCU
Aged over 1 year
   DMSA
   US
   With urinary surveillance and/or high index of suspicion
      for UTI over the following 1–2 years up to the age of 4
   Plus, perform a locally reliable test for VUR if:
      renal scar (any age)
      more than one UTI (aged under 4 years)
      family history of VUR (aged under 4 years)
   In addition:
      consider repeat DMSA scan if further UTI
         (aged under 4 years at initial investigation)
   In addition, consider performing an abdominal X-ray if:
      history suggests stones
      Proteus infection
      recurrent UTI

DMSA, dimercaptosuccinic acid; MCU, micturating cystourethrogram; UTI, urinary tract infection; VUR, vesico-ureteric reflux.

Age 0–1 year

There is general consensus about investigation of these children [9,17,106]. They should have an early ultrasound to detect anatomical detail, a MCU for detection and grading of VUR and anatomical detail of bladder and urethra, together with a DMSA scan after at least a 2-month interval for detection of renal scarring. The detection of abnormalities of the urinary tract is higher the younger the child. Very young children appear to be at highest risk of sustaining permanent renal damage. Therefore the opportunities for prevention of initial or extending damage are high.

Age 1–4 years

There is no clear consensus on investigation of this age group. The guidelines issued by the Royal College of Physicians in 1991 [17] did not give clear advice, and since then a consensus has not been established. Most centres would agree that all children in this age group with a proven UTI should be investigated, because UTI may be a marker of underlying urinary tract abnormality and is associated with renal scarring. US and DMSA are the most widely used and logical tests. Ideally, one would like to know if these children have VUR (and intrarenal reflux). However, the only test currently available which has been shown reliably to demonstrate VUR in this age group is the contrast or direct isotope cystogram. Both of these involve catheterization and thus most centres are selective, reserving it for those with recurrent UTIs or those with scarring or other abnormalities seen on DMSA or US, or those with a family history of VUR, or a personal history of antenatal renal dilatation.

This selective investigation plan has much to recommend it at the present state of knowledge. It can, however, be criticized for not identifying children at risk of scarring kidneys at a subsequent UTI. Thus, if this selective approach is adopted, it is essential that the families and their primary healthcare providers understand that they should maintain a high index of suspicion for subsequent UTI up to the age of 4 years and, if another occurs, further investigation in the form of a further DMSA and/or MCU should be considered. The younger the child, the more important it is to consider performing a MCU.

Older children

It is logical to want to know whether these children have normal urinary tracts. One of the problems in investigating older children is judging whether the first *recognized* UTI is actually the first; often it is not. In children presenting with their first diagnosed UTI, the rate of discovery of scars is similar at all ages [2]. Thus, a test for scarring would seem to be the logical starting point for investigation of these children. Many people have suggested there is only the need to perform an US; however, as already discussed, this misses scars in many situations and should not be relied on as the sole investigation [99,107]. Thus we would recommend a DMSA scan and US, unless routine US in a particular unit or centre has been shown not to miss scars. There is some evidence that if children get to the age of 4 years without scarring their urinary tracts, that they are statistically unlikely to develop first scarring after that age [65]. In older children it therefore makes sense only to look for VUR in those who have evidence of scarring. This is important because scarring may lead to local distortion of the intrarenal architecture, predisposing adjacent areas to intrarenal reflux. Thus children with renal scarring who have VUR may be at risk of extending the scar, if they develop a UTI. Even this, so far, almost universal approach is now being questioned. As the role of surgery in reflux is being increasingly reduced (see below), it could be argued that demonstrating reflux in a child with scarring does not always alter the management. In practice, before performing a MCU the question should always be asked whether the knowledge that VUR is present (or absent) alter the management of the child? Irrespective of the findings on MCUG, it could be argued that the initial management should be prevention of infection with anitbiotics (see below) and MCUG should only be performed in children who have breakthrough infections on medical management. This approach should currently not be considered in the first year of life and would also not be appropriate if there was clinical or US evidence of bladder outflow obstruction.

The child with evidence of scarring diagnosed at any age

When scarring is first detected, it is not possible to determine at what age that scar occurred. There is, as discussed above, evidence that the vast majority of novel scarring takes place within the first 4 years of life. There is also evidence that once a scar is present, progression of that scarring may develop at any age. Progression of scarring is presumed to occur because the conditions of intrarenal reflux and VUR are still present

and, in the face of infection, further renal damage may occur. In addition, scarring itself distorts the intrarenal architecture and may make it more likely that adjacent areas of kidney will have intrarenal reflux and be susceptible to scarring in the face of infection. Thus it is logical to want to know whether there is still VUR present, with the intention of trying to prevent further damage from UTI in those with VUR. However, many shy away from this approach because of the nature of current methods of assessing or testing for reflux.

What is clear is that if there was a less-invasive, low-radiation, and reliable technique for detecting VUR, children would be investigated in a more logical way, and also our knowledge about the natural history of VUR and it relationship to scarring would be improved.

The child with a family history of vesico-ureteric reflux

Vesico-ureteric reflux is a genetic disorder [73] and there is evidence of a 20–50 times increased risk of VUR in children with a family history of VUR [69,71]. Children with UTI who have a family history of VUR probably warrant more intensive investigation than those without. Routine screening for VUR in asymptomatic siblings or offspring of individuals with VUR would appear to be justified to identify those at greatest risk of subsequent renal damage. As well as offering an opportunity to prevent renal damage in this group, careful surveillance may provide further information and insight into the natural history of VUR and the relationship of UTI, VUR, and scarring. However, it remains to be shown whether screening first-degree relatives for VUR offers advantages over increasing awareness of parents and healthcare professionals that children are a high risk group in whom there should be a high index of suspicion for UTI. Given these uncertainties, there is no agreement as to the correct approach to first-degree relatives of patients with reflux. Our own current approach is to offer investigations to newborns who are first-degree relatives of patients with VUR. Such newborns are commenced on prophylactic antibiotics at birth until a MCU has been performed. Those with reflux then proceed to a DMSA scan. On current evidence we feel this approach maximizes the chance of prevention. Similarly, siblings or offspring of patients with severe renal damage from reflux are offered screening. Under 1-year-olds are investigated as for newborns. Over 1-year-olds have a DMSA scan with an ultrasound, and MCUG is reserved for those with an abnormal DMSA scan.

Timing of investigations

Ultrasound

Ultrasound can be performed in the acute phase or subsequently. Severe acute pyelonephritis may cause the kidney to appear 'bright' and/or enlarged on US. These changes may be focal.

MCUG

There is no need to delay MCUG once the initial UTI is treated. There is a suggestion, but no good evidence, that there is an increased detection of VUR at the time of UTI. Even if this hypothesis was correct, then the patient is at risk of VUR at the very time it may be important. MCUG should often be arranged before discharge in those admitted for UTI to reduce non-attendance [108].

DMSA

The question of timing of the DMSA scan is interesting. If DMSA is performed at the time of UTI then a large proportion will show some areas of reduced uptake [109–111]. However, only about 50% of those defects will be still be there more than 2 months later [109,112]. It is therefore important that the clinician is aware of the timing of the DMSA scan in relation to the acute infection in any individual case. In the piglet model of acute pyelonephritis, DMSA is highly specific and sensitive in diagnosing pathologically proven pyelonephritis [113,114]. Whereas permanent scars typically are localized to the site of the acute defect, acute defects do not predict for those with VUR, and we do not understand the factors involved in resolution of acute changes versus progression to permanent scarring. Whereas acute DMSA is clearly useful in a research setting, its place in the routine clinical investigation of children with UTI is not yet established. In order to show *permanent* scarring reliably, DMSA should be performed at least 2–3 months after a UTI, although some suggest a longer interval [115].

Long-term management

Within organizations, it is important to develop systems that empower parents. Parents generally want the best for their children and this motivation can be harnessed by increasing their understanding of the medical issues.

Information and education of families is important in suspicion and detection of UTI, and with compliance with treatment. Parents will often be more assiduous at tasks like urine collection than healthcare professionals.

Specific advice to families should include information on:

- Where and when to ring for sensitivities of a urine culture and to enquire if their child is on an appropriate antibiotic.

- What investigations are planned and how results will be conveyed.

- What follow-up is needed and why.

- What to do if they suspect a UTI in their child. This information may need to be different for children at highest risk of scarring (e.g. children with VUR), for example the use of children's assessment units or day units as a back up to primary care.

Important points about issues such as investigation plans or VUR should be backed up with written information whenever feasible, since most people absorb only a fraction of a clinic discussion.

Management of vesico-ureteric reflux

It should be remembered that both medical and surgical management strategies for VUR were introduced without controlled studies documenting long-term benefit.

Medical management

The aim in medical management of VUR, with prophylactic antibiotics, is to prevent recurrent (or sometimes first) UTI and consequent renal scarring, while waiting for the VUR to resolve with time. While there is some evidence that prophylactic antibiotics reduce the risk of repeated UTI in children, with less than 50% having a recurrence in a 5-year follow-up [55,116–119], 'methodological and applicability problems with published trials mean that there is considerable uncertainty about whether long-term low-dose antibiotic administration prevents UTI in children. Well-designed, randomized, placebo-controlled trials are still required to evaluate this commonly used intervention' [120].

While the aim of prophylaxis is to obtain high concentration of the antibiotic in the urine with minimal effect on normal body flora, there are few data on the effect of long-term antibiotic prophylaxis on bowel and peri-urethral flora or on drug resistance in the community. Trimethoprim and nitrofurantoin are the agents that have been studied most extensively. Nalidixic acid is also used but the evidence for its use is not as extensive. Cephalosporins are widely used clinically for prophylaxis, but are not as well documented (Table 11.9) [121].

Breakthrough infections may be problematic and may be due to non-compliance or true bacterial resistance. Non-compliance should be suspected when the infecting organism is sensitive to the prophylactic antibiotic prescribed. Bacterial resistance might also arise with intermittent administration of prophylactic antibiotics. Probably only between one-third and two-thirds of patients are compliant with prophylaxis [123,124]. Patient and family understanding of the underlying reasoning and purpose of prophylaxis are essential in encouraging compliance.

Optimum duration of prophylaxis is not known; some propose prophylaxis as long as VUR persists, others propose a shorter duration. There is currently neither consensus nor good evidence for either view. Small series and clinical experience suggest that antibiotic prophylaxis has been successfully discontinued in some highly selected groups of children with persistent VUR [125]. However, there is no real evidence that helps in answering the difficult and important question of how long to continue antibiotic prophylaxis when VUR does not resolve.

Chances of resolution of vesico-ureteric reflux with time

Resolution of VUR over time with medical treatment is related to the grade of VUR and the age of the patient (Fig. 11.6). In general, a lower grade of reflux has a better chance of spontaneous resolution. For grade III reflux, increasing age at presentation and bilateral reflux decreases the probability of resolution. Bilateral grade IV and V reflux has the poorest chance of resolution [79]. It is not known whether urine infection affects resolution of VUR, but in monkeys there is some evidence that it may delay normal resolution [126].

Surgical management

There are two main forms of surgical treatment of VUR: endoscopic subureteric injection and re-implantation.

Endoscopic subureteric injection. Injection of tissue-augmenting substances is done under general

Table 11.9 Dosage of antibiotics for prophylaxis against UTI [122]

Drug	Dosage	Comment
Trimethoprim	1–2 mg/kg/day	Single dose at night
Nitrofurantoin	1–2 mg/kg/day	Single dose at night
Nalidixic acid	15–20 mg/kg/day	Split into two doses
Cephalexin	10–15 mg/kg/day	Single dose at night

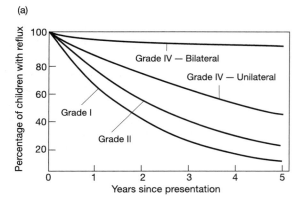

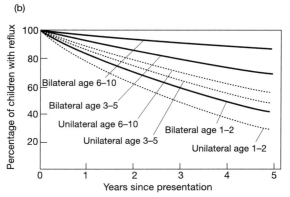

Fig. 11.6 Resolution of vesico-ureteric reflux: percentage chance of reflux persistence for 1–5 years following presentation. (a) Grades I, II, and IV reflux; (b) grade III reflux by age at presentation. (Reproduced from Elder J *et al.* Pediatric vesicoureteral reflux guidelines: panel summary report on the management of primary vesicoureteral reflux in children. J Urol 1997; 157: 1846–1851 with permission from Lippincott Williams and Wilkins.)

anaesthetic and requires only a short stay (or day case) in hospital. The success rate in abolition of VUR varies with the centre, the material used, the timing of re-evaluation, and test used in re-examination.

Use of polytetraflouroethylene (Teflon) or silicon has a success rate of 70–90% [79] and a recurrence rate of 5–10%. Use of collagen has a success rate of around 60%, and dextranomer, 60–90% [127]. The term STING (initially referring to the technique in which Teflon is injected) is frequently used generically to refer to this type of procedure. The technique is very operator dependent. There is a lack of controlled studies of the technique and studies have included large numbers of grade I and II VUR, which tend to have spontaneous resolution. This approach has been advocated as relatively non-invasive. Although clearly a single procedure is less invasive than a surgical re-implantation, this comparison becomes more difficult when account is taken of the need for repeat procedures and imaging because of the primary and secondary failure rate. There are concerns regarding long-term effects, including migration of foreign materials. The longevity of the treatment and need for repeat are not fully known.

Re-implantation. Surgical success in curing VUR with re-implantation is high, greater than 95% overall. The success rate is greater than 98% in grades of reflux I to IV, dropping to 80% with grade V [79]. This is, however, a major operation, requiring a stay of several days in hospital with the associated risks and costs. The likelihood of obstruction following re-implantation surgery is in the region of 2% [79].

Key points: Theoretical basis of medical management of VUR

- Reflux resolves with time.

- Antibiotics maintain urine sterility.

Key points: Theoretical basis of surgical treatment of VUR

- Surgery cures VUR.

- Scarring will be prevented if there is no VUR, even if infection occurs.

Comparison of medical versus surgical treatment for vesico-ureteric reflux

Two large, multicentre, prospective trials of medical versus surgical treatment for children with severe VUR do not show superiority of either treatment [74,78,118,119,128]. Neither surgical nor medical treatment appears to protect completely against progression of scarring, although apparent progression may result from contraction of a scar or a differential rate of growth of normal versus scarred kidney tissue. Although the incidence of further UTI was similar in the medically and surgically treated groups, there was a reduction in clinical pyelonephritis in the surgical group, but no difference in renal scarring. The choice of treatment therefore remains an individual judgement that will be based on a number of factors. Breakthrough infection, despite medical treatment or because of non-compliance, remains a commonly used factor for consideration of surgical treatment, as does deterioration of DMSA appearance. Whereas the question of how long antibiotic prophylaxis should continue remains unanswered, there is a finality about successful surgical treatment of VUR which is appealing if VUR does not resolve spontaneously. However, there is little evidence about whether persistence of VUR to adulthood is detrimental.

The American Urological Association convened the Pediatric VUR Guidelines Panel, who analysed the treatment outcomes in the literature from 1965 to 1994. The following recommendations were made in their report, published in 1997 [79]. For children with no scarring, surgery at initial investigation was only recommended for those with grade V reflux. For children with renal scarring, surgery was recommended for older children with grade III reflux or worse. In addition, surgery was recommended for those who, at follow-up, still had VUR persisting at grade III or above. Antibiotic prophylaxis was recommended for all others. The report also concluded that urethral dilatation and cystoscopic examination of the ureteric orifices was not beneficial. The report failed to recommend endoscopic ureteric injection for any groups of patients because of lack of United States Federal Drug Administration approval for the materials used. However, the report also states that 'given the general lack of direct evidence that any treatment option is superior to another, parent and patient preferences should generally be honoured'.

As there is lack of direct evidence for benefit of surgery, no clear guidelines can be given. Many practitioners and parents prefer to follow a much more conservative route, avoiding surgery where possible.

Key points: Vesico-ureteric reflux

- No clear advantage has been shown for medical versus surgical treatment for VUR.

- Family understanding of the need for prophylaxis and early detection and treatment of infection are essential.

- Factors advocated for consideration of surgical treatment include:
  - recurrent UTI, despite medical treatment or because of non-compliance;
  - deterioration of DMSA appearance of the kidney.

- It is not known how long antibiotic prophylaxis should continue.

Prognosis

While there is good evidence that UTI in childhood is associated with renal scarring, there is no way of quantifying the long-term risk of chronic renal failure or hypertension resulting from an individual episode of UTI. Nor is there good evidence of the long-term risk associated with minor degrees of scarring. One problem is the time scale. Children with reflux nephropathy may not present in renal failure or with hypertension until very many years later, making prospective studies difficult to perform. Many existing studies are of small numbers or are retrospective. Ideally, cohorts of children need to be followed prospectively for 40 or 50 years to determine more accurate estimates of adverse outcomes in adulthood.

Renal failure

The published incidence of ESRF secondary to renal scarring varies. In Australia and New Zealand from 1971 to 1998, reflux nephropathy was the primary diagnosis in 13% of patients entering the dialysis and transplantation programme between the ages of

5 and 44 years, with no clear trend of change [129]. In Wales between 1994 and 1997, 30% of chronic renal failure (GFR less than a third normal) in childhood has been attributed to reflux nephropathy [130]. In part of France, pyelonephritis with reflux accounted for 12% of chronic renal failure. [131]. Pyelonephritic renal scarring was reported to be the primary renal diagnosis in 39% of children undergoing renal transplantation in Ireland from 1980 to 1990 [132]. North American and European registries do not code specifically for renal scarring, thus it is difficult to distinguish between those reaching renal failure due to scarring of normal kidneys (i.e. possibly preventable reflux nephropathy) and those in whom the underlying diagnosis is reflux-associated dysplasia. Nor is it possible to discern the role of UTI in deterioration of renal function in those with dysplasia (who also have a high incidence of VUR, putting them at risk of possible damage from UTI). Hopefully, prospective studies will clarify issues. The most compelling data come from Sweden where the incidence of ESRF in childhood caused by non-obstructive reflux nephropathy has reduced from 6% in the years 1978–1985 to zero in the years 1986–1994 [7]. The Swedes suggest that increased awareness and improved diagnosis of UTI in young children has been important.

Hypertension

There are numerous retrospective and prospective studies linking the development of hypertension with renal scarring [69,133,134]. There is very good evidence that there is a substantially increased risk, which is worse for those with more severe and bilateral scarring [135]. The size and duration of risk for any individual, or for those with less severe scarring, is difficult to enumerate. The data depend on the population studied. One small population-based, follow-up study, 16–26 years after childhood UTI, found no difference in blood pressure between those with or without renal scarring [136]. What appears to be a small or scarred kidney on imaging may actually represent a number of different underlying pathologies, e.g. dysplasia or hypoplasia. Not all of these may be associated with a greater risk of hypertension, but in cases of doubt, regular long-term monitoring of blood pressure is required. It is currently recommended that children with scars have their BP monitored on a yearly basis for life, in order to detect pre-symptomatic hypertension.

Pregnancy-related complications

Pregnant women have an increased risk of cystitis and UTI if they had UTI and VUR in childhood. However ureteric re-implantation in childhood does not appear to protect against symptomatic UTI in pregnancy, and may be associated with increased risk [137]. The risk of hypertension [138] and pre-eclampsia [139] is higher in women with renal scarring. Fetal outcome is worse if the mother has renal impairment or established hypertension prior to the pregnancy [140].

In conclusion

UTI is common and may be associated with renal abnormalities and significant long-term sequelae in a minority of cases. There are many unanswered questions about the relationship between VUR, UTI, and scarring, and there is debate about the best investigation and management strategies. Since most children with scarring already have it at the time of first investigation, it is likely that the greatest potential for prevention of renal damage lies in increased awareness, better diagnosis, and management of young children with UTI in primary healthcare.

References

1. Jakobsson B, Esbjorner E, Hansson S. Minimum incidence and diagnostic rate of first urinary tract infection. *Pediatrics* 1999;104:222–226.
2. Coulthard M, Lambert H, Keir M. Occurence of renal scars in children after their first referral for urinary tract infection. *BMJ* 1997;315:918–919.
3. Wettergren B, Jodal U, Jonasson G. Epidemiology of bacteruria during the first year of life. *Acta Ped Scand* 1985;74:925–933.
4. Jodal U. The natural history of bacteruria in childhood. *Infect Dis Clin North Am* 1987;1:713–729.
5. Hellström A-L, Hanson E, Hansson S, Hjälmås K, Jodal U. Association between urinary symptoms at 7 years old and previous urinary tract infection. *Arch Dis Child* 1991;66:232–234.
6. Marild S, Jodal U. Incidence rate of first-time symptomatic urinary tract infection in children under 6 years of age. *Acta Paediatr* 1998;87:549–552.
7. Esbjorner E. Epidemiology of chronic renal failure in children: a report from Sweden 1986–1994. *Pediatr Nephrol* 1997;11:438–442.
8. Vernon S, Foo CK, Coulthard MG. How general practitioners manage children with urinary tract infection: an audit in the former Northern Region. *Br J Gen Pract* 1997;47:297–300.
9. American Academy of Pediatrics. Practice parameter: the diagnosis, treatment, and evaluation of the initial urinary tract infection in febrile infants and young children. *Pediatrics* 1999;103(4):843–852.
10. Downs SM. Technical report: Urinary tract infections in febrile infants and young children. The Urinary Tract Subcommittee of the American Academy of Pediatrics Committee on Quality Improvement. *Pediatrics* 1999;103:e54.
11. Wennerström M, Hanson S, Jodal U, Stokland E. Primary and aquired renal scarring in boys and girls with urinary tract infection. *J Pediatr* 2000;136:30–34.
12. Koff S, Wagner T, Jayanthi V. The relationship among dysfunctional elimination syndromes, primary vesicoureteral reflux and urinary tract infections in children. *J Urol* 1998;160:1019–1022.
13. Blethyn A, Jenkins H, Roberts R, Jones KV. Radiological evidence of constipation in urinary tract infection. *Arch Dis Child* 1995;73:534–535.
14. Shopfner C. Urinary tract pathology associated with constipation. *Radiology* 1968;90:865–877.
15. Dohil R, Roberts E, Verrier-Jones K, Jenkins H. Constipation and reversible urinary tract abnormalities. *Arch Dis Child* 1994;56–57.
16. Mond NC, Grüneberg RN, Smellie JM. Study of childhood urinary tract infection in general practice. *BMJ* 1970;i:602–605.
17. Royal College of Physicians Research Unit Working Group. Guidelines for the management of acute urinary tract infection in childhood. *Journal of the Royal College of Physicians of London.* 1991;25:36–42.
18. van der Voort V, Edwards A, Roberts R, Verrier-Jones K. The struggle to diagnose UTI in children under two in primary care. *Family Pract* 1997;14:44–48.
19. Ramage IJ, Chapman JP, Hollman AS, Elabassi M, McColl JH, Beattie TJ. Accuracy of clean-catch urine collection in infancy. *J Pediatr* 1999;135:765–767.
20. Macfarlane PI, Houghton C, Hughes C. Pad urine collection for early childhood urinary-tract infection. *Lancet* 1999;354:571.
21. Rees J, Vernon S, Pedler SJ, Coulthard MG. Collection of urine from washed-up potties. *Lancet* 1996;348:197.
22. Liaw LCT, Nayar DM, Pedler SJ, Coulthard MG. Home collection of urine for culture from infants by three methods: survey of parents' preferences and bacterial contamination rates. *BMJ* 2000; 320:1312–1313.
23. Taylor MRH, Dillon M, Keane CT. Reduction of mixed growth rates in urine by using a 'finger tap' method of collection. *BMJ* 1986;292:990.
24. Vernon S, Redfearn A, Pedler SJ, Lambert HJ, Coulthard MG. Urine collection on sanitary towels. *Lancet* 1994;344:612.
25. Nelson JD, Peters PC. Suprapubic aspiration of urine in premature and term infants. *Pediatrics* 1965;36:132–134.
26. Pryles CV, Atkin MD, Morse TS, Welch KJ. Comparative bacteriologic study of urine obtained from children by percutaneous suprapubic aspiration of the bladder and by catheter. *Pediatrics* 1959; 24:983–991.

27. Wettergren B, Jodal U, Jonasson G. Epidemiology of bacteriuria during the first year of life. *Acta Paediatr Scand* 1985;74:925–933.

28. Hansson S, Brandstrom P, Jodal U, Larsson P. Low bacterial counts in infants with urinary tract infection. *J Pediatr* 1998;132:180–182.

29. Aronson AS, Gustafson B, Svenningsen NW. Combined suprapubic aspiration and clean-voided urine examination in infants and children. *Acta Paediatr Scand* 1973;62:396–400.

30. Weathers W, Wenzl J. Suprapubic aspiration of the bladder: perforation of a viscus other than the bladder. *Am J Dis Child* 1969;117:590–592.

31. Edwards B, White RHR, Maxted H, Deverill I, White PA. Screening methods for covert bacteriuria in schoolgirls. *BMJ* 1975;2:463–467.

32. Jewkes FE, McMaster DJ, Napier WA *et al.* Home culture of urine specimens—boric acid bottles or Dipslides. *Arch Dis Child* 1990;65:286–289.

33. Rosenthal SL, Freundlich LF. Room temperature incubation of dipslide urine cultures. *Urology* 1976;8:251–253.

34. Watson PG, Duerden BI. Laboratory assessment of physical and chemical methods of preserving urine specimens. *J Clin Pathol* 1977;30:532–536.

35. Kass EH. Asymptomatic infections of the urinary tract. *Transactions of the Association of American Physicians* 1956;69:65–63.

36. Gore SM. Interpreting results. In *Statistics in practice*, Gore SM, Altman DG (eds). British Medical Association, London 1982, 16–20.

37. Jaeschke R, Guyatt G, Lijmer J. Diagnostic tests. In *Users' guides to the medical literature*, Guyatt G, Rennie D (eds). AMA Press, Chicago 2002, 121–140.

38. Vickers D, Ahmad T, Coulthard MG. Diagnosis of urinary tract infection in children: fresh urine microscopy or culture? *Lancet* 1991;338:767–770.

39. Hardy JD, Furnell PM, Brumfitt W. Comparison of sterile bag, clean catch and suprapubic aspiration in the diagnosis of urinary infection in early childhood. *Br J Urol* 1976;48:279–283.

40. Shannon FT, Sepp E, Rose GR. The diagnosis of bacteriuria by bladder puncture in infancy and childhood. *Austr Paediatr J* 1969;5:97–100.

41. Stansfeld JM. The measurement and meaning of pyuria. *Arch Dis Child* 1962;37:257–262.

42. Kumar RK, Turner GM, Coulthard MG. Don't count on urinary white cells to diagnose childhood urinary tract infection.*BMJ* 1996;312:1359.

43. Turner GM, Coulthard MG. Fever can cause pyuria in children. *BMJ* 1995;311:924.

44. Powell HR, McCredie DA, Ritchie MA. Urinary nitrite in symptomatic and asymptomatic urinary infection. *Arch Dis Child* 1987;62:138–140.

45. Moyer VA, Craig EJ. Acute urinary tract infection. In *Evidence based pediatrics and child health*, Moyer VA (ed.) BMJ Books, London 2000:318–325.

46. Winberg J, Anderson HJ, Bergstrom T, Jacobsson B, Larson H, Lincoln K. Epidemiology of symptomatic urinary tract infection in childhood. *Acta Paediatr Scand* 1974;Suppl:252.

47. Jodal U, Winberg J. Management of children with unobstructed urinary tract infection. *Pediatr Nephrol* 1987;1:647–656.

48. Jantunen ME, Saxen H, Lukinmaa S, Ala-Houhala M, Siitonen A. Genomic identity of pyelonephritic *Escherichia coli* isolated from blood, urine and faeces of children with urosepsis. *Pediatr Nephrol* 2000;14:C42.

49. Miller T, Phillips S. Pyelonephritis: the relationship between infection, renal scarring and antimicrobial therapy. *Kidney Int* 1981;19:654–662.

50. Ransley PG, Risdon RA. Reflux nephropathy: effects of antimicrobial therapy on the evolution of the early pyelonephritic scar. *Kidney Int* 1981;20:733–738.

51. Smellie JM, Ransley PG, Normand ICS, Prescod N, Edwards D. Development of new renal scars: a collaborative study. *BMJ* 1985;290:1957–1960.

52. Smellie J, Poulton A, Prescod N. Retrospective study of children with renal scarring associated with reflux and urinary infection. *BMJ* 1994;308(6938):1193–1196.

53. Dick P, Feldman W. Routine diagnostic imaging for childhood urinary tract infections: a systematic overview. *J Pediatr* 1996;128:15–22.

54. Bachur R. Nonresponders: prolonged fever among infants with urinary tract infections. *Pediatrics* 2000;105:1147.

55. Smellie J. Controlled trial of prophylactic treatment in childhood urinary tract infection. *Lancet* 1978; ii:175–178.

56. Jepson R, Mihaljevic L, Craig J. Cranberries for preventing urinary tract infections. *The Cochrane Library* 2000;3.

57. Loening-Bauche V. Urinary incontinence and urinary tract infection and their resolution with treatment of chronic constipation of childhood. *Pediatrics* 1997; 100:228–232.

58. Schoen E, Colby C, Ray G. Newborn circumcision decreases incidence and costs of urinary tract infections during the first year of life. *Pediatrics* 2000; 105:789–793.

59. Wiswell TE. The prepuce, urinary tract infections, and the consequences. *Pediatrics* 2000;105(4):860–862.

60. Walsh P. Editorial comment. *J Urol* 1999;162(4):1562.

61. American Academy of Pediatrics. Circumcision policy statement. *Pediatrics* 1999;103:686–693.

62. Winter AL, Hardy BE, Alton DJ, Arbus GS, Churchill BM. Acquired renal scars in children. *J Urol* 1983;129:1190–1194.

63. Stokland E, Hellstöm M, Jacobsson B, Jodal U, Sixt R. Evaluation of DMSA scintigraphy and urography in assessing both acute and permanent renal damage in children. *Acta Radiol* 1998(39):447–452.

64. Berg U, Johansson S. Age as a main determinant of renal functional damage in Urinary tract infection. *Arch Dis Child* 1983;58:963–969.

65. Vernon S, Coulthard M, Lambert H, Keir M, Matthews J. New renal scarring in children who at age 3 and 4 years had had normal scans with dimercaptosuccinic acid: follow up study. *BMJ* 1997;315:905–908.

66. Benador D, Benador N, Slosman D, Mermillod B, Girardin E. Are children at highest risk of renal sequelae after pyelonephritis? *Lancet* 1997;349:17–19.

67. Coulthard MG, Flecknell P, Manas D, O'Donnel M. Renal scarring caused by vesicoureteric reflux and urinary infection: a study in pigs. *Pediatr Nephrol* 2002;17:481–484.

68. Couthard MG. Do kidneys outgrow the risk of reflux nephropathy? *Pediatr Nephrol.* 2002;17:477–480.

69. Jacobson S, Hansson S, Jakobsson B. Vesico-ureteric reflux: occurence and long-term risks. *Acta Paediatr Suppl* 1999;431:22–33.

70. Zerin J, Ritchey M, Chang A. Incidental vesicoureteral reflux in neonates with antenatally detected hydronephrosis and other renal abnormalities. *Radiology* 1993;187:157–160.

71. Anderson N, Abbott G, *et al.* Vesicoureteric reflux in the newborn: relationship to fetal renal pelvic diameter. *Pediatr Nephrol* 1997;11:610–616.

72. Scott J, Swallow V, Coulthard M, Lambert H, Lee R. Screening of newborn babies for familial ureteric reflux. *Lancet* 1997;350:396–400.

73. Feather SA, Malcolm S, Woolf AS *et al.* Primary, nonsyndromic vesicoureteric reflux is genetically heterogeneous with a locus on chromosome 1. *Am J Hum Genet* 2000;66:1420–1425.

74. International Reflux Study Committee. Medical versus surgical treatment of primary vesico-ureteral reflux. *Pediatrics* 1981;67:392–400.

75. Hellström M, Jacobsson B. Diagnosis of vesico-ureteric reflux. *Acta Paediatr Suppl* 1999;88(431):3–12.

76. Ekman H, Jacobsson B, Koch N, Sundin T. High diuresis, a factor in preventing vesicoureteric reflux. *J Urol* 1966;95:511–515.

77. Zinner NR, Paquin AJ. Experimental vesicoureteral reflux: III. Role of hydration in vesicoureteral reflux. *J Urol* 1963;90:713–718.

78. Smellie J, Tamminem-Mobius T, Koskimies O, Olbing H, Claesson I, Wikstad I, *et al.* Five year study of medical or surgical treatment in children with severe reflux: radiological renal findings. *Pediatr Nephrol* 1992;6:223–230.

79. Elder J, Peters C, Arant B, Ewalt D, Hawtrey C, Hurwitz R, *et al.* Pediatric vesicoureteral reflux guidelines panel summary report on the management of primary vesicoureteral reflux in children. *J Urol* 1997;157:1846–1851.

80. Yeung C, Godley M, Dhillon H, Duffy P, Ransley P. Urodynamic patterns in infants with normal lower urinary tracts or primary vesico-ureteric reflux. *Br J Urol* 1998;81:461–467.

81. Sillen U. Bladder dysfunction in children with vesicoureteric reflux. *Acta Paediatr Suppl* 1999;431:40–47.

82. Sillen U, Hellstrom A, Hermanson G, Abrahamson K. Comparison of urodynamic and free voiding pattern in infants with dilating reflux. *J Urol* 1999; 161:1928–1933.

83. Chandra M, Maddix H. Urodynamic dysfunction in infants with vesicoureteral reflux. *J Pediatr* 2000; 136(6):754–759.

84. Willemsen J, Nijman R. Vesicoureteral reflux and videourodynamic studies: results of a prospective study. *Urology* 2000;55:939–943.

85. Godley M, Risdon R, Ransley P. Effect of unilateral vesicoureteric reflux on renal growth and the uptake of 99mTc DMSA by the kidney. An experimental study in the minipig. *Br J Urol* 1989;63:340–347.

86. Ransley PG, Risdon RA. Reflux and renal scarring. *Br J Radiol* 1978;51(Suppl 14):1–35.

87. Ransley P, Risdon R. Renal papillae and intrarenal reflux in the pig. *Lancet* 1974;2:1114.

88. Ransley P, Risdon R. Renal papillary morphology in infants and young children. *Urol Res* 1975;3:111–113.

89. Rolleston G, Maling T, Hodson C. Intrarenal reflux and the scarred kidney. *Arch Dis Child* 1974; 49:531–539.

90. Uldall P, Frokjaer O, Kaas K. Intrarenal reflux. *Acta Paediatr Scand* 1976;65:711–715.

91. Hinchcliffe SA, Chan Y-F, Jones H, *et al.* Renal hypoplasia and psotnatally acquired cortical loss in children with vesicoureteral reflux. *Pediatr Nephrol* 1992;6:439–444.

92. Risdon RA, Yeung CK, Ransley P. Reflux nephropathy in children submitted to unilateral nephrectomy: a clinicopathological study. *Clin Nephrol* 1993;40: 308–314.

93. Gobet R, Cisek L, Chang B, Barnewolt C, Retik A, Peters C. Experimental fetal vesicoureteral reflux induces renal tubular and glomerular damage and is associated with persistant bladder instability. *J Urol* 1999;162:1090–1095.

94. Ransley P, Risdon R, Godley M. Effects of vesicoureteric reflux on renal growth and function as measured by GFR, plasma creatinine, and urinary concentrating ability. *Br J Urol* 1987;60:193–204.

95. Rushton H, Majd M, Jantausch B, Wiedermann B, Belman A. Renal scarring following reflux and nonreflux pyelonephritis in children: evaluation with 99m technetium-dimercaptosuccinic acid scintigraphy. *J Urol* 1992;147:1327–1332.

96. Stokland E, Hellstrom M, Jacobsson B, Jodal U, Sixt R. Renal damage one year after first urinary tract infection: Role of dimercaptosuccinic acid scintography. *J Pediatr* 1996;129(6):815–820.

97. Jakobsson B, Berg U, Svensson L. Renal scarring after acute pyelonephritis. *Arch Dis Child* 1994; 70:111–115.

98. Roebuck D, Howard R, Metreweli C. How sensitive is ultrasound in the detection of renal scars? *Br J Radiol* 1999;72:345–348.

99. Smellie J, Rigdon S, Prescod N. Urinary tract infection: a comparison of four methods of investigation. *Arch Dis Child* 1995;72:247–250.

100. Tasker A, Lindsell D, Moncrieff M. Can ultrasound reliably detect renal scarring in children with urinary tract infection? *Clin Radiol* 1993;47:177–179.

101. Barry B, Hall N, Cornford E, Broderick N, Somers J, Rose D. Improved ultrasound detection of renal scarring in children following urinary tract infection. *Clin Radiol* 1998;53:747–751.

102. Poli-Merol M, Francois S, Pfliger F, Lefebvre F, Roussel B, Liehn J, *et al.* Interest of direct radionuclide cystography in repeated urinary infection exploration in childhood. *Eur J Pediatr Surg* 1998; 8:339–342.

103. Barthold J, Martin-Crespo R, Kryger J, Gonzalez R. Quantitative nuclear cystography does not predict

outcome in patients with primary vesicoureteral reflux. *J Urol* 1999;162:1193–1196.

104. Gordon I, Peters A, Morony S. Indirect radionuclide cystography: a sensitive technique for the detection of vesico-ureteral reflux. *Pediatr Nephrol* 1990; 4:604–606.

105. DeSadeleer C, DeBoe V, Kruppens F, Desprechins B, Verboven M, Piepsz A. How good is technetium-99m mercaptoacetyltriglycine indirect cystography? *Eur J Nucl Med* 1994;21:223–227.

106. Pilling D, Postlethwaite R. Clinical Opinion— Imaging in Urinary Tract Infection: British Paediatric Association Standing Committee on Paediatric Practice Guidelines, 1996.

107. Smellie J, Rigden S. Pitfalls in the investigation of children with urinary tract infection. *Arch Dis Child* 1995;72:251–258.

108. McDonald A, Scranton M, Gillespie R, Mahajan V, Edwards G. Voiding cystourethrograms and urinary tract infections: how long to wait? *Pediatrics* 2000;105:851–852.

109. Jakobsson B, Soderlundh S, Berg U. Diagnostic significance of 99mTc-dimercaptosuccinic acid (DMSA) scintigraphy in urinary tract infection. *Arch Dis Child* 1992;67:1338–1342.

110. Rosenberg A, Rossleigh M, Brydon M, Bass S, Leighton D, Farnsworth R. Evaluation of acute urinary tract infection in children by dimercaptosuccinic acid scintigraphy: a prospective study. *J Urol* 1992;148:1746–1749.

111. Stokland E, Hellstrom M, Jacobsson B, Jodal U, Lundgren P, Sixt R. Early 99mTc dimercaptosuccinic acid (DMSA) scintigraphy in symptomatic first time urinary tract infection. *Acta Paediatr* 1996; 85:430–436.

112. Benador D, Benador N, Slosman D, Nussle D, Mermillod B, Girardin E. Cortical scintigraphy in the evaluation of renal parenchymal changes in children with pyelonephritis. *J Pediatr* 1994;124:17–20.

113. Rushton H, Majd M, Chandra R, Yim D. Evaluation of [99m]technetium–dimercapto-succinic acid renal scans in experimental acute pyelonephritis in piglets. *J Urol* 1988;140:1169–1174.

114. Parkhouse H, Godley M, Cooper J, Risdon R, Ransley P. Renal imaging with Tc99m labeled DMSA in the detection of acute pyelonephritis:an experimental study in the pig. *Nucl Med Commun* 1989;10:63–70.

115. Jakobsson B, Svensson L. Transient pyelonephritic changes on 99m Technetium–dimercaptosuccinic acid scan for at least five months after infection. *Acta Paediatr* 1997;86:803–807.

116. Lohr J, Nunley D, Howards S, Ford R. Prevention of recurrent urinary tract infections in girls. *Pediatrics* 1977;59:562–565.

117. Jodal U, Koskimies O, Hanson E, *et al.* Infection pattern in children with vesicoureteral reflux randomly allocated to operation or long term prophylaxis. The International Reflux Study in Children. *J Urol* 1992;148:1650–1652.

118. Olbing H, Caesson I, Ebel K, Seppanen U, Smellie J, Tamminem-Mobius T, *et al.* Renal scars and parenchymal thinning in children with vesicoureteral reflux: a 5-year report of the International Reflux Study in Children (European branch). *J Urol* 1992;148:1653–1656.

119. Weiss R, Duckett J, Spitzer A. Results of a randomized clinical trial of medical versus surgical management of infants and children with grade III and IV primary vesicoureteral reflux (United States). *J Urol* 1992; 148:1667–1673.

120. Williams G, Lee A, Craig J. Antibiotics for the prevention of urinary tract infection in children: A systematic review of randomized controlled trials. *J Pediatr* 2001;138:868–874.

121. Bollgren I. Antibiotic prophylaxis in children with urinary tract infection. *Acta Paediatr* 1999; 431(Suppl):48–52.

122. Katz G, Smellie JM. Urinary tract infections. *J Maternal Child Health* 1976;Sept:24–27.

123. Daschner F, Marget W. Treatment of recurrent urinary tract infection in children II Compliance of parents and children antibiotic therapy regimens. *Acta Pediatr Scand* 1975;64:105–108.

124. Smyth A, Judd B. Compliance with antibiotic prophylaxis in urinary tract infection. *Arch Dis Child* 1993;68:235–236.

125. Cooper C, Chung B, Kirsch A, Canning D, Snyder H. The outcome of stopping prophylactic antibiotics in older children with vesicoureteral reflux. *J Urol* 2000;163:272–273.

126. Roberts J. Vesicoureteral reflux and pyelonephritis in the monkey: a review. *J Urol* 1992;148: 1721–1725.

127. Lackgren G, Wahlin N, Stenberg A. Endoscopic treatment of children with vesico ureteric reflux. *Acta Paediatr* 1999;431(Suppl):62–71.

128. Birmingham Reflux Study Group. Prospective trail of operative versus non-operative treatment of severe vesicoureteric reflux in children: five years' observation. *BMJ* 1987;295:237–241.

129. Craig J, Irwig L, Knight J, Roy L. Does treatment of vesicoureteric reflux in childhood prevent end-stage renal disease attributable to reflux nephropathy. *Pediatrics* 2000;105:1236–1241.

130. Imam A, Roberts R, Vernier-Jones K. Chronic renal failure in children in Wales: a prospective epidemiological study 1994–1997. *Pediatr Nephrol* 1998: C182.

131. Deleau J, Andre J-L, Briancon S, Musse J-P. Chronic renal failure in children: an epidemiological survey in Lorraine (France) 1975–1990. *Pediatr Nephrol* 1994;8:472–476.

132. Thomas G, Conlon P, Spencer S, Hickey D, Carmody M, Gill D. Paediatric renal transplantation in Ireland: 1980–1990. *Irish J Med Sci* 1992; 161:487–489.

133. Goonasekera C, Shah V, Wade A, Barratt M, Dillon M. 15 year follow up of renin and blood pressure in reflux nephropathy. *Lancet* 1996;347:640–643.

134. Goonasekera C, Dillon M. Reflux nephropathy and hypertension. *J Hum Hypertens* 1998;12:497–504.

135. Smellie J, Prescod N, Shaw P, Risdon R, Bryant T. Childhood reflux and urinary infection: a follow-up

of 10–41 years in 226 adults. *Pediatr Nephrol* 1998; 12:727–736.

136. Wennerström M, Hansson S, Hedner T, Himmelmann A, Jodal U. Ambulatory blood pressure 16–26 years after the first urinary tract infection in childhood. *J Hypertens* 2000;18:485–491.

137. Mansfield J, Snow B, Cartwright P, Wadsworth K. Complications of pregnancy in women after childhood reimplantation for vesicoureteral reflux: an update with 25 years of followup. *J Urol* 1995;154: 787–790.

138. Martinell J, Jodal U, Lindin-Janson G. Pregnancies in women with and without renal scarring and urinary infections in childhood. *BMJ* 1990;300:840–844.

139. McGladdery S, Aparicio S, Verrier-Jones K, Roberts R, Sacks S. Outcome of pregnancy in an Oxford–Cardiff cohort of women with previous bacteriuria. *Q J Med* 1992;84:533–539.

140. Jungers P, Houillier P, Chauveau D, Choukroun G, Moynot A, Skhiri H, *et al*. Pregnancy in women with reflux nephropathy. *Kidney Int* 1996; 50:593–599.

12 | *Common urological problems*

Robert J. Postlethwaite and Alan Dickson

Urological problems occur with much greater frequency than any specifically nephrological problem in children, and hence the paediatrician, specialist orgeneralist, will far more commonly be concerned with, for example, the management of antenatal hydronephrosis than nephrotic syndrome. Paediatricians, therefore, need to be familiar with the presentation and management of a range of urological problems.

The dilated urinary tract

The majority of presentations of urinary tract dilatation relate to congenital problems and few are acquired lesions. During the past 20 years the most common presentation of urinary tract dilatation has been during the antenatal period. This special clinical problem is covered specifically in Chapter 13. This chapter will therefore include discussion of some conditions, which may be suggested in the antenatal phase, but which produce serious clinical concerns in the days, months, or years after the child is born. It is a general rule that management strategies developed for patients with symptomatic disease cannot be applied to patients with asymptomatic lesions identified on screening. This largely explains the difference in emphasis in management in this chapter compared with that in Chapter 13.

Definition of hydronephrosis and obstruction

Hydronephrosis is a term that describes dilatation of the collecting system of the kidney and *hydroureter* describes dilatation of the ureter. The measurement criteria used to define hydronephrosis are discussed in Chapter 6. Neither term implies the presence of obstruction.

One of the problems in addressing the issue of the dilated urinary tract is that there is no generally accepted definition of urinary tract obstruction and even less agreement about how this is identified in clinical practice. It is also conventional to distinguish acute obstruction from chronic obstruction and complete from partial obstruction. At the extremes and in experimental animals these distinctions are clear, but in clinical practice they merge into one another. The acutely unwell child with symptoms and rapidly deteriorating hydronephrosis on imaging presents no problem in categorization, although precise diagnosis and management might be more of a debate. Problems of definition of obstructive hydronephrosis are much greater in the common situation of chronic partial obstruction. Koff's definition of obstruction as 'any restriction to urinary flow that left untreated will cause progressive renal deterioration' [1] remains the most useful concept clinically. Peter's extension of this idea to take account of the context of the developing kidney, defining obstruction as 'a condition of impaired urinary drainage which, if uncorrected, will limit the ultimate functional potential of a developing kidney', is a useful development [2]. Although this is particularly relevant to the issue of antenatal hydronephrosis, it is of general applicability in paediatrics, where possible effects of 'obstruction' on renal growth bring a new dimension to the problem which is not present in the adult situation. This issue is reviewed by Chevalier [3] and Peters [2].

Definition of presence of obstruction, its degree and chronicity depend on integration of information available from clinical and radiological assessment. Ultrasound can and should measure the amount of hydronephrosis and hydroureter. Radio-isotope imaging can measure differential renal function and generate curves which may be non-obstructive, equivocal, or obstructive; they do not in isolation, however, define obstruction. Clinically we find that an accurate description of the actual imaging findings is far more helpful than the use of such terminology as 'partial pelvi-ureteric junction obstruction'.

Causes of a dilated urinary system

Obstruction

This may result from either a physical anatomical lesion (e.g. stones, see Chapter 4; posterior urethral valves) or component dysfunction (e.g. pelvi-ureteric obstruction, neuropathic bladder, see Chapter 10).

Reflux

Reflux (see Chapter 11) generally results from primary anatomical abnormality and dysfunction of the uretero-vesical valve, but can be secondary to dysfunction of other components (e.g. neuropathic bladder, see Chapter 10) or to lower urinary tract obstruction (e.g. posterior urethral valves).

Non-obstruction non-reflux

This results from primary abnormality of the structure and/or function of components of the urinary tract (e.g. prune belly syndrome, primary congenital megaureter). Mild non-obstructive dilatation is sometimes seen in conditions with high urinary flow rates, such as diabetes insipidus. This might also explain the mild dilatation sometimes seen in single kidneys.

Obstruction and reflux

This most commonly occurs in a complete duplex system where the upper pole ureter is subject to an obstructive lesion (e.g. ureterocele) and the lower pole ureter is subject to reflux due to its very short course through the bladder wall.

Key points: Definition of hydronephrosis

- Hydronephrosis describes dilatation of the renal pelvis.

- There are non-obstructive causes of hydronephrosis, including:
  – reflux;
  – non-obstruction, non-reflux (e.g. prune belly syndrome);
  – obstruction and reflux (e.g. duplex system with ureterocele).

- Diagnosis of obstruction depends on integration of clinical, functional, and imaging information.

Pathophysiology of obstruction

The urinary tract is effectively a pumping system and conduit for the transport of urine from the kidneys to outside the body. The system includes reservoirs, tubes, and valves and, as with any dynamic system, will dysfunction if any of these components fail or malfunction. The first effect of such dysfunction is dilatation of part or all of the urinary tract, dependent on the site of the problem. Urine is first collected in the collecting system and pelvis of the kidney and is then pushed by active peristalsis through the pelvi-ureteric junction and ureter through the one-way-valve, uretero-vesical junction into the bladder (Fig. 12.1). There, urine is stored until voluntary (or automatic in the infant) emptying is initiated by complex neurological control mechanisms, resulting in the unobstructed flow of urine through the relaxed muscle sphincter continence complex and urethral conduit. Normal urine transport is vulnerable both to anatomical abnormalities throughout the urinary tract and malfunction of its active components. In summary, however, these two areas converge to produce a series of pathological lesions, all of which lead to dilatation, clinical symptoms, and renal injury.

Urinary tract obstruction leads to renal injury that may be irreversible. Initially there is an increase in pressure proximal to the obstruction due to continued glomerular filtration [4]. This rise in pressure results in dilatation of the collecting system and is also transmitted back to the proximal tubule and glomerulus, with consequent reduction in glomerular filtration rate (GFR). The mechanisms of this reduction in GFR are complex but the net effect is that the ensuing chronic reduction in GFR is primarily due to a decrease in renal perfusion. The tubular damage is due to direct effects of raised intratubular pressure, ischaemia due to reduced perfusion, and inflammatory cell infiltrate. Over time this leads to irreversible injury which does not recover when the obstruction is resolved.

The major functional effects of these changes are reduced GFR (of a single kidney; overall GFR if the obstruction is bilateral), polyuria, sodium wasting, and type I renal tubular acidosis with hyperkalaemia.

The renal prognosis after relief of urinary tract obstruction depends upon the severity and the duration of the obstruction. With total ureteral obstruction there is evidence that relatively complete recovery of glomerular filtration rate can be achieved

Urinary Tract
Urine flow - areas of dysfunction

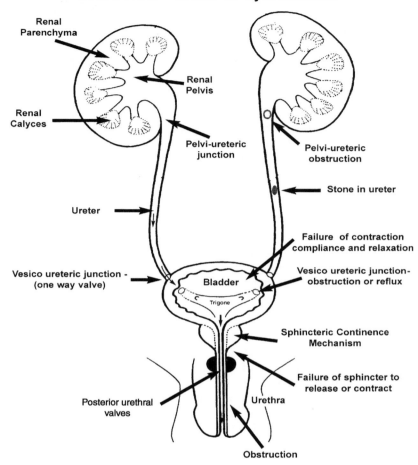

Renal
Parenchyma

Renal
Pelvis

Renal
Calyces

Pelvi-ureteric
junction

Pelvi-ureteric
obstruction

Stone in ureter

Ureter

Failure of contraction
compliance and relaxation

Vesico ureteric junction -
(one way valve)

Bladder

Trigone

Vesico ureteric junction-
obstruction or reflux

Sphincteric Continence
Mechanism

Failure of sphincter to
release or contract

Posterior urethral
valves

Urethra

Obstruction

Fig. 12.1 Diagrammatic representation of urine flow and sites of dysfunction where this can be interrupted.

if obstruction is relieved within 1 week, while little or no recovery occurs after 12 weeks of obstruction [5]. Measurement of GFR probably overestimates recovery, and even with good recovery of GFR problems with polyuria and renal tubular acidosis may remain.

There are a number of characteristic patterns of urine output in urinary tract obstruction (UTO). Complete bilateral UTO results in absolute anuria. Partial obstruction, however, is characterized by normal or generally increased urine output because of the tubular effects of UTO. Typically, after relief of bilateral UTO, there is a diuresis that might be of massive proportions. It is always important to monitor for

this. In the authors' experience this diuresis is almost always inappropriate in children and should be replaced ml for ml. Half-normal saline (in glucose) is the most appropriate initial replacement fluid. Bicarbonate and/or potassium may need to be added, depending on the biochemistry.

Hypertension is occasionally induced by UTO. It most commonly occurs with acute UTO, either bilateral or unilateral [6]. The hypertension is caused by activation of the renin-angiotensin system because of reduced renal perfusion. With chronic UTO, hypertension is not common; the salt wasting and polyuria that occur may explain this observation.

Key points: Pathophysiology of obstruction

- Major functional effects are:
  - reduced GFR;
  - polyuria, sodium wasting, and renal tubular acidosis;
  - hypertension (particularly with acute obstruction).

- Renal recovery after relief of the obstruction depends on the severity and duration of obstruction.

- Acute obstruction leads to anuria (if bilateral or in a single system).

- Patients with chronic obstruction usually have polyuria.

- Massive polyuria typically occurs after relief of bilateral urinary tract obstruction.

Clinical presentation of urinary tract obstruction

The clinical manifestations of UTO vary with the site, the degree, and the rapidity of onset of the obstruction. *Acute urinary obstruction* will almost immediately produce problems. The problems are particularly acute in upper tract obstruction. There will be dilatation of the urinary tract proximal to the level of the obstruction. The stretching of the walls of any part of the urinary tract will cause pain, which is classically colicky in nature. The site of the obstruction determines the location of the pain. Upper ureteral or renal pelvic lesions lead to flank pain or tenderness. Lower ureteral obstruction causes pain that may radiate to the ipsilateral testis or labia. In the upper urinary tract hydronephrosis and/or hydroureter will develop, dependent on the site of the obstruction, and pressure will eventually rise within the kidney. Clinically, the kidney will enlarge and may become palpable and tender. Renal perfusion is likely to decrease and, as a result, the systemic blood pressure is liable to rise. The kidney itself will rapidly develop irreversible damage and nephron loss (see above) and it is therefore clear that acute renal obstruction is an emergency situation. If the obstruction is bilateral or occurs in a single system, the problems of acute renal failure are rapidly increased.

Chronic obstruction implies incomplete obstruction, where urine is able to drain but only at the expense of high intra-urinary tract pressure above the obstruction. Pain is typically absent and the kidney non-palpable. The diagnosis of chronic urinary tract obstruction is easy in the presence of obvious lesions (e.g. stone or neuropathic bladder) but is often difficult, and in particular, the areas of uretero-vesical obstruction, post-operative pyeloplasty and ureteric re-implantation provide the most controversy. Serious functional deterioration in chronic obstruction occurs when there are other factors present, particularly infection.

Vesico-ureteric reflux (see Chapter 11) has long been recognized as a clinical problem. Its implications depend on its degree. It is likely to lead to urinary infection due to the urinary stasis that it causes. It produces urinary tract dilatation by transfer of intravesical pressures into the upper urinary tract. Mild reflux may not cause any dilatation, but these levels of reflux are rarely troublesome. At the severe end of the spectrum, the ureter becomes dilated and perhaps tortuous, the kidney becomes hydronephrotic and hugely enlarged and the renal parenchyma is thinned. Changes indistinguishable radiologically from parenchymal scarring can occur before birth, but the most significant risk of scarring is in the early years of life if infected urine refluxes into the renal tissue through compound papillae in the renal calyces.

Chronic UTO in children may present in numerous ways and the symptoms depend on the site of obstruction. Hydronephrosis may be identified when an abdominal ultrasound is done for some unrelated reason or for a reason of doubtful relation to the hydronephrosis (e.g. abdominal pain). Imaging performed for other reasons, for example radio-isotope imaging for skeletal problems, may coincidentally identify an hydronephrosis. Wetting problems, usually diurnal, occur as a consequence of polyuria or bladder outflow obstruction. Polyuria, proteinuria, and hypertension are also occasional presenting features. Progressive decline in renal function with failure to thrive and other manifestations of chronic renal insufficiency also rarely occur with bilateral UTO.

Imaging in the diagnosis of obstruction

The common dilemma facing the clinician presented with a dilated urinary system is to decide whether the

Key points: Clinical presentation of urinary tract obstruction

- The more acute the obstruction, the more severe the symptoms.

- Acute obstruction is an emergency situation because of rapid decline in renal function.

- The kidney is typically not palpable in chronic obstruction.

dilatation is indicative of obstruction. There are occasional situations in which severe obstruction may be present without dilatation on imaging. The most important is sudden acute obstruction, when it may take 1–3 days for dilatation to develop. The second, even more rare situation is when the kidney is surrounded by fibrous tissue. The only situation in which this is likely to occur in paediatric practice is in an obstructed renal transplant.

A number of tests have been proposed in the evaluation of urinary tract dilatation (see also Chapter 6). Although the micturating cystourethrogram does not define obstruction, it is an important part of the evaluation of hydronephrosis, as reflux is an important cause of non-obstructive hydronephrosis. It sometimes gives additional information, such as indicating the presence of ureterocele or suggesting a duplex kidney.

Intravenous urography does not show abnormalities specific for obstruction and is not now a primary investigation in these children. It still provides a very good visual image of the kidney and even now is sometimes invaluable as a secondary investigation in difficult cases to define the anatomy or help in the adjudication of equivocal cases.

Resistive indices on Doppler ultrasound have been explored but do not have a major role in the diagnosis of obstruction [7].

The three major imaging techniques for assessing the dilated urinary system are ultrasonography, renography, and the Whitaker test. All the tests are subject to false positives and, much more rarely, false negatives. To interpret them, the clinician must appreciate the pathophysiology of obstruction and understand the workings of these tests and possible inaccuracies. Additionally, the significance depends on the natural history of the situation being studied and the clinical context.

Ultrasonography is excellent at detecting dilatation but gives little information about the functional consequences of the dilatation. Good correlation between the antero-posterior (AP) diameter of the renal pelvis and the likelihood of obstruction has now been shown in infants [8], but similar correlations and measurements are not available for older children. In this case, only a qualitative statement about the degree of dilatation can be made. Significant increase in AP diameter of the renal pelvis on serial measurement, which is not explained by growth of the child, is highly suggestive of obstruction.

Dynamic renography has superseded all other modes of assessment of obstruction, as it produces measurable information about differential renal function of the two kidneys and urinary drainage. The technique is discussed in Chapter 6. In adults, approximately 50% of patients with an obstructive diuretic renogram eventually require surgery, either for pain or for progressive parenchymal loss [9]. The significance of the obstructed renogram in different situations in children will be discussed in the next section of this chapter and Chapter 14.

Typically, children with pelvi-ureteric obstruction presenting with clinical symptoms, do not give rise to any difficulty with diagnosis based on ultrasound and renography. Ultrasound will usually show a marked hydronephrosis; dynamic renography will show an obstructive curve with probable loss of differential function in the affected kidney. Intravenous urography, if performed, will show a delayed nephrogram, marked intrarenal and extrarenal hydronephrosis, and failure to demonstrate the ureter.

The same, however, cannot be said of vesico-ureteric obstruction. Ultrasonography and pyelography will demonstrate hydronephrosis and hydroureter, which becomes more dilated towards the level of the bladder. Unfortunately, dynamic renography does not reliably give clear evidence of obstruction. The underlying reason for this failure of clear renographic diagnosis is the huge capacity of the collecting system and hydroureter into which the kidney has to drain before the obstructed vesico-ureteric junction has its effect on renal clearance of the isotope. In some situations it has proved useful to resort to the use of antegrade perfusion pressure tests (Whitaker test, see Chapter 6). This investigation also allows direct infusion of contrast to allow clear imaging of the single system down to the bladder. However, the procedure is invasive, requires general anaesthesia in children, has potential complications, and, like dynamic renography, can give equivocal results. The Whitaker test is therefore not widely used. Most surgeons would accept the presence of related symptoms, the loss of function on renography, or increasing dilatation of the urinary tract as indications for surgery.

Key points: Imaging in the diagnosis of urinary tract obstruction

- Rarely, urinary tract dilatation may be absent despite the presence of severe obstruction.

- All imaging tests in the assessment of obstruction give rise to false positives and negatives.

- To interpret these tests it is important to understand:
  – the pathophysiology of obstruction;
  – the possible inaccuracies in the test;
  – the clinical context.

- Ultrasound and the diuretic renogram are the mainstays of diagnosis.

- Pressure-flow studies may resolve equivocal cases.

Clinical acute urinary tract obstruction

This is an unusual event in children's practice, occurring much less commonly than in adults. It can be classified clinically into:

- unilateral upper tract obstruction;

- lower urinary tract obstruction.

Acute upper tract obstruction

This has three causes in children (Table 12.1). The most common is a calculus impacted somewhere in the ureter, either at the pelvi-ureteric junction or the uretero-vesical junction, or, most commonly, in the pelvic ureter itself.

Acute presentation of pelvi-ureteric junction obstruction is probably almost as common as

Table 12.1   Causes of acute upper tract obstruction

Impacted renal calculus
Acute pelvi-ureteric junction obstruction
Acute uretero-vesical obstruction

ureteric stones. Most will present with acute onset of renal colic and only a few present in Dietl's crisis, when the kidney is so tense that the child presents with an acute peritonitic abdomen. In Dietl's crisis situations, the diagnosis is sometimes made at laparotomy for peritonitis. The acute onset in this situation is sometimes related to infection or injury but this is not always so and it may remain unclear exactly what has initiated the obstruction.

Acute uretero-vesical obstruction is rare and in the authors' experience only occurs in the presence of infection. Sometimes the organisms involved are unusual, including staphylococci and streptococci. The presentation in this situation is more of acute pyelonephritis than ureteric obstruction.

Initial management of acute unilateral obstruction is conservative if the diagnosis has not been made at laparotomy. Conservative management includes resuscitation, bed rest, analgesia, antibiotics, and, in the case of ureteric stones, a forced diuresis. The majority of children will settle surprisingly rapidly within 12–24 hours. Active intervention is required if there is evidence of pyonephrosis or if conservative management fails. Deteriorating renal function is also an indication for active intervention. It generally arises when there is acute obstruction in a single kidney. Pathology can occasionally be bilateral with, for example, calculi in both ureters in metabolic conditions such as cystinuria. In the majority of situations it is possible to produce acute relief by achieving renal drainage using a percutaneous nephrostomy. This is not difficult to achieve because the kidney is usually enlarged and easily palpable, except in a very obese child. The technique is assisted by ultrasound identification of the distended renal pelvis.

The majority of obstructing calculi will pass themselves without any intervention. Those that do not may require open ureterolithotomy, but there are now minimally invasive modalities that are applicable to obstructing stones. These include extracorporeal shock-wave lithotripsy (ESWL) and ureteroscopy/laser lithotripsy.

All acutely presenting pelvi-ureteric and uretero-vesical obstructions require surgical management.

However, this is best achieved on a semi-urgent basis rather than in the emergency phase. After the acute problem has settled and any infection has been controlled, assessment of the function of the kidney and the anatomical site of obstruction can be achieved using ultrasound scanning, renography, and, if necessary, intravenous urography. The occasional kidney with poor function should be removed but, in general, reconstructive pyeloplasty or ureteric re-implantation will relieve the obstruction and ensure excellent functional recovery.

Key points: Acute upper urinary tract obstruction

- Acute presentation of pelvi-ureteric junction obstruction and ureteric stones are equally common causes.

- Rarely may present with an acute peritonitic abdomen (Dietl's crisis).

- Acute uretero-vesical junction obstruction is rare and usually associated with infection.

- Initial management is conservative.

- Indications for active intervention include:
  – deterioration in individual renal function;
  – pyonephrosis;
  – failed conservative management.

- All acutely presenting PUJ obstructions require surgical intervention.

Acute lower urinary tract obstruction

Acute lower urinary tract obstruction in children is equally as uncommon as upper tract obstruction and presents as acute retention of urine (Table 12.2).

The acute retention which results from the two most common problems (Table 12.2) is benign in nature and will resolve rapidly following treatment of the primary problem. It is generally unusual to have to resort to catheterization in such children. The retention associated with gross constipation will be relieved by the use of enemas. The retention associated with local genital problems will usually resolve following administration of adequate analgesia and local soothing applications. These patients do not really require significant urological investigation. There are much more serious urological problems which can cause

Table 12.2 Causes of acute urinary retention in children

Commonest
  Gross constipation
  Local problem with external genitalia or vaginitis
Uncommon
  Posterior urethral valves (male)
  Hydrocolpos (females)
  Prolapsing ectopic ureteroceles
  Pelvic tumours (e.g. rhabdomyosarcoma of
    bladder and prostate)
  Neuropathic bladder
  Pelvic trauma
  Meatal stenosis
  Bladder calculi

acute retention and which require immediate intervention to relieve the obstruction (Table 12.2). These can present at any age in childhood.

Acute lower urinary tract obstruction related to these pathologies is an emergency situation. Failure to relieve such obstruction, particularly in infants, can lead to serious infection extending into the kidneys and septicaemia. In the worst situations this can even lead to the death of the child and in other situations is likely to lead to permanent renal scarring.

In general, the majority of children presenting with serious urinary retention can be drained following passage with a urethral catheter. In general a silastic 8 French gauge Foley catheter should be utilized for this purpose but in the small male infant it may sometimes only be possible to pass a 5 French gauge feeding tube. Occasionally, a suprapubic catheter may need to be used and various kits are available that allow passage of a retaining catheter through a trocar. Great care has

---

Key points: Acute lower urinary tract obstruction

- Presents as retention of urine.

- Catheterization is rarely required for the two most common problems (see Table 12.2).

- With the uncommon urological causes of acute retention, immediate intervention will be required.

- Intervention in urological causes will usually be urethral catheterization but occasionally a suprapubic catheter will be required.

to be taken using a trocar-introducing set when the bladder is small, as is often the case in small infants. On some occasions the only method of entry into a bladder is to pass a fine 4 French gauge feeding tube through a wide intravenous catheter introduced percutaneously into the bladder cavity.

The definitive management of these conditions will be discussed later in the chapter, although the treatment of pelvic tumours is not included.

Specific causes of urinary tract dilatation in children

Posterior urethral valves

Posterior urethral valves is a condition that affects male children only. The valves may develop in two forms:

(1)   valve leaflets, rather like venous valves, coming off the verumontanum in the distal posterior urethra;

(2)   a circular diaphragm in the urethra, just below the verumontanum but above the bulb of the urethra.

The frequency of these two forms is equal.

Posterior urethral valves are a congenital malformation that occurs during development of the urethra. Posterior urethral valves begin to show effects on the developing urinary tract early in the second trimester of development. The back pressure produced by the valves results in vesico-ureteric reflux, hydronephrosis, renal dysplasia, and impaired renal function. The effect on renal function is variable, with some children eventually having normal renal function and others proceeding to a total loss of renal function and renal failure.

The children often present in the antenatal phase based on antenatal maternal ultrasound scans. The classical features on antenatal scanning include oligohydramnios, bilateral hydronephrosis and hydroureter, a thick-walled bladder, and a dilated posterior urethra. The oligohydramnios may result in marked pulmonary hypoplasia, which can be problematical and sometimes fatal after birth. Not all fetuses with posterior valves survive pregnancy and some die *in utero*.

When a male newborn is found to have bilateral hydronephrosis and hydroureter, he should be regarded as having posterior urethral valves until proved otherwise. Any concern regarding lung function takes precedence over the urinary tract, which can be managed by catheter drainage and fluid replacement unless renal failure has set in. Those children who escape antenatal detection usually present in early postnatal life with severe urinary tract infection, failure to thrive or even renal failure. When a diagnosis is suspected, a size 5 French gauge feeding tube should be passed urethrally or a size 4 French gauge feeding tube should be inserted suprapubically through a wide intravenous cannula into the bladder. This will have the result of draining the obstructed system, reducing the possibility of infection and thereby reducing the opportunity for further renal damage. The children should be commenced immediately on intravenous broad-spectrum antibiotics, as infection occurring within the closed system of posterior urethral valves can be lethal. All such infants should be transferred to the care of a paediatric urologist and paediatric nephrologist.

After relief of the obstruction there will often be a diuretic phase, resulting in salt and water loss, which will require careful replacement and monitoring for some days. If the child is well enough, a MCU is performed to demonstrate the diagnostic massive posterior urethral dilatation.

Key points: Initial management of posterior urethral valves

- Majority are now detected antenatally.

- Bilateral hydronephrosis and hydroureter in a male infant should always be assumed to be posterior uretheral valves until proved otherwise.

- Respiratory problems (if present) take precedence over surgery for the valves.

- Establish drainage with a catheter urethrally or suprapubically.

- Cover with broad-spectrum antibiotics after instrumentation.

- Monitor for diuresis following relief of obstruction.

- Perform MCUG to confirm valves if the patient is well enough.

Definitive treatment of posterior urethral valves is dependent on the situation of each child. In general, the intention would always be to attempt to ablate the valves as soon as possible after the diagnosis was made. Unfortunately some children have impaired renal function or difficulties with infection that necessitate a diversion of the upper urinary tract to achieve reliable drainage. The author's preferred method [10] for dealing with posterior urethral valves is the Whitaker hook, which allows insulated diathermy disruption of the valves without any risk of burning extending to the adjacent urethral wall and subsequent stricture. Our results with this technique have been excellent and urethral injury has been avoided.

In those infants who have been unsuitable for early valve disruption, urinary diversion is required and planned surgical treatment of the valves is usually delayed until the age of 1 year. After the valves have been disrupted, the diversion can be closed to allow normal passage of urine to be achieved.

Follow-up of children with posterior urethral valves is extremely important. There are several important clinical problems which may develop and that will require management. Details are shown in Tables 12.3 and 12.4 [11–13]. The somewhat surprising finding that early presentation was an adverse prognostic factor has been confirmed by other studies. Indeed, in one later study comparing 1969–1978 to 1979–1992, a marked reduction in the age at diagnosis and at valve resection was associated with earlier onset of end stage renal failure. The authors speculated that this paradoxical finding was due to earlier detection of severe forms of posterior urethral valves [12]. A number of studies have suggested that

either the nadir plasma creatinine in the first year of life or the creatinine within 5 days of relief of obstruction are predictive of later renal function [13,14]. A figure of less than 80 μmol/l has generally indicated a good prognosis. This might be useful in planning further management and discussions with parents. The following issues are important in follow-up:

1. In patients with chronic renal failure, optimal management of renal failure will hopefully slow the progression to ESRF (see Chapter 23).

2. Monitoring for proteinuria is important. Development of this heralds declining renal function and dietary and drug therapy is likely to have a major impact (see Chapter 23).

3. Urinary incontinence beyond the age of 5 years should prompt evaluation of bladder function. Again, management of any bladder problem should retard the development of long-term problems. Personal experience suggests that severe bladder problems are a particular problem in patients with early onset renal failure, with recurrence of the obstructive nephropathy in the transplanted kidney. Bladder studies should therefore be undertaken in patients with early renal failure.

4. Urinary tract infection and hypertension, if it arises, should be treated aggressively.

Table 12.3 Outcome of posterior urethral valves [11]

Died during first hospital admission	4%
Died of CRF in childhood	6%
ESRF programme	16%
CRF ($P_{Cr} > 150$ μmol/l)	6%
Good outcome	68%

CRF, chronic renal failure; ESRF, end stage renal failure; P_{Cr}, plasma creatinine.

Table 12.4 Factors predicting poor long-term outcome in posterior urethral valves [11]

Early presentation
Daytime incontinence after the age of 5 years
Proteinuria aged 5 years
Plasma creatinine <80 μmol/l after catheterization [12,13]

Key points: Follow-up of posterior urethral valves

- Optimal management of:
  – urinary tract infection;
  – hypertension;
  – chronic renal impairment.

- Monitor for development of proteinuria.

- Bladder function studies if daytime wetting >5 years of age.

Pelvi-ureteric obstruction and vesico-ureteric obstruction

As with all dilating urinary tract anomalies, pelvi-ureteric obstruction and vesico-ureteric obstruction present now in two different ways. These diagnoses are both easily suggested on antenatal maternal ultrasound scans, and should be investigated and managed according to a protocol. This aspect of pelvi-ureteric obstruction and vesico-ureteric obstruction is covered in Chapters 13 and 14.

However, both conditions can slip the antenatal screening net and present with clinical problems postnatally, as was the typical situation in all children with these conditions prior to the advent of ultrasound scans. The children who present virtually all come to surgical correction of their lesion, if for no other reason than that they have symptoms that require relief.

The diagnosis of obstruction in these situations can, however, be difficult, particularly in the vesico-ureteric lesion. The basis of diagnosis is ultrasound and dynamic renography and, to a lesser degree, conventional pyeloureterography.

Pelvi-ureteric junction obstruction

Pelvi-ureteric junction obstruction is due to a functional obstruction of the junction between the renal pelvis and the ureter. The majority of children with this condition now present following maternal scans (see Chapter 14). Some, however, still present clinically with a mass or episodes of renal pain such as recurrent colic. A few will appear acutely with very acute renal pain (Dietl's crisis), pyelonephrosis, post-traumatic renal injury, or even following development of a renal calculus. In the presence of pyonephrosis, it may be necessary to insert a percutaneous drain to relieve sepsis and allow the assessment of renal function prior to considering surgery.

Surgical intervention is indicated because the children present with symptoms. The controversy about management of asymptomatic neonates with pelvi-ureteric junction obstruction identified *in utero* on ultrasound is discussed in Chapter 14. Surgical options in this condition include nephrectomy and pyeloplasty. Nephrectomy is performed when the potential function of the kidney after relief of the obstruction does not warrant reconstruction. In chronic obstruction, an obstructed kidney's potential function can be determined by employing a DMSA renal isotope scan preoperatively [15]. If the kidney's differential function is less than 15%, nephrectomy is then indicated.

Corrective surgery involves the well-accepted Anderson–Hynes pyeloplasty. The kidney can be exposed through a standard loin incision, an anterior muscle-split extraperitoneal approach, or a posterior lumbotomy. Although laparoscopic pyeloplasty has been described in children, the method has not yet found wide acceptance and has not yet been validated.

At operation, the kidney is found to have a tense hydronephrosis and in about 25% of patients there is an aberrant lower pole renal artery traversing the pelvi-ureteric junction. It is unclear how much contribution this artery makes to the obstruction and, even when it is present, pyeloplasty should be performed allowing the vessel to fall behind the renal pelvis. The operation on the kidney comprises three separate parts. First, resection of the pelvi-ureteric junction; second, the renal pelvis is also significantly resected to reduce ongoing postoperative urinary stasis; third, the pelvi-ureteric junction is reconstructed to provide a wide patent pathway for the drainage of urine. Although there does remain controversy about the drainage of kidneys following pyeloplasty, increasing numbers of surgeons are using internal JJ stents to carry urine from the kidney to the bladder during the healing phase. The authors' experience of this technique has allowed the earlier discharge of patients from hospital, with the mean hospital stay reduced to 3 days.

Pyeloplasty is a very effective operation and reliably resolves the obstruction with resulting improvement in the kidney's function. In our own series of over 100 cases, the only significant complications have been related to external drainage catheters. Follow-up after pyeloplasty involves ultrasound in the first 2 months, after which the JJ stent is removed, and thereafter diuresis renography 6–12 months after operation. Our postoperative assessments show significant improvement in the function of the kidney in 97% of patients and no loss of function in any.

Key points: pelvi-ureteric junction obstruction

- Usually diagnosed antenatally.

- Postnatal presentations:
  – abdominal pain;
  – Dietl's crisis;
  – abdominal mass;
  – infection (pyonephrosis);
  – post-traumatic.

- Pyeloplasty is very effective.

Uretero-vesical junction obstruction

This is a much rarer condition than its counterpart at the top of the ureter. In uretero-vesical junction obstruction there is a functional obstruction. The ureter is not found to be completely closed, but rapidly tapers from a very dilated distal ureter to a tiny lumen through the bladder wall.

The most common presentation of this condition postnatally is pyelonephritis or pyonephrosis, and the child can be extremely ill. Acute management involves drainage of the kidney and ureter with a percutaneous drain and appropriate antibiotics. Prior to surgery, the functional contribution of the kidney should be assessed by dynamic renography and DMSA renal scan to allow accurate assessment of the long-term function of the kidney (as described above in relation to the pelvi-ureteric junction obstruction).

Surgical correction requires reimplantation of the ureter. This involves mobilization and resection of the narrowed uretero-vesical junction, and some form of narrowing procedure to the lower ureteric segment which is to be reimplanted back into the bladder in a non-refluxing way. The authors' preference and the most commonly employed method is tapering of the dilated lower ureter by resection of its posterior wall.

The results of this surgical procedure are difficult to assess, for the same reasons as in the preoperative situation, the problem being the ongoing large capacity of the collecting system. Usually, however, although the ultrasound scan and the renogram will show no improvement after surgery, particularly during the first 12–24 months, the child's symptoms do resolve. Longer-term follow-up is required before the reassuring reduction in hydroureteronephrosis is observed on ultrasound scan. The overall results of this surgery are good, and very few children require further interventions.

abnormality within the structure of the urinary tract. Some people have found the term offensive and/or trivializing and, hence, other names have arisen.

Prune belly syndrome is a congenital disorder defined by a characteristic clinical triad (Table 12.5).

Renal abnormalities are the major determinants of survival. They consist of dysplasia with the added features of damage from hydronephrosis and infection. The ureters are grossly dilated and tortuous due to replacement of smooth muscle with fibrous tissue. Ureteral stenoses may occur due to kinking of the ureters, and peristalsis is ineffective or lacking. Ureteric reflux is present in 75% of cases. The bladder is usually enlarged with a thickened wall but not trabeculated. A hallmark of prune belly syndrome is a markedly hypoplastic prostate which leads to dilatation of the prostatic urethra. Cryptorchidism is seen universally in boys with prune belly syndrome, the gonads characteristically being above the level of the iliac vessels. The germ cells are markedly reduced in number, appear atypical, and may predispose to malignant tumours later in life [18]. A constant feature of prune belly syndrome is partial aplasia or hypoplasia of the abdominal musculature.

Virtually all the babies with prune belly syndrome are now diagnosed antenatally. In the small number of cases that are not detected antenatally, the syndrome is usually recognized at birth or in early childhood because of the appearance of the abdominal wall, recurrent urinary tract infections, and varying degrees of renal insufficiency. There are occasional reports of prune belly syndrome presenting as end stage renal failure in the adult [19].

Key points: Uretero-vesical junction obstruction

- Much rarer than pelvi-ureteric junction obstruction.

- Commonly presents with infection.

- Results of surgery are difficult to assess.

Prune belly syndrome (Eagle–Barrett syndrome, triad syndrome)

Prune belly syndrome [16–18] is the best example of hydronephrosis and hydroureter due to intrinsic

Table 12.5 Features of prune belly syndrome [16–18]

Triad of:
   Severe urinary tract abnormalities
   Abdominal muscle deficiency
   Bilateral cryptorchidism in males
Other organ systems involved in 65–73%:
   Cardiopulmonary
   Gastrointestinal
   Skeletal
   Developmental problems
Incidence 1 in 35 000 to 50 000 births
97% of cases are male
Pathogenesis:
   Bladder outlet obstruction
   Mesenchymal defect theory
Occasionally associated with chromosomal abnormalities

The syndrome presents a wide spectrum of pathology and urinary tract disorder. In older reports, 20% of affected children were said to be stillborn and 50% did not survive to the age of 2 years [20]. Maintenance haemodialysis or peritoneal dialysis is possible in these children [21] and the results of renal transplantation are also encouraging [22]. Thus the prognosis for these children should have improved significantly and it should be possible to offer treatment to all, except those dying of severe respiratory problems in the newborn period.

In patients surviving the newborn period without the need for dialysis, about 25–30% will develop renal failure. A nadir plasma creatinine above 62 μmol/l and episodes of clinical pyelonephritis (but not non-febrile urinary tract infections) predict for renal failure in the long term [23].

The appearance on imaging is a very poor guide to renal function; it has long been recognized that grossly dilated urinary systems in this condition can have surprisingly good renal function.

Clinically, three groups can be delineated. Group 1 are the most seriously affected and include the lethal variant, suffering urethral obstruction, renal failure, and pulmonary hypoplasia secondary to oligohydramnios. There are occasional reports of such babies dying *in utero* and others die in early life because of lung and kidney failure. Group 2 are babies with mild to moderate renal failure and pulmonary hypoplasia. Group 3 are babies who have the syndrome but with only modest loss of renal function.

The prognosis for Groups 2 and 3 is quite favourable, provided proper care is instituted. When the babies are born, the most striking feature is the thick, leathery, soft, abdominal wall. Sometimes there may be a patent urachus draining urine through the umbilicus, and in such cases there is often great difficulty in initiating normal micturition through the urethra. In others, the urinary tract is intact and urine drains satisfactorily.

In the ideal situation, best management is to do nothing surgically. Prophylactic antibiotics are indicated because of the high degree of urinary stasis. Indications for intervention include:

- failing renal function;

- troublesome urinary infection;

- inability to void.

The patients in Group 3 do not tend to have these problems and have stable renal function and general well-being in spite of having grossly abnormal megacystis, megaureter, and megahydronephrosis.

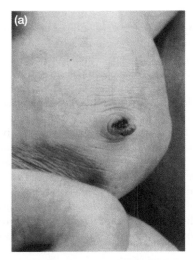

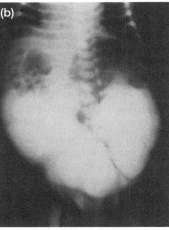

Fig. 12.2 (a) Appearance of abdominal wall in prune belly syndrome (b) Micturating cystourethrogram appearances in prune belly syndrome showing megacystis and megaureter. From Clinical Paediatric Nephrology 2/e by RJ Postlethwaite. Reprinted with permission of Elsevier Science.

The Group 2 children who require surgical intervention present very challenging management problems. On some occasions it is necessary to formalize the patent urachus as a vesicostomy, and in other situations ureterostomies may be required. The difficulty with these diversions in prune belly syndrome is in establishing indications for undiversion and thereafter maintaining satisfactory renal and bladder function. If at all possible, diversion should be avoided, as reconstitution of the intact functioning urinary tract proves difficult.

Some authorities have advised complete tailoring of the urinary tract, involving massive reduction in the size of the collecting systems, ureters, and bladder. The theory behind this is to reduce the capacity of the urinary tract, reduce urinary stasis, and improve urinary drainage. These techniques have been widely discussed but have not gained wide support throughout the world of paediatric urology and there has been no real documented objective evidence of benefit to patients from this major intervention.

There is wide clinical variability in the degree of abdominal wall laxity [17]. The wrinkled appearance is often lost, leaving a smooth potbelly, and the appearance in adulthood is also remarkably varied (see ref. 20 for pictures). Complications of the abdominal wall problems are surprisingly minimal, but include difficulty with coughing, micturition, defaecation, and posture. This variability makes selection for abdominal surgery difficult, but excellent outcomes have been reported [24,25].

Sexual function in males with prune belly syndrome appears to be intact, as the majority can achieve normal erections and orgasm. There is, however, no recorded fertility in prune belly syndrome. Some testes have been described as having normal germinal epithelium and showing spermatogenesis and, with the advance in fertility medicine, it is possible that some of these patients in the future will achieve fertility. The high intra-abdominal undescended testes thus pose a management problem. The management of such testes is covered later in this chapter.

Key points: Prune belly syndrome

- End stage renal failure management is possible in these patients.

- Imaging gives a very poor indication of renal function.

- The role of surgery in management of the renal problems is very limited.

- Complications of the abdominal wall problems are surprisingly few, and surgery is helpful in those in whom they occur.

- Sexual function is maintained but not fertility. This might change with improvements in fertility medicine.

- Because of the malignant risk, and with the possibility of fertility in the future, orchidopexy should not be delayed.

Renal agenesis, ectopia, and fusion

For renal agenesis, ectopia, and fusion anomalies, the same algorithm can be used for evaluation (Fig. 12.3). All these lesions are associated with a large number of chromosomal syndromes, non-chromosomal syndromes, and unclassified malformations, although the precise pattern varies for the individual lesion. Baseline renal function should be established and, as a minimum, should consist of plasma creatinine and urinalysis (1). Clinical evaluation as set out in Chapter 19 should be undertaken (2). If other congenital anomalies are identified, further investigation will depend on the specific diagnosis (3). Even in the absence of a recognized syndrome, all these lesions are associated with a high incidence of other urological abnormalities, particularly reflux and hydronephrosis (4). If the ultrasound has shown hydronephrosis, a mercaptoacetyltriglycine (MAG3) renogram is probably the preferred radio-isotope investigation. Otherwise a dimercaptosuccinic acid (DMSA) scan may be more informative. The radio-isotope imaging will also help to establish if there is an ectopic kidney present if there is apparently a single kidney; in this case, the radiologist must be informed of the possibility, so that appropriate views can be taken. Additionally, the initial ultrasound can be used to look for Müllerian duct abnormalities, which are common in unilateral renal agenesis. Subsequent follow-up will depend on the findings at this stage.

Bilateral renal agenesis

Bilateral renal agenesis results in severe oligohydramnios during intrauterine life. The baby is born with typical Potter's facies and is either stillborn or dies shortly after birth. There are a number of syndromes associated with bilateral renal agenesis. Interestingly 5% of first-degree relatives of patients with bilateral renal agenesis have unilateral renal agenesis (URA) [26].

Unilateral renal agenesis

The reported incidence of unilateral renal agenesis (URA) varies from 1 in 500 to 1 in 3200 [27]. It cannot be assumed that this necessarily results from a failure of development of the metanephros, as it is clear that entities such as regression of multicystic dysplastic kidney can result in the same appearance [28]. Thus the pathogenesis of URA is multifactorial.

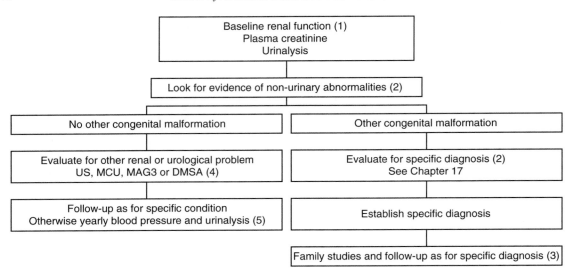

Fig. 12.3   Evaluation of the patient with renal agenesis, renal ectopia or fusion.

This problem is now usually identified on routine antenatal ultrasound. The only important differential diagnosis is of an unrecognized ectopic kidney, and identification of a possible URA should lead to a search for a possible ectopic kidney.

Associated renal anomalies are present in at least 48% of children with URA [29]. Vescio-ureteric reflux is the most common abnormality.

In non-syndromal URA, families with autosomal dominant, autosomal recessive, and X-linked inheritance have been reported. Nine per cent of first-degree relatives of a patient with URA have a related urogenital anomaly [26]. Ultrasound examination of first-degree relatives is, therefore, indicated. For non-syndromic renal agenesis, in which renal anomalies have been excluded in first-degree relatives, the empiric risk of recurrence is 3% [30]. Seventy per cent of patients with URA have major or minor genital anomalies. In girls this is usually an abnormality of the Müllerian structures, and assessment of these should be included in the ultrasound examination.

In addition to counselling about the recurrence risk, it is important to ensure that the family has a realistic understanding of the risks posed by the single kidney. Questions about diet and physical contact sports are almost invariably asked, and on occasion children have been subjected to quite unreasonable restrictions as a consequence of URA. In the authors' view, notwithstanding the concerns about long-term renal function set out below, there is no indication for any dietary restriction in these children, while, of course, healthy eating with moderate protein and salt intake should be advocated. Similarly, active sports are beneficial for all children and there is no evidence of major risk from sporting activities for these children. While it is probably wise to advise against high physical contact sports, such as rugby or judo, there is no evidence base for this and certainly other sports with less physical contact must be advocated.

Long-term prognosis remains a matter of great debate. There has been a long debate about the possible risks of renal ablation in adults and the additional risk from 'second hits' in the presence of reduced nephron numbers. This has been summarized recently [31]. Argueso *et al.* reviewed 157 patients with URA [32]. Mean age at diagnosis was 37 years. Six patients had died of renal failure, hypertension was present in 47%, proteinuria in 19%, and reduced renal function in 13%. This contrasts with the reports of Wikstad *et al.* [33] and Baudoin *et al.* [34] Although the report of Wikstad *et al.* did emphasize some potentially worrying features, GFR in patients followed for 26–40 years was 104.6 ± 2.3 ml/min/1.73 m^2 [33] and Baudouin *et al.* found, on average, that GFR was 75% of a reported two-kidney value after follow-up of 18–56 years [34]. It is also noteworthy that none of the 132 patients in these two series developed renal failure.

Both these latter series selected patients on the basis of a normal contralateral kidney and this probably explains the difference from the report of Argueso *et al.* In the authors' view, in patients with a normal contralateral kidney on imaging and normal renal function, the risk of long-term problems is very low and families should be counselled accordingly. Yearly blood pressure measurement and urinalysis, with the occasional measurement of plasma creatinine, should identify the occasional patient at risk of declining renal function.

Renal fusion and ectopia

Renal fusion [35] most commonly occurs at the poles of the kidneys but can rarely be complete, forming a single renal mass. There are syndromal associations of all types of renal fusion and a high incidence of associated urological anomalies (see above).

Horseshoe kidney

This is the classical example of polar fusion of the kidney, and is the most common renal fusion anomaly (1:400 to 1:500 live births) [35]. The lower poles are fused across the midline by an isthmus of functioning tissue. The kidneys lie slightly more caudal than usual, with the lower poles adjacent to the spine. Intravenous urography shows diagnostic features of rotation of the calyces in an antero-medial direction, but does not usually show the isthmus. The isthmus is well demonstrated on a DMSA scan (see Fig. 12.4).

Ninety per cent of horseshoe kidneys cause no problem and are found incidentally. The most common presentation is with urinary tract infection (UTI), other presentations being with an abdominal mass, haematuria, or abdominal pain. Horseshoe kidneys are rare in females; one of the associations is with Turner's syndrome and some authorities suggest that females with horseshoe kidney should be

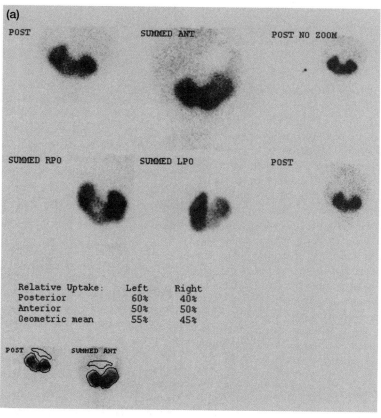

Fig. 12.4　DMSA scan appearances of horseshoe kidney.

considered for a karyotype [35]. Vesico-ureteric reflux is present in 50%. Some have associated pelvi-ureteric obstruction and the isthmus occasionally produces obstruction as the ureter passes over it; on those occasions, it requires division along with obligatory pyeloplasty. There is an increased incidence of renal calculi. Wilms' tumour in children and transitional cell carcinoma in adults is seen with increased frequency in horseshoe kidneys [35].

Crossed renal ectopia

Crossed renal ectopia (Fig. 12.5) occurs where there is upper to lower pole fusion, and in this situation the crossed kidney lies below and medially to the normally sited one and is abnormally rotated. The ureter from the ectopic kidney crosses the midline and passes to the appropriate side of the bladder. The kidneys are not usually normal and are often associated with ureteric or lower tract lesions, causing secondary renal problems. The abnormality is also seen in relation to other distal congenital abnormalities, most notably cloacal and anorectal anomalies. Most patients with this condition will eventually require renal and/or lower urinary tract surgery.

Ectopic kidney

The ectopic kidney derives from an error of ascent. Ectopic kidneys occur anywhere in the abdomen or thorax but most commonly in the pelvis. They are generally of abnormal shape and contribute less than the normal 50% differential renal function, although on some occasions they can be the only functioning renal tissue in the body. Some present antenatally, whilst others present as a pelvic mass, which may initially be thought to be a tumour. Others present with associated pelvi-ureteric obstruction or vesico-ureteric reflux and accompanying infection. Associated renal anomalies are common: 56% are hydronephrotic, moderate to severe reflux is present in 26%, and 22% have a dilated extrarenal pelvis with malrotation, suggesting apparent pelvi-ureteric junction obstruction [36]. The prognosis relates to the underlying urological disease. Surgical reconstruction, when required, is often technically difficult because of the unusual anatomy and blood supply.

Complete renal fusion

Complete renal fusion is rare. The single mass is disc-shaped and, again, is most commonly found in the

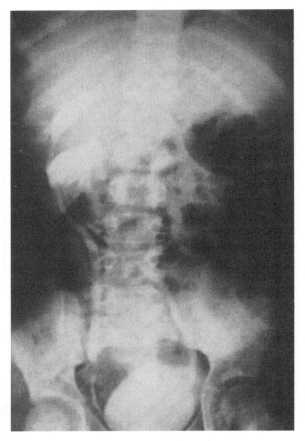

Fig. 12.5 Left crossed renal ectopia showing polar fusion and abnormal rotation. The ureter from the ectopic kidney crosses the midline to drain into the appropriate side of the bladder. From Clinical Paediatric Nephrology 2/e by RJ Postlethwaite. Reprinted with permission of Elsevier Science.

pelvis overlying the sacrum. Such presentations are essentially similar to a single pelvic kidney.

Key points: Renal agenesis and renal fusion

- Both syndromal and non-syndromal associations are common.

- Associated renal and urological problems are common and imaging should be performed routinely.

- Counselling of the family about the recurrence risk and lifestyle decisions is important.

Duplication of the upper urinary tract

Duplication is one of the most frequent urinary tract anomalies (0.8% in unselected autopsy studies [35]) but is usually asymptomatic. Unilateral duplication is five to six times more common than bilateral duplication [36]. It arises as the end result of the development of an accessory ureteric bud. The condition occurs in a number of syndromes. Additionally it carries a familial incidence. It occurs predominantly in females.

The diagnosis and assessment of duplications, ectopic ureters, and ureteroceles demand the use of all available urinary tract imaging and often cystoscopy as well. Ultrasound allows the initial identification of the collecting system and ureteric dilatation and ureteroceles. Intravenous urography displays characteristic diagnostic signs of the drooping flower appearance, caused by a tense dilated but non-functioning upper pole moiety pushing down a functioning lower moiety that is dilated due to reflux. The intravenous urogram will also show features of a ureterocele in the bladder (Fig. 12.6). Micturating cystography is essential because vesico-ureteric reflux is so common and it also demonstrates the ureterocele. Radio-isotope scanning is extremely useful in assessing the function of the respective moieties of a duplex kidney, thereby giving direction regarding management and surgical treatment. As the majority of patients with duplications are asymptomatic, they do not require investigation, neither does a duplex kidney identified coincidentally on imaging (usually ultrasound). Unless there is a clinical problem plausibly related to the duplex or potential for prevention of complications, further imaging is not indicated to confirm or refute the presence of duplex. Patients should be informed of the possible finding.

Duplication may be partial or complete. When the duplication is incomplete, the ureters may join at any point along their length but most commonly over the sacro-iliac joint. These systems almost always function as single systems and there is little evidence that their distal single ureters and vesico-ureteric junctions are more liable to pathology than a normal entire single system. Yo-yo reflux has been postulated in the past, implying some disorder of ureteric peristalsis allowing urine to reflux from one moiety's ureter back upwards into the other's, rather than down towards the bladder. There is little evidence for this fanciful concept and it should be discounted as a cause of clinical problems.

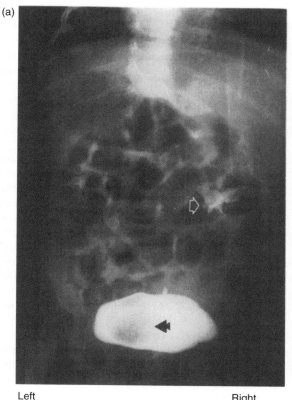

(a)

Left   Right

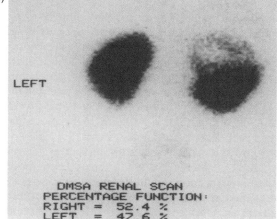

(b)

Fig. 12.6 Duplication of urinary tract with ureterocele. IVU shows 'drooping flower' appearance (arrowed) (a) and filling defect in bladder caused by ureterocele. The poorly functioning upper moiety is not visualised on the IVU but is shown on the DMSA scan (b) From Clinical Paediatric Nephrology 2/e by RJ Postlethwaite. Reprinted with permission of Elsevier Science.

When the ureteric junction is at a higher level, just below the kidney, there can be obstruction to one moiety as its ureter joins its partner. This will show as hydronephrosis of that moiety on ultrasound scan. Such a situation will present during follow-up of antenatal hydronephrosis or with classical pelvi-ureteric obstruction. Surgical reconstruction of this anomaly is challenging and demands careful consideration at operation to prevent complications affecting both moieties.

Complications of duplication in the upper urinary tract are most commonly seen when there is complete duplication, with both ureters extending down to the bladder. When duplication is complete, both ureters enter the bladder, with the ureter from the upper renal moiety opening lowermost and more medially on the trigone. Reflux is the most common complication and affects the lower moiety ureter because of its short intramural tunnel as it traverses the bladder wall. The upper pole is more likely to be associated with obstructive lesions, including ureteroceles or stenosis at the uretero-vesical junction. Developmental dysplastic changes and scarring in the renal parenchyma often accompany primary reflux and obstruction in this duplication situation. Severe scarring in the lower pole of a kidney should always alert the doctor to investigate for a duplex kidney with accompanying lower pole reflux.

The diagnosis of reflux into the lower pole of a duplicated system was at one time thought to be an indication for early surgical management by reimplantation. Several recent studies have demonstrated that the rate of resolution of low-grade to moderate-grade reflux (I–III) into duplicated systems is not dissimilar to the spontaneous resolution rate for reflux of similar grade in single systems; however, reflux into duplex systems does seem to be more severe than that observed in single systems [35].

Thus, the considerations about surgery for reflux in duplex systems are no different from those in single systems and would depend on the severity of the reflux and the risk of renal damage from further infections. Obstructive lesions are always an indication for surgery. If the renal moieties are well preserved, reconstructive procedures are rarely indicated. Generally the indications for surgery include severe scarring and loss of function in the moiety, when heminephroureterectomy is therefore required. In the unusual situation where there is a ureterocele partially obstructing the upper pole ureter and the upper moiety function is therefore well preserved, the obstruction can be relieved by endoscopic incision of the ureterocele through the cystoscope. This may result in eventual vesico-ureteric reflux into the upper pole, necessitating further management.

Sometimes, the upper pole ureter enters the lower urinary tract in a very ectopic position, even outwith the bladder itself. It may come to open in the bladder neck area or urethra, or into the Wolffian duct derivatives in the male or Müllerian duct derivatives in the female. Some ectopic orifices in the bladder neck may allow reflux and lead to infection but this is not common. If the ectopic ureter enters the lower urinary tract or the genital system, the urine from that ureter is obviously outside the continence mechanism, and the effect will include dribbling incontinence and often urinary tract infection. Vaginal discharge is another rare presentation of ectopic ureter and should be included in the differential diagnosis of this problem. These situations can only be resolved by surgical intervention, usually upper polar heminephroureterectomy or very occasionally reimplantation of the ureter into the bladder or into its partner when the upper pole function is worth preserving.

> # Key points: Duplication of the upper urinary tract
>
> - A common anomaly, but mostly asymptomatic.
> - Investigations should be determined by the clinical context.
> - Vesico-ureteric reflux is the most common association and can be managed using standard guidelines.
> - Hydronephrosis is always an indication for surgery.
> - Continuous dribbling and, rarely, copious vaginal discharge suggest an ectopic ureter.
> - Ureterocele is the most serious complication.

The most serious complication of duplication is when an ectopic ureterocele arises from the upper pole ureter. In this situation the ureterocele can extend into the bladder neck and urethra and cause obstruction of the bladder outlet, producing an emergency situation requiring rapid relief. Ureteroceles can also traverse the trigone and produce obstruction of the contralateral system, another emergency. Large ureteroceles can leave wide defects in the base of the bladder and can result in unusual neuropathic bladder dysfunction.

Management of ureteroceles is discussed in Chapter 14. Some authorities claim that there is significant recoverable function in these moieties in spite of the demonstration by Gough *et al.* [37] that the upper poles are completely dysplastic and grossly abnormal when examined following removal.

Anomalies of the male external genitalia

Hypospadias

Hypospadias is a common anomaly in boys, with an incidence of about 1 : 130 to 1 : 200 live births. The incidence is increasing, particularly the more minor forms, and although the underlying reasons for this are unclear, there are concerns that it might be due to feminising influences appearing due to pollution in the environment. Two such sources have been suggested. First, the widespread use of the contraceptive pill and its subsequent excretion; secondly, possible by-products from various industrial chemical processes.

Hypospadias itself describes the ventral situation of the external urethral meatus which can open anywhere on the under surface of the penis from the glans to the perineum (Fig. 12.7). However, the abnormality is almost always associated with a hooded foreskin, which gives the hypospadiac penis its characteristic appearance. Rotational torsion of the penis will often coexist due to abnormal skin and scrotal attachments to the penis. In the more severe proximal hypospadias anomalies, there is usually ventral chordee present, which is ventral curvature of the erect penis. This occurs due to replacement of the corpus spongiosum tissue by firm fibrous tissue. In its most severe forms, perineal and scrotal hypospadias, care should be taken to exclude female pseudohermaphroditism. At all levels of hypospadias, the external urethral meatus may be severely stenotic and require dilatation or meatotomy in the weeks after birth.

Initial assessment of hypospadias is often poorly performed. The shortening effect of chordee can often allow the meatus to reach the glans of the penis and this confuses the observer into believing that the lesion is less severe. After chordee is released and the

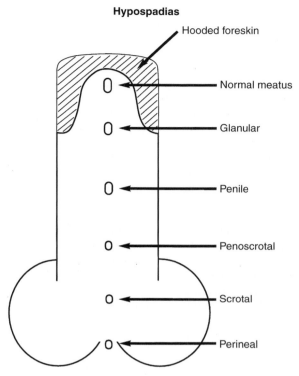

Fig. 12.7 Diagrammatic representation of ventral view of penis with sites of hypospadias.

penis lengthened, the meatus can fall back to a much more proximal position. Doctors assessing newborn babies should be aware of this kind of pitfall, which often results in the parents receiving inaccurate information about future treatment and expectations. There are some important points to note when assessing a hypospadiac penis. First, the doctor should note the size of the external penis. If the external penis is small, almost certainly the true hypospadias defect will be severe, even though the position of the external meatus may appear distal. This is an extremely important point. Parents should be warned that it is likely that the penis will require a major reconstructive procedure with greater risk of complications. If the external penis is within normal limits, the degree of severity can be determined more accurately by the position of the external meatus. If the meatus is on the distal shaft or glans, it is unlikely that there will be any chordee, and successful repair should almost always be achieved. If the meatus is more proximal, clearly the situation is more complex and more likely to have complications following surgery.

There is an uncommon association between hypospadias, undescended testes, and persistent Müllerian remnants attached to the posterior urethra, and any boy with hypospadias and an undescended testis should be investigated by ultrasound specifically to exclude this possibility. It is important to diagnose and manage these Müllerian lesions prior to reconstruction of the penis, as they will undoubtedly cause serious clinical problems after the urethra is complete. Penile and glanular hypospadias are not associated with internal urinary anomalies [38]. Urological assessment is required, however, in the context of scrotal and perineal hypospadias, as coexisting anomalies may occur.

In hypospadias, the urethral abnormality is due to failure of fusion of the urethral folds on the ventral aspect of the penis. The ventral chordee is due to bands of firm fibrous tissue (replacing the absent urethra and corpus spongiosum anterior to the urethral orifice) lying centrally and expanding laterally and distally towards the glans over the ventral surface of the corpora cavernosum.

Hypospadias causes several problems:

1. The penis has a very abnormal appearance and is generally cosmetically unacceptable to a developing adolescent and adult.

2. The urinary stream is usually diverted posteriorly because of the ventral situation of the orifice and often also because a bar of mucosa situated on the distal edge of the meatus. This leads to the child being unable to void into a toilet when standing and causes him to have to urinate in a sitting position. This causes severe embarrassment for the boy at school. The diversion of the urinary stream also affects the seminal stream and may lead to difficulties with ejaculation, impregnation, and even fertility.

3. The presence of chordee during erection may significantly affect sexual intercourse in later life.

4. The primary abnormality, if left untreated, may lead to psychological problems. Psychological problems can also follow if the boy requires multiple operative interventions during his childhood.

The management plan commences with early detection of the condition and parental counselling and reassurance. Investigations, if indicated, should be arranged as soon as possible to determine any important coexisting problems.

Definitive management is clearly surgical and should be planned for the early part of the second year of life. This allows for the surgery and any follow-up procedure to be completed before the child has any long-term memory, thereby minimizing psychological sequelae. The surgical procedure required is determined by the position of the meatus, the quality of the distal urethra, and the presence or absence of rotation or chordee.

There have been many operations described for hypospadias over the past 100 years. The art of surgery has developed considerably in the past 15 years so that good cosmetic results and excellent function can be expected for the majority of children.

In general, paediatric surgeons and urologists favour single-stage procedures, whereas plastic surgeons favour staged reconstructions.

There are currently four procedures widely practised by paediatric urologists. In all these procedures the foreskin is either utilized in the urethroplasty or to help cover the shaft of the penis with skin. Parents should always be advised to avoid having the child undergo circumcision, as the foreskin is likely to be required for the reconstruction. This is particularly important when dealing with Muslim or Jewish babies. Muslims are not required to have circumcision performed immediately after birth and such parents are usually very happy if they are informed that the circumcision will be performed during the hypospadias operation. The Jewish faith requires circumcision to be performed on the eighth day of life and the situation is therefore more complicated. In general, most Jewish Moyels and doctors agree to only a very minor procedure being performed in order to respect the law but not compromise the eventual reconstruction of the penis. The remains of the foreskin will always be removed during the operation to leave the appearance of a normal circumcised penis.

Operations

1. The MAGPI operation (meatal advancement and glanuloplasty incorporated) is a useful manipulation of the glans in glandular hypospadias. It is a minor procedure commonly performed as a daycase with excellent results. However, it is critical that patients are correctly selected on the basis of the quality of the glans, distal urethra and the absence of chordee. In

appropriate patients a surgeon can expect greater than 95% success with this procedure.

2. Meatal-based skin flaps, raised from the proximal ventral surface of the penis and sutured to the distal urethral plate, have long been employed to lengthen the urethra. The Mathieu procedure is the most commonly used procedure utilizing this approach. The glans is reconstructed around the distal neo-urethra to give a reasonable final appearance. In the authors' experience, less than 3% of patients undergoing Mathieu repair require any further procedure.

3. Urethral plate urethroplasties have gained favour during the past 10 years. In these operations the urethral plate is tubularized over a catheter. The urethral plate can be incised in the midline to allow a tension-free repair, as described by Snodgrass [39]. These procedures allow almost anatomical reconstruction of the glans and give the best cosmetic results. Unfortunately there appears to be a higher rate of complication (particularly strictures) than with the Mathieu-type procedures. However, the procedure can be applied to more proximal hypospadias and success rates of 90% are reported.

4. The transverse preputial island flap (Duckett) operation can be applied if the meatus is off the penis, if there is chordee, or if the distal urethra is of poor quality. This operation utilizes the mucosa from the inner aspect of the foreskin, which is mobilized and maintained on a vascular pedicle. The neo-urethra is constructed as a tube from this mucosa or by suturing it to the urethral plate as an onlay graft. The cosmetic results of this procedure are the poorest, but mainly because of the poor original condition of the glans. Nevertheless the final appearance is usually acceptable and overall success is reported in between 70 and 85% of cases.

The staged approaches usually involve primary grafting of skin into the glans and penis to allow secondary, easy tension-free repair. The protagonists for these operations believe that they give better cosmetic results and have fewer long-term complications in adult life, although there is little objective evidence to support either.

Circumcision

Comprehensive information about circumcision can be obtained from the American Academy of Pediatrics website (http://www.aap.org/visit/circumcision.htm). Available at this site are 'Care of the uncircumcised penis'; 'Circumcision: Information for Parents'; and 'Circumcision Policy Statement' [40].

Circumcision has long been the most common operation practised by humans. Religious and cultural circumcision is still widely performed, often by non-medical personnel, even in Western countries. There seems to be little in the way of acute complications which subsequently present to hospital. Nevertheless, serious acute problems have been reported, including haemorrhage, glandular injury, denuding of penile skin, and urethral trauma. In the long term, meatal stenosis commonly complicates neonatal circumcision due to local trauma from napkin rubbing and constant exposure to urine.

Attitudes to medical circumcision of boys have altered significantly during the past decade. These changes have occurred in two respects: first, there has been an increased awareness of the changes that occur to the normal foreskin in childhood, but secondly, there has been increased concern about increased risk to the uncircumcised male, particularly of urinary tract infection (UTI) but also of penile carcinoma and sexually transmitted disease.

The most significant realization has been that almost all foreskins are tight and non-retractile in early life, no doubt to prevent damage to the glans and meatus while the child remains in nappies. This tightness often results in ballooning of the foreskin during micturition, due to the space within the prepuce filling with urine before being eventually released. The normal foreskin naturally opens up over time to provide a soft, supple,

---

Key points: Hypospadias

- Incidence 1:130 to 1:200, but incidence is increasing.

- In severe cases exclude female pseudohermaphroditism.

- Circumcision is contraindicated.

- Chordee can lead to underestimation of severity of the hypospadias.

- Ultrasound should be performed to exclude Müllerian duct abnormality if there is undescended testis.

- Surgery should be planned for after one year of age.

retractile foreskin by puberty, at which time retractability is essential. The typical asymptomatic tight foreskin (Fig. 12.8) is not a phimosis and not an indication for circumcision. Ballooning of the foreskin during micturition is not an indication for circumcision. Many innocent foreskins have parted company with their children because of failure of doctors to realize the true natural history of foreskin development during childhood.

Most of the discussion about the risks to the uncircumcised male have focused on the risk of UTI and all the studies that have examined the association between UTI and circumcision status show an increased risk in uncircumcised males, with the greatest risk in infants less than 1 year of age. The magnitude of the effect varies between studies. Using the numbers from the literature, one can estimate that 7–14 of 1000 uncircumcised males will develop a UTI in the first year of life, compared with 1–2 of 1000 circumcised male infants. Although the relative risk of UTI in the uncircumcised male compared with the circumcised male is increased from four- to as much as tenfold during the first year of life, the absolute risk of developing a UTI in an uncircumcised male infant is low (at most about 1%) [41]. Using similar data, Craig *et al.* [42] estimated that 99 circumcisions need to be performed to prevent one UTI, and 'in a cohort of 100 boys circumcised to prevent one UTI, 0.2 to 5 boys will have complications, albeit usually of a minor nature, in addition to the cost and discomfort of the procedure'. Furthermore, a three fold reduction in risk of developing UTI can be derived from breast feeding [43]. Studies indicate that penile cancer is increased threefold in uncircumcised males, but the disease is so rare (9–10 cases per year per million men in the USA) that the risk, even for uncircumcised males, is extremely low [41]. Similarly, it was concluded that 'behavioural factors continue to be far more important in determining a person's risk of contracting sexually transmitted diseases than circumcision status' [40].

For these reasons among others, the American Academy of Pediatrics came to the conclusion that 'Existing scientific evidence demonstrates potential medical benefits of new-born male circumcision; however, these data are not sufficient to recommend routine neonatal circumcision' [41]. Interestingly, they state that 'it is legitimate for the parents to take into account cultural, religious, and ethnic traditions, in addition to medical factors, when making this choice'. Practice in the USA, therefore, differs from that in the United Kingdom, where the majority of specialists restrict circumcision to medical indications.

Studies have shown that hygiene can significantly decrease the incidence of phimosis, adhesions, and inflammation [41]. It is important to ensure that parents have good advice about penile care. Detailed advice is available at the website above, but the important message is **never try to forcibly retract the foreskin**.

Medical indications for circumcision

Balanitis xerotica obliterans (BXO) is probably the single absolute indication for circumcision. BXO is a primary, non-infective, aggressive inflammation of

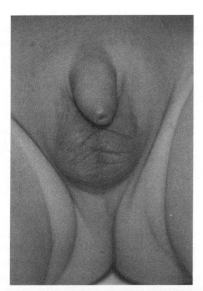
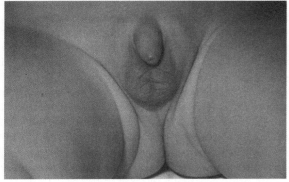

Fig. 12.8   The normal tight non-retractile foreskin.

the foreskin, which results in hard, fibrotic, true phimosis of the prepuce and its meatus. The condition can also extend into the distal urethra, causing serious stricture formation. The condition causes local pain, which is often extreme during voiding and sometimes may also lead to obstruction to micturition. Local therapies have not been found to be effective and circumcision is the treatment of choice.

All other indications for medical circumcision in boys are relative rather than absolute. These include:

1. *Balanitis*: this is infection of the foreskin and penis, the infection having arisen from within the foreskin. Generally this manifests a very dramatic appearance and causes severe discomfort and concern to both parent and child. Fortunately, it is not commonly a recurrent condition and often just happens once during childhood and rarely, if ever, has long-term effects. A single episode is never an indication for circumcision and recurrent episodes should initially stimulate more careful local hygiene rather than circumcision. Prolonged applications of local steroid cream will often render the previously non-retractile tight foreskin supple and moveable within 2–3 months. If the foreskin remains non-retractile because of underlying prepucial adhesions to the glans, these are easily separated under general anaesthetic to provide subsequent easy retraction. Once the foreskin is retractile and good local hygiene is maintained, then infection is a rare event.

2. *Paraphimosis*: this is a most unpleasant and painful acute condition, caused by retracting a tight foreskin over the glans so that the ring of the foreskin meatus acts as a partial tourniquet around the base of the glans. This causes glanular oedema and swelling, making reduction of the foreskin extremely painful and very difficult. If the foreskin proves impossible to reduce, then general anaesthesia is required and most surgeons would opt to perform circumcision then rather than risk further complication. Those paraphimosis foreskins that do reduce can develop fibrous changes necessitating eventual circumcision, but some return to normal and eventually become normally retractile in time.

3. *Recurrent local foreskin discomfort*: some boys appear to suffer ongoing irritation and discomfort for long periods of time. Generally these children are managed with local care, but some continue to have difficulty. If conservative options are exhausted, circumcision is a reasonable course to follow in such instances and invariably produces relief of the problem.

4. *Prevention of urinary tract infections*: routine circumcision to prevent UTI has been discussed above. There may be some benefit from circumcising boys who suffer urinary infection and have underlying conditions which are known to predispose to urinary infection, such as vesico-ureteric reflux. Circumcision in these circumstances can produce quite dramatic improvement.

Key points: Circumcision

- Despite benefits, routine circumcision is not justified.

- Penile hygiene can reduce penile problems, and parents should be instructed in this.

- Familiarity with normal changes in the foreskin in childhood is important.

- A tight, adherent foreskin is often normal and not an indication for circumcision.

- Ballooning of the foreskin is not an indication for circumcision.

- There are few medical indications for circumcision.

- Hypospadias is a contraindication to circumcision.

Undescended testis (cryptorchidism)

The testis develops on the posterior abdominal wall close to the mesonephric ridge. Between the seventh and ninth months of intrauterine life, it passes from an intra-abdominal position through the inguinal canal to lie in the scrotum. The incidence of undescended testes varies with gestational and postnatal age (Table 12.6).

Table 12.6 Prevalence of cryptorchidism by age [45]

Age	Prevalence
Preterm	30.3%
Full term	3.4%
1 year	0.7–0.8%
School age	0.76–0.95%
Adulthood	0.7–1.0%

All testes that are impalpable in the scrotum are not necessarily undescended. Retractile testes are a common variant of normal in which the testis is pulled up out of the scrotum by the cremasteric reflex to reside in the inguinal region. This effect can continue all through childhood and the testis does not settle in the scrotum in some boys until puberty. *The retractile testis can be clearly differentiated from the true undescended testis because it can be manipulated with ease into the body of the scrotum.* If this occurs, the testis will generally eventually fix in the scrotum. If there is tension and the testis immediately pulls back into the groin, then the testis is not retractile but undescended and needs surgery. More recently it has become clear that some retractile testes, possibly as many as 2%, do eventually become undescended during the course of childhood [44]. This is believed to occur because of shortening of the remnant of the processus vaginalis. For this reason it is advisable for retractile testes to be followed up until they fix in the scrotum.

The true undescended testis is thought to be held up in its normal path of descent. It may lie intra-abdominally, in the inguinal canal, or outside the external inguinal ring. A few testes are found in slightly ectopic positions, particularly towards the perineum, the base of the penis, and the femoral area. Undescended testes are almost invariably associated with a hernia and absence of such at the orchidopexy procedure begs the question whether the testis was truly undescended.

Normally descended and undescended testes usually have identical histology until 1 year of age. Thereafter the undescended testis begins to undergo progressive deterioration with a diminishing number of germ cells, abnormal Leydig cells, and peritubular fibrosis [46,47]. When the cryptorchidism remains uncorrected, as many as 40% of the contralateral descended testes show germ cell loss and consequent infertility [48] (Table 12.7).

The reported risk for malignancy with undescended testis is 48.9 per 100 000, which is 22 times higher than in the general population. The risk for an intra-abdominal testis if six times higher than for an undescended testis in another location [44]. There is little evidence that orchidopexy does anything to reduce this risk, but a scrotal testis is more available for assessment than an undescended one. Orchidopexy therefore allows easier identification of testicular swellings and hopefully earlier diagnosis of tumours.

In the United Kingdom, all children undergo many routine examinations during childhood, commencing

Table 12.7 Age at orchidopexy and subsequent fertility [48]

Age	Fertility
1–2 years	90%
2–3 years	50%
5–8 years	40%
9–12 years	30%
>15 years	15%

at birth, then at 6 weeks, and later again during the first year of life and at school. Despite this, many boys still present in mid to late childhood with their undescended testes. The reasons for this are unclear but must include errors on the part of the examining doctors. The assessment of a small child's scrotum is a difficult clinical examination and all doctors who have the responsibility of care for children should be well acquainted with the accepted procedures for this examination. It is most unfortunate when an undescended testis appears in teenage boy, because at that stage there is little hope of achieving fertility from that testis.

Physical examination of the undescended testis

First, the examiner must determine whether the testis is impalpable or palpable. The management of these two clinical findings is completely different, as described below. If the testis is palpable, it must be carefully assessed to determine whether it is retractile or undescended. The boy should be in a warm environment and the examiner should have warm hands to avoid stimulating cremasteric contraction and retraction of the testis. The flat pulps of the fingers are used to manipulate the testis, sweeping firmly down the length of the groin from the anterior superior iliac spine to the neck of the scrotum, thus pushing the testis distally. The retractile testis will manipulate to the most dependent part of the scrotum and remain there for at least a few seconds before the cremasteric reflex is seen to carry it back to the inguinal region. The undescended testis is diagnosed normally because it cannot be induced into the scrotum or, more occasionally, cannot be pushed into the lower scrotum without tension.

The management of the undescended testis is essentially surgical. There is little place for stimulation by chorionic gonadotrophin or luteinizing hormone releasing hormone in the true undescended testis, but their administration in an equivocal retractile testis

Table 12.8 Some endocrine causes of impalpable testes

Kallman's syndrome
Prader–Willi syndrome
Pituitary hypoplasia
Anorchia
Wolffian duct anomalies
MIF deficiency
Androgen insensitivity syndrome
Persistent Müllerian duct disorder
Testicular feminization
Reifenstein's syndrome

may clarify the situation. Orchidopexy is now thought to be best performed at the age of 1 year, for reasons described above. However, the surgical procedure at this age is technically demanding and should only be undertaken by experienced surgeons. There is a risk to the vital structures in the spermatic cord, the vessels, and vas deferens, because of their fine nature and fragility. The procedure involves careful dissection of the cord, herniotomy, and placement of the testis in a subdartos pouch in the scrotal wall.

The impalpable testis is a different problem from a palpable undescended testis. The possibility of an endocrine disorder should be considered (Table 12.8). If a testis is impalpable, it is essential to determine if and where it exists. Routine management of an impalpable testis commences with laparoscopy, which allows identification of either a testis in the abdomen, or the vas and vessels entering the internal inguinal ring into the inguinal canal or, rarely, blind-ending vessels in the pelvis. The findings on laparoscopy determine further management. In the rare situation of blind-ending vessels in the pelvis, no further treatment is required. If the vas and vessels are seen to enter the inguinal canal, then groin exploration is indicated to allow removal of the impalpable testicular remnant. If there is an intra-abdominal testis, then management must be carefully discussed with the parents. There is no sure method of achieving a scrotal testis is from an intra-abdominal position, and all approaches risk loss of the testis. One option is to remove the testis altogether, if the contralateral testis is normal. This removes the malignant risk and avoids the need for complex surgical procedures. The most favoured management option is a staged Fowler-Stephens orchidopexy. The first stage involves *in situ* division of the testicular vessels, nowadays usually through the laparoscope. The testis is left for several months to develop a collateral blood supply along the vas and the overlying peritoneum. The second stage is performed 3–6 months later, when it is usually possible to achieve scrotal placement.

Key points: Undescended testis

- A retractile testis should be followed until it is stable in the scrotum.

- Almost invariably there is an associated hernia.

- Malignant risk is not reduced by orchidopexy.

- Orchidopexy should be performed at 1 year of age.

- Urological problems are uncommon and routine screening is not indicated.

- The presence of hypospadias gives a 27% chance of intersex disorder.

- The impalpable testis needs a different investigation and management plan.

The acute scrotum

The acute scrotum is one of the most common causes of emergency surgical admission of boys to hospital. Some common causes are given in Table 12.9.

Various methods have been employed to identify loss of perfusion in acutely swollen testicles, in order to diagnose torsion of the testis and avoid unnecessary exploration for non-torsions. Doppler ultrasound scans and isotope scans have both been utilized for this purpose but have both been responsible for producing false-negative scans, thereby running the risk of leaving genuine torsions without exploration. The only sure way of excluding torsion of the testis remains exploration of the scrotum.

Table 12.9 The acute paediatric scrotum

Painful and swollen	Not painful and swollen
Testicular torsion	Acute idiopathic scrotal
Epididymo-orchitis	oedema
Mumps orchitis	Hydrocele
Torsion of appendix testis	Reducible inguinal hernia
Trauma	Varicocele
Haemorrhage into tumour	Testicular tumour
Incarcerated inguinal hernia	
Acute hydrocele	
Vasculitis	

Torsion of the testis occurs most commonly around puberty, the twist occurring inside the tunica vaginalis (intravaginal). The onset of symptoms can be either quite acute or quite gradual. The pain may begin in the scrotum or abdomen and soon becomes very severe. The testis becomes ischaemic and congested and, if left, will undergo infarction. In general, it is felt that a testis can only survive up to 6 hours of torsion and ischaemia before infarction sets in. For this reason the acute scrotum should be explored urgently to avoid missing an early twisted testis that could be saved. At operation the testis is untwisted and warmed to see if recovery is possible. If so, the testis is fixed to the scrotal septum to avoid recurrent torsion but if the testis remains non-viable, it should be removed to prevent secondary sepsis. Since the underlying anatomical abnormality which allows torsion is bilateral, the contralateral testis must always be fixed to the scrotum.

Torsion may also occur in the perinatal phase, usually before the child is born. This torsion occurs extravaginally outside the tunica and sometimes occurs bilaterally. Perinatal cases are usually asymptomatic but the scrotum is swollen and blue in colour, and the testis hard. The differential diagnosis includes an incarcerated inguinal hernia. The testis is always dead so that treatment is confined to orchidectomy and fixation of the other testis.

Acute epididymo-orchitis is rare in children but more common in adolescence. It is sometimes secondary to either an abnormality of the lower urinary tract, such as urethral stricture or posterior urethral valves, or just urinary tract infection. All boys who present with unexplained acute epididymo-orchitis should therefore have their urinary tract assessed. There are several clinical situations which are known to predipose to epididymo-orchitis, including recent instrumentation of the lower urinary tract such as cystoscopy or urethral dilatation. Risks of such infective complications can be significantly reduced by administration of appropriate prophylactic antibiotics. Recurrent acute epididymo-orchitis may occur in boys on intermittent catheterization. If this situation is seen to be developing, consideration should be given to performing vasectomy in order to protect the testicle from permanent damage resulting in impaired spermatogenesis. No such boy should be allowed to have more than one episode of epididymo-orchitis before vasectomy is performed.

Torsion of the testicular appendage, most commonly the hydatid of Morgagni, an embryological remnant, can present with either just minor local inflammation or a much more florid, red, swollen hemiscrotum. Often, the typical diagnostic small black nodule is apparent on careful inspection through the scrotal skin attached at the upper pole of the testis. Even if the diagnosis is clear and torsion of the testis has been positively excluded, it is probably still wise to operate and remove the appendage as conservative watching tends to be associated with persistent local discomfort.

Acute idiopathic scrotal oedema is a scrotal rather than testicular condition and is usually easily diagnosable as such. The important feature is that the scrotal wall, but not the testis, is very swollen, oedematous, and tender and these changes extend into the groin and perineum. The condition probably has an allergic basis, resulting from some unknown stimulus. Insect bites have been suggested but this is quite unsupported by evidence. The condition is self-limiting within 48–72 hours and there is no specific treatment, except analgesia. The use of antihistamine drugs has been recommended but it is difficult to discern whether these hasten the resolution of the symptoms.

Key points: Acute scrotum

- The only way of excluding torsion of the testis is surgical exploration.

- Torsion occurs most commonly around puberty.

- Testes can only survive 6 hours ischaemia, therefore the need for urgent exploration.

- Torsion may occur in the perinatal phase, when the testis is not usually salvageable.

- Unexplained acute epididymo-orchitis in childhood is an indication for evaluation of the urinary tract.

Anomalies of the female external genitalia

Vulvovaginitis

Vulvovaginitis is generally considered to be the most common gynaecological problem in premenarchal girls. The incidence is unknown, but an impression of the frequency of the problem is provided by the observation that 200 girls were seen with this problem at a paediatric accident and emergency department in under 3 years [49]. In a later study, 50% of control patients reported that they had experienced genital irritation at some stage and 30% of them had mild introital redness at the time of examination [50]. Predisposing factors are thought to include: less protective covering of the introitus by the labia majora; low oestrogen concentrations, leaving the vaginal mucosa susceptible to irritation and infection; exposure to irritants (such as bubble bath); poor hygiene; and infection by specific pathogens. Clinical features are given in Table 12.10.

Given the frequency with which vulvovaginitis occurs, it is not surprising that it is a more common cause of dysuria and frequency than UTI. In one study of adolescent girls with dysuria and frequency, 41% had vaginitis, 25% other local causes, and only 17% UTI [51]. Clinical experience would suggest that this holds true at all other ages in childhood.

The data from Jaquiery *et al.* [50] suggest that the majority (80%) of vulvovaginitis is not due to infective causes. Some common causes of non-infectious vulvovaginitis are given in Table 12.11.

A wide range of pathogens may cause infective vulvovaginitis (Table 12.12). Despite this long list of pathogens, the majority of pathogens isolated in the series referred to above were *Candida* or commensal organisms [49,50]. Additionally, *Enterobius vermicularis* was isolated in 21.5% of patients in one study [49]. Infective cases have more visible vaginal discharge and more extensive redness in the genital area [50].

An ever-present concern of the doctor, and often of parents, when faced with a child with vulvovaginitis is the possibility of sexual abuse. Sexual abuse was not identified in any of the 250 cases in the series we have referred to [49,50]. Furthermore, on physical findings alone sexual abuse is difficult to distinguish from vulvovaginitis due to other causes. Additionally, physical findings are often absent in sexual abuse even when the perpetrator admits to penetration of the child's genitalia [52]. Thus in the absence of more specific findings on examination

> # Key points: Vulvovaginitis
>
> - Most common gynaecological problem in premenarchal girls.
>
> - A more common cause of dysuria and frequency than urinary tract infection.
>
> - Sexual abuse is rare but should always be considered.
>
> - In the majority of cases an infectious cause cannot be identified.
>
> - Infection is suggested by significant vaginal discharge and extensive vulval redness.
>
> - Antibiotics and antifungals should only be used if a definite pathogen is isolated.

Table 12.10 Clinical features of vulvovaginitis [49]

Symptoms		Signs	
Soreness	54%	Genital redness	84%
Discharge	52%	Visible discharge	33%
Dysuria with or without frequency	51%	Perianal soiling	18%
Itch	40%	Specific skin lesion	14%
Abdominal pain	26%	None	2.4%
Bleeding	19%		

Table 12.11 Some common causes of non-infectious vulvovaginitis

Condition	Historical clues
Poor hygiene	Infrequent bathing, hand washing, and clothing changes; soiled underwear, toilet independence
Frictional trauma	Tight clothing, nylon underwear, leotards, wet bathing suits, obesity, sports, masturbation, or sexual abuse
Chemical irritants	Bubble bath, perfumed or harsh soaps, detergents, powder, water softeners, feminine hygiene products
Medication related	Topical antibiotic, steroid or hormone creams, chemotherapy
Contact dermatitis	Topical creams or ointments, poison ivy
Generalized skin disorder	History of pruritis, chronic skin lesions, prior diagnosis
Rare conditions	Vaginal foreign body, anatomic anomalies (vesicovaginal fistulas, rectovaginal fistulas, ectopic ureters), neoplasms, systemic diseases (Stevens–Johnson syndrome), Crohn's disease

Table 12.12 Infectious causes of prepubertal and pubertal vulvovaginitis

Non-sexually transmitted	Sexually transmitted
Bacterial skin pathogens	Bacterial pathogens
Group A beta-haemolytic streptococci[a]	*Chlamydia trachomatis*[a]
Streptococcus pneumoniae[a]	*Gardnerella vaginalis*
Haemophilus influenzae[a]	*Neisseria gonorrhoeae*[a]
Neisseria meningitidis	Genital mycoplasmas
Staphylococci	*Treponema pallidum*
Viral pathogens	Protozoa
Varicella-zoster virus	*Trichomonas vaginalis*[a]
Herpes simplex types 1 and 2	*Viral pathogens*
Adenoviruses[a]	Herpes simplex types 1 and 2
Echoviruses[a]	Human papilloma virus
Measles virus	Parasites
Gastrointestinal pathogens	*Pthirus* (lice)
Candida species[a]	*Sarcoptes scabiei*
Shigella species[a]	
Enterobius vermicularis	
Yersinia species	

[a] Pathogens associated with prominent vaginal discharge.

Table 12.13 Diagnostic considerations in sexual abuse (AAP guidelines) [52]

Concerning findings	More concerning findings
Abrasions or bruising on inner thighs and genitalia	Scarring, tears, or distortion of hymen
Scarring or tears of labia minora	Decreased amount of, or absent, hymen
Enlargement of hymenal opening	Scarring of the fossa navicularis
	Injury to, or scarring of, the posterior fourchette
	Anal lacerations

Table 12.14 Implications of commonly encountered sexually transmitted diseases for diagnosis of sexual abuse in infants and prepubertal children [52]

Gonorrhoea[a]	Diagnostic
Syphilis[a]	Diagnostic
HIV[b]	Diagnostic
Chlamydia[a]	Diagnostic
Trichomonas vaginalis	Highly suspicious
Condylomata acuminata[a] (anogenital warts)	Suspicious
Herpes (genital location)	Suspicious
Bacterial vaginosis	Inconclusive

[a] If not perinatally acquired.
[b] If not perinatally or transfusion acquired.

(Table 12.13), sexually transmitted organisms on culture (Table 12.14), concerns about the child's behaviour or social conditions, or a disclosure by the child, it is impossible to make a diagnosis of sexual abuse on the basis of the finding of a non-specific vulvovaginitis.

Management of vulvovaginitis consists of reassurance of the parents about the benign and self-limiting nature of the problem and avoidance of obvious precipitants such as bubble bath. Antibiotics should only be prescribed on the basis of positive bacteriology. If the problems are particularly troublesome and infectious, and other causes have been excluded, local oestrogen cream applied for 8 weeks often improves the situation.

Labial adhesions

Labial adhesions are a common problem. Fusion of the labia minora across the midline, obscuring the vaginal orifice and sometimes partially extending across the external urethral meatus, most often occurs congenitally but is usually noticed by the parents some time after birth. The problem often causes high anxiety for the parents who fear that their daughter has no vagina. This is not helped by the failure of doctors to recognize the simplicity of the condition and reassure the parents that behind the adhesions lies a normal vaginal orifice. Sometimes, the problem is not noted until it presents in other ways, which include dysuria, diversion of the urinary stream, and wetting or even unusual bubbling feelings in the vagina. Occasionally, similar labial adhesions may develop after local vulval or vaginal infection.

Although the natural history of such adhesions is to open up spontaneously in time, parental concerns and pressure or local symptoms generally dictate that something needs to be done. The adhesions can be opened physically with ease but this is usually painful and causes distress to the child and mother, so that it generally has to be done under general anaesthetic. Application of local lubricating creams to the adherent labia are often effective at opening them up, but this takes time and requires multiple daily treatments for a prolonged period. This repeated manoeuvring around the perineum in the older toddler or infant is often also unacceptable to the parents and is therefore often discontinued. Local oestrogen creams have long been recommended as producing rapid and reliable resolution of the problem, but this has never been objectively confirmed and the authors' experience has been variable. There is no doubt that the adhesions can recur following any of these above treatments. If separation needs to be achieved, the best management is probably local physical separation with or without general anaesthesia as required, followed by occasional application of Vaseline to prevent re-adhesion. Parents are generally just relieved to see the normal vaginal orifice after the adhesions have been opened.

Key points: Labial adhesions

- Labial adhesions are common.

- They are easily distinguished clinically from imperforate hymen and congenital absence of the vagina.

- They always resolve spontaneously before puberty.

- Treatment is with oestrogen cream or physical separation under general anaesthesia.

Hydrocolpos and hydrometrocolpos

Hydrocolpos and hydrometrocolpos are rare problems which are usually encountered at birth. There are two congenital abnormalities of the vagina that can result in obstruction of the vagina in spite of normal Müllerian differentiation. These conditions are imperforate hymen and a transverse vaginal septum situated at a higher level. Girls with these lesions have normal labia majora and minora, and these conditions should not be confused with persistent urogenital sinus abnormalities.

The imperforate hymen situation is easily recognized after birth, when a tense lower abdominal swelling is associated with a bulging interlabial membrane. In the transverse vaginal septum situation, the external appearance is normal and the site of the obstructing membrane is not apparent on external assessment. Vaginoscopy is required for diagnosis. Septal vaginal obstruction has a familial incidence, the anomaly being inherited as an autosomal recessive disorder.

In these conditions, the vagina and, less frequently, the uterus and Fallopian tubes are distended with mucinous female genital secretions from the vagina and uterus of the fetus, due to stimulating circulating maternal oestrogens. The lesions are nowadays sometimes predicted on maternal scans. Postnatal ultrasound of the baby confirms a midline cystic mass behind the bladder extending into the abdomen. If the obstruction is not recognized, the mass will often shrink by reabsorption and not present again until puberty with amenorrhoea, lower abdominal pain, and bilateral lower limb pain.

Imperforate hymen is easily managed by incision of the bulging thin membrane, which releases surprisingly large volumes of fluid. The management of higher vaginal septal obstructions is more difficult and care must be taken not to damage adjacent structures. It should still be possible, however, to deal with this lesion transvaginally.

Key points: Hydrocolpos

- Rare, usually encountered at birth.

- Imperforate hymen is easily recognized.

- Transverse vaginal septum requires vaginoscopy for diagnosis.

Urogenital sinus abnormalities

In this condition the urethra and vagina share a common terminal channel, with a single opening at the vulva. Urogenital sinus stenosis is not uncommon and is associated with massive hydrocolpos and urinary tract obstruction. This anatomical situation is common to a number of diverse conditions. The most common lesion producing this effect is congenital adrenal hyperplasia with virilization of the female fetus. Other more complex abnormalities, such as cloacal anomalies, include similar urogenital sinus situations.

The basic principles behind surgical reconstruction are the same as for the anomalies, and include separation of the vagina from the urethra and bladder, preserving the urogenital sinus as urethra, and bringing the vagina to the perineum. If the vagina does not reach the perineum, a piece of colon or small bowel can be utilized to achieve this. However, enterocystoplasties are often complicated by prolapse and constant drainage of secretions and are best avoided if possible.

Recently Pena [53] has suggested total mobilization of the urogenital complex into the perineum in order to produce normally appearing and normally functioning tissues.

Key points: Urogenital sinus abnormalities

- Urethra and vagina have a common opening on the vulva.

- Present with hydrocolpos and urinary obstruction.

- Management is surgical.

Bladder exstrophy

Bladder exstrophy has an incidence of between 1:10 000 and 1:50 000 live births and is twice as common in males [54]. The aetiology of this condition is unknown. There seems to be a failure of invasion of the cloacal membrane by mesoderm, so that the ectoderm and the endoderm are in abnormal contact in the developing lower abdominal wall. The unstable membrane subsequently disintegrates, so that the anterior pelvic viscera are laid open on the abdominal surface.

At birth, the pubic symphysis is completely diastased and this is associated with an anterior lower abdominal wall muscular defect, the rectus muscles being pulled apart by the pelvic diastasis. The anterior

bladder and urethral walls are deficient, including the bladder neck and external urethral sphincter. The penis or clitoris is therefore epispadiac and the margin of the posterior bladder wall is continuous with the edges of the anterior abdominal wall defect. The umbilical cord is displaced inferiorly and is adherent to the superior margin of the bladder. The posterior bladder wall herniates outwards through the muscular defect on the anterior abdominal wall as a large bulge. The penis is epispadiac and the urethra is represented only by a strip of mucosa on the dorsum of the severely upturned penis (dorsal chordee) which has a broad splayed glans and an incomplete ventral foreskin. The scrotum is wide and shallow, separated from the penis, usually with descended testes but sometimes herniae. In the female, there is a hemiclitoris on each side, the vaginal opening is pulled anteriorly and the labia are widely separated. The anus is displaced anteriorly in both sexes.

Historically, the results of bladder exstrophy surgery have been very poor. Typically, the child would have failed closures requiring multiple procedures both to the bladder and genitalia, with the eventual end point including renal dysfunction, urinary incontinence, genital disfigurement, and corporal dysfunction. Because of the rare nature of the condition, surgeons gained sparse experience.

During the past decade however, some units around the world have built up specific experience in this condition, and significant knowledge and understanding have been gained. More recently, the National Health Service in England has determined through the National Specialist Commissioning Advisory Group (NSCAG) that only two specialist hospitals should look after this condition with a view to concentrating experience and facilitating audit. Furthermore, these patients require specialist input of other health professionals with experience of bladder exstrophy. The contribution of nephrologists, nurse specialists, psychologists, and other support staff cannot be underestimated in achieving optimal outcomes.

Aims of treatment include preservation of renal function, urinary incontinence, sexual function, and acceptable cosmetic appearance. Current management protocols vary, but typically include neonatal closure of the bladder defect facilitated by pelvic bone osteotomy, followed by combined epispadias repair and bladder neck reconstruction, with ureteric reimplantation when the bladder has an appropriate capacity. However, many children will require bladder augmentation surgery, continent diversions, and occasionally even artificial urinary sphincters in order to achieve a satisfactory result.

References

1. Koff SA. Problematic UPJ obstruction. J Urol, 1987, 138, 390.
2. Peters CA. Urinary tract obstruction in children. J Urol, 1995, 154, 1874–1883.
3. Chevalier RL, Gomez RA. Obstructive Uropathy: Physiology. In Pediatric Nephrology, 4th Edition. Barratt TM, Avner ED, Harmon WE (eds). Lippincott, Williams and Wilkins, 1999, 873–885.
4. Klahr S. New Insights into the consequences and mechanisms of renal impairment in obstructive nephropathy. Am J Kidney Dis, 1991, 18, 689.
5. Better OS, Arieff AI, Massry SG et al. Studies on renal function after relief of complete unilateral obstruction of three months' duration in man. Am J Med, 1973, 54, 234.
6. Weidemann P, Beretta-Picoli C, Hisrh D et al. Curable hypertension with unilateral hydronephrosis. Ann Int Med, 1977, 87, 437.
7. Koff SA. Obstructive Uropathy: Clinical. In Pediatric Nephrology, 4th Edition. Barratt TM, Avner ED, Harmon WE (eds). Lippincott, Williams and Wilkins, 1999, 887–896.
8. Subramaniam R, Kouriefs C, Dickson AP. Antenatally detected pelviureteric obstruction: concerns about conservative management. BJU Int 1999, 84, 335–338.
9. Lupton EW, Testa HJ. The obstructive renogram: an appraisal of the significance. J Urol, 1992, 147, 981.
10. Whitaker RH. The Whitaker Test. Urol Clin North Am, 1979, 6, 529.
11. Parkhouse HF, Barratt TM, Dillon MJ, Duffy PG et al. Long-term outcome of boys with posterior urethral valves. Br J Urol, 1988, 62, 59–62.
12. Drozdz D, Drozdz M, Gretz N et al. Progression to end stage renal disease in children with posterior urethral valves. Pediatr Nephrol, 1998, 12, 630–636.
13. Denes ED, Barthold JS, Gonzalez R. Early prognostic value of serum creatinine levels in children with posterior urethral valves. J Urol, 1997, 157, 1441–1443.
14. Onuora VC, Mirza K, Koko AH et al. Prognostic factors in Saudi children with posterior urethral valves. Pediatr Nephrol, 2000, 14, 221–223.
15. Thompson A, Gough DC. The use of renal scintigraphy in assessing the potential for recovery in the obstructed renal tract in children. BJU Int 2001, 87, 853–856.
16. Sutherland RS, Mevorach RA, Kogan BA. The prune-belly syndrome: current insights. Pediatr Nephrol, 1995, 9, 770–778.
17. Jennings RW. Prune Belly Syndrome. Semin Pediatr Surg, 2000, 9, 115–120.
18. Massad CA, Cohen MB, Kogan BA et al. Morphology and histochemistry of infant testes in the prune belly syndrome. J Urol, 1991, 146, 1598.
19. Wallner M, Kramar R. Detection of prune-belly syndrome in a 35-year-old man: a rare cause of end-stage failure in an adult. Am J Nephrol, 1990, 10, 413.
20. Duckett JW. The Prune Belly Syndrome. In Clinical Pediatric Urology, Kelelalis PP, King LR (eds). Saunders, Philadelphia, 1976.
21. Crompton CH, Balfe JW, Khoury A. Peritoneal dialysis in the prune belly syndrome. Perit Dial Int, 1994, 14, 17.
22. Fontaine E, Salomon L, Gagnadoux MF et al. Long-term results of renal transplantation in the prune belly syndrome. J Urol, 1997, 158, 892.
23. Noh PH, Cooper CS, Winkler AC et al. Prognostic factors for long-term renal function in boys with prune-belly syndrome. J Urol, 1999, 162, 1399–1401.
24. Furness PD, Cheng EY, Franco I, Firlit CF. The prune-belly syndrome: a new and simplified technique of abdominal wall reconstruction. J Urol, 1998, 160, 1195–1197.
25. Ger R, Coryllos EV. Management of the abdominal wall defect in the prune belly syndrome by muscle transposition: an 18-year follow-up. Clin Anat, 2000, 13, 341–346.
26. Roodhooft AM, Birnholz JC, Holmes LB. Familial nature of congenital absence and severe dysgenesis of both kidneys. N Eng J Med, 1984, 310, 1341–1345.
27. Robson WLM, Leung AKC, Rogers RC, Unilateral renal agenesis. In Advances in Pediatrics, Barness LA, DeViro DC, Kaback MM, et al. (eds), Vol 42. Mosby, 1995, 575–592.
28. Mesrobian HG, Rushton HG, Bulas D. Unilateral renal agenesis may result from in utero regression of multi-cystic renal dysplasia. J Urol, 1993, 150, 793–794.
29. Cascio S, Paran S, Puri P. Associated urological anomalies in children with unilateral renal agenesis. J Urol, 1999, 162, 1081–1083.
30. Limwongse C, Clarren SM, Cassidy S. Syndromes and malformations of the urinary tract. In Pediatric Nephrology, 4th edition. Barratt TM, Avner ED, Harmon WE (eds). Lippincott, Williams and Wilkins, 1999, 427–452.
31. Vesselin DN, Taal MW, Sakharova OV, Brenner BM. Multi-hit nature of chronic renal disease. Curr Opin Nephrol Hypertens, 2000, 9, 85–97.
32. Argueso LR, Ritchley ML, Boyle ET et al. Prognosis of patients with renal agenesis. Pediatr Nephrol, 1992, 6, 412–416.
33. Wikstad I, Celsi G, Larsonn L, Herin P, Aperia A. Kidney function in adults with unilateral agenesis or nephrectomized in childhood. Pediatr Nephrol, 1988, 2, 177–182.
34. Baudoin P, Provoost AP, Molenaar JC. Renal function up to 50 years after unilateral nephrectomy in childhood. Am J Kidney Dis, 1993, 21, 603–611.
35. Decter RM. Renal duplication and fusion anomalies. Ped Clin N Amer, 1997, 44, 1323–1340.
36. Gleason PE, Kelalis PP, Husmann DA, Kramer SA. Hydronephrosis in renal ectopia: incidence, etiology and significance. J Urol, 1994, 151, 1660–1661.
37. Abel C, Lendon M, Gough DC. Histology of the upper pole in complete urinary duplication – does it affect surgical management? Br J Urol, 1997, 80, 663–665.

38. Davenport M, MacKinnon AE. The value of ultrasound screening of the upper urinary tract in hypospadias. Br J Urol, 1988, 62, 595–596.

39. Snodgrass W. Tubularized, incised plate urethroplasty for distal hypospadias. J Urol, 1994. 151. 464–465.

40. *http://www.aap.org/visit/circumcision.htm*

41. American Academy of Pediatrics: Circumcision policy statement. Pediatrics, 1999, 103, 696–693.

42. Craig JC, Knight JF, Sureshkumar P, Mantz E, Roy LP. Effect of circumcision on incidence of urinary tract infection in preschool boys. J Pediatr, 1996, 128, 23–27.

43. Pisacane A, Graziano L, Mazzarella G *et al.* Breastfeeding and urinary tract infection. J Pediatr, 1992, 120, 87–89.

44. Gill B, Kogan S. Cryptorchidism: current concepts. Pediatr Clin N Am, 1997, 44, 1211–1228.

45. Scorer GC, Farrington GH. Congenital deformities of the testis and epipidymis. London, Butterworths, 1971.

46. Hadziselimovic F. Cryptorchidism. In Adult and Pediatric Urology, Gillenwater JY, Grayhack JPT, Howards SS *et al.* (eds). St Louis, CV Mosby, 1991, 2217–2228.

47. Hadziselimovic F, Herzog B, Buser M. Development of cryptorchid testes. Eur J Pediatr, 1987, 146 (suppl l2), 8.

48. Ludwig G, Potempa J. Der optimale zeitpunct der behandling der kryptorchismus. Dtsch Med Wochenshr, 1975, 100, 680.

49. Pierce AM, Hart CA. Vulvovaginitis: causes and management. Arch Dis Child, 1992, 67, 509–512.

50. Jaquiery A, Stylianopoulos A, Hogg G, Grover S. Vulvovaginitis: clinical features, aetiology, and microbiology of the genital tract. Arch Dis Child, 1999, 81, 64–67.

51. Demetriou E, Emans SJ, Masland RP. Dysuria in adolescent girls: urinary tract infection or vaginitis. Pediatrics, 1982, 70, 299–301.

52. American Academy of Pediatrics. Guidelines for the evaluation of sexual abuse of children: subject review. Pediatrics, 1999, 103, 186–191.

53. Pena A. Total urogenital mobilzation – an easier way to repair cloacas. J Pediatr Surg, 1997, 32, 263–267.

54. Lattimer JK. Exstrophy closure: a follow-up of 70 cases. J Urol, 1966, 95, 356.

13 | *Antenatal detection of renal anomalies*

Malcolm A. Lewis

Introduction

Second trimester, high-resolution, two-dimensional ultrasound scanning has opened up a whole new world with regard to the diagnosis of fetal anomalies. Over the next few years, the addition of three-dimensional ultrasound scanning and magnetic resonance imaging will improve the ability to detect and define structural fetal anomalies. Ultrasound can detect anomalies in most organ systems, but the contrast between solid organ appearance and fluid makes ultrasound particularly informative with regards to renal anomalies. As a result, renal anomalies account for about 20% of all significant abnormalities found on detailed scanning at 18–20 weeks' gestation [1]. The frequency of detection of renal anomalies makes the need for counselling in this area great. It must always be remembered when undertaking this, however, that renal anomalies can coexist with other anomalies, and these may not all be as apparent on ultrasound scanning [2, 3]. Thus any advice given is based on what can be seen—there will always remain an element of doubt about what cannot be seen.

Types of abnormality detected antenatally

The abnormalities that can be detected fall into four groups, although these are not mutually exclusive:

1. abnormalities in the size of the kidneys;
2. abnormalities in the texture of the renal parenchyma;
3. the presence of visible cysts;
4. the presence of hydronephrosis.

In addition, it is important to remember the bladder and ureters, as abnormalities seen in relation to these structures are important in formulating a diagnosis.

Ultrasound allows the definition of structure but it does not allow the definition of function. The placenta is responsible for providing clearance during pregnancy. Thus, the only non-invasive marker of function available is the volume of amniotic fluid. This can be normal, increased, or decreased.

Renal size

The normal kidney grows steadily throughout gestation and centile charts exist for renal size at any particular gestational age [4]. As a rule of thumb, the normal kidney has a length of about 1.1 mm/week of gestation. Causes of large and small kidneys on antenatal ultrasound examination are shown in Table 13.1.

Renal parenchymal texture

The assessment of renal parenchymal texture is very much dependent upon the settings of the ultrasound machine and the experience of the operator. Comparison can be made with the liver, although in both the fetus and the newborn infant, the normal kidney appears somewhat 'brighter' than in the older child. In clinical practice, renal parenchymal texture can be divided into two groups—normal and obviously echobright. The brightness of a structure on ultrasound depends upon the extent of the reflection of ultrasound waves from the structure. Reflection of

Table 13.1 Causes of abnormally sized kidneys on antenatal ultrasound

Large kidney(s) on antenatal US
   Hydronephrosis
   Polycystic kidney disease
   Multicystic dysplastic kidney
   Cystic dysplasia (occasionally)
   Congenital nephrotic syndrome
   Renal tumour
   Compensatory hypertrophy
Small kidney(s) on antenatal US
   Renal dysplasia/hypoplasia
   Damage from obstructive uropathy

ultrasound waves takes place when the beam meets a surface of a different density to the one through which it is travelling. If a kidney is found to be echobright, then there must be multiple surfaces for the reflection of sound. This may indicate the presence of vast numbers of microcysts, which are so small that they are beyond the resolution of the scanner. Causes of echobright kidneys on antenatal ultrasound examination are shown in Table 13.2.

Macrocysts

Macrocysts (visible cysts) occur in several conditions (Table 13.3) and are visualized as distinct spherical areas within the renal parenchyma containing fluid. Care needs to be taken to differentiate between cysts and the somewhat less echogenic areas that represent the medullary pyramids. Equally, it is possible to mistake dilated calyces for cysts and vice versa.

Hydronephrosis

Hydronephrosis is defined as separation of the calyces and dilatation of the renal pelvis. The fetus is in a continuous state of diuresis to maintain amniotic fluid volume and dilatation may occur secondary to this high flow rate. Under normal circumstances, one would not expect the renal pelvis to have a transverse diameter in excess of 5 mm. When the transverse pelvic diameter is above this, then a search for a cause is indicated (see Chapter 14). Hydronephrosis occurs in dysplastic conditions where there is unilateral or bilateral distension of the renal pelvis with or without ureteric dilatation. It occurs without ureteric dilatation in pelvi-ureteric junction obstructions and with ureteric dilatation in vesico-ureteric junction obstructions. Vesico-ureteric

Table 13.2 Causes of echobright kidneys on antenatal ultrasound

---

Polycystic kidney disease (all forms)
Cystic dysplasia
Damage from obstructive uropathy
Glomerulocystic disease
Congenital nephrotic syndrome

Table 13.3 Causes of renal macrocysts on antenatal ultrasound

---

Autosomal dominant polycystic kidney disease
Polycystic kidney disease in tuberous sclerosis
Multicystic dysplastic kidney
Cystic dysplasia

---

reflux may cause unilateral or bilateral hydronephrosis. Bladder outlet obstructions usually lead to bilateral ureteric and renal pelvic dilatation. Where there is severe obstruction, a hydronephrotic kidney can rupture, leading to the formation of a urinoma around the kidney or urinary ascites. A localized urinoma can be difficult to differentiate from severe calyceal dilatation associated with a duplex system.

The bladder

The bladder is a dynamic organ, filling and emptying continuously from the time urine production commences. With the high rate of urine production in the fetus it is, therefore, unusual not to see the bladder during the course of a detailed scan. The bladder can appear absent in conjunction with oligohydramnios, where there is renal agenesis bilaterally or renal failure secondary to parenchymal renal disease, such as polycystic kidney disease. Similarly, in bladder outlet obstruction it is possible for the bladder to appear empty if there has been a bladder rupture and urinary ascites is present. The bladder can appear large where there is a bladder outlet obstruction, and often there is coned dilatation of the posterior urethra in association with this. Occasionally, a dilated urachus can be seen superior to the bladder in cases of obstructive uropathy. Neuropathic bladder rarely manifests as apparent obstructive uropathy, alhtough the author has observed this in two cases. The bladder in the fetus with a neural tube defect does not appear sonographically abnormal *in utero* and appears to function well independent of the spinal cord until birth. Where dilatation of any part of the renal tract is observed in a fetus with a neural tube defect, it is therefore more likely to be secondary to renal dysplasia [5] or an accompanying defect, such as a cloacal anomaly.

The ureters

The normal ureter is not visible on antenatal scanning. Dilatation occurs in vesico-ureteric junction obstruction and with bladder outlet obstruction. Non-obstructive causes of dilatation include vesico-ureteric reflux and dysplasia with or without severe reflux. Due to the proximity of the aorta, inferior vena cava (IVC) and pelvic vessels to the kidneys and bladder, it is always worthwhile confirming that a dilated structure is not vascular, using Doppler flow studies. Similarly, the hypoechoic psoas muscle can sometimes be mistaken for a dilated ureter.

Key points: Causes of dilated ureters on antenatal ultrasound

- Non-obstructive:
  – vesico-ureteric reflux;
  – dysplasia ± vesico-ureteric reflux.

- Obstructive:
  – vesico-ureteric junction obstruction;
  – bladder outlet obstruction.

Amniotic fluid volume

Over the first 10–14 weeks of pregnancy, amniotic fluid is produced by the placenta. Renal anomalies do not therefore present with oligohydramnios at this stage. Between 14 and 16 weeks there is a watershed, when production is by both the fetal kidney and the placenta. After 16 weeks' gestation, amniotic fluid is produced predominantly by the fetal kidneys. In the absence of a rupture of the amniotic membranes, oligo- or anhydramnios represents failure of urine excretion, due either to obstruction to urine outflow, failure of the kidneys to produce urine, or both. Polyhydramnios can be secondary to the fetus being in a polyuric state, but can also be secondary to failure of reabsorption of amniotic fluid in fetuses with swallowing problems or upper intestinal atresias. This is important to remember as some syndromes, e.g. VACTERAL (see Chapter 17), are associated with both renal anomalies and upper intestinal atresias, and in these circumstances amniotic fluid volume may be maintained even in the presence of poorly functioning kidneys.

The assessment of amniotic fluid volume is subjective. Anhydramnios is usually clear-cut, although judging the degree of oligohydramnios is difficult. Amniotic fluid volumes normally reduce as the third trimester of pregnancy progresses, and so deciding whether any reduction is excessive and because of failing kidneys can be difficult. Measurement of the amniotic fluid index (AFI); the sum of the lengths of the largest free pocket of amniotic fluid in each of the four quadrants of the uterus has been used to quantify the volume of amniotic fluid present, although most experienced antenatal radiologists find this no better than clinical observation of the scan [6]. When observing amniotic fluid pockets it is important to use Doppler flow studies as umbilical cord can be mistaken for a fluid collection.

The main consequence of oligohydramnios is pulmonary hypoplasia. Expansion and development of the lungs *in utero* is secondary to the balance of pressures between the amniotic fluid and the lung fluid being produced by the developing lungs [7]. Added to this are the changes in pressure from fetal breathing movements. Where there is severe oligohydramnios before 24 weeks gestation, there is almost always critical pulmonary hypoplasia, leading to death in the early newborn period through pulmonary insufficiency. There are, however, exceptions, and occasional babies are born where there has been severe oligohydramnios from an early stage in gestation but the lungs appear normal. Where oligohydramnios develops later in pregnancy, the chances of there being critical pulmonary hypoplasia are less. What needs to be established is whether the severity of pulmonary hypoplasia is related to the underlying pathology. The author's experience has suggested that taking into account the degree of oligohydramnios, pulmonary outcome is worse in fetuses with intrinsic defects of renal parenchymal development, such as polycystic kidney disease, when compared to those with 'acquired' renal disease from obstructive uropathy. The question arises as to whether this is secondary to some physiological stimulus to pulmonary development that is not produced by the intrinsically abnormal kidney. The alternative explanation is that these intrinsically abnormal kidneys are frequently very large, with a resultant combined effect of oligohydramnios plus diaphragmatic compression.

Key points: Abnormalities of amniotic fluid volume

- Causes of oligohydramnios include:
  – rupture of the amniotic membranes;
  – failure of urine excretion: obstruction to urine outflow, failure of the kidneys to produce urine, or both.

- Causes of polyhydramnios include:
  – polyuric fetus;
  – failure of reabsorption of amniotic fluid: swallowing problems or upper intestinal atresias.

- Where there is severe oligohydramnios before 24 weeks' gestation, there is almost always critical pulmonary hypoplasia, leading to early neonatal death.

Renal conditions detectable on antenatal scans

Table 13.4 shows the conditions that can be detected antenatally, together with details of the corresponding appearances of the kidneys, ureters, bladder, and amniotic fluid volume. It can be seen that few appearances are exclusive to one condition, and making a diagnosis is dependent upon combining the sonographic abnormalities detected with a detailed family history in all cases, and scans of the parent's kidneys where echobright or cystic kidneys are detected in the fetus. The measurement of maternal serum α-fetoprotein or amniotic fluid α-fetoprotein is indicated where congenital nephrotic syndrome is a possibility. As more genetic markers become available, the

use of chorionic villous biopsy in informative families with known conditions will become more common (see Chapter 16).

Unilateral hydronephrosis

Hydronephrosis is the most commonly diagnosed fetal renal abnormality [8]. The discovery of unilateral hydronephrosis is rarely of great significance to the fetus but can be a great source of anxiety for the prospective parents. Unilateral hydronephrosis can be due to pelvi-ureteric junction obstruction, vesico-ureteric junction obstruction, vesico-ureteric reflux, or dysplasia with or without accompanying non-obstructive ureteric dilatation or reflux. It is important to note whether the distribution of the hydronephrosis

Table 13.4 Conditions that can be detected antenatally, with details of the corresponding appearances of the kidneys, ureters, bladder, and amniotic fluid volume

Condition	Kidney(s)	Ureter(s)	Bladder	Amniotic fluid volume
Pelvi-ureteric junction obstruction	Hydronephrosis on the affected side	Not seen	Normal	Normal unless severe bilateral disease
Vesico-ureteric junction obstruction	Hydronephrosis on the affected side	Can be seen on the affected side	Normal	Normal unless severe bilateral disease
Vesico-ureteric reflux	Variable hydronephrosis	Visible if severe	Normal	Normal
Bladder outlet obstruction	Variable bilateral hydronephrosis; occasional urinomas	Usually dilated bilaterally	Distended, posterior urethra visible	Oligohydramnios or anhydramnios
Megacystis, megaureter	Bilateral hydronephrosis	Bilateral dilatation	Enlarged, but posterior urethra not prominent	Normal or sometimes reduced
Duplex system	Normal or hydronephrotic upper or lower pole	Dilated to one or both moieties	Normal or ureterocele visible	Normal
Renal agenesis	Absent on affected side (beware adrenal gland)	Not seen	Normal (unless bilateral)	Normal (unless bilateral)
Renal dysplasia	Normal or echobright, small, normal or large, occasional visible macrocysts	Not seen, sometimes dilated with reflux	Normal	Normal, oligohydramnios, occasionally polyhydramnios
Multicystic dysplastic kidney	Large macrocysts replacing kidney	Not seen	Normal	Normal unless bilateral disease present
Dominant PKD	Large echobright kidneys, occasionally visible macrocysts	Not seen	Normal or small	Range from normal to absolute oligohydramnios
Recessive PKD	Large echobright kidneys, occasionally visible macrocysts	Not seen	Normal or small	Range from normal to absolute oligohydramnios
Congenital nephrotic syndrome	Large echobright kidneys	Not seen	Normal	Polyhydramnios

PKD, polycystic kidney disease.

within the kidney is asymmetrical, suggesting the presence of a duplex kidney. Where duplex kidneys are associated with concomitant structural abnormalities, they are usually associated with vesico-ureteric reflux and/or pelvi-ureteric junction obstruction in the lower pole. The upper pole is most frequently associated with a ureterocele within the bladder or, less often, with an ectopic ureter. Noting the presence of a ureterocele is important, partly for making the diagnosis but predominantly because a ureterocele can change during the course of the pregnancy. It can cause variable distortion of the bladder anatomy and either obstruction to the lower pole ureter, obstruction to the contralateral ureter, or bladder outlet obstruction. Where a ureterocele is seen antenatally, close observation with monthly scans is indicated, as bladder outlet obstruction and bilateral severe hydronephrosis can ensue. Unilateral hydronephrosis where there is contralateral renal agenesis is clearly a more worrying problem. It must be remembered that the high urine flow to maintain amniotic fluid volumes can itself cause mild dilatation in a single system. Abnormalities of the kidney are more common where the contralateral kidney is absent, but these usually take the form of vesico-ureteric reflux or renal dysplasia, and rarely are severe obstructive lesions present in the single kidney.

Bilateral hydronephrosis

The potential causes of bilateral hydronephrosis are the same as those of unilateral hydronephrosis. In addition, it is important to consider bladder outlet obstruction, as discussed below. Even where hydronephrosis is bilateral, it is unusual to find the lesions on both sides are so severe as to cause oligohydramnios. Most bilateral lesions are secondary to vesico-ureteric reflux or dysplasia without there being a physical obstruction to flow. However, where severe bilateral hydronephrosis (transverse pelvic diameters >15 mm) is found, it is necessary to follow the patient with monthly scans, as if oligohydramnios were to develop, then consideration would need to be given to either nephrostomy drainage into the amniotic cavity or early delivery, depending on the gestation of the fetus. Nephrostomy drainage in these circumstances is still an experimental technique [9]. Early delivery can be considered beyond 32 weeks' gestation after the administration of corticosteroids to the mother to minimize the risk of surfactant deficiency lung disease in the infant. Close collaboration between the nephrologist or paediatrician and the obstetrician is required.

Bladder outlet obstruction

Bladder outlet obstruction is the most frequently antenatally diagnosed severe renal tract abnormality. The causes of bladder outlet obstruction are listed in Table 13.5.

Table 13.5 Causes of bladder outlet obstruction

Posterior urethral valves
Urethral atresia/duplication
VATER/VACTERAL anomalad (usually with recto-vesical fistula and urethral stricture)
Cloacal anomaly
Prolapsed ureterocele
Neuropathic bladder (exceptionally rare)
Megacystis megaureter (usually no physical obstruction but apparent bladder outlet obstruction)
Megacystis microcolon (usually no physical obstruction, microcolon only evident after birth)
Hydrometrocolpos (it is easy to mistake a dilated uterus for a bladder)

Key points: Antenatal hydronephrosis

- Causes of unilateral hydronephrosis include pelvi-ureteric junction obstruction, vesico-ureteric junction obstruction, vesico-ureteric reflux, or dysplasia with or without accompanying non-obstructive ureteric dilatation or reflux.

- Causes of bilateral hydronephrosis include all of the above plus bladder outlet obstruction.

- Posterior urethral valves are the most common cause of bladder outlet obstruction.

- The diagnosis of posterior urethral valves is a presumptive one based upon the sex of the infant and the finding of an enlarged bladder and the absence of other visible anomalies.

Posterior urethral valves are the most common cause of bladder outlet obstruction. The variability of the antenatal sonographic appearance of this condition is tremendous, ranging from an apparently normal 18–20-week scan to severe bilateral hydronephrosis and hydroureter with renal parenchymal loss and oligohydramnios. The diagnosis of posterior urethral valves is a presumptive one based upon the sex of the infant and the finding of an enlarged bladder and the absence of other visible anomalies. This always needs to be taken into account when counselling parents.

Once bladder outlet obstruction has been diagnosed, monitoring ought to be undertaken with monthly ultrasound scans. Where there is no detectable amniotic fluid (absolute oligohydramnios or anhydramnios) before 24 weeks' gestation, the prognosis is exceptionally poor [10] and many parents will opt for termination. Where amniotic fluid volumes fall on follow-up and/or upper tract changes develop (increasing renal pelvis dilatation, echobright kidneys, or urinoma), many would advocate intervention. At present, there is no good test that will determine potential renal function in the fetus. Some advocate the measurement of the electrolytes in fetal urine [11]. Although these show some correlation with renal outcome, the problem arises as to when the urine sampled was produced. To assess fetal urine quality accurately entails fetal bladder puncture, drainage of the urinary tracts and then sampling of the fetal urine once the bladder has refilled. Even in this situation it is not certain as to whether the fetal urinary electrolytes will be altered by the decompression of the system. The assumption that falling amniotic fluid volumes represent worsening obstruction is questionable. Intrinsic renal failure due to secondary renal dysplasia is a more likely cause in most. If this is the case, then intervention is unlikely to improve outcome.

Intervention can take the form of regular bladder drainage by bladder aspiration, the insertion of a vesico-amniotic shunt [12], the *in utero* fulgarization of the valves through the passage of a scope into the fetal bladder and then down into the posterior urethra, or other definitive drainage surgery in the fetus [13]. The latter has only been performed late in the third trimester and it is uncertain as to whether this technique, with its inherent risks to both the mother and the fetus, offers any advantage at this stage of pregnancy. Vesico-amniotic shunts have been frequently used, although there is no controlled evidence to show a better outcome than with no intervention [8]. The risks to the fetus of vesico-amniotic shunting are the induction of premature labour, infection and failure of the catheter to drain. This latter complication can be through catheter slippage or secondary vesico-ureteric junction obstruction once the empty bladder contracts. Regular bladder drainage will potentially relieve pressure on the kidneys but involves multiple interventions for the mother, increasing the risks of the induction of labour. It does nothing for the oligohydramnios and, if pulmonary hypoplasia is to be prevented, it would therefore need to be coupled with regular amnio-infusions [14], another unproven technique.

When considering any form of antenatal intervention, one has to balance the potential benefits to the fetus against the potential harm to both the fetus and the mother, both in the short term and in the long term through uterine trauma. On balance, the author does not advocate any of the above procedures. Fetal surgery in particular is of dubious value and may have long-term implications for the mother in future pregnancies.

Where amniotic fluid volume is maintained, it is important not to intervene. In these cases there is even less evidence of benefit and many cases turn out postnatally to have non-obstructive causes of renal tract dilatation such as megacystis megaureter (with or without prune belly syndrome). Where there is a megacystis it is important to remember the association of megacystis and microcolon, as this only becomes apparent after birth [15].

Key points: Antenatal interventions

- Antenatal interventions for bladder outlet obstruction include:
  – regular bladder aspiration;
  – *in utero* fulgurization of posterior urethral valves;
  – insertion of vesico-amniotic shunt.

- None of these therapies have an evidence base.

- Risks to the fetus include induction of premature labour and infection.

- Risks to the mother include uterine trauma.

Renal dysplasia

Renal dysplasia takes numerous forms. At one end of the spectrum is renal agenesis, where no kidney is formed at all. If this is bilateral, it leads to Potter's syndrome. Bilateral renal agenesis is usually easily diagnosed after detailed scanning because of anhydramnios. It is easy to miss unilateral renal agenesis as the adrenal gland on the affected side flops down and can be mistaken for a kidney.

The multicystic dysplastic kidney is a large, non-functioning kidney, where the whole of the renal substance is replaced with macrocysts of variable size. They are most commonly unilateral, although they may be bilateral, a generally fatal condition. Multicystic dysplasia can occur in conjunction with ureteric atresia on the affected side, critical pelvi-ureteric junction obstruction, or an orthotopic ureterocele. Only the latter is ever of clinical significance as the ureterocele itself may prolapse and cause bladder outlet obstruction. Multicystic dysplastic kidneys can regress and disappear during pregnancy or grow to enormous sizes. Rarely, they will reach a size great enough to obstruct labour. Multicystic dysplasia can occur in one moiety of a duplex system, giving rise to an unusual appearance with clear macrocysts but also some apparently normal renal tissue.

Cystic renal dysplasia is very variable in its presentation. Affected kidneys usually appear echobright and sometimes have visible cysts of 1–2 mm diameter within them. Most of these kidneys are small, although occasionally they can be large. Some are abnormal bilaterally and some are associated with evidence of lower renal tract dysplasia and renal pelvic or ureteric dilatation. Presentation in family members can be variable. The author has recently seen a family where the first child had a multicystic dysplastic kidney on the left and severe cystic dysplasia with marked ureteric dilatation on the right. Postnatal examination demonstrated grade IV reflux on the right. Renal function was moderately impaired. In the second pregnancy bilateral multicystic dysplastic kidneys were identified at 20 weeks' gestation and there was anhydramnios. The pregnancy was terminated and post-mortem examination confirmed the diagnosis. At this stage investigation of the parents showed the mother to have normal kidneys but the father to have small kidneys with a few small discrete cortical cysts within them. He gave a history of mild polyuria throughout his life and noted that his own father, then in his 70s, had also had polyuria throughout his life. In the third pregnancy the fetus has normal amniotic fluid volumes, mild bilateral ureteric and renal pelvic dilatation and bilateral echobright kidneys with occasional macrocysts within them. The kidneys are of a normal size and the picture suggests diffuse bilateral cystic dysplasia.

Glomerulocystic kidney disease is a distinct histological entity that most commonly presents antenatally with very enlarged, diffusely echobright kidneys, which are indistinguishable from the changes seen in polycystic kidney disease. In non-inherited forms, this and other dysplastic conditions can be a part of other syndromic diagnoses, making close examination of the rest of the fetus and the sampling of amniotic fluid (if present) for chromosomal analysis important [16].

Polycystic kidney disease

Inherited polycystic kidney disease frequently presents antenatally. Both the 'infantile' recessive form (ARPKD) and the 'adult' dominant form (ADPKD) can be detected on the 18–20 week antenatal scan [17]. ARPKD typically presents as bilaterally enlarged, echobright kidneys with oligohydramnios. The distension of the fetal abdomen can be so great as to obstruct labour and require a Caesarean section. Where this occurs, there is almost always critical pulmonary insufficiency with early neonatal death. Other cases have smaller (but still enlarged) echobright kidneys, sometimes with an occasional visible cyst 1–2 mm in diameter. There is less severe oligohydramnios. These fetuses do better after birth, though renal failure will ensue at some point in the majority. On the whole, families tend to have infants that follow a similar clinical pattern, so those who have had a baby with a severe neonatal presentation may well have others affected in the same way [18]. This is important for counselling purposes, as the potential exists for early antenatal diagnosis in informative families using chorionic villous biopsy. In non-informative families, the diagnosis rests on a further 18-week scan. Clearly, where mothers have had to have a Caesarean section, only to deliver a child who dies in the neonatal period, early diagnosis and the option of a termination of pregnancy is important.

ADPKD has an incidence in the population 40 times greater than that of ARPKD. It is clear that some patients with ADPKD present in fetal life. ADPKD can present in fetal life with an identical picture to that seen in ARPKD. Where there are massively enlarged kidneys, the prognosis is poor, as with ARPKD. In other cases, however, there is moderate enlargement of the kidney, perhaps with one or two visible cysts and a normal amniotic fluid volume. These patients do well after birth, although some have early onset hypertension. The long-term prognosis for this group is uncertain. Although reports have suggested that 20% of children with early onset ADPKD will progress to renal failure in the first decade [19], this figure may fall as an increased number of possibly milder cases are diagnosed early through antenatal scanning. Recognizing dominant rather than recessive disease is important, as this increases the recurrence risk quoted to families from 25% to 50%. Wherever large, echobright kidneys are seen on the antenatal scan, both parents should be offered renal ultrasound scanning. Following this principle, four of the last five cases seen by the author with presumed ARPKD turned out to be ADPKD. In three of these cases, there was no previous diagnosis of ADPKD in the family. The reason why some patients will form cysts in childhood but not present until adulthood (if at all), whereas others with the same disease will present with a severe neonatal presentation is unclear. One suggestion is that the *PKD1* and *PKD2* gene mutations lead to the production of cysts but that there are 'modifier' genes that determine the rate of production of these cysts [20]. This may explain why there is so much variation in the offspring of parents with ADPKD, with some children within the same kindred having an early onset of clinical problems and others having late-onset disease like their parents. Unfortunately, this precludes exact prediction of outcome following antenatal diagnosis, unless there is severe oligo- or anhydramnios and massive renal enlargement before 24 weeks' gestation, where the outcome is known to be almost uniformly fatal.

Key point

- Wherever large, echobright kidneys are detected on an antenatal scan, both parents should be offered renal ultrasound scanning to look for evidence of autosomal dominant polycystic kidney disease.

Tuberous sclerosis can also present in the antenatal period. When abnormal, the kidneys are most frequently significantly enlarged with macrocysts within the parenchyma, similar to the appearances seen in ADPKD. Microcystic disease of the glomerulocystic variety is also recognized. The renal outcome with the former presentation is usually good through early childhood, although hypertension can be a problem soon after birth. Clearly, it is important in these cases to look for cardiac or cerebral markers of the condition on the detailed scan.

Congenital nephrotic syndrome

Congenital nephrotic syndrome is discussed in Chapter 19. Congenital nephrotic syndrome of the Finnish type is the most common variety in the Caucasian population. In this autosomal recessive condition, there is massive proteinuria with its onset during fetal life. The kidneys appear somewhat enlarged and echogenic on scan, but unlike polycystic kidney disease, there is usually polyhydramnios. Due to the heavy fetal proteinuria, both the maternal serum α-fetoprotein and the amniotic fluid α-fetoprotein levels are massively elevated. The ultrasound and α-fetoprotein changes, taken in conjunction with a detailed scan showing no open neural tube defect (confirmed, if an amniocentesis has been performed, by a normal acetylcholinesterase level), are generally sufficient to make a diagnosis [21]. The outlook for patients with congenital nephrotic syndrome is poor, although increasing success is being reported with early bilateral nephrectomy followed by dialysis and transplantation [22]. In view of the inevitability of having to lead a life of end stage renal failure management, many families will opt for a termination of pregnancy following an antenatal diagnosis [21].

Tumours detected antenatally

Renal tumours detected antenatally are rare [23]. Many masses turn out to be suprarenal in origin, neuroblastoma or adrenal haemorrhage being likely diagnoses [24]. The antenatal detection of Wilms' tumour is exceptionally rare [23] and most intrinsic renal masses turn out to be benign mesoblastic nephromas [25]. Where a renal mass is detected antenatally, no intervention is usually required before delivery, although advice ought to be sought from a centre with paediatric nephro-urological and oncological expertise.

Termination of pregnancy

In the United Kingdom, the Abortion Act permits termination of pregnancy up to 24 weeks' gestation for a variety of indications. After 24 weeks' gestation, termination of pregnancy is only permitted if the fetus has a serious congenital abnormality. 'Serious' is not defined precisely. The advantage of late termination is that in some cases it spares a family anguish when a mother is carrying a fetus that will inevitably die. More importantly, late termination may spare a mother the need for a Caesarean section. Wherever possible, termination of a pregnancy ought to take place before 24 weeks, but where a diagnosis is made late or circumstances change as the pregnancy progresses, late termination is an option. One problem with late termination is that a fetus is born that might breathe, and in these circumstances it can prove difficult not to offer this infant neonatal intensive care. For this reason, when a termination is undertaken after 22 weeks' gestation, most specialist centres offer the parents the choice of the fetus having an intracardiac injection of potassium chloride prior to the induction of labour. Parents, doctors, and other health professionals have widely divergent views on the ethics of this practice.

Counselling families

Antenatal diagnosis of renal anomalies is an imprecise science and there is therefore frequently room for doubt. When counselling families, it is important to present the facts in terms of the most likely diagnosis and the likely outcome. Where the abnormality involves the bladder as well as the kidneys, details of outcome with regard to this also need to be given. Similarly, in cases where there are multiple congenital anomalies, other specialists and geneticists may need to be involved. It is helpful to follow a consultation with a letter detailing all that has been discussed. Where parents are contemplating a termination of pregnancy, more than one meeting in close succession may be required and these meetings can be lengthy and repetitive as parents come to terms with the problem. Some parents will opt for termination when there is a possibility of a good outcome, whereas others will opt to carry on with the pregnancy despite the certain death of the fetus upon delivery. There are no correct answers for any one condition, though families clearly need to be reassured that the decision that they have made is the correct one. Families need to be encouraged to think about the effects upon themselves, any other children, and any future children when making this decision.

Delivery of the fetus with an antenatally detected renal anomaly

The vast majority of fetuses that have antenatally detected renal anomalies can be delivered in their local hospital and further investigation undertaken after birth. Fetuses with oligohydramnios and the likelihood of renal failure in the newborn period

should be delivered, wherever possible, at a unit capable of delivering full respiratory support, including high-frequency oscillatory ventilation and inhaled nitric oxide. Such a unit should have a paediatric nephrologist in attendance if early dialysis is contemplated. Where other or multiple congenital anomalies are noted antenatally, decisions about the site of delivery need to be taken in conjunction with the other paediatric medical and surgical specialists involved.

Key points: Delivery of the fetus with an antenatally detected renal anomaly

- Delivery should take place in a centre where all modalities of respiratory support are available.

- A paediatric nephrologist should be available if early dialysis is contemplated.

References

1. Smith NC, Hau C. A six year study of the antenatal detection of fetal abnormality in six Scottish health boards. *Br. J. Obstet. Gynaecol.* 1999;106:206–12.
2. Stoll C, Alembik Y, Dott B, Meyer MJ, Pennerath A, Peter MO *et al.* Evaluation of prenatal diagnosis of congenital heart disease. *Prenat. Diagn.* 1998;18:801–7.
3. Stoll C, Alembik Y, Dott B, Roth MP. Evaluation of prenatal diagnosis of congenital gastro-intestinal atresias. *Eur. J. Epidemiol.* 1996;12:611–16.
4. Cohen HL, Cooper J, Eisenberg P, Mandel FS, Gross BR, Goldman MA *et al.* Normal length of fetal kidneys: sonographic study in 397 obstetric patients. *Am. J. Roentgenol.* 1991;157:545–8.
5. Whitaker RH, Hunt GM. Incidence and distribution of renal anomalies in patients with neural tube defects. *Eur. Urol.* 1987;13:322–3.
6. Magann EF, Sanderson M, Martin JN, Chauhan S. The amniotic fluid index, single deepest pocket, and two-diameter pocket in normal human pregnancy. *Am. J. Obstet. Gynaecol.* 2000;183:1581–8.
7. Laudy JA, Wladimiroff JW. The fetal lung. 1: Developmental aspects. *Ultrasound Obstet. Gynecol.* 2000;16:284–90.
8. Dillon E, Ryall A. A 10 year audit of antenatal ultrasound detection of renal disease. *Br. J. Radiol.* 1998; 71:497–500.
9. Pinckert TL, Kiernan SC. In utero nephrostomy catheter placement. *Fetal Diagn. Ther.* 1994;9:348–52.
10. Coplen DE. Prenatal intervention for hydronephrosis. *J. Urol.* 1997;157:2270–7.

11. Nicolaides KH, Cheng HH, Snijders RJ, Moniz CF. Fetal urine biochemistry in the assessment of obstructive uropathy. *Am. J. Obstet. Gynecol.* 1992;166:932–7.

12. Szaflik K, Korarzewski M, Adamczewski D. Fetal bladder catheterization in severe obstructive uropathy before the 24th week of pregnancy. *Fetal Diagn. Ther.* 1988;13:133–5.

13. Holmes N, Harrison MR, Baskin LS. Fetal surgery for posterior urethral valves: long term postnatal outcomes. *Pediatrics* 2001:108:E7.

14. Cameron D, Lupton BA, Farquharson D, Hiruki T. Amnioinfusions in renal agenesis. *Obstet. Gynaecol.* 1994;83:872–6.

15. McHugo J, Whittle M. Enlarged fetal bladders:aetiology management and outcome. *Prenat. Diagn.* 2001; 21:958–63.

16. Nicolaides KH, Cheng HH, Abbas A, Snijcers RJ, Gosden C. Fetal renal defects: associated malformations and chromosomal defects. *Fetal Diagn. Ther.* 1992;7:1–11.

17. Michaud J, Russo P, Grignon A, Dallaire L, Bichet D, Rosenblatt D *et al.* Autosomal dominant polycystic kidney disease in the fetus. *Am. J. Med. Genet.* 1994;51:240–6.

18. Deget F, Rudnik-Schoneborn S, Zerres K. Course of autosomal recessive polycystic kidney disease (ARPKD) in siblings: a clinical comparison of 20 sibships. *Clin. Genet.* 1995;47:248–53.

19. Fick GM, Johnson AM, Strain JD, Kimberling WJ, Kumar S, Manco-Johnson ML *et al.* Characteristics of very early onset autosomal dominant polycystic kidney disease. *J. Am. Soc. Nephrol.* 1993;3:1863–70.

20. Wu G. Current advances in molecular genetics of autosomal-dominant polycystic kidney disease. *Curr. Opin. Nephrol. Hypertens.* 2001;10:23–31.

21. Hogge WA, Hogge JS, Schnatterly PT, Sun CJ, Blitzer MG. Congenital nephrosis:detection of index cases through maternal alpha-fetoprotein screening. *Am. J. Obstet. Gynecol.* 1992;167:1330–3.

22. Holmberg C, Antikainen M, Ronnholm K, Ala HM, Jalanko H. Management of congenital nephrotic syndrome of the Finnish type. *Pediatr. Nephrol.* 1995; 9:87–93.

23. Ritchey ML, Azizkhan RG, Beckwith JB, Hrabovsky EE, Haase GM. Neonatal Wilms' tumor. *J. Pediatr. Surg.* 1995;30:856–9.

24. Brame M, Masel J, Homsy Y. Antenatal detection and management of suprarenal masses. *Urology* 1999; 54:1097.

25. Irsutti M, Puget C, Duga I, Sarramon MF, Guitard J. Mesoblastic nephroma: prenatal ultrasonographic and MRI features. *Pediatr. Radiol.* 2000;30:147–50.

14 | Antenatal renal problems: management in the postnatal period

Mark Woodward and David Frank

Introduction

The detection of renal abnormalities with antenatal ultrasonography was first reported in the 1970s [1]. Since then, the increasing use of ultrasound has allowed an appreciation of the true incidence of urological abnormalities, the most common of which is hydronephrosis, and has identified a large number of patients who require reassessment postnatally.

The major limitation of antenatal identification of urinary tract dilatation, which will clearly give rise to parental anxiety, is that hydronephrosis does not necessarily imply obstruction nor give any indication of function of an affected kidney. It has become increasingly apparent that the natural history of many antenatally detected renal abnormalities is for spontaneous improvement or resolution without the need for surgical intervention. It is therefore essential that potential diagnoses should be clearly explained to parents and the postnatal management should be logical, efficient, and cost-effective.

In this chapter we define antenatal hydronephrosis, discuss the incidence of this and other antenatally diagnosed renal abnormalities, and provide accurate information for parental counselling. We also present an investigation algorithm and discuss a number of the potential diagnoses in more detail.

Definitions

The most common renal abnormality detected antenatally is hydronephrosis. Large numbers of publications have been generated discussing diagnosis, outcome, and management of antenatal hydronephrosis (ANH), but unfortunately there is no universal classification system with which to compare them. The two main systems currently in use either grade

the severity of the hydronephrosis according to the ultrasonographic appearances of the renal parenchyma and pelvicalyceal system (Society of Fetal Urology grading system, see Table 14.1) or use various measurements taken from the kidney.

A number of different measurements have been used in the literature to define ANH, including the length of the renal pelvis and the ratio of renal pelvic anteroposterior (AP) diameter to the renal length. Currently the most generally accepted measurement is the *maximum AP diameter of the renal pelvis (RPD)* (see Fig. 6.8), although the precise point above which the RPD has been considered to be abnormal has also varied in the literature (see Table 14.2).

Grignon *et al.* [2] initially suggested that a RPD above 10 mm should be considered to be pathological, as 28 of 29 fetuses with a RPD below 10 mm showed complete resolution postnatally, although their evaluation of the patients postnatally was related to the identification of potential obstructive uropathy. Owen *et al.* [3] subsequently suggested that a RPD below 5 mm at 18 weeks gestation, below 8 mm at 34 weeks gestation, and below 10 mm at

Table 14.1 Society of Fetal Urology grading system for antenatally detected hydronephrosis

Grade	Central renal complex = Pelvis	Renal parenchymal thickness
0	Intact	Normal
I	Mild splitting = dilatation	Normal
II	Moderate splitting, but complex confined within renal border	Normal
III	Marked splitting, pelvis dilated outside renal border, and *calyces dilated*	Normal
IV	Further pelvicalyceal dilatation	Thin

Table 14.2 Cumulative outcome data from 15 published series demonstrating final diagnoses in antenatally diagnosed hydronephrosis

	Definition of hydronephrosis	Transient hydro-nephrosis	Large/extra-renal pelvis (idiopathic dilatation)	PUJ obstruction	VUR	VUJ obstruction/megaureter	PUV/bladder outflow obstruction	MCDK	Duplex/ureterocele	Renal agenesis/dysplasia/cyst	Lost to follow-up/others	Total
Ahmed et al., 1988	Not defined	24	28	40	8	9	5	6	16	6	6	148
Anderson et al., 1997	>4 mm	202		22	33	3	1		3			264
Dremsek et al., 1997	>5 mm	26		1	1	1	1					30
Dudley et al., 1997	≥5 mm	36	43	3	12	3		2	1			100
Gruenewald et al., 1990	≥10 mm	2		16	5	7	3		2			35
Gunn et al., 1995	Length	216	14	16	14	7	3	8		3	28	309
Jaswon et al., 1999	≥5 mm	43	30	4	23					4		104
Johnson et al., 1992	Length	30	5	7	3	1	1	6		3		56
Kitagawa et al., 1998	≥4 mm if <33/40; ≥7 mm if >33/40	15	51	4	7	4	3		7	3	12	103
Lam et al., 1993	>10 mm	16	7	5	5	2		3		2	2	42
Livera et al., 1989	≥10 mm	37	17	12	2	4	2		2	11	5	92
Owen et al., 1996	≥10 mm		16	6	4			5			4	35
Paduano et al., 1991	Not defined	28	5	12	10	8		3		2	5	73
Stocks et al., 1996	≥4 mm if <33/40; ≥7 mm if >33/40	8	7	6	6							27
Thon et al., 1987	Not defined	18		8		3	2		1	6	4	42
Total		701	223	162	133	52	21	33	32	37	66	1460
Percentage of total		48.0	15.3	11.1	9.1	3.6	1.4	2.3	2.2	2.5	4.5	

PUJ, pelvi-ureteric junction; VUR, vesico-ureteric reflux; VUJ, vesico-ureteric junction; PUV, posterior urethral valves; MCDK, multicystic dysplastic kidney.

term should be accepted as normal, as a reasonable proportion of the patients (22/57 = 39%) subsequently showed no significant postnatal urological abnormality, although this proportion would be considered by many to be unacceptable.

Siemens *et al.* [4] used very similar measurements of below 6 mm, below 8 mm, and below 10 mm at less than 20, 20–30, and more than 30 weeks of gestation, and concluded that these had a 95% positive predictive value in predicting 'insignificant' postnatal pelviectasis. However, they defined 'insignificant' as 'no or minimal renal pelvic splitting' (Society for Fetal Urology grade 0 or I) and did accept that this would exclude a number of children with non-dilating vesico-ureteric reflux (VUR) as they did not routinely assess the patients postnatally with micturating cystourethrography (MCUG). Indeed 2 of the 46 patients in their series subsequently progressed to significant hydronephrosis (grade II), although none required surgery.

Ouzounian *et al.* published outcome data from antenatal screening over a one-year period, in which they identified 98 hydronephrotic kidneys in 84 patients using a RPD $\geqslant$ 4 mm [5]. They constructed receiver–operating characteristic curves and with this discovered that a RPD $\geqslant$ 5 mm was 100% sensitive and 24% specific in predicting subsequent hydronephrosis, and they therefore recommended that this be used as the threshold for postnatal investigation.

The current local policy in Bristol is for postnatal investigation to be performed on the basis of a RPD $\geqslant$ 5 mm [6] and this threshold has been accepted by a number of other authors [7,8], although data from another group using a RPD $\geqslant$ 4 mm have also been reported [9].

Incidence

The majority of renal abnormalities are detected between 18 and 20 weeks gestation at the routine anomaly scan and clearly the precise incidence depends on the definition of ANH. The Bristol group published prospective data from scans on 18 766 pregnant women (with hydronephrosis defined as RPD $\geqslant$ 5 mm) and detected hydronephrosis in 100 cases (0.59%), which was bilateral in 46% [6]. A second large prospective study from Stoke on Trent published data from 6292 antenatal scans and showed hydronephrosis (RPD > 10 mm) in 92 (0.65%) [10].

Similar figures have been produced from other centres [4], although Anderson *et al.* [9] demonstrated hydronephrosis in 426 fetuses (4.3%) from a total of 9800 scans using the more stringent cut-off of a RPD $\geqslant$ 4 mm at any stage after 16 weeks gestation.

Parental counselling

In order to be able to counsel parents appropriately regarding the significance of ANH and other renal abnormalities, it is necessary to have a clear idea as to the range of potential differential diagnoses and likely outcomes. Jaswon *et al.* [8] have also demonstrated that the uptake of postnatal investigations is increased by antenatal counselling—only 10% of parents in a counselled group failed to attend for postnatal investigations, compared with 20% of non-counselled parents.

The degree of hydronephrosis, renal size and parenchymal thickness, the presence or absence of ureteric and/or bladder dilatation, and the volume of amniotic fluid are all key features of the antenatal ultrasound scan which will help suggest a diagnosis. The most common renal diagnoses and a number of rarer non-renal causes of ANH are set out in Table 14.3. The antenatal ultrasound scan may also identify or suggest other associated abnormalities, including cardiac and neurological, which will have implications for antenatal management.

Table 14.3 Causes of antenatal hydronephrosis (most of which can cause bilateral hydronephrosis)

Renal
    Physiological/transient hydronephrosis
    PUJ obstruction (Fig. 14.1)
    Vesico-ureteric reflux
    Posterior urethral valves (Fig. 14.2)
    Megaureter (obstructed or non-obstructed)
    Multicystic dysplastic kidney (Fig. 14.3)
    Ureterocele
    Ectopic ureter
    Prune belly
    Urethral atresia
    Renal cysts
    Urachal cyst
Non-renal
    Ovarian cyst
    Hydrocolpos
    Sacrococcygeal teratoma
    Enteric duplication
    Duodenal atresia
    Meningocele

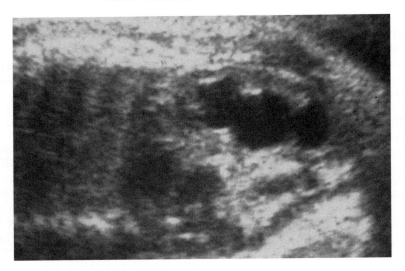

Fig. 14.1   Antenatal ultrasound revealed hydronephrosis with no evidence of ureteric dilatation and postnatal investigations confirmed PUJ obstruction. (Reproduced with permission of Miss Pippa Kyle, Consultant in Fetal Medicine, Bristol.)

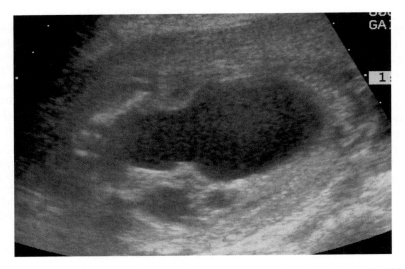

Fig. 14.2   Antenatal ultrasound demonstrated oligohydramnios, a large distended thick-walled bladder (shown), and bilateral dysplastic kidneys, compatible with posterior urethral valves. (Reproduced with permission of Miss Pippa Kyle, Consultant in Fetal Medicine, Bristol.)

A number of different groups have published their outcome data in ANH, and we have combined these in Table 14.2 to give an indication of the relative frequencies of each condition in a cumulative series of almost 1500 patients, which can be used for counselling purposes.

It is possible to make two broad generalizations with regards to diagnosis and outcome with ANH.

First, Grignon *et al.* [2] and others have demonstrated that the likelihood of a patient having a significant postnatal renal abnormality is proportional to the severity of the ANH. In their series, if the RPD was greater than 20 mm, then 94% of the patients had a significant abnormality requiring surgery or long-term follow-up; if the RPD was 10–15 mm, then 50% had an abnormality; and if the RPD was less

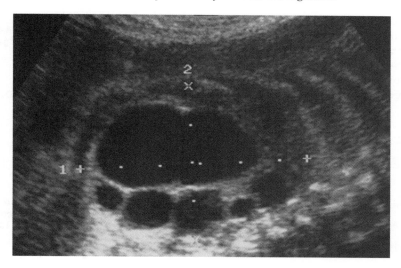

Fig. 14.3 Antenatal ultrasound of multicystic dysplastic kidney (MCDK), with multiple fluid-filled cysts and absent renal cortex. (Reproduced with permission of Miss Pippa Kyle, Consultant in Fetal Medicine, Bristol.)

than 10 mm, then only 3% had an abnormality. Second, the actual postnatal diagnosis relates to the degree of ANH. In mild hydronephrosis (RPD 5–9 mm) the most likely diagnosis is VUR, whereas pelvi-ureteric junction (PUJ) obstruction is the most common cause of more marked hydronephrosis (RPD>10 mm, and especially if >15 mm) [11].

The following are common points that may need to be considered during parental counselling.

What if the hydronephrosis resolves antenatally?

Antenatal resolution of hydronephrosis is recognized; however, these patients must still undergo postnatal ultrasound investigation as it is well documented that the hydronephrosis can recur [12]. Resolution of ANH was seen in 15 patients in the Bristol series, of whom seven were shown subsequently to have postnatal hydronephrosis (two had reflux and one a duplex system) [6].

How many babies will have normal postnatal scans?

This again depends largely on the definition of ANH but overall 36% of babies in the Bristol study had normal postnatal scans [6], and in our combined series approximately 50% of postnatal scans were normal (Table 14.2). The likelihood of a normal scan postnatally is increased if the ANH is mild—in one

reported series 100% of babies with RPD 6–10 mm were normal postnatally [13]. The controversial issue of whether babies with normal postnatal ultrasound scans should undergo further postnatal investigation will be discussed later in this chapter.

How many babies will have no urological problem?

The most common diagnoses in our combined series were transient hydronephrosis and a large non-obstructed renal pelvis and/or extrarenal pelvis, which accounted for approximately 63% of cases overall.

How many babies may need surgery?

Published data suggest that between approximately 15 and 40% of patients with ANH require surgery at some stage. In Ouzounian *et al.*'s series [5], 13/84 (15.4%) needed surgery, all of which were pyeloplasties, and in Gruenewald *et al.*'s publication [13], 14/34 (41%) were managed surgically.

However, conservative management has evolved for a number of urological conditions in recent years. The only condition that definitely requires surgery from our combined series is PUV (posterior urethral valves) (only 1.4% of cases). There are a number of conditions in which surgery is possibly indicated [PUJ obstruction, vesico-ureteric junction (VUJ) obstruction, multicystic dysplastic kidney (MCDK), vesico-ureteric reflux (VUR), duplex], which account for 28% of cases in our series overall, but a significant proportion of these will be successfully managed non-operatively. On the basis of this, we would estimate that currently only approximately 5% of patients with ANH will ultimately need surgery.

Key points: Definition and epidemiology

- A definition of ANH of ≥5 mm RPD is adopted in this chapter.

- Incidence of ANH is 1 : 188.

- Approximately 50% of antenatal scans are normal postnatally.

- Possible indication for surgery in 28%.

- Probably about 5% ultimately require surgery.

- Posterior urethral valves account for 1.4%, and are the only definite indication for surgery.

Postnatal investigations

Initial assessment of a neonate with documented ANH includes physical examination, looking specifically for the presence of an abdominal mass (possible PUJ obstruction or MCDK), deficient abdominal wall musculature with undescended testes (prune belly syndrome) or a palpable bladder (possible PUV). Our policy locally is to organize subsequent investigations according to the protocol outlined in Fig. 14.4, initially with ultrasound scans at 1 and 6 weeks. A number of local units do not have the necessary resources to perform all 1-week scans, and an acceptable alternative, if the initial RPD is 6–10 mm, is to only perform a 6-week scan. The first postnatal scan is deliberately delayed for a week to avoid the false-negative results that may be produced by scanning within the first 24–48 h, when the baby is relatively oliguric. Blood is taken and initial investigations are performed urgently (within 48 h) if unilateral hydronephrosis is seen in a solitary kidney, or if the bladder is distended or a ureterocele is suspected in cases of bilateral hydronephrosis (Table 14.4). A second scan at 6 weeks is necessary because initial scans, even if delayed for 48 h, may be normal and subsequent scans may show postnatal hydronephrosis. Dejter *et al.* [14]

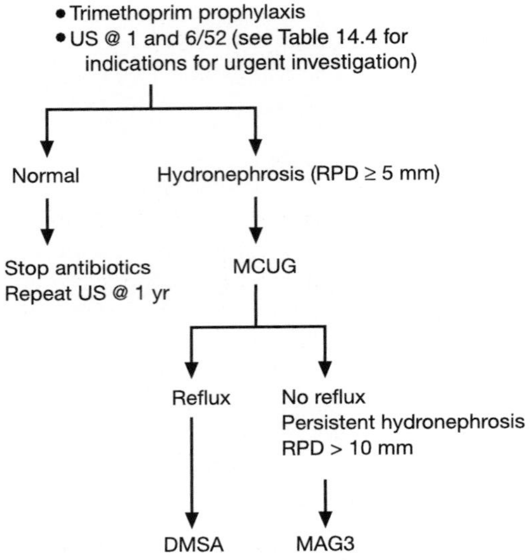

Fig. 14.4 Local investigation algorithm used for antenatally detected hydronephrosis [6]. Persistent hydronephrosis with renal pelvic diameter (RPD) <10 mm is followed up with repeat ultrasound at 1 year. Isotope scans are performed to look for obstruction if RPD >10 mm, even in the presence of vesico-ureteric reflux (VUR), as it is recognized that VUR can coexist with pelvi-ureteric junction (PUJ) obstruction in 8–14% of cases. MCUG, micturating cystourethrography; DMSA, dimercaptosuccinic acid scan; MAG3, mercaptoacetyltriglycine scan.

Table 14.4 Indications for urgent investigation, which include ultrasound and micturating cystourethrography (MCUG) within 48 hours

Bilateral hydronephrosis
  + distended bladder (posterior urethral valves, prune belly syndrome)
  + ureterocele
Unilateral hydronephrosis
  + solitary kidney

---

reported five neonates in whom initial scans had been normal and repeats at 6–8 weeks showed hydronephrosis with final diagnoses of PUJ obstruction (three), obstructed megaureter (one), and VUR (one). It has been demonstrated that efficient use of algorithms such as this reduces the number of follow-up outpatient appointments that are necessary for parents [3].

Ultrasound is also the initial investigation of choice in all other published series and a number support our postnatal investigation algorithm [3,7]. However, the timing and indications for further investigation vary, with certain groups recommending *dynamic renography* to look for obstruction prior to performing MCUG [13,15] and others restricting investigation with MCUG to those patients with evidence of ureteric dilatation [16].

Antibiotic prophylaxis

The importance of postnatal antibiotic prophylaxis in ANH has never been examined in the context of a trial and there are currently no published data to suggest that prophylaxis is associated with a better outcome. Until such data are available, our recommendations are that all infants are routinely commenced on prophylactic antibiotics (trimethoprim 2 mg/kg once daily) postnatally.

Micturating cystourethrography

MCUG is performed in all patients with persistent hydronephrosis demonstrated on postnatal ultrasound. It remains the definitive diagnostic test for assessment of VUR and the key investigation for the detection of posterior urethral valves. It is essential to prepare the parents and they are provided with information sheets prior to the investigation and, in addition, the trimethoprim is increased to a treatment dose (4 mg/kg twice daily) for 48 h starting immediately before MCUG. A urethral catheter is passed and contrast instilled into the bladder, followed by intermittent fluoroscopic monitoring during filling and voiding. The procedure is usually well tolerated in infants, and adverse effects such as irritative symptoms or urinary tract infection (UTI) are rare. Fluoroscopic exposure is kept as brief as possible, although there is an inevitable radiation dose to the gonads, particularly the ovaries.

Dynamic renography: diuretic renograms

Diuretic renograms are performed in order to help determine whether urinary tract obstruction is present in patients with persistent hydronephrosis in the absence of VUR, or if the RPD > 10 mm even in the presence of VUR. Obstruction is rarely complete, which would cause severe renal dysplasia, and has been best defined as any restriction to urinary outflow that, left untreated, would cause progressive renal deterioration. Newborns and infants are examined using $^{99}T_c^m$–mercaptoacyltriglycerine (MAG3), which has very high protein binding and renal extraction, and appears to give more accurate assessment of both function and drainage than $^{99}T_c^m$–diethylenetriaminepentaacetic acid (DTPA). See Chapters 6 and 12 for discussion of interpretation of dynamic renography.

The renogram requires careful interpretation, particularly in the neonate, as the results can easily be affected by the level of hydration of the patient, the regions of interest drawn by the radiologist, the failure of the immature neonatal kidney to respond to the diuretic, and by the presence or absence of reflux. Gordon recently described a theoretical model of the infant kidney and elegantly demonstrated that simple alterations in kidney function, tubular reabsorption, and pelvic size could produce dramatically different renographic curves [17]. The 'well-tempered renogram' (i.v. hydration and urethral catheter) has been described which is supposed to eliminate some of the above variables; however, this then becomes an invasive study without any definite increase in its ability to define obstruction accurately.

Although a non-obstructed curve is an important result to obtain from renography, a significant proportion of apparently 'obstructed' renograms do not appear to predict renal damage. Gordon *et al.* [18] presented retrospective data from 266 renograms in 69 children presenting with apparent PUJ obstruction between 1980 and 1987 from Great Ormond Street Hospital and clearly showed that renography was unreliable for positively identifying obstruction. Although approximately 32% of the renograms in a group treated non-operatively were defined as 'obstructive', their renal function did not deteriorate and, therefore, by definition, true obstruction could not have been present. These acknowledged limitations have led to differential renal function being recognized as a more dependable parameter for management decisions in this population [19].

Key points: Postnatal investigations

- Indications for urgent investigations (within 48 hours) are given in Table 14.4.

- US at 1 week can be omitted in mild hydronephrosis (<10 mm RPD).

- Urinary prophylaxis should be routinely offered (no evidence base).

- Antibiotics should be increased to therapy doses for 48 hours for MCUG.

Investigation of mild hydronephrosis (5–9 mm)

The importance of postnatal investigation of mild hydronephrosis, which is most commonly due to VUR, remains controversial. A number of centres, including Bristol, maintain that investigation with MCUG, if the hydronephrosis persists postnatally, is vital as it allows early identification of VUR and initiation of treatment prior to development of UTI and/or reflux nephropathy [6,9].

In support of this, McIlroy et al. [20] screened patients with RPD greater than 4 mm and demonstrated 69 cases of VUR of which 60 were in patients with mild hydronephrosis. Although the majority had low-grade reflux (43/60), there was no cut-off point that would predict high-grade reflux, which was associated with renal damage. Similarly, Pal et al. [21] looked specifically at the use of MCUG in 65 patients with mild hydronephrosis (defined by them as 5–15 mm) and showed VUR in 14/65 (21.5%), which included 3/19 (15.8%) with a RPD below 10 mm. Marra et al. [22] also performed cystography on 47 patients with mild hydronephrosis and demonstrated VUR in 14 (29.7%), which is a much higher incidence than the incidence estimated in the general population, of 0.4–1.8%.

The argument against full investigation of mild hydronephrosis is that it is often physiological and transient and does not justify the potential risks of MCUG. Dremsek et al. [7] concluded that there was no evidence that UTI could be predicted by detection of ANH, as during their study period 17 infants presented to their hospital with UTI, of whom seven were subsequently shown to have VUR, but unfortunately none had been shown to have hydronephrosis either antenatally or postnatally.

More recently, Harding et al. [12] published results from a study of 65 subjects with mild hydronephrosis, which resolved spontaneously in 28 (43%). They identified 12 patients with coexistent ureteric and/or calyceal dilatation postnatally, who were much more likely to have underlying pathology than a group with isolated renal pelvis dilatation. They therefore suggested that only this group should be referred for further investigation, and that patients with isolated renal pelvis dilatation should be followed up with serial ultrasound without cystography. They accepted that a small number of non-physiological cases would be missed but felt that the benefits in terms of a reduction in parental anxiety and the elimination of unnecessary investigations outweighed this risk. However, it should be noted that the incidence of UTI was higher in this study group than in controls. It would be essential that the parents should be made aware of the presenting symptoms and risks of UTI secondary to undiagnosed VUR, and it is difficult to be certain how much anxiety this in itself would induce.

Investigation when hydronephrosis resolves postnatally

There is increasing evidence to support investigation of all children with ANH with MCUG, as the presence of a normal postnatal scan does not necessarily exclude VUR, although this is not currently our local policy. This would clearly have enormous logistic and financial implications, as reference to Table 14.3 reveals that 48% of patients with ANH have normal postnatal scans and are currently not investigated. Pal et al. [21] showed that 11/41 (26.8%) normal kidneys (on a second follow-up scan) refluxed and similarly Jaswon et al. [8] reported that the postnatal ultrasound was normal in 14/23 (61%) of neonates with VUR. Tibballs et al. [23] also clearly demonstrated that the postnatal ultrasound appearances correlated poorly with the presence and degree of VUR in children with ANH. In their series of 177 patients, approximately 25% of normal kidneys on postnatal ultrasound had grade III–V VUR on MCUG.

Key points: Investigation of mild hydronephrosis

- This is most commonly due to VUR.
- Investigation remains controversial.
- This is even more the case when the hydronephrosis has resolved antenatally.

Causes of antenatal hydronephrosis

Transient hydronephrosis

Approximately 50% of patients with ANH will have normal postnatal scans and would not routinely be investigated further in the neonatal period. The aetiology of the ANH is uncertain but it may occur because of insufficient maturation of the PUJ or VUJ, coupled with increased fetal urinary output, fetal ureteral folds, or indeed, as discussed previously, may indicate VUR. Gunn *et al.* [24] demonstrated transient hydronephrosis in 216/298 (72%) patients, 53 of whom were followed up at 2–3 years. In that period, only one patient had presented with a UTI (at 20 months) and was found to have grade I reflux and they concluded that no serious urinary tract pathology was missed in this situation. In the Bristol series, 36 babies were shown to have no evidence of postnatal hydronephrosis at 1 or 6 weeks and, of the 28 available for study at 1 year, none had evidence of hydronephrosis.

Persistent hydronephrosis without obstruction

Hydronephrosis without evidence of obstruction is demonstrated postnatally in approximately 15% of patients. Dudley *et al.* [6] followed up 34/43 infants with non-obstructive postnatal hydronephrosis and showed that 20 (46.5%) had completely resolved by 12 months, whereas 14 persisted. Thus, repeat US at 1 year of age is indicated (Fig. 14.4).

Najmaldin *et al.* [25] described 6-year follow-up of 42 renal units with so-called 'PUJ hydronephrosis' and demonstrated that two units progressed to obstruction, one of which required pyeloplasty, although these units had actually had equivocal diuretic renogram curves initially. Overall, 27 (64%) kidneys had not changed and 13 (31%) had improved, and they concluded that 'PUJ hydronephrosis' was a benign condition but one that merited long-term follow-up. Thus infrequent US (we recommend at 3, 5, 10, and 15 years) is indicated, with dynamic renography being added if there is increasing hydronephrosis not explained by renal growth.

In addition, these infants are at increased risk of urinary stone formation. Rickwood and Reiner [26] reported four children with upper urinary tract dilatation not associated with VUR or with obstruction who presented with calculi at 2–5 years of age, often following *Proteus* urinary infections.

Pelvi-ureteric junction obstruction

PUJ obstruction occurs in approximately 1 in 2000 children, with a male:female ratio of 3:1 and is bilateral in 20–25% of cases. The obstruction is usually caused by intrinsic stenosis/valves (75%), an insertion anomaly of the ureter (often high and oblique, but this may be a secondary phenomenon), peripelvic fibrosis, or crossing vessels (20% of cases are associated with an accessory renal artery). The diagnosis is generally suspected antenatally in a fetus with hydronephrosis without ureteric dilatation, and with a normal bladder and normal amniotic fluid volume (see Fig. 14.1).

The degree of ANH gives some indication of the likelihood of PUJ obstruction. Dudley *et al.* [6] found that 3/4 fetuses with a RPD greater than 15 mm were diagnosed postnatally with PUJ obstruction, compared with none of 70 fetuses with a RPD below 15 mm. Similarly, Podevin *et al.* [11] showed that 7/11 fetuses with a RPD greater than 15 mm had PUJ obstruction, compared with 2/15 with a RPD of 11–15 mm and only 1/18 with a RPD less than 11 mm. Postnatally, the majority of mild to moderate PUJ obstructions will tend to deteriorate within the first 6 months of life as a result of maturational changes in GFR (which increases from 23 ml/min/1.73 m^2 at birth, to 88 ml/min/1.73 m^2 at 4 months, 100 ml/min/1.73 m^2 at 6 months, and 120 ml/min/1.73 m^2 at 1 year) occurring before maturation of the PUJ.

Diagnosis

The diagnosis of PUJ obstruction is currently confirmed using dynamic renography. As discussed previously (Chapters 6 and 12), these investigations are subject to large number of variables and may not necessarily identify those patients who have true obstruction. A more useful measure is an estimate of differential renal function, which is usually considered to be significant if the renal function is depressed to less than 35% [27] or 40% [28] of the total.

As has been discussed in Chapters 6 and 12 a number of other investigations have been described that may facilitate the diagnosis of obstruction. A particular consideration in an infant is that an intravenous urogram (IVU) is rarely used in the initial assessment of suspected PUJ obstruction, although it may help to distinguish an extrarenal pelvis without calyceal dilatation (requiring no further evaluation) from mild PUJ obstruction in the older child.

Animal studies have demonstrated that renal obstruction results in increased renal vascular resistance, which results in an altered waveform with Doppler ultrasound. The renal resistive index (RI) is defined as (peak systolic velocity – end diastolic velocity)/peak systolic velocity. The ranges for adults have been fairly well defined, with an RI greater than 0.7 representing the upper limit of normal. RI in children does appear to correlate well with results from traditional diuretic renography and Andriani *et al.* [29] have recently published normal ranges for last trimester fetuses and infants up to 6 months of age, which will permit further studies to be undertaken.

The ejection fraction (EF) is defined as the percentage uptake of a radionucleotide by the kidney 2–3 min after injection of isotope, and is an alternative method of determining differential renal function. The normal EF in the newborn is 1.5% by each kidney, increasing to 2.5% by end of the first year of life. The correlation of EF with GFR is good (coefficient 0.92) but normal ranges in children aged 1–2 years have been incompletely defined, which currently limits its use.

The measurement of increasing length in the contralateral kidney has also been described as a method of diagnosing PUJ obstruction. Koff *et al.* [30] demonstrated 'renal counterbalance' in normal kidneys opposite a unilateral hydronephrotic kidney, and proposed that plotting serial measurements of normal renal length could facilitate the diagnosis of obstruction. They subsequently produced a renal growth–renal function chart for this purpose, although other centres have not, in fact, found a correlation between the findings on the normal and affected sides.

Indications for surgery

The practice of routine dismembered pyeloplasty for PUJ obstruction was initially questioned by Ransley and Manzoni [19]. They suggested that drainage curves on dynamic renography were unreliable indicators of obstruction and pioneered the use of differential renal function, reserving surgery for kidneys with loss of function.

In their original series of 112 patients (142 kidneys), they classified the kidneys as having poor (<20%), moderate (20–39%) and good (≥40%) differential function on isotope scans at 1 month [28]. They followed patients with good renal function (100/106) with an annual scan and did not operate unless renal function deteriorated (<40%). The patients were followed up to 6 years and by then only 23% had undergone pyeloplasty (generally by age 3), usually because of deterioration of renal function. Interestingly, no patient with a RPD below 12 mm underwent pyeloplasty. Patients with moderate function (27) were generally treated with pyeloplasty

(23), although the renal function in those patients treated non-operatively (four) improved spontaneously to good function. Patients with poor function (nine) had a percutaneous nephrostomy inserted to see if the renal function improved sufficiently to merit pyeloplasty (3/9 improved to >10%).

A number of other groups have also reported their data following similar protocols. Madden *et al.* [31] described 53 patients (63 kidneys) of whom 39 were managed non-operatively and only eight (21%) required pyeloplasty. The remaining patients (31) continued to be managed non-operatively and showed improved appearance on US (16/31) and improved drainage (8/17).

Similarly, Cartwright *et al.* [27] reported a series of 39 neonates with PUJ obstruction with good differential renal function (>35%) who were managed non-operatively and only six (15%) required surgery because of decreased function, UTI, or pain. Reassuringly, their renal function returned to the initial level postoperatively and their differential function was ultimately no different from that of a similar group who had undergone early pyeloplasty.

The proponents of early surgery suggest that a partially obstructed renal unit is denied the opportunity to recover if the obstruction is not relieved, although there is no good evidence to support this view. A number of cases have been cited in the literature in which the renal unit was lost when surgery was delayed, but in fact the initial function of these kidneys was very poor (<20% in six and <10% in two) [32]. There has also been a failure to consider the normal neonatal increase in GFR in the literature. King *et al.* [33] reported 11 patients below 3 months of age who underwent immediate pyeloplasty, and compared the relative increase in their renal function with that of older children also undergoing pyeloplasty. The mean increase was 18.9% in younger patients and only 4.6% in older, but the final relative function values of 36.5% and 32.5% were not significantly different. It could therefore be concluded that the larger increase in the younger group was only that expected with normal age-related maturation of renal function.

Koff and Campbell [34] described an extended use of non-operative management, which included even moderate or poorly functioning kidneys. They reported 104 consecutive neonates with non-operatively managed unilateral hydronephrosis, with a follow-up to 5 years. Overall, only seven (7%) patients underwent pyeloplasty, because of reduced differential function (>10%) or progressive hydronephrosis, and postoperatively their function returned to pre-deterioration levels. A total of 16 patients were identified with reduced renal function initially (mean 26%, range 7–40%) of whom 15 improved (mean 48%, range 32–57%) and only one deteriorated (from 38 to 20%, returning to exceed 40% post-pyeloplasty).

Randomized controlled trials

Long-term follow-up results from an ongoing randomized trial at Great Ormond Street are awaited with interest. Recently data have become available from the Society for Fetal Urology, who recruited 32 infants (across 10 centres) with grade III or more hydronephrosis, obstruction, and greater than 40% differential function [35]. The group randomized to surgery, not surprisingly, had improved drainage and reduced hydronephrosis postoperatively, whereas their differential renal function remained stable. Renal function deteriorated in 25% of the children in conservative arm, sufficient to require surgery, but remained stable in the other 75%.

Overall, these studies support non-operative management for neonates with a suspected unilateral PUJ obstruction and a good functioning kidney. Our local policy is to monitor these children with ultrasound every 3 months initially, and isotope renograms every 6–12 months. Surgery is reserved for those cases with reduced function initially (<40%) or those that show a later deterioration (decrease in differential function by >10% or to <40%). In the case of bilateral PUJ obstruction, management decisions cannot be supported by differential function and pyeloplasty is usually performed at 3 months on the most dilated side, or on the kidney that appears to be working less well. The long-term outcome of conservatively treated PUJ obstruction in terms of the incidence of symptoms, UTI, stones, and decreased function at any stage in the future remains uncertain and we await the results of ongoing studies with interest.

Vesico-ureteric reflux

Vesico-ureteric reflux is detected postnatally in approximately 9% of neonates overall with antenatal hydronephrosis. In the Bristol series, 18/70 with an RPD below 15 mm were shown to have VUR (in fact all cases had RPD < 10 mm) [6]. As discussed previously, VUR may exist even in the presence of normal postnatal scans and some authors have argued that postnatal scans should not be used to direct investigations for reflux. Jaswon *et al.* [8] specifically investigated all neonates with RPD greater than 5 mm with MCUG, irrespective of postnatal scans, and showed reflux in 14/57 (24.6%) of those with a normal postnatal scan.

Most series demonstrate a preponderance of males, and the reflux is usually dilating (at least grade III—see Fig. 11.3). In clinical practice, VUR is found at least as often in girls. Anderson *et al.* [9] hypothesized that the cut-off RPD of greater than 10 mm, used in many series as the threshold for investigation, may be too high, and subsequently performed MCUG on 264 infants with ANH with RPD ≥ 4 mm, even if the postnatal ultrasound was normal. Interestingly, they identified primary VUR in 13% overall, with a sex ratio (17 girls and 16 boys) that compared with the ratio seen in infants below 1 year of age presenting with UTI. They also confirmed that 23% of patients with a normal postnatal ultrasound had VUR.

A number of authors have suggested that VUR in males arises as a result of transient fetal urethral obstruction (see Fig. 14.5). For example, Avni *et al.* [36] reported bladder or urethral abnormalities (which most commonly included a dilated posterior urethra) on MCUG in 15/25 baby boys with VUR. They hypothesized that dilatation of the posterior urethra (secondary to a variety of developmental anomalies) resulted in an oblique 'flap-valve' insertion of the distal membranous urethra. Bladder outflow obstruction (between 9 and 13 weeks) with secondary VUR was a possible consequence and the degree of VUR could be related to the degree and duration of this obstruction.

A number of studies have demonstrated that renal damage is often present in neonates with VUR at their initial evaluation, prior to the occurrence of infection, which would clearly not be preventable by postnatal screening. Crabbe *et al.* [37] showed impaired function (global parenchymal loss) in 4/20 children with VUR at a mean age of 34 days. Similarly Najmaldin *et al.* [38] showed reduced function (9–41%) in 9/14 patients examined with sterile VUR and Anderson and Rickwood [39] demonstrated that 60% of refluxing units were abnormal with DMSA assessments prior to infection.

The majority of neonates with VUR are managed non-operatively with simple antibiotic prophylaxis. Overall, 64/98 (65%) of refluxing units resolve

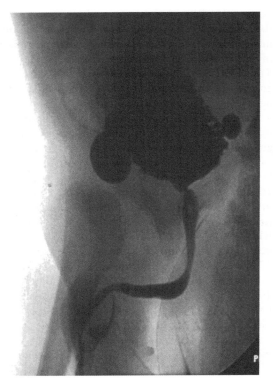

Fig. 14.5 Micturating cystourethrography in a neonate with bilateral ANH demonstrated a normal urethra but numerous bladder diverticulae, which may have been produced by the presence of transient fetal urethral obstruction.

within 2 years, which includes 20% of those infants with more severe grade IV or V reflux [40]. Interestingly, Godley *et al.* [41] recently demonstrated that those infants with VUR and bilateral renal abnormalities at initial investigations were likely to have persistent VUR at 16 months and abnormal bladder function (in 90%), whereas if the infants had normal kidneys at birth, then the VUR was likely to resolve and bladder function was usually normal (in 71%).

Vesico-ureteric junction obstruction

Shokeir and Nijman [42] recently produced an excellent review discussing primary megaureter (PM) and VUJ obstruction. In the described classification, megaureters can be considered to be refluxing, obstructed, non-refluxing and non-obstructed, or both refluxing and obstructed. PM is a compound term including both obstructed and non-obstructed

PM and, as with PUJ obstruction, the main management difficulty is the ability to differentiate one from the other.

An obstructed PM is produced by an aperistaltic segment of distal ureter at the VUJ, has a male:female ratio of 4:1, is bilateral in 25%, and is more common in left ureters. For completeness, a refluxing megaureter occurs because of a short or absent intravesical ureter or other derangement of VUJ; a refluxing and obstructed megaureter is seen in 2% of refluxing megaureters and is produced when the distal ureteric segment has an inadequate intramural tunnel but also has ineffective peristalsis; and a non-refluxing non-obstructed megaureter is probably produced by the relatively high fetal urine flow rates or by transient anatomical obstructions such as fetal folds.

Diagnosis

The diagnosis is suspected when ultrasound shows a dilated ureter (>7 mm) and renal pelvis with variable renal parenchymal atrophy, and the MCUG shows no reflux. Dynamic renography and differential renal function are used to differentiate obstructed from non-obstructed megaureters, but the same arguments apply as for PUJ obstruction. Ipsilateral PUJ obstruction can be seen in up to 13% of primary megaureter, and this may be suspected from renography. IVU provides useful anatomical information and may identify those patients in whom both reflux and obstruction coexist, as poor drainage of upper tracts on a delayed IVU film would suggest associated obstruction.

Indications for surgery

The traditional surgical approach for the obstructed VUJ would involve excision of the distal ureteric segment, tapering of the ureter, and reimplantation; however, the overall complication rate in neonates is high. Open insertion of a JJ stent as a temporizing procedure in infants with VUJ obstruction and recurrent UTIs despite antibiotic prophylaxis, has been reported with excellent results [43]. The encouraging results of endopyelotomy for PUJ obstruction have also recently prompted the description of endoureterotomy in five adults, with encouraging results up to 4 years [44], although there are no published descriptions of this procedure in children.

Non-operative treatment is being described increasingly, applying similar management protocols to those used in PUJ obstruction. The Philadelphia group reported 35 renal units associated with primary obstructive megaureter detected by prenatal ultrasound and only two (6%) required an operation for diminishing renal function [45]. The majority showed decreased dilatation on sequential scans and the group only recommended surgery when the relative renal function decreased to below 35%, or if the patients developed UTI in spite of antibiotic prophylaxis. More recently they described follow-up of 25 patients (of whom 17 had presented antenatally) to a mean of 7.3 years [46]. None of the patients had had problems with stones, pain, or UTI. In addition, the urinary tract dilatation had improved (12/18 who had IVU) or had remained static (6/18) and there had been no deterioration in differential function on renogram. Oliveira *et al.* [47] followed up eight infants non-operatively over a 6-year period and documented that the ureteric dilatation improved (>13 mm to 8 mm) and renal function and renograms

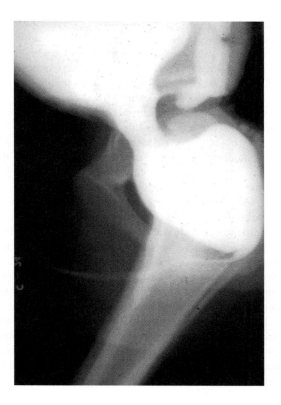

Fig. 14.6 Micturating cystourethrography demonstrates the classical appearance of PUV with a markedly dilated posterior urethra.

were stable throughout, and similar experiences have been reported from other groups.

Posterior urethral valves

Posterior urethral valves are the most common cause of severe obstructive uropathy, occurring in approximately 1 in 8000 newborns and accounting for approximately 1.4% of cases in the combined series. Suspicious features on antenatal ultrasound include progressive bilateral hydronephrosis and the presence of a large, thick-walled bladder with diverticulae and poor emptying (see Fig. 14.6). Similar appearances can also be produced by massive vesico-ureteric reflux and also by the prune belly syndrome. Elevated fetal urinary Na, Cl, and β_2-microglobulin are recognized as antenatal predictors of poor outcome, but the volume of amniotic fluid remains an important prognostic feature.

Postnatally, neonates with severe bilateral renal dysplasia may present with associated pulmonary hypoplasia. In all suspected cases, a urethral catheter should be passed, and an ultrasound and MCUG organized urgently (within 48 h) (see Table 14.4). Postnatal management and prognosis are discussed in detail in Chapter 12.

Ureterocele

A ureterocele is a cystic dilatation of the intravesical ureter, occurring in 1 in 5000 neonates, with a male : female ratio of 1 : 3–5. They are commonly associated with duplicated collecting systems (80–90%), are bilateral in 10–20% of patients, and are associated with ectopic insertion of the ureter into bladder in up to 75% of cases. Ureteroceles may remain entirely within the bladder (intravesical) or extend through the bladder neck (ectopic). Single-system ureteroceles are commonly associated with multicystic dysplastic kidney.

In a duplex system, the ectopic ureter drains the upper pole moiety, entering the bladder wall medial and inferior to the normal lower pole ureter, and may be obstructed by the ureterocele, resulting in upper pole hydronephrosis. A large ureterocele may also obstruct the contralateral ureteric orifice, or the bladder neck, resulting in bilateral obstruction (Fig. 14.7), which merits urgent postnatal investigation. It is usually possible to identify the duplicated collecting system and ureterocele with postnatal ultrasound. MCUG is necessary to demonstrate whether reflux exists into the lower pole or the ectopic ureter, and a MAG3 renogram is also performed to look at function, although there is often very little in the upper pole.

Shankar *et al.* [48] recently reported the Liverpool experience of 52 consecutive patients with ante-natally detected duplex system ureterocele. Surgery was reserved for patients with breakthrough UTI, useful upper pole renal function (>10%), lower pole obstruction or VUR greater than grade III, or bladder outflow obstruction secondary to the ureterocele. Definitive surgical treatment usually comprised upper pole hemi-nephroureterectomy; however, transurethral endoscopic incision of the ureterocele was often performed as an initial intervention. Although a minimally invasive procedure resulting in immediate relief of the obstruction, endoscopic uretero-cele incision is rarely a definitive procedure, is unlikely to result in a significant improvement in upper pole function, [16] and can result in upper pole moiety reflux in up to 30% of cases. The Liverpool series included 14 patients who were managed expectantly

with regular ultrasound and prophylactic antibiotics until completion of toilet training, or until the age of 5. During the follow-up period (median 8 years), none of these patients developed symptoms or UTI, and there was evidence of resolution of the hydronephrosis and ureterocele collapse in a proportion of cases.

Key points: Ureterocele

- Commonly associated with duplex kidney.

- In the duplex kidney the ureterocele is usually associated with the upper moiety but can obstruct the lower moiety.

- A large ureterocele may:
  – obstruct the contralateral kidney;
  – obstruct the bladder neck.

Multicystic dysplastic kidney

Multicystic dysplastic kidney is a developmental anomaly in which the renal parenchyma is completely replaced by multiple, tense, non-communicating cysts of varying sizes, with no discernable renal cortex (see Chapter 6 and Fig. 14.8). The proximal ureter is atretic or non-patent and the kidney is non-functioning on isotope scan. The incidence of MCDK has been reported to vary between 1 in 2400 [49] and 1 in 4300 [50] with a male:female ratio of 2 : 1 and is bilateral in 10% of cases. Although traditionally described as the most common cause of abdominal mass in the neonate, MCDK is usually detected antenatally (see Fig. 14.3) and in one series only 10/23 (43%) were palpable [50]. MCDK is not inherited, unlike polycys-tic disease, and is occasionally confused with PUJ obstruction. The diagnosis is confirmed postnatally with ultrasound and DMSA at 1 month. MCUG is also performed because contralateral renal anomalies are seen in approximately 25%, which include renal agenesis, PUJ obstruction, and VUR (in 20–25%).

Postnatal management of MCDK depends on the presence of symptoms. Nephrectomy is recom-mended for symptomatic masses and also if infection occurs. Urinary tract pathology (e.g. VUR) should be excluded in a patient presenting with infection, because the MCDK itself is unlikely to be the cause as it is usually isolated from the lower urinary tract by a non-patent ureter. The management of asymptomatic MCDK remains very controversial as the incidence of

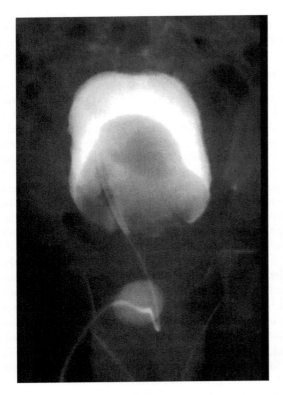

Fig. 14.7 Large ureterocele demonstrated on micturating cystourethrography, which was obstructing bladder out-flow and causing bilateral hydronephrosis.

short-term complications is very low and disappearance of MCDK, both clinically and on ultrasound, is seen in most patients by the age of 5 years [51].

Conservative management

Gordon *et al.* [50] presented a series of 25 cases of MCDK from Leeds, in which 14 were managed conservatively. Follow-up ultrasound in 11 (2 disappeared, 6 were smaller, and 3 were static) suggested that the natural history was towards spontaneous involution, and none of these patients developed symptoms or hypertension, which supported conservative treatment. In their discussion they reviewed the arguments for removal of MCDK, which include the risks of hypertension and malignancy.

MCDK can occasionally give rise to renin-dependent hypertension but they considered the risk of this to be low. They found only nine cases of hypertension in the literature, of whom three responded to nephrectomy, and they also cited several series of children with surgical causes of hypertension, none of whom had MCDK. In addition, they found only six cases of malignancy, including a 68-year-old adult, in the literature, when there are approximately 1000 new cases of MCDK per annum.

Rickwood *et al.* [52] also reported conservative management of 39/44 infants with MCDK and found no evidence of hypertension with a mean follow-up of 3 years, concluding that routine nephrectomy was not necessary. This approach is supported by the MCDK registry, established by American Academy of Paediatrics [51], who have a database of 441 patients registered from 49 centres in the US and Canada, of whom 260 have been managed non-operatively and there have been no nephrectomies performed for hypertension or malignancy.

Surgical management

Webb *et al.* [53] presented data from Manchester supporting nephrectomy at 3 months. They report three children with hypertension secondary to MCDK, one of whom had been discharged elsewhere because of disappearance of the cystic kidney. All the children were normotensive following nephrectomy, although one child may have actually had renal dysplasia rather than MCDK. They argued that resolution of MCDK cysts does not mean resolution of risks of hypertension, as stromal tissue may still be present, and support early nephrectomy before hypertension damages the contralateral kidney, resulting in the disappointing surgical results that may be seen in older children. In fact, closer inspection of the MCDK registry reveals four children who developed hypertension, which may have been related to the MCDK [51].

Although it has been estimated that it would be necessary to remove between 1600 [54] and 8000

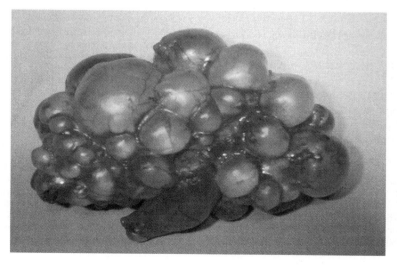

Fig. 14.8 Appearance of MCDK post-nephrectomy. (Reproduced with permission of Mr Mike O'Brien, Specialist Registrar in Paediatric Surgery, Bristol.)

[51] MCDKs to prevent one Wilms' tumour, Webb _et al._ [53] also argued that malignant transformation may be difficult to detect in adult life as the residual tissue may not be visible on ultrasound, and haematuria and/or positive cytology is unlikely to be detectable because of the atretic ureter. In support of surgery, in their series 49/62 (79%) underwent nephrectomy with no perioperative complications.

Local approach

Our approach currently is to make the diagnosis postnatally with ultrasound and DMSA and also to perform MCUG to investigate contralateral reflux. Nephrectomy is performed if there is a large mass, if the MCDK fails to involute by 1 year, and also at parental request. Conservative management is fairly intensive, including an ultrasound and blood pressure check every 3–6 months in infancy and annually thereafter. We would strongly support the pleas of previous authors for the setting up of a national registry in the United Kingdom.

Key points: Multicystic dysplastic kidney

• MCUG is performed because contralateral VUR is present in 20–25%.

• If symptoms are present, nephrectomy is indicated.

• Management of asymptomatic cases is controversial:
  – the majority view prefers a conservative approach;
  – a minority advise nephrectomy even if cysts have regressed because of a small chance of late complications.

References

1. Garrett WJ, Grunwald G, Robinson DE. Prenatal diagnosis of fetal polycystic kidney by ultrasound. _Aust N Z J Obstet Gynaecol_ 1970;10(1):7–9.
2. Grignon A, Filion R, Filiatrault D, Robitaille P, Homsy Y, Boutin H, _et al._ Urinary tract dilatation _in utero_: classification and clinical applications. _Radiology_ 1986;160(3):645–7.
3. Owen RJ, Lamont AC, Brookes J. Early management and postnatal investigation of prenatally diagnosed hydronephrosis [see comments]. _Clin Radiol_ 1996; 51(3):173–6.
4. Siemens DR, Prouse KA, MacNeily AE, Sauerbrei EE. Antenatal hydronephrosis: thresholds of renal pelvic diameter to predict insignificant postnatal pelviectasis. _Tech Urol_ 1998;4(4):198–201.
5. Ouzounian JG, Castro MA, Fresquez M, al-Sulyman OM, Kovacs BW. Prognostic significance of antenatally detected fetal pyelectasis. _Ultrasound Obstet Gynecol_ 1996;7(6):424–8.
6. Dudley JA, Haworth JM, McGraw ME, Frank JD, Tizard EJ. Clinical relevance and implications of antenatal hydronephrosis. _Arch Dis Child Fetal Neonatal Ed_ 1997;76(1):F31–4.
7. Dremsek PA, Gindl K, Voitl P, Strobl R, Hafner E, Geissler W, _et al._ Renal pyelectasis in fetuses and neonates: diagnostic value of renal pelvis diameter in pre- and postnatal sonographic screening. _Am J Roentgenol_ 1997;168(4):1017–19.
8. Jaswon MS, Dibble L, Puri S, Davis J, Young J, Dave R, _et al._ Prospective study of outcome in antenatally diagnosed renal pelvis dilatation [see comments]. _Arch Dis Child Fetal Neonatal Ed_ 1999;80(2):F135–8.
9. Anderson NG, Abbott GD, Mogridge N, Allan RB, Maling TM, Wells JE. Vesicoureteric reflux in the newborn: relationship to fetal renal pelvic diameter. _Pediatr Nephrol_ 1997;11(5):610–16.
10. Livera LN, Brookfield DS, Egginton JA, Hawnaur JM. Antenatal ultrasonography to detect fetal renal abnormalities: a prospective screening programme. _BMJ_ 1989;298(6685):1421–3.
11. Podevin G, Mandelbrot L, Vuillard E, Oury JF, Aigrain Y. Outcome of urological abnormalities prenatally diagnosed by ultrasound. _Fetal Diagn Ther_ 1996;11(3):181–90.
12. Harding LJ, Malone PS, Wellesley DG. Antenatal minimal hydronephrosis: is its follow-up an unnecessary cause of concern? _Prenat Diagn_ 1999;19(8):701–5.
13. Gruenewald SM, Cohen RC, Antico VF, Farlow DC, Cass DT. Diagnosis and treatment of antenatal uropathies. _J Paediatr Child Health_ 1990;26(3):142–7.
14. Dejter SW, Jr., Gibbons MD. The fate of infant kidneys with fetal hydronephrosis but initially normal postnatal sonography. _J Urol_ 1989;142(2 Pt 2):661–2; discussion 667–8.
15. Lam BC, Wong SN, Yeung CY, Tang MH, Ghosh A. Outcome and management of babies with prenatal ultrasonographic renal abnormalities. _Am J Perinatol_ 1993;10(4):263–8.
16. Kitagawa H, Pringle KC, Stone P, Flower J, Murakami N, Robinson R. Postnatal follow-up of hydronephrosis detected by prenatal ultrasound: the natural history. _Fetal Diagn Ther_ 1998;13(1):19–25.
17. Gordon I. Diuretic renography in infants with prenatal unilateral hydronephrosis: an explanation for the controversy about poor drainage. _BJU Int_ 2001;87(6):551–5.
18. Gordon I, Dhillon HK, Gatanash H, Peters AM. Antenatal diagnosis of pelvic hydronephrosis:

assessment of renal function and drainage as a guide to management. *J Nucl Med* 1991;32(9):1649–54.

19. Ransley P, Manzoni G. Extended role of DTPA scan in assessment of function and PUJ obstruction in neonates. *Dialogues in Paediatric Urology* 1985;8:6–8.

20. McIlroy PJ, Abbott GD, Anderson NG, Turner JG, Mogridge N, Wells JE. Outcome of primary vesico-ureteric reflux detected following fetal renal pelvic dilatation. *J Paediatr Child Health* 2000;36(6):569–73.

21. Pal CR, Tuson JR, Lindsell DR, McHugh K, Hope PL, Ives K. The role of micturating cystourethrography in antenatally detected mild hydronephrosis. *Pediatr Radiol* 1998;28(3):152–5.

22. Marra G, Barbieri G, Moioli C, Assael BM, Grumieri G, Caccamo ML. Mild fetal hydronephrosis indicating vesicoureteric reflux. *Arch Dis Child Fetal Neonatal Ed* 1994;70(2):F147–9; discussion 149–50.

23. Tibballs JM, De Bruyn R. Primary vesicoureteric reflux—how useful is postnatal ultrasound? *Arch Dis Child* 1996;75(5):444–7.

24. Gunn TR, Mora JD, Pease P. Antenatal diagnosis of urinary tract abnormalities by ultrasonography after 28 weeks' gestation: incidence and outcome. *Am J Obstet Gynecol* 1995;172(2 Pt 1):479–86.

25. Najmaldin AS, Burge DM, Atwell JD. Outcome of antenatally diagnosed pelviureteric junction hydro-nephrosis. *Br J Urol* 1991;67(1):96–9.

26. Rickwood AM, Reiner I. Urinary stone formation in children with prenatally diagnosed uropathies. *Br J Urol* 1991;68(5):541–2.

27. Cartwright PC, Duckett JW, Keating MA, Snyder HMD, Escala J, Blyth B, et al. Managing apparent ureteropelvic junction obstruction in the newborn. *J Urol* 1992;148(4):1224–8.

28. Ransley PG, Dhillon HK, Gordon I, Duffy PG, Dillon MJ, Barratt TM. The postnatal management of hydronephrosis diagnosed by prenatal ultrasound. *J Urol* 1990;144(2 Pt 2):584–7; discussion 593–4.

29. Andriani G, Persico A, Tursini S, Ballone E, Cirotti D, Lelli Chiesa P. The renal-resistive index from the last 3 months of pregnancy to 6 months old. *BJU Int* 2001;87(6):562–4.

30. Koff SA, Peller PA, Young DC, Pollifrone DL. The assessment of obstruction in the newborn with unilateral hydronephrosis by measuring the size of the opposite kidney. *J Urol* 1994;152(2 Pt 2):596–9.

31. Madden NP, Thomas DF, Gordon AC, Arthur RJ, Irving HC, Smith SE. Antenatally detected pelvi-ureteric junction obstruction. Is non-operation safe? *Br J Urol* 1991;68(3):305–10.

32. Perez LM, Friedman RM, King LR. The case for relief of ureteropelvic junction obstruction in neonates and young children at time of diagnosis. *Urology* 1991;38(3):195–201.

33. King LR, Coughlin PW, Bloch EC, Bowie JD, Ansong K, Hanna MK. The case for immediate pyeloplasty in the neonate with ureteropelvic junction obstruction. *J Urol* 1984;132(4):725–8.

34. Koff SA, Campbell KD. The nonoperative management of unilateral neonatal hydronephrosis: natural history of poorly functioning kidneys. *J Urol* 1994;152(2 Pt 2):593–5.

35. Palmer LS, Maizels M, Cartwright PC, Fernbach SK, Conway JJ. Surgery versus observation for managing obstructive grade 3 to 4 unilateral hydronephrosis: a report from the Society for Fetal Urology. *J Urol* 1998;159(1):222–8.

36. Avni EF, Schulman CC. The origin of vesico-ureteric reflux in male newborns: further evidence in favour of a transient fetal urethral obstruction. *Br J Urol* 1996;78(3):454–9.

37. Crabbe DC, Thomas DF, Gordon AC, Irving HC, Arthur RJ, Smith SE. Use of 99mtechnetium-dimercaptosuccinic acid to study patterns of renal damage associated with prenatally detected vesi-coureteral reflux. *J Urol* 1992;148(4):1229–31.

38. Najmaldin A, Burge DM, Atwell JD. Reflux nephropathy secondary to intrauterine vesicoureteric reflux. *J Pediatr Surg* 1990;25(4):387–90.

39. Anderson PA, Rickwood AM. Features of primary vesicoureteric reflux detected by prenatal sonography. *Br J Urol* 1991;67(3):267–71.

40. Elder JS. Commentary: importance of antenatal diagnosis of vesicoureteral reflux. *J Urol* 1992;148(5 Pt 2):1750–4.

41. Godley ML, Desai D, Yeung CK, Dhillon HK, Duffy PG, Ransley PG. The relationship between early renal status, and the resolution of vesico-ureteric reflux and bladder function at 16 months. *BJU Int* 2001;87(6):457–62.

42. Shokeir AA, Nijman RJ. Primary megaureter: current trends in diagnosis and treatment. *BJU Int* 2000;86(7):861–8.

43. Shenoy MU, Rance CH. Is there a place for the insertion of a JJ stent as a temporizing procedure for symptomatic partial congenital vesico-ureteric junction obstruction in infancy? *BJU Int* 1999;84(4):524–5.

44. Bapat S, Bapat M, Kirpekar D. Endoureterotomy for congenital primary obstructive megaureter: preliminary report. *J Endourol* 2000;14(3):263–7.

45. Keating MA, Escala J, Snyder HMD, Heyman S, Duckett JW. Changing concepts in management of primary obstructive megaureter. *J Urol* 1989;142(2 Pt 2):636–40; discussion 667–8.

46. Baskin LS, Zderic SA, Snyder HM, Duckett JW. Primary dilated megaureter: long-term followup. *J Urol* 1994;152(2 Pt 2):618–21.

47. Oliveira EA, Diniz JS, Rabelo EA, Silva JM, Pereira AK, Filgueiras MT, et al. Primary megaureter detected by prenatal ultrasonography: conservative management and prolonged follow-up. *Int Urol Nephrol* 2000;32(1):13–18.

48. Shankar KR, Vishwanath N, Rickwood AM. Outcome of patients with prenatally detected duplex system ureterocele; natural history of those managed expectantly. *J Urol* 2001;165(3):1226–8.

49. Liebeschuetz S, Thomas R. Unilateral multicystic dysplastic kidney. *Arch Dis Child* 1997;77(4):369.

50. Gordon AC, Thomas DF, Arthur RJ, Irving HC. Multicystic dysplastic kidney: is nephrectomy still appropriate? *J Urol* 1988;140(5 Pt 2):1231–4.

51. Wacksman J, Phipps L. Report of the Multicystic Kidney Registry: preliminary findings. *J Urol* 1993;150(6):1870–2.

52. Rickwood AM, Anderson PA, Williams MP. Multicystic renal dysplasia detected by prenatal ultrasonography. Natural history and results of conservative management. *Br J Urol* 1992;69(5):538–40.

53. Webb NJ, Lewis MA, Bruce J, Gough DC, Ladusans EJ, Thomson AP, *et al*. Unilateral multicystic dysplastic kidney: the case for nephrectomy. *Arch Dis Child* 1997;76(1):31–4.

54. Beckwith JB. Should asymptomatic unilateral multicystic dysplastic kidneys be removed because of the future risk of neoplasia? *Pediatr Nephrol* 1992;6(6):511.

15 | *The neonate with renal disease*

Jean-Pierre Guignard and Alfred Drukker

Introduction

The care of the healthy and sick newborn infant requires a thorough understanding of fetal development and of the major physiological changes that take place just prior to, at the time of, and immediately after birth. Paediatricians need to be aware of the normal physiological balance of the neonate, which is easily disturbed by disease or iatrogenic intervention. This chapter describes the special pathophysiological aspects of renal function and dysfunction in the human fetus and neonate, and describes renal disease states specific to the newborn period.

Embryology

Nephrogenesis in the human starts at 5 weeks of gestation. The primary final kidney, the metanephros, develops through partially functioning stages, the pro- and mesonephros. The metanephros will only be formed when clusters of the metanephric blastema come into contact with a tube growing upwards from the cloacal region, the ureteric bud. After this induction, a vesicle is formed which transforms into an S-shaped body. Following in-growth of endothelial cells, the precursors of small vessels, a primitive glomerulus is formed. Glomerular development commences at approximately 9 weeks of gestation. The urine collecting system is formed by elongation and tree-like division of the ureteric bud ('branching') and the transformation of cells of the metanephric mesenchyme into renal epithelial cells. A large network of capillaries generates an ever-growing filtration surface; larger vessels provide afferent and efferent renal blood flow.

The first circumstantial evidence that a humoral factor was involved in nephrogenesis was presented by Grobstein when studying the very specific reciprocal inductive processes of the metanephric mesenchyme and ureteric bud [1]. This is still one of the keystones of understanding kidney development. Our present knowledge implicates many factors in this primary inductive process, including tissue inhibitor of matrix metalloproteinase-2 (TIMP-2), the angiotensin-1 and -2 receptors (AT_1, AT_2), integrins, fibroblast growth factor-2 (FGF-2), *Pax-2* and *Pax-8*, and the *RET* gene. The entire process of renal embryology has, in recent years, been shown to be controlled and regulated by many genes (and gene products) as well as a variety of cytokines and growth factors. An in-depth description of these processes is presented in recent reviews [2–4].

There are a number of situations in which abnormalities in the expression of these key nephrogenesis genes have been shown to be associated with the development of clinical renal disease [5–10].

One kidney was generally thought to contain approximately one million nephrons. Recent evidence, however, indicates that this number is rather variable. More importantly, it has been shown that the endowment of nephrons at birth has a major impact on the general health of the individual later in life. Individuals born with a low nephron number appear to be at increased risk of subsequent hypertension, heart disease, and renal impairment [11].

Perinatal and postnatal renal function

Renal function *in utero*

During pregnancy, fetal body fluid homeostasis is controlled and maintained by the very effective bidirectional exchange between mother and fetus across the placental barrier. It could therefore be argued that fetal renal excretory function is superfluous. This is not the case. Fetal urine is produced from approximately the 10th week of gestation. By 22 weeks, the fetal urine production is 2–5 ml/h, rising to 25–40 ml/h at term. This is significantly more than in the immediate postnatal period (1–3 ml/h). Fetal urine is a major constituent of amniotic fluid contributing up to 60% of total volume at birth. Disturbances of the fetal cycle of swallowing amniotic fluid, upper gastrointestinal reabsorption, and renal excretion may lead to oligohydramnios (less than the expected amount of amniotic fluid at any specific stage of gestation) or polyhydramnios (>2 litres of amniotic fluid). The former is seen in renal agenesis and urinary tract obstruction, for example with posterior urethral valves. Pronounced oligohydramnios is responsible for the 'fetal compression' syndrome, most pronounced in renal agenesis, with the so-called Potter facies [12]. Polyhydramnios is caused either by primary overproduction of amniotic fluid, upper gastrointestinal obstruction, or fetal polyuria (diabetes insipidus, Bartter's syndrome) [13].

Because of the free passage of small chemical particles across the placenta, the *milieu intérieur* of the baby at the time of birth is basically identical to that of the mother. An example of this is that the plasma creatinine of the mother and the fetus during the second half of pregnancy equilibrate at all maternal plasma creatinine levels [14]. This balance is obviously disturbed when the umbilical cord is severed, after which the newborn baby will, in due time, reach a new steady state, based on independent neonatal factors.

Renal function in the newborn

Overall renal function at birth, both glomerular and tubular, is deficient in absolute as well as relative terms (corrected for $1.73 \, m^2$ body surface area) in comparison with late childhood or adult values [15]. Nevertheless, from the moment of birth the kidneys are very well equipped to deal with the

physiological burden of the neonate and are able to sustain normal development and maturation. The kidneys are, however, severely limited in their adaptive response to stress, be this due to disease or iatrogenic manipulations. When this limiting factor is not recognized, life-threatening situations may ensue. An overview of the major renal functional changes during the first year of life is presented in Table 15.1.

Renal blood flow

The kidneys of the newborn baby receive only 15–20% of the cardiac output, in contrast to the 25% observed in the adult. Most of the blood reaching the kidneys of the newborn immediately after birth is directed to the most mature sodium and water conserving nephrons, located deep in the renal cortex (juxtamedullary nephrons). The high renal vascular resistance, typical for the fetus and the newborn, and the initial pattern of intrarenal blood flow distribution change within days, results in a better overall renal perfusion, ultimately preferential to the nephrons in the outer cortex. A variety of vasoactive factors, including the renal nerves, adenosine, vasopressin, atrial natriuretic peptide, nitric oxide, endothelin, eicosanoids, the kallikrein–kinin system, and the renin–angiotensin axis are all involved in regulating these changes [16]. Many of these factors are also involved in the postnatal regulation of blood pressure (BP) and water and sodium homeostasis.

Glomerular filtration rate

At birth, systemic BP is low and the intravascular resistance extremely high, resulting in a very reduced driving force for filtration. In addition, at this early

Table 15.1 Normal values of renal function during infancy

	Premature infant	Term infant			
	First 3 days	First 3 days	2 weeks	8 weeks	1 year
Daily excretion of urine					
ml/kg/24 h	15–75	20–75	25–120	80–130	40–100
% of fluid intake	40–80	40–80	50–70	45–65	40–60
Maximal urine osmolality (mOsm/kg H_2O)	400–500	500–600	700–800	1000–1200	1200–1400
Glomerular filtration rate (ml/min/1.73 m^2)	10–15	15–20	35–45	75–80	90–110

age the filtration surface is severely limited. These are the main reasons why the glomerular filtration rate (GFR) at birth is very low, even when corrected for body surface area. The low GFR severely limits *all* renal functions, particularly with regard to water and electrolyte homeostasis and the excretion of waste products. This is particularly true for the premature infant. During the first month of life GFR increases rapidly, due to a rise in systemic BP, a concomitant fall in renal vascular resistance and enlargement of the filtration surface. GFR reaches stable adult levels at approximately 1 year of age. Autoregulation of GFR, that is maintenance of glomerular filtration when BP falls precipitously, is less efficient in the neonate than in the adult, which may predispose the kidneys of the newborn to hypovolaemic injury.

Neonatal fluid homeostasis

It has long been recognized that at birth the total body water (TBW) content of the term neonate is high (~75% of total body mass), most of which (~40% of total body mass) is extracellular fluid (ECF). Within days, the total amount of water starts to decrease and at the same time a shift of fluids between compartments commences; the ECF space contracts and water enters the cells, which increase in number and size. The intracellular fluid space (ICF) at 2 months of age comprises approximately 43% and the ECF 30% of body weight. By 9 months of age TBW is 62%, ICF 35%, and ECF 27% of body weight.

It is a well-known clinical observation that in the first days after birth, full-term infants lose 5–10% of their birthweight and that this percentage is somewhat higher in premature babies. This fluid loss comes primarily from the extra cellular space [17]. The total blood volume of the neonate immediately after birth (80–100 ml/kg) is largely dependent on the placental transfusion of whole blood, which is itself related to the time of clamping of the cord and the positioning of the baby in relation to the placenta at that time.

One of the characteristics of neonatal renal physiology is that most membranes are leaky, including those of the vasculature. When i.v. non-colloid fluids, such as saline or Ringer solution, are given, a large proportion will end up in the interstitial space. This, together with the low GFR, explains the low and delayed urinary excretion of such a load at this young age [18].

Urine concentrating and diluting capacity

The neonatal kidney has a low urinary concentrating capacity. One important consequence of this is that in the event of water depletion, such as is seen in severe vomiting, diarrhoea, fever, or phototherapy for hyperbilirubinaemia, the neonatal kidney will continue to produce an obligatory, dilute urine. Dehydration may ensue. Although the renal concentration mechanism is not well developed at birth (it matures rapidly within a month or two), the neonatal kidney is well attuned to dilute the urine adequately, a much older physiological mechanism in evolutionary terms [18]. This does not, however, mean that the infant can excrete a water load efficiently. This function is again limited, mainly by the low GFR of the newborn.

Acid–base balance

In all mammals the tight regulation of acid–base homeostasis is achieved through extra- and intracellular buffer systems and appropriate respiratory and, particularly, renal adaptations. At birth these buffers are well developed and the respiratory regulatory responses of a spontaneously breathing and neurologically intact newborn are good, although impaired in premature infants with respiratory problems. The renal compensatory mechanisms are slow and limited because of the low neonatal GFR and the not yet well developed tubular transport systems for bicarbonate and hydrogen ions. The available ammonia and neutral phosphate will bind hydrogen ions to form ammonium and acid phosphates ('titratable acid'), which are excreted in the urine.

The renal threshold for bicarbonate at birth in the full-term newborn infant is approximately 18–20 mmol/l, compared with 24–26 mmol/l in the adult, a level which is only reached at approximately 1 year of age. Premature infants may have a bicarbonate threshold as low as 14 mmol/l. This low threshold is responsible for the physiological metabolic acidosis of the newborn [19]. Disease (asphyxia, sepsis, volume depletion) or drug therapy may greatly aggravate this situation, leading to a pronounced metabolic acidosis, generally with an increased anion gap.

Key point

- In the newborn period, the glomerular filtration rate is low and the urine concentrating ability is limited.

Clinical and laboratory presentation of renal disease in the newborn

Antenatal evaluation

Recent years have seen tremendous strides in the evaluation of the unborn baby, to achieve better obstetric management and for the purpose of early diagnosis of disease in the fetus. In both instances the intrauterine evaluation consists of ultrasound (US) imaging of the position and the maturity of the fetus, its gender, as well as a review of fetal organs and estimation of the amount of amniotic fluid. Abnormalities of the urogenital system are the most frequently observed antenatal congenital abnormalities (unilateral or bilateral renal agenesis, urinary tract obstruction with hydronephrosis, cyst formation, renal masses, malinsertion of ureters), followed by cardiac and central nervous system problems. Antenatally detected hydronephrosis needs frequent follow-up by US with measurement of the renal and pelvic diameters, for which normal values are available [20] (see Chapter 14). US information on the volume of amniotic fluid can provide insight into possible renal impairment. When severe hydronephrosis is found, the obstetrician is faced with having to decide between advising *in-utero* intervention or proceeding with careful conservative follow-up until delivery. The amount of amniotic fluid is an all-important index to be followed, since impaired fetal urine flow (fetal oliguria) may result in oligohydramnios. Intrauterine hydronephrosis with oligohydramnios is therefore an ominous sign.

Intrauterine surgical intervention for hydronephrosis in the fetus has unfortunately been disappointing with regard to both renal outcome and the incidence of significant complications. The advantages of early delivery to hasten postnatal management of the renal disease have to be weighed very carefully against the dangers of extreme prematurity. 'Wait and see' still seems the wisest course to be taken, with careful obstetric follow-up together with nephro-urological consultations. In early pregnancy an abortion can be performed on a severely affected fetus. This is discussed in more detail in Chapter 13.

Postnatal evaluation

Clinical

One of the difficulties in treating neonates is the paucity of organ-specific symptoms of disease. This holds true for neonatal renal disorders. Many kidney diseases of the newborn may (initially) have no, or very few, renal signs and symptoms, and often the only manifestations are hypothermia instead of fever, listlessness, feeding difficulties, vomiting, diarrhoea, poor growth, jaundice, convulsions, and respiratory distress. Under these conditions the diagnostic acumen of the physician is severely tested and has to rely mainly on a good physical examination combined with a few basic laboratory investigations and a high index of suspicion for an underlying renal disorder. A thorough ante– and postnatal history of mother and child (and family) with, in addition, results of previous antenatal US examination, if available, are indispensable. Information should be obtained about familial renal disease such as renal malformations or the much rarer autosomal recessive or dominant polycystic kidney disease, congenital nephrotic syndrome, or diabetes insipidus. The paediatrician should enquire whether the pregnancy and delivery were normal (infections, medications, ultrasonographic screening, results of α-fetoprotein testing, amount of amniotic fluid, position and weight and size of the placenta, Apgar score, number of umbilical vessels). The course of previous pregnancies needs to be known.

Inspection of the neonate may indicate a renal disorder. The following findings may indicate renal disease: a single umbilical artery (congenital renal malformations), eye abnormalities such as aniridia, ear deformities, peri-auricular pits, branchial fistulas and cysts (congenital renal malformations), Potter facies consisting of a beaked nose, wide-set eyes with a prominent fold arising from the inner canthus and low-set ears (bilateral renal agenesis), heart failure (hypertension), absence or deficiency of abdominal muscles with cryptorchidism (the so-called prune belly triad when combined with megacystis–megaureter), deformities of lumbar or sacral spine (meningomyelocele) and other skeletal problems (renal malformations), imperforate anus, bladder extrophy, and genital abnormalities including epi- or hypospadia and meatal stenosis (renal malformations). A long list of well-known and relatively easily recognizable congenital or inborn paediatric syndromes have renal involvement. These are discussed in Chapter 17.

Peripheral oedema is not rare in newborns, particularly in premature infants. The cause of this generally temporary physiological finding is unclear, but may be due to changes in distribution of body fluids and possibly 'leaky' neonatal membranes and/or vitamin E deficiency. Oedema may also be due to heart failure and a wide variety of kidney diseases, e.g. congenital nephrotic syndrome, as well as iatrogenic fluid overload. The finding of generalized oedema and ascites (hydrops or anasarca) was in the past almost a sine qua non for erythroblastosis due to blood-group incompatibility; nowadays this is fortunately a very rare occurrence. Other causes of ascites and oedema are liver disease, leakage of bile or lymph (chylous ascites), and gastrointestinal or urinary tract obstruction (urinary ascites).

Observing urine output

When a renal disorder is suspected, urine voiding patterns have to be evaluated. Normally, more than 90% of newborns pass urine within 24 hours. If after 48 h no urine has been passed, nephro-urological investigations are indicated. Estimation of the urine flow rate should be undertaken with a small catheter draining into a 'sterile' urine bag. It has to be realized that even under the best of circumstances such a collection is rarely accurate. The normal urine volume of neonates varies between 1–3 ml/kg/h. Oliguria in the newborn is defined as a urine output of less than 1 ml/kg/h. A poor urinary stream and dribbling may indicate obstruction of the lower urinary tract (e.g. posterior urethral valves) or other abnormality, and warrants further investigation, initially with ultrasound examination. Polyuria (urine flow rate greater than 3 ml/kg/h) is best followed with frequent weighing of the infant. Weight loss in significant excess of 10% of total body weight in a term infant needs to be carefully investigated by estimation of fluid intake and output, urine osmolality (or specific gravity, SG) and blood and urinary electrolytes, as well as exclusion of an osmotic diuresis secondary to glycosuria. Such a postnatal weight loss in a healthy, breast- or formula-fed baby with a urine osmolality below 200 mosm/kg H_2O (SG < 1.005) may be the first sign of diabetes insipidus. This necessitates evaluation of the maximal urine concentration capacity after stimulation with 1-deamino-8-D-arginine vasopressin (DDAVP®). It has to be remembered that premature infants may have a temporary polyuric phase due to relative fluid overload that needs to be excreted.

Palpation of abdomen

On examination the emphasis, from a renal point of view, is on palpation of the abdomen, unless obvious other lesions are present. In the healthy neonate both kidneys can easily be felt; their size is approximately 4.5×2.5 cm. Familial genetic or congenital renal cystic disease is generally associated with easily palpable, large kidneys. Such a finding has to be differentiated from other abdominal masses that can be found in 1% of newborns. This should preferably be done by abdominal US or, when necessary, with other imaging techniques. The differential diagnosis of a palpable abdominal mass is shown in Table 15.2.

Laboratory tests

In the newborn one should strive—more than at any other age—to perform the minimum number of preferably non-invasive laboratory tests necessary to confirm a clinical diagnosis.

The urine of the newborn is dilute alkaline, and often contains a small amount of protein during the first days of life, particularly in premature infants. Proteinuria varies with gestational and postnatal ages and is slightly higher in premature neonates than in term neonates. Transient, physiological proteinuria may be observed during the first days of life (mean on day 1, 500 mg/l; mean on day 4, 200 mg/l, both with a large range; by 2 weeks of life, it decreases to 50 mg/l or below) [21]. Persistent heavy proteinuria (>100 mg/mmol creatinine) is rare, but when present necessitates further evaluation, in particular for infectious diseases (toxoplasmosis, cytomegalovirus, HIV), nephrotoxic medications (antibiotics, mercury

Table 15.2 Causes of abdominal masses in the neonate

Type of mass	Percentage of total
Renal	55
Hydronephrosis	
Multicystic dysplastic kidney	
Polycystic kidney disease	
Mesoblastic nephroma	
Renal ectopia	
Renal vein thrombosis	
Nephroblastomatosis	
Wilms' tumour	
Genital	15
Hydrometrocolpos	
Ovarian cyst	
Gastrointestinal	15
Non-renal retroperitoneal	10
Hepato-spleno-biliary	5

Table 15.3   Causes of proteinuria in the newborn

Physiological proteinuria
Vascular disorders
   Renal venous thrombosis
   Corticomedullary necrosis
Congenital nephrotic syndrome
   Hereditary diseases
      Finnish type
      Onycho-osteodysplasia (nail–patella syndrome)
      Severe infantile sialidosis
Infectious diseases
   Syphilis
   Toxoplasmosis
   Cytomegalovirus
   HIV
Medications
   Mercury compounds
   Other nephrotoxic compounds

Table 15.4   Major causes of haematuria in the newborn

Bleeding tendency
Vascular disorders
   Acute tubular necrosis
   Corticomedullary necrosis
   Renal venous thrombosis
   Adrenal haemorrhage
Cystic diseases
   Autosomal recessive polycystic kidney disease
   Autosomal dominant polycystic kidney disease
   Cystic dysplasia
   Multicystic dysplastic kidney
Tumours
   Wilms' tumor
   Mesoblastic nephroma and fetal hamartoma
   Angioma
Trauma
Obstructive/refluxing uropathy
Nephritides
   Pyelonephritis
   Interstitial nephritis (drugs)
   Glomerulonephritis

compounds), congenital nephrotic syndrome, renal venous thrombosis, or acute renal insufficiency with tubular necrosis (Table 15.3). Gross haematuria is rare and should be differentiated from the so-called 'red diaper syndrome' caused by discoloration of the urine due to urate crystals or *Serratia marcescens*. Mild temporary glucosuria is not uncommon and results from low glucose thresholds in short and immature tubuli. The urine sediment may contain a few (3–10) red and 25 (males) to 50 (females) white blood cells per high-power field. The various causes of significant haematuria are given in Table 15.4. Significant pyuria is seen in acute urinary tract infections as well as systemic infections often occurring simultaneously. Urine cultures taken by sterile bags are notoriously unreliable in both sexes. When urinary tract infection (UTI) is suspected, for example in septicaemia of the newborn, urine should be obtained by a suprapubic aspiration of the bladder, together with a blood culture. In the newborn period it is impossible to obtain an accurately timed urine collection without bladder catheterization. Therefore, chemical analysis of spot urine samples is often expressed as urine solute to creatinine ratios. These ratios are, however, unreliable in the newborn period, mainly because of great variations in urinary creatinine concentrations at this young age [22].

Few blood tests are required. For evaluation of renal disease, the acid–base status of the baby, a blood count, a blood culture, viral serology, as well as plasma creatinine and electrolyte levels, should generally suffice. Plasma creatinine at the time of birth reflects the maternal plasma creatinine level. Surprisingly, plasma creatinine rises after birth in very low birthweight infants: the more premature the infant, the higher the creatinine level [14]. This is probably due to the tubular reabsorption of creatinine, in contrast to the tubular secretion of creatinine seen at all other ages. Tubular reabsorption of creatinine is probably due to the back-diffusion of creatinine across leaky immature tubules [23]. It should therefore be realized that during the first 2–3 weeks of life, high plasma creatinine levels are physiological and not a reflection of possible renal insufficiency. Once the plasma creatinine stabilizes, the GFR can be estimated by a formula devised by Schwartz *et al.* [24,25] based on plasma creatinine (μmol/l) and the length (cm) of the infant (child), with a special correction factor, K, for full-term infants ($K = 33$) [24] and low birthweight babies ($K = 24$) [25]:

$$\text{GFR (ml/min/1.73 m}^2) = K \frac{\text{length (cm)}}{\text{creatinine } (\mu\text{mol/l})}.$$

Creatinine output per unit body weight increases steadily during growth as a function of muscle mass. Creatinine excretion correlates with gestational age, body length, and body weight, the best correlation being observed with the latter: creatinine output $= 71 \pm 10 \, \mu$mol/kg per 24 h [26].

Key points

- On inspection of the neonate, certain external abnormalities may suggest renal disease.

- The plasma creatinine concentration is elevated at birth, and further increases transiently in very premature infants.

- More than 90% of newborns will pass urine within the first 24 hours of life: investigations are indicated in those who have not passed urine by 48 hours of age.

Congenital renal diseases in the neonate

Congenital nephrotic syndrome

The clinical picture of congenital nephrotic syndrome consists of a severe, steroid-resistant proteinuria leading to excessive oedema formation shortly after birth [27]. This is discussed in more detail in Chapter 19.

Bartter's syndrome

In 1962, Bartter and colleagues described a clinical entity consisting of failure to thrive, mental retardation, hypokalaemic alkalosis, and normotensive hyperaldosteronism, generally presenting within the first 2 years of life. There are several forms of neonatal Bartter's syndrome due to defective genes (*SLC12A1* on 15q15–21 in type 1, *KCNJ1* on 11q24–25 in type 2, *CLCNKB* on 1p36 in type 3, and *SLC12A3* on 16q13 in Gitelman syndrome) [28]. The neonatal forms of Bartter's syndrome are characterized by polyhydramnios (fetal polyuria), premature birth, severe polyuria with polydipsia (difficult to assess in the newborn period), and even dangerous dehydration due to impaired tubular water conservation. Hypercalciuria and early onset nephrocalcinosis are common. The disease, differential diagnoses, and management are discussed in more detail in Chapter 5.

Nephrogenic diabetes insipidus

The polyuria of nephrogenic diabetes insipidus (NDI) starts before birth and can cause polyhydramnios, probably the first sign of the disease on an antenatal

US examination. The disease is caused by a hereditary defect causing distal tubular insensitivity to arginine vasopressin, the antidiuretic hormone [29]. The most common X-linked recessive form of the disease is due to a mutation of the vasopressin-2 (V2) receptor gene, whereas the rare autosomal recessive and dominant forms are caused by a defect in the water channel gene, aquaporin 2 (*AQP2*). The polyuria is not readily recognized after birth and therefore the non-specific symptoms of significant weight loss (>10% of body weight) and 'unexplained' fever should arouse suspicion. Another non-specific sign of the disease is failure to thrive, probably due to insufficient calorie intake because of the polydipsia. Hydronephrosis is not uncommon. Severe hypernatraemia can cause cerebral bleeding and should be avoided. These episodes of haemorrhage followed by cerebral calcification have been cited as the cause of mental retardation observed in this disease. The diagnosis of NDI will rest on the finding of a low urine osmolality ($U_{osm} < 200$ mosm/kg H_2O or urine SG < 1.005) with failure to increase after the administration of DDAVP®. Treatment consists of the administration of adequate quantities of low-osmotic, low-sodium fluids (comparable to maternal milk), combined with the use of thiazide diuretics such as hydrochlorothiazide (2–4 mg/kg/24 h). By contracting the extracellular space, and consequently stimulating proximal sodium reabsorption, the diuretic paradoxically induces water conservation. Prostaglandin synthesis inhibitors such as indometacin (2 mg/kg/24 h) have been used concomitantly, with encouraging results, but not without risk! Indometacin may indeed alter renal function and produce adverse haematopoietic reactions as well as gastrointestinal bleeding. Careful clinical and laboratory monitoring is thus mandatory. With the advances in the genetic background of the disease, new treatment modalities can be expected.

Oligonephropathy

In 1962, Royer *et al.* [30] were the first to describe a rare form of (bilateral) renal hypoplasia with few, enlarged nephrons, ultimately leading to renal insufficiency in early childhood. The condition was termed oligomeganephronia. Interest in this condition increased following two independent observations. The first showed that in experimental animal models, reduction of the number of nephrons leads to generalized and glomerular hypertension, burdening each remaining nephron with an increased work load ('hyperfiltration') and progressive nephrosclerosis with chronic renal insufficiency [31,32]. The other observation was an epidemiological survey showing a high incidence of hypertension (and later also of chronic renal insufficiency and diabetes) in human adults born prematurely, with a reduced number of nephrons [11]. The number of nephrons at birth is not only dependent upon the length of gestation but is also controlled by many genetic as well as environmental factors, including intrauterine nutrition (impaired placental transport, protein and vitamin A deficiency) [33], drug administration (gentamicin, ciclosporin A), and irradiation. Various diseases associated with a low birthweight and the associated low complement of nephrons in humans (hypertension, diabetes) are major causes of morbidity and mortality in the adult population when not treated appropriately, thus posing a significant public health problem. In practice, all the paediatrician/neonatologist can do is to help and promote optimal nutrition in pregnant women and emphasize the risk of drugs given to the expectant mother, as well as the long-term effect of significant premature delivery. Blood pressure should be measured throughout childhood in children born prematurely. The latter information should accompany the child/adolescent when he/she is transferred to the care of the general practitioner or a specialist in internal medicine. These physicians will rarely enquire about the length of gestation and the birthweight of the individual!

Key points

- Congenital diseases such as congenital nephrotic syndrome, Bartter's syndrome, and nephrogenic diabetes insipidus may be suspected before birth.

- A reduced nephron number at birth is associated with significant long-term renal and cardio-vascular morbidity.

Acquired renal diseases

Acute renal failure

Acute renal failure (ARF) is one of the most serious renal disorders of the newborn. It is generally accompanied by oligo- or anuria, although in some cases of severe ARF, no significant fall in urine output is observed, so-called non-oliguric ARF. This is most commonly, though not exclusively, seen in association with drug toxicity, particularly with aminoglycosides [34,35]. Causes of ARF in the neonatal period are shown in Table 15.5.

For diagnostic and therapeutic purposes ARF is divided into three somewhat overlapping categories: pre-renal, intrinsic renal, and post-renal ARF. The most easily identifiable and treatable causes of ARF are the pre-renal and post-renal categories.

Table 15.5 Aetiology of neonatal renal failure

Antenatal vascular damage
    Maternal treatment: non-steroidal anti-inflammatory
      drugs, angiotensin converting enzyme inhibitors
    Twin–twin transfusion
    Co-twin death
    Neonatal renal failure associated with intrauterine
      growth retardation and severe oligohydramnios
Primary renal and urological diseases
    Congenital bilateral obstructive uropathies (posterior
      urethral valves)
    Polycystic kidney disease
    Renal dysplasia/hypoplasia
    Multicystic dysplasia
    Renal agenesis
    Rarely:
      Renal tubular dysgenesis
      Idiopathic diffuse mesangial sclerosis
      Neonatal renal failure with glomerular immaturity
      Finnish-type congenital nephrotic syndrome
Acquired postnatal renal diseases
    Shock
    Dehydration
    Perinatal haemorrhage (i.e. abruptio placentae)
    Necrotizing enterocolitis
    Heart failure
    Cardiopulmonary bypass; extracorporeal
      membrane oxygenation
    Disseminated intravascular coagulation
    Vascular thrombosis (artery, vein)
    Perinatal asphyxia
    Haemolytic uraemic syndrome
    Isoimmune haemolytic diseases with
      massive haemoglobinuria
    Myoglobinuria, haemoglobinuria,
      uric acid nephropathy
    Infection: pyelonephritis, syphilis,
      toxoplasmosis, candidiasis
    Bilateral fungal bezoar
    Closure of congenital abdominal wall defects
    Nephrotoxic drug administration: non-steroidal
      anti-inflammatory drugs (indometacin); converting
      enzyme inhibitors (captopril, enalapril); contrast
      media; amphotericin B; aminoglycosides; vancomycin

Pre-renal ARF is generally caused by a failure of the systemic circulation in the course of fluid loss due to diarrhoea, vomiting, haemorrhage, high environmental temperature, sudden compartmental fluid shifts, e.g. during cardiac surgery, and rarely in the course of prolonged phototherapy for jaundice. The aetiology of individual cases of pre-renal ARF is generally clearly apparent. Early diagnosis and rapid fluid replacement can often prevent pre-renal ARF or greatly improve its outcome. In the majority of cases, the prognosis is favourable; even in the face of prolonged oligo- or anuria the kidneys tend to eventually 'open-up' spontaneously. Complete clinical recovery is generally the rule. Until that time, conservative therapeutic measures need to be taken, aimed at preventing disturbances in water and electrolyte balance. These are discussed in more detail in Chapter 22. If these do not suffice, temporary renal replacement therapy may be necessary (see below).

The causes of *post-renal ARF* are less obvious and will generally only be detected when an US examination of the entire urogenital tract and the abdomen is undertaken. It is for this reason that this investigation should be performed as soon as possible in all infants with ARF, even in those with an apparent cause of their renal failure. In most cases of post-renal ARF, a bilateral urinary tract obstructive lesion will be detected, though this may occasionally be unilateral with a non-functioning or absent contralateral kidney. With temporary drainage or surgical repair of the obstructed urinary tract, reasonably good short-term results can be obtained. The ultimate prognosis in babies with post-renal ARF will, however, depend on the extent of the renal parenchymal damage sustained during antenatal and early postnatal life.

Intrinsic renal ARF carries the worst prognosis. Its causes are acute vascular events, such as renal venous thrombosis (traumatic delivery, child of diabetic mother) or renal artery stenosis (following umbilical catheterization for fluid management in neonatal intensive care units), congenital, familial nephritides, including congenital nephrotic syndrome, acute interstitial nephritis (drug allergy), or, very rarely, renal deposition of large amounts of bilirubin, uric acid, calcium, oxalate, or haemoglobin/myoglobin.

Clinical

The clinical signs of ARF are a combination of the symptoms associated with the underlying disease and that of the renal insufficiency, which may cause disturbances in water, electrolyte and acid–base homeostasis, hypertension, and uraemia.

Laboratory

Proteinuria, haematuria, and an active urinary sediment with red cells, casts, and debris are very suggestive of intrinsic ARF. Chemical analysis of urine (only drops are needed) is the easiest, least expensive, and most helpful way to distinguish between the pre-renal and intrinsic forms of ARF (Table 15.6). These chemical tests are based on the assumption that previously healthy kidneys respond to acute hypoperfusion by maximally conserving water and electrolytes. In contrast, an intrinsically damaged kidney will not be able to do so, because with renal parenchymal damage the renal concentrating capacity is one of the first renal functions to be affected. Therefore, a urinary osmolarity (U_{osm}) greater than 400 mosm/kg H_2O, a urinary sodium concentration (U_{Na}) less than 40 mmol/l and a fractional excretion of sodium (FE_{Na}) below 2% suggest a pre-renal problem, whereas a U_{osm} of less than 400 mosm/kg H_2O, a U_{Na} greater than 40 mmol/l and a FE_{Na} above 2.5% indicate intrinsic renal ARF. The calculation of FE_{Na} is more reliable than the U_{Na} values. It has to be realized that these indices are only valid in the early stages of ARF, before volume expanders and/or diuretics are given. In addition, caution should be exercised when applying these indices to very premature, salt-losing neonates with 'normal' FE_{Na} values sometimes in excess of 5%.

Imaging studies

In complex cases of ARF, invasive imaging studies may be indicated. We re-emphasize, however, that it is

Table 15.6 Diagnostic indices in neonates with acute oliguria

	Acute pre-renal failure	Acute intrinsic renal failure
U_{osm} (mosm/kg H_2O)	>400	<400
U_{Na}, (mmol/l)	<40	>40
U/P urea	>20	<10
U/P osm	>1.3	<1.0
FeNa%	<2	>3

FeNa: fractional excretion of sodium: (U/PNa)/(U/Pcreatinine)

prudent to make maximal use of US-Doppler facilities. All other imaging studies (except perhaps MRI) employ contrast media, which should be avoided in any form of ARF when possible, particularly in the newborn period.

Treatment

The treatment of ARF depends upon the underlying cause. In pre-renal ARF, the first phase of the treatment schedule consists of a rapid correction of the fluid deficit with isotonic saline, saline–glucose, or Ringer solutions containing 20–25 mmol/l of sodium bicarbonate. When no urine flow results, this initial therapeutic step should be followed by the administration of 20–25 ml/kg plasma and 2–5 mg/kg of a loop diuretic (furosemide). The use of intravenous mannitol is not recommended because of the risk of intracerebral haemorrhage as a consequence of a brisk increase in plasma osmolality. When the above measures fail, it has to be assumed that intrinsic renal damage has occurred, which necessitates a different, far more conservative therapeutic approach. This consists mainly of maintaining fluid and electrolyte homeostasis. Fluid restriction is indicated; the amount of fluids administered will have to be based on insensible fluid losses (0.7 ml/kg/h in full-term neonates, higher in low birthweight infants and depending on many factors, such as whether the babies have fever or if phototherapy is needed) and gastrointestinal and urinary losses (Table 15.7). Acidosis, hyperkalaemia, hyperphosphataemia, and hypocalcaemia need to be controlled, while restricting fluid intake to insensible losses plus urine output. When prescribing fluid replacement, it has to be realized that most babies with pre-renal ARF, certainly after unsuccessful fluid resuscitation, are volume expanded. These calculations have to be performed on a 3-hourly, rather than a daily, basis. Often only minimal volumes of fluids can be given, and great care must be taken to maintain normoglycaemia. This requires a very careful approach, with frequent weighing (which is associated with significant practical difficulties in the sick neonate) and monitoring of BP, heart, and pulmonary function in a neonatal intensive care setting. If these latter measures also fail, some form of acute renal replacement therapy must be considered, such as continuous arteriovenous haemofiltration/ haemodialysis (CAVH/CAVHD) [36] or peritoneal dialysis (PD) [37] (see Chapter 22).

Table 15.7 Normal fluid losses in the neonate

	Birth weight		
	<1500 g	1500–2500 g	>2500 g
Fluid losses (ml/kg/24h)			
Basal insensible fluid	30–60	15–35	15–25
Stool	5–10	5–10	5–10
Urine[a]	50–100	50–100	50–100
Increment for phototherapy	20	20	20

[a] Urinary fluid loss is calculated as the amount of water needed at a urine osmolality of 150–300 mosm/kg H_2O when renal solute excretions equal 15 mosm/kg birth weight per day.

In intrinsic ARF, the therapeutic approach is as above but generally without the initial active phase of restoring fluid balance. In post-renal (obstructive) ARF, a surgical approach is often needed, augmented with some of the above measures if renal function remains impaired after adequate drainage of the urinary tract. In the recovery phase of pre-renal ARF and after relief of long-standing urinary tract obstruction, the urine output may be large with the danger of non-recognized secondary hypovolaemia. Urine output and body weight monitoring is mandatory.

Complications

The major complication of any form of ARF is iatrogenic infection. It must therefore be stressed that during all stages of the management of the sick baby with ARF, strict sterility and hygiene should be maintained. The fewer bladder and i.v. catheters, the better. Aggressive empirical antibiotic treatment is often necessary.

Outcome

Promptly treated pre-renal ARF has a good renal prognosis. When acute tubular necrosis ensues, a prolonged period of anuria/oliguria (2–3 weeks) can be expected with a good chance of eventual recovery. The outcome of intrinsic ARF depends somewhat on the underlying cause, but may be good in those without significant extrarenal morbidity [38]. In post-renal ARF, the extent of the renal parenchymal damage is the major predictor of long-term outcome;

where there has been prolonged severe obstruction to the urinary tract with significant parenchymal loss, e.g. after posterior urethral valves, the outcome is less good. Even with the most up-to-date therapeutic measures, the overall mortality of ARF is still high. Intrinsic renal failure has indeed been associated with high mortality, ranging from 20 to 75%, with survival relating to the reversibility of the underlying condition (hypoxia, asphyxia, shock, infection, cardiac failure).

Key points

- Acute renal failure is usually functional and reversible.

- Intrinsic causes of acute renal failure are associated with a less favourable outcome.

- Although technically difficult, dialysis can be performed in the newborn period.

Renal vascular thrombosis

Renal venous thrombosis

Renal venous thrombosis predominantly affects male infants (male:female ratio ~2/1) of diabetic and pre-diabetic mothers, and is seen more frequently after traumatic deliveries. It is more common in infants with a thrombotic tendency due to haemoconcentration, hyperviscocity or hypovolaemia, whatever their cause [39]. Protein C deficiency and homocystinuria, both rare hereditary diseases, are associated with hypercoagulability and need to be considered in the differential diagnosis of renal venous thrombosis. The thrombosis generally starts in the arcuate and/or interlobular vessels and extends into the main renal veins; the entire venous drainage system of the kidney(s) can be affected and the thrombus sometimes extends into the neighbouring vessels, such as the suprarenal vein or the vena cava. When the latter is affected, oedema may be seen in the lower extremities. The diagnosis of renal venous thrombosis should be suspected in every neonate with haematuria (often macroscopic), reduced urinary output, and decreased renal function. In the acute stages hypertension is often absent. The affected kidney becomes swollen and enlarged and can generally be easily palpated. Anaemia, thrombocytopenia, fragmented red blood cells, and increased levels of fibrinogen degradation products can be detected. A thorough US-Doppler examination can show the obstructive lesion(s) and provide information on renal venous blood flow. A non-functioning kidney on [^{99}Tc]DTPA scan indicates absent perfusion. The treatment of renal venous thrombosis is the subject of some debate. Some advocate a conservative approach, hoping for recanalization of the thrombus, while others recommend a very active therapeutic strategy with the i.v. administration of a thrombolytic agent such as urokinase. This requires very careful monitoring of the coagulation status of the neonate and is not without danger, particularly in premature infants at high risk of intraventricular haemorrhage. The intermediate approach, recommended in most cases, consists of systemic heparinization, preferably with low molecular weight heparin in a dose (100 IU/kg 'stat' and 25 IU/kg/h thereafter) to achieve a bleeding time of 240–300 s or an activated partial thromboplastin time (PTT) of 1.5–2 times normal. Recent experience indicates that recombinant human tissue plasminogen activator may be a good alternative (Table 15.8). Adequate nutrition and the general measures of 'intrinsic' ARF are indicated. The prognosis of renal venous thrombosis depends on the extent of the lesion and whether the lesion is uni- or bilateral. The latter will often lead to chronic renal insufficiency. When the vena cava is affected, subsequent obliteration of its lumen and extensive collateral circulation can be observed. Significant hypertension is one of the most important long-term complications of renal venous thrombosis and all survivors should have their BP measured on a regular basis. Following an acute episode of thrombosis, all neonates should be screened for coagulation disorders, such as protein C deficiency or factor V Leiden mutation.

Key point

- Renal venous thrombosis affects infants of diabetic mothers and infants with a thrombotic tendency due to haemoconcentration, hyperviscosity, or hypovolaemia.

Table 15.8 Thrombolysis with recombinant tissue-type plasminogen activator (r-TPA) in neonates with renal vascular thrombosis (vein or artery ± aorta)

Obtain parental consent
r-TPA administration
   Heparin is stopped 3 h before the r-TPA is administered
   r-TPA is infused in an indwelling vascular catheter
   r-TPA: 0.1 mg/kg over a 10-min period followed by
      0.3 mg/kg per hour over a 3-h period
   Additional r-TPA infusions at intervals of 12–24 h
      if revascularization is not complete
      (colour-flow Doppler imaging). The r-TPA dose can be
      increased up to 0.4 mg/kg/h
   Arterial punctures, urinary catheterizations, subcutaneous,
      or intramuscular injections are not allowed
   Maintain the fibrinogen concentration ⩾1.5 g/l
      during r-TPA administration
Heparin administration
   Heparin is initiated at the end of the r-TPA infusion
   Initial heparin dose is 100 U/kg/day
   Adjustment of heparin dose with activated PTT or
      anti-factor Xa concentration
Contraindications to r-TPA administration
   Absolute
      Major surgery during the past 10 days
      Pre-existing intracranial haemorrhage or
         cerebral ischaemia
      A history of severe bleeding (pulmonary,
         gastrointestinal)
   Relative (to correct before
      thrombolysis therapy is performed)
      Platelet count <100 000/mm^3
      Fibrinogen concentration <1 g/l
      Severe coagulation factor deficiency
      Arterial hypertension

PTT, partial thromboplastin time.

Renal artery thrombosis

Renal artery thrombosis is seen most frequently in neonates who have been administered high osmotic fluids via the umbilical artery, where the tip of the aortic catheter is placed in the region of the renal artery. This has become one of the most frequent causes of hypertension in the neonate (see below), which needs to be treated aggressively because of the possible complications of congestive heart failure and/or intracranial haemorrhage.

Urinary tract infection

Clinical

The incidence of neonatal UTI is 0.7% in full-term neonates and almost 3% in premature infants. The first month of life is the only time when there is a clear male preponderance of the incidence of UTI (male:female, 5:1). The increased susceptibility of premature babies continues during the entire first year of life [40]. A high incidence of UTI has been noted in children with urinary tract malformations [41], immediately following circumcision, and, for unknown reasons, also in those exposed to cocaine *in utero* and in the postnatal period. The most common invading organism in the neonatal period is *Escherichia coli*, followed by *Klebsiella pneumonia, Proteus mirabilis*, coliform bacteria, *Pseudomonas aeruginosa*, enterococci, staphylococci, streptococci group B, and *Candida albicans* (in premature infants). The clinical manifestations of UTI are atypical, sometimes with hypothermia instead of fever, irritability, poor feeding, and vomiting [42]. Unexplained jaundice should raise the suspicion of urosepsis.

Laboratory

Sterile urine collection is extremely difficult in the neonate. Bag specimens of urine are unreliable, both in male and female babies. Urine culture samples should therefore be obtained exclusively by percutaneous suprapubic aspiration or bladder catheterization. The latter should be performed with a small-sized sterile feeding tube and not with a Foley catheter.

The immediate evaluation of a baby with UTI includes a careful sepsis work-up, ultrasound examination of the entire urinary tract, and probably a micturating cystourethrogram once the infection is under control. The diagnosis and investigation of UTI is discussed in detail in Chapter 11.

Treatment

The treatment of neonatal UTI should not be postponed. Once infection is suspected and reliable blood and urine cultures have been obtained, treatment should be started immediately. The choice of the antibiotic(s) will depend on many factors, including local knowledge of the most common invading organisms and their antibiotic sensitivities. The most commonly accepted initial treatment of neonatal UTI is still based on i.v. amoxicillin (50–100 mg/kg/24 h) and gentamicin (3.5–7.5 mg/kg/24 h) for approximately 10 days, with constant monitoring of gentamicin (and creatinine) blood levels. Once the urine culture results have been obtained, the treatment can be adjusted according to the sensitivity of the cultured micro-organism.

Key point

- A high incidence of urinary tract infection is present in newborn infants with urinary tract malformations.

Arterial hypertension

Hypertension in the healthy newborn is rare. The offspring of hypertensive parents (especially where both parents are hypertensive) will, from as early as the newborn period, have a slightly higher blood pressure (BP) than babies with normotensive parents [43]. Hypertension is not, however, rare (1–2%) in sick neonates and this is particularly so in babies treated in neonatal intensive care units. It is one of the more significant complications of catheterization of the umbilical arteries for fluid administration including parenteral feeding. Other causes of hypertension at this age are shown in Table 15.9. With modern Doppler techniques, which are available in all modern newborn nurseries, there should nowadays be no problem measuring BP in any neonate [44]. Doppler measurements are reliable and reproducible, in comparison to direct intra-arterial readings. The cuff should cover at least 50% of the circumference of one of the upper extremities while the infant is relatively quiet (preferably not during feeding). Ausculatory BP measurements are possible but cumbersome, requiring much patience on the part of the doctor, nurse, and mother. Normal data for BP of male and female neonates of all birth weights are now available (Tables 15.10 and 15.11) [45–47]. Following birth, the BP rises by 1–2 mmHg/day during the first week and thereafter by 1–2 mmHg/week until 2 months of age. Hypertension is defined, as in older children, by the finding of repeated BP readings (on at least three different occasions) above the 95th percentile for age, weight, and gender.

In the newborn with hypertension, coarctation of the aorta should be excluded by palpation of the femoral pulses and BP measurements in all four extremities (see normal values in Tables 15.10 and 15.11). If suspected clinically, imaging techniques should be performed, including abdominal US-Doppler examination and eventually aortography. The latter is not easy at this young age. When BP can be controlled with drug therapy, invasive imaging

Table 15.9 Main causes of hypertension in the newborn

Vascular
　Renal artery hypoplasia/stenosis/thrombus
　Coarctation of the aorta
　Aortic/renal thrombus secondary to umbilical artery
　　catheterization
Renal
　Polycystic kidney disease
　Multicystic dysplasia/hypoplastic kidney(s)
　Obstructive uropathy
　Acute and chronic renal failure
Tumours
　Neuroblastoma
　Mesoblastoma
　Phaeochromocytoma
Endocrine
　Congenital adrenal hyperplasia
　Cushing's syndrome
　Thyrotoxicosis
Central nervous system
　Raised intracranial pressure
　Meningitis
　Convulsions
Respiratory
　Bronchopulmonary dysplasia
Miscellaneous
　Drugs: phenylephrine eye drops (10% solution)
　Infants of drug-taking mothers
　Adrenal haemorrhage with renal artery compression
　Closure of abdominal wall defects
　Idiopathic (in premature infants)
　Increased cardiac output and/or peripheral resistance
　Blood hyperviscosity
　Hyperactive sympathetic nervous system
　Severe hypercalcaemia

Table 15.10 Range of systolic and diastolic BP (mmHg ± SD) in healthy premature infants (below 2000 g) in the first week of life

Age (days)	Systolic		Diastolic	
	Minimum	Maximum	Minimum	Maximum
1	48 ± 9	63 ± 12	25 ± 7	35 ± 10
4	57 ± 10	71 ± 11	32 ± 8	45 ± 10
7	61 ± 7	74 ± 12	34 ± 9	46 ± 10

Table 15.11 Systolic BP (mmHg ± SD)[a] of healthy newborn infants, in relation to postnatal age and level of consciousness

State of animation	3 days	6 days	8–10 days	6 weeks
Awake	72 ± 6	77 ± 10	88 ± 17	96 ± 11
Asleep	68 ± 7	72 ± 9	75 ± 9	89 ± 11

[a] Measured by the Doppler technique (mean ± SD).

techniques should be deferred until a later date. Renal artery stenosis can sometimes be diagnosed by the auscultation of an abdominal 'bruit'. Endocrine causes of hypertension may be detectable at birth, for example adrenogenital syndrome. Hypertension is often seen after surgical repair of large abdominal defects.

Symptoms of hypertension

Symptoms of hypertension are non-specific and include failure to thrive, lethargy, convulsions (hypertensive encephalopathy), and cardiac failure. Hypertensive retinopathy is not often found, but if present can be completely reversible. Once hypertension has been diagnosed in a neonate, a very aggressive therapeutic approach is indicated. There is a very high morbidity and mortality if untreated. Severe hypertension should be managed in a neonatal intensive care setting, where agents such as sodium nitroprusside can be given without danger. In moderate to severe hypertension, calcium-channel blockers (e.g. nifedepine) and angiotensin converting enzyme inhibitors (e.g. captopril) can be used, whereas in mild hypertension, diuretics, a vasodilator (hydralazine) or beta-blocker (propranalol) may be appropriate [48]. Newborn infants require somewhat large doses of antihypertensives relative to their body weight. Frequently used medications for the treatment of hypertension in the neonatal period are summarized in Table 15.12. All neonates with hypertension need careful long-term follow-up.

Key point
• Symptoms of arterial hypertension in the neonate are non-specific and include failure to thrive, lethargy, convulsions, and cardiac failure.

Chronic and end-stage renal failure

Chronic and end-stage renal failure are rare in the neonatal period. Far more common are renal conditions with parenchymal lesions that will ultimately progress to chronic and/or end-stage renal failure in later childhood. An example of this course of events is residual renal parenchymal injury after ARF with tubular necrosis, or after severe bilateral renal venous thrombosis.

The major causes of chronic and end-stage renal failure in the neonatal period are severe bilateral renal dysplasia and cystic malformation, unilateral renal agenesis/dysplasia with disease (obstruction) in the contralateral kidney, the neonatal form of nephronophthisis, or very early onset of diffuse renal oxalate deposition in primary hyperoxaluria. Primary glomerulonephritides are rare at this age and generally do not cause chronic renal failure in early infancy.

The management of chronic and, in particular, end-stage renal failure at this very young age is a major medical, socio-economic, and ethical problem. Such

Table 15.12 Dosage and route of administration of the most commonly used antihypertensive drugs in the neonate

Agent	Starting dose	Interval	Maximum recommended dose	Route
Furosemide	1 mg/kg	Every 4–6 h	5 mg/kg/dose	o/i.v.
Hydrochlorothiazide	1 mg/kg	Every 8 h	3 mg/kg/dose	o
Propranolol	0.25 mg/kg/dose	Every 6–8 h	5 mg/kg/dose	o/iv
Atenolol	0.5 mg/kg/dose	Every 12–24 h	4 mg/kg/dose	o
Labetolol	0.5 mg/kg/dose	Every 1–4 h	2 mg/kg/dose	i.v.
Sodium nitroprusside	0.5 µg/kg/min	—	6 µg/kg/min	i.v.
Captopril	0.1 mg/kg/dose	Every 8–12 h	0.5 mg/kg/dose	o
Enalapril	5 µg/kg/dose	Every 8–24 h	20 µg/kg/dose	i.v.
Nifedipine	0.5 mg/kg/dose	Every 4–6 h	2 mg/kg/dose	o

o, Oral; i.v., intravenous.

treatment necessitates the involvement of a paediatric nephrologist in close co-operation with his or her multi-professional team and many other consultants. Since most of the disorders causing chronic and end-stage renal failure in the very young are not amenable to specific therapies, only symptomatic treatment is available. This involves the conservative management of the uraemic state with control of hypertension when present (dysplastic kidneys are often salt-losing states and the renal insufficiency of such a condition is often normotensive), avoiding or treating disturbances in fluid, electrolyte, and acid–base homeostasis, prevention of uraemic osteodystrophy with active vitamin D preparations and oral calcium-salt supplements, prevention and treatment of anaemia with erythropoietin and iron supplements, and, above all, sufficient caloric intake. These are difficult, although achievable, goals [49]. When end-stage renal failure occurs, renal replacement therapy with dialysis and/or renal transplantation is indicated. These treatment modalities are beyond the scope of the present chapter; it should be stressed that all dialysis modalities are technically possible in the neonate, although associated with an increased incidence of complications compared with older children [50].

Key point

- The major causes of end-stage renal failure in the neonate are severe hypoplasia and renal dysplasia secondary to urinary tract malformations.

Drugs and the neonatal kidney

Pharmacokinetics

The rapid changes in GFR and tubular function after birth necessitate that the dosage of drugs that are eliminated by glomerular filtration or tubular secretion be adjusted according to the level of renal function [51]. For drugs eliminated by glomerular filtration, the correct dosage can be calculated according to the standard recommendations for older children with varying degrees of renal failure (see Chapter 26). Toxic plasma drug levels may ensue if these precautions are not recognized and the drug

dosage is not reduced, relative to the low GFR of the newborn. This is one possible cause of renal toxicity. The other is that the management of very sick neonates often does not leave the treating paediatrician an alternative but empirically to employ potent drugs that can impair renal function. It is therefore imperative that the drug plasma trough levels be monitored frequently. We will discuss in some detail medications given to mothers during pregnancy and commonly used drugs in the treatment of the sick newborns (in neonatal units) that are known to interfere with renal function. The mode of action of most of these drugs will be well known.

Drugs given during pregnancy

Angiotensin converting enzyme inhibitors

These rapidly cross the placental barrier. By inhibiting angiotensin II formation and prostaglandin synthesis in both the mother and the fetus, these agents affect placental perfusion and fetal GFR. Their deleterious effects include: oligohydramnios, intrauterine growth retardation, premature labour, fetal and neonatal ARF, bony malformations, limb contractures, patent ductus arteriosus, pulmonary hypoplasia, prolonged hypotension, and even neonatal death [52]. These agents are clearly contraindicated throughout pregnancy. The same applies to specific angiotensin II receptor-antagonists.

Non-steroidal anti-inflammatory drugs

According to clinical observations and experiments in laboratory animals, indometacin given during pregnancy may cause renal hypoperfusion and ARF associated with a reduction in urine flow rate. This results in oligohydramnios, disturbances in renal maturational processes, and the appearance of glomerular cysts. Irreversible neonatal renal failure has also been observed in infants whose mother had been given indometacin in the days or weeks before birth [53]. When used as a tocolytic agent (reducing uterine contractions), indometacin may adversely affect fetal renal function and cause prenatal and postnatal renal failure.

Drugs given to neonates

Furosemide

Furosemide is excreted by glomerular filtration and secreted in the tubules by a weak organic acid tubular transport mechanism, both of which function at a low level in the neonate. Furosemide not only promotes natriuresis and diuresis but also causes increased urinary calcium excretion. Prolonged furosemide administration (at least 2 mg/kg/day for ⩾12 days) has therefore been associated with renal stone formation or nephrocalcinosis [54]. Urinary tract infection seems to increase the risk of renal calcification. In the past it was claimed that chlorothiazide could prevent or cure renal calcium deposition, though recent data are not confirmative. Long-term administration of furosemide to preterm infants has been reported to be associated with secondary hyperparathyroidism and bone disease.

Dopamine

The renal effects of dopamine in newborn infants have not been well established. It was claimed that dopamine, given to premature infants in an i.v. dose of 0.5–2.0 µg/kg/min, significantly increased urine flow, creatinine clearance, and urinary sodium excretion [55]. Dopamine does not, however, consistently improve renal function; from a purely renal viewpoint the benefit of dopamine in high-risk neonates therefore remains questionable.

Tolazoline

Tolazoline is an α-adrenergic blocking agent, sometimes used as a pulmonary vasodilator in persistent pulmonary hypertension of the newborn. It also has histamine-like properties and a direct non-adrenergic relaxant effect on smooth muscles. The high renal vascular resistance responsible for the decreased renal perfusion seen in all neonates (rats, rabbits, piglets, humans) is aggravated when tolazoline is given; this is due to its partial α-agonist action [56].

Indometacin

Inhibition of prostaglandin synthesis with indometacin is used in premature infants for the pharmacological closure of the ductus arteriosus. When indometacin was given twice in a dose of 0.1–0.2 mg/kg at 8 or 24-h intervals, a variable decrease in urine flow rate, GFR, free-water clearance, and urinary electrolyte excretion was noted, without changes in arterial BP [57]. These effects are transient, and the altered functions return to pretreatment values within 1–2 weeks after discontinuation of the drug. Similar effects are likely to occur with other NSAIDs such as ibuprofen [58].

Aminoglycosides

Aminoglycosides are mainly excreted by glomerular filtration and their dosages therefore have to be adjusted to the low level of GFR present at birth, as emphasized above. Since GFR increases very rapidly during the first month of life, an aminoglycoside dosage that may be toxic at birth may become sub-therapeutic after a few weeks. The half-life of gentamicin has an inverse correlation to gestational age, so that conceptional age rather than postnatal age must be considered when adjusting the dose [51].

Contrast agents

The use of hypertonic radiographic contrast material in infants has been associated with major renal side-effects, such as renal artery thrombosis, medullary necrosis, ischaemia, and renal insufficiency. The usual dose of these contrast agents, which generally have an osmolality of 1300–2000 mosm/kg H_2O, can cause an abrupt rise in the plasma osmolality (20–110 mosm/kg H_2O) of newborn infants and cause intraventricular haemorrhage, particularly in premature babies. Radiographic studies requiring contrast media should be performed with the utmost caution during the neonatal period and only after adequate hydration of the infant. The use of non-ionic contrast agents, with osmolalities of approximately 450 mosm/kg H_2O, markedly reduces the risk of toxicity, and is now standard practice in most paediatric radiology departments.

Key point

- Drugs given to the mother (angiotensin converting enzyme inhibitors, non-steroidal anti-inflammatory drugs) or to the neonate (indometacin, aminoglycosides, tolazoline, dopamine, furosemide) can severely compromise neonatal renal function.

References

1. Grobstein C. Trans-filter induction of tubules in mouse metanephric mesenchyme. Exp Cell Research 1956;10:424–440.
2. Dressler G. Genetic control of kidney development. Adv Nephrol Necker Hosp 1997;26:1–17.
3. Orellana SA, Avner ED. Cell and molecular biology of kidney development. Semin Nephrol 1998;18:233–243.
4. Burrow CR. Regulatory molecules in kidney development. Pediatr Nephrol 2000;14:240–253.
5. Piscione TD, Rosenblum ND. The malformed kidney: disruption of glomerular and tubular development. Clin Genet 1999;56:341–356.
6. Pope IV JC, Brock III JW, Adams MC, Stephens FD, Ichikawa I. How they begin and how they end: classical and new theories for the development and deterioration of congenital anomalies of the kidney and urinary tract, CAKUT. J Am Soc Nephrol 1999;10:2018–2028.
7. Zerres K, Mucher G, Becker J, Steinkamm C, Rudnik-Schoneborn S, Heikkila P, Rapola J, Salonen R, Germino GG, Onuchic L, Somlo S, Avner ED, Harman LA, Stockwin JM, Guay-Woodford LM. Prenatal diagnosis of autosomal recessive polycystic kidney disease (ARPKD); molecular genetics, clinical experience and fetal morphology. Am J Med Genet 1998;76:137–144.
8. Kömhoff M, Wang JL, Cheng HF, Langenbach R, McKanna JA, Harris RC, Breyer MD. Cyclooxygenase-2-selective inhibitors impair glomerulogenesis and renal cortical development. Kidney Int 2000;57:414–422.
9. Kaplan BS, Restaino I, Raval DS, Gottlieb RP, Bernstein J. Renal failure in the neonate associated with in utero exposure to non-steroidal anti-inflammatory agents. Pediatr Nephrol 1994;8:700–704.
10. Peruzzi L, Gianoglio B, Porcellini MC, Coppo R. Neonatal end-stage renal failure associated with maternal ingestion of cyclo-oxygenase-type-2 selective inhibitor nimesulide as tocolytic. Lancet 1999; 354:1615.
11. Barker DJP, Osmond C, Golding J, Kuh D, Wadsworth MEJ. Growth in utero, blood pressure in childhood and adult life, and mortality from cardiovascular disease. BMJ 1989;298:564–567.
12. Thomas IT, Smith DW. Oligohydramnios, cause of the nonrenal features of Potter's syndrome, including pulmonary hypoplasia. J Pediatr 1974;84:811–815.
13. Brace RA. Physiology of amniotic fluid volume regulation. Clin Obstet Gynecol 1997;40:280–289.
14. Guignard JP, Drukker A. Why do newborn infants have a high plasma creatinine? Pediatrics 1999; www.pediatrics.org/cgi/content/full/103/4/e49
15. Guignard JP, Torrado A, Da Cunha O, Gautier E. Glomerular filtration rate in the first three weeks of life. J Pediatr 1975;87:268–272.
16. Semama DS, Thonney M, Guignard JP. Role of endogenous endothelin in renal haemodynamics of newborn rabbits. Pediatr Nephrol 1993;7:886–890.
17. Coulter DM. Postnatal fluid and electrolyte changes and clinical implications. In Fetal and Neonatal Body Fluids, the Scientific Basis for Clinical Practice, Brace RA (ed), Itheca NY, Perinatology Press, 1989.
18. Chevalier RL. The moth and the aspen tree: sodium in early postnatal development. Kidney Int 2001;59:1617–1625.
19. Brewer ED. Disorders of acid–base balance. Pediatr Clin North Am 1990;37:429–447.
20. Blachar A, Blachar Y. Congenital Evaluation: follow-up and clinical outcome. In Pediatric Nephrology, Drukker A, Gruskin AB (Eds), Pediatr Adolesc Med, Basle, Karger, 1994, vol 5, pp. 141–154.
21. Karlsson FA, Hardell LI, Hellsing K. A prospective study of urinary proteins in early infancy. Acta Paediatr Scand 1979;68:663–667.
22. Matos V, Drukker A, Guignard JP. Spot urine samples for evaluating solute excretion in the first week of life. Arch Dis Child Fetal Neonatal Ed 1999;80:F240–F242.
23. Matos P, Duarte-Silva M, Drukker A, Guignard JP. Creatinine reabsorption by the newborn rabbit kidney. Pediatr Res 1998;44:639–641.
24. Schwartz GJ, Feld LG, Langdorf DJ. A simple estimate of glomerular filtration rate in full-term infants during the first year of life. J Pediatr 1984;104:849–854.
25. Brion LP, Fleischman AR, McCarton C, Schwartz GJ. A simple estimate of glomerular filtration rate in low birth weight infants during the first year of life: non-invasive assessment of body composition and growth. J Pediatr 1986;109:698–707.
26. Sutphen J-L. Anthropometric determinants of creatinine excretion in preterm infants. Pediatrics 1982; 69:719–723.
27. Holmberg C, Antikainen M, Ronnholm K, Ala Houhata M, Jalanko H. Management of congenital nephrotic syndrome of the Finnish type. Pediatr Nephrol 1995;9:87–93.
28. Zelikovic I. Molecular pathophysiology of tubular transport disorders. Pediatr Nephrol 2001;16:919–935.
29. van Lieburg AF, Knoers NVAM, Monnens LAH. Clinical presentation and follow-up of 30 patients with congenital nephrogenic diabetes insipidus. J Am Soc Nephrol 1999;10:1958–1964.
30. Royer P, Habib R, Mathieu H, Courtecuisse V. L'hypoplasie rénale bilatérale congénitale avec réduction du nombre et hypertrophie des néphrons chez l'enfant. Ann Pédiatr 1962;38:133–146.
31. Brenner BM, Garcia DL, Anderson S. Glomeruli and blood pressure. Less of one, more of the other? Am J Hypertens 1988;1:335–347.
32. Brenner BM, Lawler EV, Mackenzie HS. The hyperfiltration theory: a paradigm shift in nephrology. Kidney Int 1996;49:1774–1777.
33. Gilbert T, Merlet-Bénichou C. Retinoids and nephron mass control. Pediatr Nephrol 2000;1137–1144.
34. Stapleton FB, Jones DP, Green RS. Acute renal failure in neonates: incidence, etiology and outcome. Pediatr Nephrol 1987;1:314–320.
35. Karlowicz MG, Adelman RD. Nonoliguric and oliguric acute renal failure in asphyxiated term neonates. Pediatr Nephrol 1995;9:718–722.
36. Latta K, Krull F, Wilken M, Burdelski M, Rodeck B, Offner G. Continuous arteriovenous haemofiltration in critically ill children. Pediatr Nephrol 1994;8:334–337.
37. Blowey DL, McFarland K, Alon U, McGraw-Houchens M, Hellerstein S, Warady BA. Peritoneal

dialysis in the neonatal period: outcome data. J Perinatol 1993;13:59–64.

38. Chevalier RL, Campbell F, Brenbridge AN. Prognostic factors in neonatal acute renal failure. Pediatrics 1984;74:265–272.

39. Brun P, Beaufils F, Pillion G, Schlegel N, Loirat C. Thrombose des veines rénales du nouveau-né: traitement et pronostic à long terme. Ann Pediatr (Paris) 1993;40:75–80.

40. Mitchell CK, Franco SM, Vogel RL. Incidence of urinary tract infection in an inner-city outpatient population. J Perinatol 1995;15:131–134.

41. El-Dahr SS, Lewy JE. Urinary tract obstruction and infection in the neonate. Clin Perinatol 1992; 19:213–222.

42. Hellerstein S. Urinary tract infections. Old and new concepts. Pediatr Clin North Am 1995; 42:1433–1457.

43. Singh HP, Hurley RM, Meyers TF. Neonatal hypertension. Incidence and risk factors. Am J Hypertens 1992;5:51–55.

44. Dweck HS, Reynolds DW, Cassady G. Indirect blood pressure measurement in newborns. Am J Dis Child 1974;127:492–494.

45. Guignard JP, Gouyon JB, Adelman RD. Arterial hypertension in the newborn infant. Biol Neonate 1989;55:77–83.

46. De Swiet M, Fayers P, Shinebourne EA. Systolic blood pressure in a population of infants in the first year of life: the Brompton study. Pediatrics 1980;65:1028–1035.

47. Hegyi T, Carbone MT, Anwar M, Ostfeld B, Hiatt M, Koons A, Pinto-Martin J, Paneth N. Blood pressure ranges in premature infants. I. The first hours of life. J Pediatr 1994;124:627–633.

48. Gruskin AB, Dabbagh S, Fleishmann LE, Atiyeh BA. Application since 1980 of antihypertensive agents to treat pediatric disease. J Human Hypertens 1994; 8:381–388.

49. Ledermann SE, Shaw V, Trompeter RS. Long-term enteral nutrition in infants and young children with chronic renal failure. Pediatr Nephrol 1999;13:870–875.

50. Coulthard MG, Sharp J. Haemodialysis and ultrafiltration in babies weighing under 1000 g. Arch Dis Child Fetal Neonatal Ed 1995;73:F162–F165.

51. Assael BM. Pharmacokinetics and drug distribution during postnatal development. Pharmacol Ther 1982;18:159–197.

52. Shotan A, Widerhorn J, Hurst A, Elkayam U. Risks of angiotensin-converting enzyme inhibition during pregnancy: experimental and clinical evidence, potential mechanisms, and recommendations for use. Am J Med 1994;96:451–456.

53. Van der Heijden BJ, Carlus C, Narcy F, Bavoux F, Delezoide AL, Gubler MC. Persistent anuria, neonatal death, and renal microcystic lesions after prenatal exposure to indomethacin. Am J Obstet Gynecol 1994;171:617–623.

54. Downing GJ, Egelhoff JC, Daily DK, Alon U. Furosemide-related renal calcifications in the premature infant. A longitudinal ultrasonography study. Pediatr Radiol 1991;21:563–565.

55. Seri I, Rudas G, Bors Z, Kanyicska B, Tulassay T. Effects of low-dose dopamine infusion on cardiovascular and renal functions, cerebral blood flow, and plasma catecholamine levels in sick preterm neonates. Pediatr Res 1993;34:742–749.

56. Trompeter RS, Chantler C, Haycock GB. Tolazoline and acute renal failure in the newborn. Lancet 1981;1:1219.

57. Catterton Z, Sellers B Jr, Gray B. Inulin clearance in the premature infant receiving indomethacin. J Pediatr 1980;96:737–739.

58. Chamaa NS, Mosig D, Drukker A, Guignard JP. The renal hemodynamic effects of ibuprofen in the newborn rabbit. Pediatr Res 2000;48:600–605.

16 | *Inherited renal disease and genetic counselling*

Nine V.A.M. Knoers and Leo A.H. Monnens

Introduction

Genetics remains one of the most rapidly advancing fields of medical science. The past two decades have witnessed an explosion in molecular technology, which has enabled the identification of genes for an increasing number of inherited single-gene disorders. An important sequel of this advancement in molecular science is the availability of genetic tests for diagnostic purposes in these disorders.

It is expected that within the next few years the pace of this progress will further increase. Earlier than expected, in autumn 2000, the first draft ('working draft') of the human genome sequence was delivered as a result of the efforts of the Human Genome Project, and marked a milestone in the fields of molecular biology and medicine [1,2]. Although the precise implications of the availability of the entire human genome sequence cannot be fully foreseen, it will inevitably be of great importance. The information on gene structure will allow molecular analysis not only in any single-gene disease, but also in the more common multifactorial or complex disorders, such as hypertension, diabetes, myocardial infarction, cancer, and others. In addition, the availability of the complete human genome sequence will also significantly facilitate molecular studies of individual variation in the response to drugs (pharmacogenetics). Genetic testing in complex diseases and pharmacogenetics will not provide a diagnosis but, rather, will give evidence of individual susceptibility.

Together with the development of powerful, high-throughput technologies to exploit its use, the complete DNA sequence information will also increase our insight into the function of the proteins encoded by the genes, their biological interactions, and their role in normal development and in disease. In the long term, this knowledge may provide a framework for the development of new therapeutic strategies.

One of the most promising new technologies for large-scale sequence analysis, mutation detection, and gene expression is the oligonucleotide microarray or DNA chip [3–5].

The use of genetic tests for diagnostic purposes is becoming increasingly commonplace in clinical practice and it is therefore important that clinicians are aware of the technical and ethical implications of these methods. At present, genetic tests are available for a significant number of renal genetic disorders (Table 16.1). The purpose of this chapter is to give an overview of the uses and restrictions of currently used genetic tests for the diagnosis, prenatal assessment, carrier detection, and pre-symptomatic testing of hereditary renal disorders. We will additionally discuss genetic counselling and ethical aspects of prenatal and presymptomatic diagnosis. The clinical details, natural history, and treatment of these disorders are described in other chapters.

The use of genetic tests in the diagnosis of patients with clinical renal disease

In general there are two major approaches to the molecular diagnosis of single-gene disorders: indirect diagnosis through linkage with DNA polymorphisms and direct diagnosis of the disease-causing mutations. In the following we will explain these two approaches in more detail.

Indirect linkage-based testing

Linkage-based testing was historically the first type of DNA diagnosis to be widely used. This approach is useful where the gene of interest has not been cloned, where mutations are difficult to find, where

Table 16.1 Single-gene renal disorders and syndromes with mainly renal abnormalities for which genetic testing is available

Disease	Mode of inheritance	Gene locus	Gene	Protein	Type of testing: linkage-based (*li*)/mutation analysis (*ma*)
ADPKD	AD	16p13.3 4q22	*PKD1* *PKD2*	Polycystin-1 Polycystin-2	*li* preferred; *ma* in *PKD2* (and in some cases in *PKD1*) possible but not routinely deployed
ARPKD	AR	6p21.1	*PKHD1*	Fibrocystin	*li*; *ma*
Alport S	XLD	Xq22.3	*COL4A5*	α5 chain type IV collagen	*li* preferred; *ma* in isolated cases
Alport S	AR (AD)	2q36–q37	*COL4A3* *COL4A4*	α3 chain and α4 chain type IV collagen	*li* preferred; *ma* in isolated cases
Bartter S	AR	15q15-q21 11q24 1p36	*SLC12A1* *KCNJ1* *CLCNKB*	NKCC2 ROMK ClC-kb	*ma* *ma* *ma*
Bartter S with sensorineural deafness	AR	1p31	*BSND*	Barttin	*li*
Branchio-oto-renal S	AD	8q13.3	*EYA1*	Eyes absent-like protein 1	*ma*
Renal-coloboma S	AD	10q24	*PAX-2*	Paired-box transcription factor	*ma*
Cystinosis	AR	17p13	*CTNS*	Cystinosin	*ma*[a]
Cystinuria type I	AR	2p16.3	*SCL3A1*	r-BAT	*ma*
Cystinuria type II and III	AR (incompletely)	19q13	*SLC7A9*	B(o,+)AT	*ma*
Dent's disease	XLR	Xp11.22	*ClCN5*	Renal voltage-dependent chloride channel	*ma*
Denys–Drash S	AD	11p13	*WT-1*	Wilms' tumour suppressor	*ma*
Frasier S	AD	11p13	*WT-1*	Wilms' tumour suppressor	*ma*
Fabry's disease	XLR	Xq22	*GLA*	α-Galactosidase	*ma*
Fanconi–Bickel S	AR	3q26.1–q26.3	*GLUT-2*	Liver-type facilitative glucose transporter	*ma*
Gitelman S	AR	16q13	*SLC12A3*	NCCT	*ma*
Familial benign hypocalciuric hypercalcaemia	AD	3q13.3–q21	*CaSR*	Extracellular calcium-sensing receptor (loss of function)	*ma*
Neonatal severe hyperparathyroidism	AR	3q13.3–q21	*CaSR*	Extracellular calcium-sensing receptor (loss of function)	*ma*
Familial hypercalciuric hypocalcaemia	AD	3q13.3–q21	*CaSR*	Extracellular calcium-sensing receptor (gain of function)	*ma*

Table 16.1 Continued

Disease	Mode of inheritance	Gene locus	Gene	Protein	Type of testing: linkage-based (*li*)/mutation analysis (*ma*)
Hypophosphataemic (Vitamin D-resistant) rickets	XLD	Xp22.2–p22.1	*PHEX*	Type II integral membrane protein (endopeptidase)	*ma*
Hypophoshataemic rickets	AD	12p13.3	*FGF23*	Fibroblast growth factor 23	*ma*
Hyperoxaluria type I	AR	2q36–q36	*AGXT*	Alanine-glyoxalate aminotransferase	*ma*
Hyperoxaluria type II	AR	9p11–q11	*GRHPR*	D glycerate dehydrogenase glyoxylate reductase	*ma*
Hypomagnesaemia/ hypocalciuria	AD	11q23	FXYD2	γ-subunit Na/K ATPase	*ma*
Hypomagnesaemia/ hypercalciuria	AR	3q27	*PCLN1*	Claudin 16	*ma*
Liddle S	AD	16p13–p12	E-NaC	Epithelial sodium channel (activating mutations)	*ma*
Oculocerebro-renal syndrome of Lowe S	XLR	Xq24–q26	*OCRL-1*	Inositol-polyphosphate-5-phosphatase	*ma*
Nail-Patella S	AD	9q34	*LMX1B*	LIM-homeodomain transcription factor-1	*ma*
NDI	XLR	Xq28	*AVPR2*	Vasopressin type 2 receptor	*ma*
NDI	AR AD	12q13	*AQP2*	Vasopressin-regulated aquaporin-2 water channel	*ma*
Nephronophthisis, juvenile	AR	2q12–q13	NPH1	Nephrocystin	*ma*[b]
Nephronophthisis, infantile	AR	9q22–q31	Unknown	Unknown	*li*
Nephronophthisis, adolescent	AR	3q21–q22	Unknown	Unknown	*li*
MCKD1	AD	1q21	–	–	*li*
MCKD2	AD	16p13	–	–	*li*
Nephrotic syndrome (Finnish type)	AR	19q13.1	NPHS1	Nephrin	*ma*
Nephrotic syndrome (steroid resistant)	AR	1q25–31	NPHS2	Podocin	*ma*
Familial focal segmental glomerulo-sclerosis type I	AD	19q13.1	*ACTN4*	α-actinin-4	*ma*
Familial focal segmental glomerulosclerosis type II	AD	11q21–q22	Unknown	Unknown	*li*
PHA type Ia	AR	16p13–p12	*ENaC*	Epithelial sodium channel (loss of function)	*ma*

Table 16.1   Continued

Disease	Mode of inheritance	Gene locus	Gene	Protein	Type of testing: linkage-based (*li*)/mutation analysis (*ma*)
PHA type Ib	AD	4q31.1	*MLR*	Mineralocorticoid receptor	*ma*
PHA type II	AD	1q31–42	Unknown	Unknown	*li*
		17p11–q21	*WNK4*	WNK kinase 4	*ma*
		12p13.3	*WNK1*	WNK kinase 1	*ma*
AME1	AR	16q22	HSD11B2	11β-hydroxysteroid dehydrogenase type II	*ma*
RTA (proximal) with ocular abnormalities	AR	4q21	*SLC4A4*	Na/HCO3 co-transporter	*ma*
RTA (combined proximal and distal) with osteopetrosis	AR	8q22	*CA2*	Carbonic anhydrase II	*ma*
RTA (distal) with deafness	AR	2cen–q13	*ATP6B1*	β1 subunit of hydrogen ATPase	*ma*
RTA (distal) without deafness	AR	7q33–q34	*ATP6N1B*	N1 subunit of hydrogen ATPase	*ma*
RTA (distal) without deafness	AD	17q21–q22	*SLC4A1*	Band 3 anion exchange protein 1 (AE1)	*ma*
Townes–Brocks S	AD	16q12.1	*SALL1*	Zinc-finger domain-rich transcription factor	*ma*

AD, autosomal dominant; ADPKD, autosomal dominant polycystic kidney disease; AME1, apparent mineralocorticoid excess type I; AR, autosomal recessive; ARPKD, autosomal recessive polycystic kidney disease; B(o,+)AT, light chain of basic amino-acid transporter; ClC-kb, renal chloride channel; MCKD, medullary cystic kidney disease; NCCT, thiazide-sensitive sodium-chloride co-transporter; NDI, nephrogenic diabetes insipidus; NKCC2, bumetanide-sensitive sodium-potassium-2 chloride co-transporter; PHA, pseudohypoaldosteronism; r-BAT, heavy chain of basic amino-acid transporter; ROMK, ATP-sensitive inwardly rectifying potassium channel; RTA, renal tubular acidosis; S, syndrome; XLD, X-linked dominant; XLR, X-linked recessive.
[a] 40% of patients carry homozygous deletions.
[b] 66% of patients harbour large homozygous deletions.

mutations are scattered widely over a large gene, and where mutation detection has been unsuccessful. In linkage-based testing, markers linked to the locus of interest are used in family studies to determine whether or not the patient has inherited the disorder in question. To perform the test it is necessary that the gene responsible for the disorder has been mapped on the genome and that one or more detectable polymorphic loci reside in its vicinity. DNA polymorphisms are sequence variants that are known to exist in the general population. They are defined as the presence of two or more alleles, which each have a frequency of at least 1% in the population. The different alleles of a polymorphism are a means of labelling the two copies of a chromosome of an individual and following how

these chromosome copies are transmitted to the next generation. Where a polymorphism is in close proximity to a disease locus, the inheritance of the disease gene in the family can be tracked. The principle of linkage-based testing is exemplified in Fig. 16.1 for a family with autosomal dominant polycystic kidney disease (ADPKD).

The first generation of polymorphisms were the so-called restriction fragment length polymorphisms (RFLPs) [6], but nowadays microsatellite polymorphisms, which present a large number of alleles [7], are the most widely used. These microsatellite markers are detected by using the polymerase chain reaction (PCR), which is an *in vitro* method for producing large amounts of a specific DNA fragment

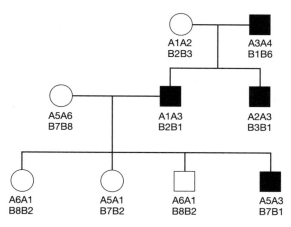

Fig. 16.1 A family with ADPKD. The disorder is segregating with the A3 and B1 alleles of two closely linked flanking polymorphic microsatellite markers.

of defined length and sequence from small amounts of complex template [8]. There are some important limitations to the use of linkage for diagnostic purposes. First, a linkage-based method is only possible where a number of affected individuals from a family are available for testing. Secondly, there is the chance of genetic recombination and loss of linkage between the disease locus and the marker, resulting from crossing-over between chromatids of paired chromosomes during meiosis. The probability of recombination is generally a function of the distance between the two loci; the further the polymorphic marker is from the gene of interest, the greater will be the chance of recombination between these loci and thus an incorrect prediction of the disease status of the individual in question. Therefore, the accuracy of indirect linkage-based testing can never be 100%. With the use of very closely linked markers, preferably with a recombination rate of less than 1%, or by using two polymorphic markers that flank the disease gene, the risk of an incorrect diagnosis can be minimized. For many diseases with known genes it is nowadays possible to use an intragenic marker, such as a microsatellite polymorphic marker within an intron of the gene, which significantly reduces the chance of recombination.

A third limitation to the use of linkage is genetic locus heterogeneity. For instance, ADPKD can be caused by mutations in at least two genes: *PKD1*, encoding polycystin-1 located at chromosome 16p13 [9] and *PKD2*, encoding polycystin-2 at chromosome 4q22 [10]. Although there are some clinical differences between

patients with mutations in *PKD1* and those with mutations in *PKD2*, these differences do not allow a reliable clinical distinction between both entities. Therefore, there is no way to determine *a priori* which of the two genes is involved in a certain family with ADPKD. If a marker for *PKD1* is used and the disease is caused by mutations in the *PKD2* gene, the results will be meaningless. Therefore, before proceeding to diagnosis, it is necessary to first establish whether the disease in the family is linked to markers in the vicinity of *PKD1* or *PKD2*.

Another important renal disorder which is genetically heterogeneous is Alport syndrome, which is known to be transmitted through X-linked, autosomal recessive and patterns of autosomal dominant inheritance [11]. Linkage-based testing in relatives of patients is only possible if the mode of transmission of the disorder in the patient has been determined; in many situations this is not clear from the pedigree. Absence of epidermal basement membrane expression of the α5 chain of type IV collagen is diagnostic of X-linked Alport syndrome and therefore may assist the clinician where uncertainty regarding mode of inheritance exists [12,13]. This is a very elegant means of diagnosis which obviates the need for renal biopsy. However, it does not give completely interpretable results in all cases.

Finally, there are situations in which a polymorphic marker is not informative, meaning that a person is homozygous for the alleles of that marker, rendering it impossible to determine which allele segregates with the disease. With the use of the many highly polymorphic microsatellite markers, this problem can nowadays be easily overcome in most cases.

Key points

- Indirect linkage-based testing for single gene disorders:
  - is only possible where a number of affected individuals from a family are available for testing;
  - is useful where the gene of interest has not been cloned, where mutations are difficult to find, where mutations are scattered widely over a large gene, and where mutation detection has been unsuccessful;
  - can never be 100% accurate because of genetic recombination and loss of linkage.

Direct mutation analysis

For an increasing number of diseases, including many inherited renal disorders (Table 16.1), it is possible to target the causative mutation directly. There are different classes of mutations: deletions of the entire gene, smaller deletions or insertions, splice-site mutations, and single nucleotide substitutions. The latter are further classified into:

(a) nonsense mutations, which are mutations resulting in replacement of a codon specifying an amino acid, by a stop-codon, thus terminating translation of the protein;

(b) missense mutations, which are mutations resulting in an altered codon specifying a different amino acid; and

(c) silent mutations, which are mutations resulting in no change in amino acid.

The latter mutations are single-base substitutions, often, but not always, occurring at the third position of a codon, which alter the codon but not the amino acid encoded. For instance, when a G is substituted for the third A from codon 'AAA', which encodes lysine, the resulting codon 'AAG' still codes for lysine.

There are many different techniques that can be used for mutation analysis. Methods for the identification of single-base substitutions are all based on amplification of the region surrounding the mutation by PCR. After amplification, different methods of mutation analysis, such as single-strand conformational analysis (SSCA), direct sequencing, restriction digestion, or the oligonucleotide ligation assay can be applied [14].

The approach for direct analysis is not identical in all cases but depends on the disease gene involved. In some disorders, one or a limited number of specific mutations account for the majority of patients and therefore a mutation analysis technique which only screens for these frequently occurring mutations may be used in the first instance. Good examples of this are the Fin_{major} and Fin_{minor} mutations in the *NPHS1* gene encoding for nephrin, which together are found in more than 90% of Finnish patients with the Finnish-type congenital nephrotic syndrome [15]. Other examples are cystinosis, where 40% of patients are homozygous for a particular deletion [16] and nephronophthisis, where the majority of patients have a homozygous large deletion [17,18]. In other disorders, multiple types of mutations, located at different sites in a gene, have

been identified. This allelic heterogeneity complicates direct testing since it necessitates screening of the whole gene in every patient. Screening of the total gene can be a very difficult and time-consuming task, especially when the genes involved are very large; the *COL4A5* gene, for instance, has 51 exons and it has been shown that X-linked Alport syndrome is caused by a very broad spectrum of mutations [19,20]. Another important example is ADPKD; although both *PKD1* and *PKD2* genes have been identified, direct mutation analysis is not a routine diagnostic method. This is mainly due to the fact that the *PKD1* gene, responsible for ADPKD in 85% of cases, is very large (46 exons) and mutations have, as yet, only been found in 30% of ADPKD patients [21].

For certain renal disorders, direct mutation analysis is relatively simple and therefore the method of choice in all cases. An illustrative example is nephrogenic diabetes insipidus (NDI). In 1992, the vasopressin type 2 receptor (V2R) gene was identified and shown to be responsible for the X-linked form of NDI [22–24]. Although X-linked NDI is also subject to allelic heterogeneity, the molecular analysis is based on direct sequencing of the V2R gene. This is mainly due to the fact that this gene is very small. For the same reason, the aquaporin-2 (*AQP2*) gene, encoding the vasopressin-sensitive water channel of the renal collecting duct, and shown to underlie both the autosomal recessive and the autosomal dominant forms of NDI [25,26], is also always directly sequenced in patients.

In familial cases of NDI, the transmission of the disorder in the pedigree will serve as a clear guide to determine which gene needs to be sequenced first. However, in isolated cases, both genes are possible candidates. Since the majority (90%) of cases of NDI are X-linked, the V2R gene is usually screened first, followed by sequencing of the *AQP2* gene if V2R mutations are not detected. The only exception to this rule is the situation in which the isolated patient is the child of a consanguineous relationship. In such cases, the *AQP2* gene is the most likely candidate.

Although, in general, direct mutation analysis is to be preferred to linkage-based testing, it can be concluded that mutation analysis is not possible in all cases, and even when technically possible, may not always be practical in the context of a routine diagnostic service (see also Table 16.1).

In direct analysis it is necessary to determine whether the mutation detected is indeed pathogenic as opposed to being an innocuous polymorphism.

Nonsense mutations are almost always deleterious for the function of the protein. Smaller deletions and insertions usually result in an alteration of the normal translational reading frame of the DNA sequence (frame-shift), which results in a truncation of the protein. Splice-site mutations lead to shorter mRNAs due to incorrect splicing in most cases.

For missense mutations, however, the situation is not always clear. In such situations, screening of control individuals, analysis of the conservation of the mutated amino acid in different species, and, if possible, functional analysis of the mutant in an *in vitro* expression system will answer the question whether the identified mutation is indeed likely to be pathogenic. In situations where there are more than one affected individuals within any single family, co-segregation of the mutation with the disease provides further evidence for the pathogenicity of any mutation.

For some disorders, diagnosis by means of mutation analysis can be important for predicting the severity of the disorder in an individual patient. For instance, in X-linked Alport syndrome it has been shown that deletions and frame-shift mutations in the *COL4A5* gene are often associated with a severe phenotype in males, including end stage renal disease at a young age and early deafness, whereas missense mutations may be associated with a milder clinical picture [20]. In other disorders, including NDI, there are no indications of any genotype–phenotype correlation.

It is evident that antenatal diagnosis, carrier- or pre-symptomatic analysis in family members is only reliable when it has been substantiated that the mutation identified in the patient is indeed pathogenic.

Key points

- Direct mutation analysis is most easily performed where a single mutation is responsible for the majority of affected individuals, e.g. the Fin_{major} and Fin_{minor} mutations in the *NPHS1* (nephrin) gene.

- Where multiple mutations have been identified, the entire gene needs to be screened: this is only feasible where the gene is small, e.g. the V2R gene which is responsible for X-linked nephrogenic diabetes insipidus.

Antenatal diagnosis

The use of ultrasonography for antenatal monitoring has increased significantly in the past decade and this has had a profound influence on medical practice. Genitourinary abnormalities are detected in up to 0.5% of fetuses assessed. Situations warranting antenatal intervention are, however, exceedingly rare. If contemplated seriously, these interventions have to be performed in a specialized centres where experience can accumulate [27]. Guidelines for the management of antenatally diagnosed urinary tract dilatation are emerging [28] (see Chapters 13 and 14), but are not definitive, as the long-term history of these disorders needs to be clarified.

A molecular antenatal diagnosis is usually performed on fetal tissue obtained by chorionic villus sampling at 10–12 weeks of gestation. The major advantages of chorionic villus sampling are that it offers prenatal diagnosis in the first trimester and that villi provide a rich source of DNA. The disadvantage is that even in experienced hands this procedure has a 1–2% risk of causing miscarriage. Although molecular analysis from amniotic fluid is also possible, it is less preferable, since amniocentesis is performed later in pregnancy (around 15 weeks' gestation) and the period needed for amniotic cells to grow before enough cells are obtained for DNA studies is at least 21 days. However, the risk of miscarriage associated with amniocentesis is only 0.5 % [29].

Key points

Chorionic villus sampling
- Is performed in the first trimester and therefore offers early diagnosis.
- Villi produce a rich source of DNA.
- Risk of miscarriage is 1–2%.

Amniocentesis
- Performed at around 15 weeks' gestation.
- Cells obtained need to grow for 21 days to obtain enough DNA.
- Risk of miscarriage is 0.5%.

In general, an antenatal diagnosis of hereditary disease affecting the kidney is most often requested and performed when the disease is severe; because of rapid progression to end stage renal disease and/or development of disabling extrarenal manifestations. Examples are autosomal recessive polycystic kidney disease (ARPKD), the congenital nephrotic syndromes, and some cases of Alport syndrome. In these disorders, a very early diagnosis has important practical consequences. We believe that an antenatal diagnosis of nephrogenic diabetes insipidus (NDI) should not be performed, since an early molecular diagnosis from cord blood taken directly after birth will ensure early treatment and a favourable prognosis, with adequate growth and normal psychomotor development [30].

An antenatal diagnosis of the Finnish type of congenital nephrotic syndrome, based on α-fetoprotein determination in amniotic fluid or, preferably, on the demonstration of a mutation in the *NPHS1* gene in a chorionic villus biopsy, will offer the parents the choice of continuation or termination of the pregnancy at a relatively early stage. α–fetoprotein concentrations of homozygotes and heterozygotes are in the same range.

Antenatal diagnosis of hereditary disorders may allow a well-considered plan for treatment. We will illustrate this with the following case.

Case 1

A 24 year old woman was referred to a paediatric nephrologist following an antenatal diagnosis of polycystic kidney disease, based on the ultrasound finding of enlarged kidneys with poor differentiation between cortex and medulla. Because both parents had normal kidneys on ultrasound examination and polycystic disease was not known in the family, it was thought most likely that the polycystic kidney disorder in the fetus was of autosomal recessive inheritance. Since oligohydramnios was present, a poor prognosis due to pulmonary hypoplasia could be predicted. We agreed with the parents that, if required, we would treat the child postnatally with artificial ventilation for at least 4 weeks before withdrawing from treatment. The newborn female infant had to be ventilated for one week after which she did well with a slight respiratory acidosis and remarkably well-preserved renal function.

An alternative to conventional antenatal diagnosis is pre-implantation genetic diagnosis (PGD), a method which detects the presence of an inherited disorder in an *in vitro* fertilized conceptus before reimplantation [31]. PGD has the advantage that, by selecting only those embryos identified as unaffected for replacement into the uterus, couples know from the start that any pregnancy should be unaffected. This therefore avoids the possibility of having to decide whether or not to terminate an established pregnancy diagnosed as affected at a more advanced stage of gestation. The disadvantages of PGD are related to the *in vitro* fertilization (IVF) procedure, with a low pregnancy rate (about 35%) and the risk of twin or triplet pregnancies. PGD is still a developing field; in previous years the method was only used for disorders with a severe decrease of life expectancy, such as cystic fibrosis and Duchenne muscular dystrophy. Nowadays, the number of disorders for which PGD is requested and performed is rapidly expanding. This list includes several renal disorders, such as X-linked Alport syndrome and Fabry's disease for which pre-implantation sexing is available. Because of the complexity of PGD, both in terms of techniques and counselling of couples, the method should only be performed in experienced clinics with a specialized team of clinical geneticists, molecular biologists, gynaecologists, and psychologists.

Pre-symptomatic diagnosis

Although conventional antenatal diagnosis and PGD could be viewed as providing a pre-symptomatic diagnosis, the term 'pre-symptomatic or predictive testing' is, in general, more strictly used for those situations in which a person at risk of developing a late-onset genetic disorder is examined at a time when this individual is completely healthy. The results of this genetic test will predict whether or not this person will become ill later in life. One of the first disorders in which pre-symptomatic diagnosis was performed was Huntington's disease. The detailed guidelines elaborated for pre-symptomatic testing in Huntington's disease have served as a model for other disorders in which predictive testing is possible [32]. These guidelines include pre-test counselling, disclosure of results in person, and the availability of post-test psychosocial support.

It is generally accepted that predictive testing for late-onset disorders should not be performed in healthy children, unless a delay in diagnosis would be harmful, for instance when an early diagnosis would improve the outcome of the disorder, as illustrated in the following case history.

Case 2

R was referred to a paediatric nephrologist immediately after birth because his brother, C, was known to have cystinosis with mild chronic renal failure. Blood was collected in order to determine the cystine content in granulocytes, since an early diagnosis of cystinosis for R would be important (see Chapter 5). Early diagnosis would guarantee an early treatment with cysteamine, which has been shown to have a beneficial effect on long-term outcome [33].

The agreement not to test children is based on the principle that the child, and not their parents, has the right to decide whether they want to know whether they are at risk. The law in the United Kingdom states that to be able to independently make this decision, a person has to be 16 years of age. Moreover, there are risks of what has been called genetic discrimination, for example the inability to obtain health or life insurance or employment because of one's genotype.

Key points

- Pre-symptomatic (predictive) testing for late-onset disorders (e.g. autosomal dominant polycystic kidney disease) should not be performed in healthy children, unless a delay in diagnosis would be harmful, for instance when an early diagnosis would improve the outcome of the disorder.

Potential for treatment

It is well recognized that supportive conservative therapies (e.g. those for bone disease, hypertension, etc.) remain the mainstay of treatment for many hereditary disorders that result in renal disturbances. There are, however, a number of hereditary diseases where specific treatment modalities improve outcome.

Based on the principles proposed by Dent and Senior [34], an adequate but demanding treatment for the prevention of stones in patients suffering from cystinuria has been described [35]. Mental retardation in nephrogenic diabetes insipidus can be prevented by adequate fluid supply and the early application of hydrochlorothiazide/indometacin in infancy [30]. An alternative to liver transplantation in hereditary tyrosinaemia type I, one of the causes of Fanconi syndrome (see Chapter 5), is the inhibition of 4-hydroxyphenylpyruvate dioxygenase [36]. Enzyme supplementation is a promising form of treatment for Fabry's disease [37]. An interesting potential treatment for the future is the use of pharmacological chaperones. Morello *et al.* have recently shown that small cell-permeable vasopressin type-2 antagonists are able to rescue the cell-surface expression of eight distinct misfolded V2R mutants [38], providing great hope for the management of NDI, where a high number of misfolded, intracellularly retained, but functional mutants are found.

Where hereditary disorders result in end stage renal failure, renal transplantation allows restoration of normal or near normal renal function. This is most effective when the life-threatening symptoms are predominantly caused by renal abnormalities, examples being Alport syndrome and congenital nephrotic syndrome. However, new problems may become evident after transplantation. Alport syndrome is characterized by the absence of $\alpha3$, $\alpha4$, and $\alpha5$ chains of type IV collagen: transplantation of an organ with normal type IV collagen expression results in the formation of alloantibodies in all patients [39], with up to 5–10% developing an acute anti-glomerular basement membrane nephritis. Similar problems develop in patients with the Finnish type of congenital nephrotic syndrome due to mutations in the *NPHS1* gene encoding nephrin, a transmembrane protein present at the slit membrane of podocytes. In around one-third of the patients the nephrotic syndrome recurs after transplantation, due to alloantibody formation against nephrin expressed in the donor kidney.

In primary hyperoxaluria, overproduction of oxalate leads to nephrocalcinosis and development of end stage renal disease in most patients. Renal transplantation alone does not cure the metabolic abnormality and the disease will recur in the transplanted kidney. However, a liver transplantation preceding the renal transplantation, or a combined liver/kidney transplantation at a later stage, will produce excellent results [40].

Although the results of early gene therapy studies were met with great enthusiasm, gene transfer into the kidney remains a great experimental challenge. Gene therapy in the kidney is especially difficult because cell-specific targeting of gene transfer is needed. Further developments in gene-transfer vectors and gene-delivery techniques are required before the therapeutic potential of gene therapy in renal disease can be fully assessed [41].

Genetic counselling

Genetic counselling is defined as a communication process, which is meant to assist a patient and/or their relatives to:

(1) comprehend the diagnosis, probable cause of the disorder, and management;

(2) appreciate the risk of recurrence;

(3) deal with this recurrence risk;

(4) choose the most appropriate course of action in view of risks and family goals;

(5) make the best possible adjustment to the disorder [42].

During a counselling session, the questions and concerns of the patient or their relatives are clarified, and the counsellor provides information in the five aforementioned areas.

Although it is commonly stated that genetic counselling should in principle be non-directive, it has been clearly substantiated that in general practice non-directive genetic counselling is in fact impossible to achieve [42,43]. The case we describe below provides an example of genetic counselling of a complicated case of Alport syndrome. The case clearly shows the difficulties encountered at the various stages of counselling and the possible influences of non-directive counselling in connection to antenatal diagnosis.

Case 3

A young woman with Alport syndrome was referred for genetic counselling. The diagnosis had been made when she was 13 years old. At that time she suffered from haematuria and proteinuria; glomerular basement membrane abnormalities compatible with Alport syndrome were found on renal biopsy. Urinalysis of samples from her parents and two siblings showed no abnormalities, indicating that she was the only person in the family with the disease. It was therefore impossible to determine whether her Alport syndrome was X-linked or autosomal. DNA analysis with an intragenic polymorphic marker in the COL4A5 gene showed that she and her two brothers had all received the same allele from their mother, indicating that the X-linked form was unlikely, unless her disease was due to a new mutation. The autosomal recessive type of Alport syndrome could not be excluded. In order to solve this problem, mutation analysis of the genes involved in Alport syndrome was planned, starting with the COL4A5 gene, in

view of the fact that the X-linked form of Alport syndrome is the most prevalent. It was explained to the young woman that it would take a very long time before the results of the mutation analysis would become available. While waiting for these results, the usefulness of a skin biopsy for the diagnosis of the different genetic forms of Alport syndrome was substantiated by several research studies [12,13]. A skin biopsy from our patient revealed a mosaic expression of the COL4A5 chain in the epidermal basal membrane, indicative of X-linked Alport syndrome.

At the time that the inheritance pattern of the disease in our patient became clear, she informed us that she was pregnant and asked about the possibilities of antenatal diagnosis. We informed her that this was technically impossible; the mutation in the COL4A5 gene was not known and since she was the only person with Alport syndrome in her family, an indirect antenatal diagnosis by linkage analysis was not possible either. Her first child was a girl. Urinalysis on three subsequent occasions did not reveal haematuria or proteinuria. A few years later the causative mutation in the COL4A5 gene was identified in the young woman. We explained to her that this mutation was predicted to cause a severe juvenile phenotype in males with Alport syndrome.

One year later she informed us that she was pregnant once again. She did not wish to pursue antenatal diagnosis because she was reassured by the outcome of her first pregnancy and was confident that things would turn out well again. During the counselling session, we once again reminded her of the consequences of the mutation for males. This information resulted in her changing her mind. Antenatal ultrasonography revealed that she was carrying twins, which further complicated the situation. The counsellee and her husband were informed in detail about the difficulties of prenatal diagnosis in twins, emphasizing the possibility that only one of the twins might be affected. Antenatal diagnosis showed that one of the twins was a boy who carried the mutation and the other was a girl. After disclosure of these results to the parents and careful genetic counselling the parents requested a selective termination of the pregnancy.

Conclusions and future prospects

The number of hereditary renal disorders that can be diagnosed by means of DNA analysis is rapidly increasing. It is to be expected that genetic tests for diagnostic purposes will become more and more integrated into the clinical practice of paediatric and adult nephrologists. It is important to be aware of both the potential and limitations of these genetic tests, and to be able to interpret the results of DNA analysis. In addition, the clinician should always pay close attention to the ethical and social aspects of a DNA diagnosis, since there is always the potential for harm to be done to the patient and/or their family members by third parties such as insurance companies.

We are entering a very exciting era in which the genes for all single-gene defects and susceptibility genes for complex disorders will be identified within a short period of time. This will not only increase the potential for the diagnosis of genetic renal disorders, but will ultimately fundamentally improve our insight into their pathogenesis, resulting in increased possibilities for the development of specific therapies.

References

1. Dunham I. Genomics—the new rock and roll? Trends Genet 2000;16:456–460.
2. Butcher J. 'Working' draft of human genome completed. Lancet 2000;356:47.
3. Hacia JG, Collins FS. Mutational analysis using oligonucleotide microarrays. J Med Genet 1999; 36:730–736.
4. Lipshutz RJ, Fodor SPA, Gingeras TR, Lockhart DJ. High density synthetic oligonucleotide arrays. Nat Genet 1999;21(1 Suppl):20–24.
5. Young RA. Biomedical Discovery with DNA arrays. Cell 2000;102:9–15.
6. Botstein D, White RL, Skolnick M, Davis RW. Construction of a genetic linkage map using restriction fragment length polymorphisms. Am J Hum Genet 1980;32:314–331.
7. Weissenbach J. A second generation linkage map of the human genome based on highly informative microsatellite loci. Gene 1993;135:275–278.
8. White TJ, Arnheim N, Erlich HA. The polymerase chain reaction. Trends Genet 1989;5:185–189.
9. European Polycystic Kidney Disease Consortium. The polycystic kidney disease 1 gene encodes a 14 kb transcript and lies within a duplicated region on chromosome 16. Cell 1994;77:881–894.
10. Mochizuli T, Wu G, Hayashi T, Xenophontos SL, Veldhuisen B, Saris JJ, Reynolds DM, Cai Y, Gabow PA, Pierides A, Kimberling A, Breuning MH, Constantinou-Deltas C, Peters DJM, Somlo S. PKD2, a gene for polycystic kidney disease that encodes an integral membrane protein. Science 1996;272:1339–1342.
11. Kashtan C. Alport syndrome: an inherited disorder of renal, ocular and cochlear membranes. Medicine 1999;78:338–360.
12. Kashtan CE, Kleppel MM, Gubler MC. Immunohistological findings in Alport syndrome. Contrib Nephrol 1996;117:142–153.
13. Van der Loop FT, Monnens LA, Schroder CH, Lemmink HH, Breuning MH, Timmer ED, Smeets HJ. Identification of COL4A5 defects in Alport's syndrome by immunohistochemistry of skin. Kidney Int 1999;55:1217–1224.
14. Strachan T, Read A (eds). Human Molecular Genetics, Oxford, BIOS Scientific Publishers Ltd. 1996, pp. 427–434.
15. Kestila M, Lenkkeri U, Manniko M, Lamerdin J, McCready P, Pataala H, Ruotsalainen V, Morita T, Nissmen M, Herva R, Kashtan CE, Peltonen L, Holmberg C, Olsen A, Tryggvason K. Positionally cloned gene for a novel glomerular protein—nephrin—is mutated in congenital nephrotic syndrome. Mol Cell 1998;1:575–582.
16. Town M, Jean G, Cherqui S, Attard M, Forestier L, Whitmore SA, Callen DF, Gribouval O, Broyer M, Bates GP, van't Hoff W, Antignac C. A novel gene encoding an integral membrane protein is mutated in nephropathic cystinosis. Nat Genet 1998;18:319–324.
17. Konrad M, Saunier S, Heidet L, Silbermann F, Benessy F, Caledo J, Le Paslier D, Broyer M, Gubler MC, Antignac C. Large homozygous deletions of the 2q13 region are a major cause of juvenile nephronophthisis. Hum Mol Genet 1996;5:367–371.
18. Hildebrandt F, Otto E, Rensing C, Nothwang HG, Vollmer M, Adolphs J, Hanush H, Brandis M. A novel gene encoding an SH3 domain protein is mutated in nephronophthisis type 1. Nat Genet 1997;17:149–153.
19. Knebelmann B, Breillat C, Forestier L, Arrondel C, Jacassier D, Giatas I, Drouot L, Deschenes G, Grunfeld JP, Broyer M, Gubler MC, Antignac C. Spectrum of mutations in the COL4A5 gene in X-linked Alport syndrome. Am J Hum Genet 1996;59:1221–1232.
20. Lemmink HH, Schroder C, Monnens LAH, Smeets HJM. The clinical spectrum of type IV collagen mutations. Hum Mutat 1997;9:477–499.
21. Watnick T, Germino GG. Molecular basis of autosomal dominant polycystic kidney disease. Semin Nephrol 1999;19:327–343.
22. Van den Ouweland AMW, Dreesen JCM, Verdijk M, Knoers NVAM, Monnens LAH, Rocchi M, van Oost BA. Mutations in the vasopressin type-2 receptor gene (AVPR2) associated with nephrogenic diabetes insipidus. Nat Genet 1992;2:99–102.
23. Pan Y, Metzenberg A, Das S, Jing B, Gitschier J. Mutations in the V2 vasopressin receptor gene are associated with nephrogenic diabetes insipidus. Nat Genet 1992;2:103–106.
24. Rosenthal W, Seiblod A, Antamarian A, Lonergan M, Arthus M, Hendy GN, Birnbaumer M, Bichet DG. Molecular identification of the gene responsible for congenital nephrogenic diabetes insipidus. Nature 1992;359:233–235.
25. Deen PMT, Verdijk MAJ, Knoers NVAM, Wieringa B, Monnens LAH, van Os CH, van Oost BA. Requirement of human renal water channel aquaporin-2 for vasopressin-dependent concentration of urine. Science 1994;264:92–95.
26. Mulders SM, Bichet DG, Rijss JP, Kamsteeg EJ, Arthus MF, Lonergan M, Fujiwara M, Morgan K, Leijendekker P, van der Sluijs P, van Os CH, Deen PM. An aquaporin-2 water channel mutant which causes autosomal dominant nephrogenic diabetes insipidus is retained in the golgi complex. J Clin Invest 1998;102:57–66.
27. Herndon CDA, Ferrer FA, Freedman A, McKenna PHMC. Consensus on the prenatal mangement of

antenatally detected urological abnormalities. J Urol 2000;164:1052–1056.

28. Fanos V, Agostiniani R, Cataldi L. Pyelectasis and hydronephrosis in the newborn and infact. Acta Pediatr 2000;89:900–904.

29. Stranc LC, Evans JA, Hamerton JL. Chorionic villus sampling and amniocentesis for prenatal diagnosis. Lancet 1997;349:711–714.

30. Knoers NVAM, Monnens LAH. Nephrogenic diabetes insipidus. Sem Nephrol 1999;19:344–352.

31. Wells D, Sherlock JK. Strategies for preimplantation genetic diagnosis of single gene disorders by DNA amplification. Prenat Diagn 1998;18:1389–1401.

32. Went L. Guidelines for the molecular genetics predictive test in Huntington's disease. J Med Genet 1994;31:555–559.

33. Markello TC, Bernardini IM, Gahl WA. Improved renal function in children with cystinosis treated with cysteamine. N Engl J Med 1993;328:1157–1162.

34. Dent CE, Senior B. Studies on the treatment of cystinuria. Br J Urol 1995;27:317–332.

35. Monnens L, Noordam K, Trybels F. Necessary practical treatment of cystinuria at night. Pediatr Nephrol 2000;14:1128–1149.

36. Lindstedt S, Holme E, Lock EA, Hjalmarson O, Strandvik, B. Treatment of hereditary tyrosinemia type I by inhibition of 4-hydroxyphenylpyruvate dioxygenase. Lancet 1992;340:813–817.

37. Schiffmann R, Murray GJ, Treco D, Daniel P, Sellos-Moura M, Myers M, Quirk JM, Zirzow GC, Borowski M, Loveday K, Anderson T, Gillespie F, Oliver KL, Jeffries NO, Doo E, Liang TJ, Kreps C, Gunter K, Frei K, Crutchfield K, Seldem RF, Brady RO. Infusion of α-galactosidase A reduces tissue globotriaosylceramide storage in patients with Fabry disease. Proc Natl Acad Sci USA 2000; 97:365–370.

38. Morello JP, Salahpair A, Laperriere A, Bernier V, Arthus MF, Lonergan M, Petaja-Repo U, Angers S, Morin D, Bichet DG, Bouvier M. Pharmacological chaperones rescue cell-surface expression and function of misfolded V2 vasopressin receptor mutants. J Clin Invest 2000;105:887–895.

39. Kalluri R, Torre A, Shield CF, Zambrosky ER, Werner M, Suchin E, Wolf G, Helmchen W, van den Heuvel L, Grossman R, Aradhye S, Neilson ZS. Identification of α3, α4, and α5 chains of type IV collagen as alloantigens for Alport posttransplant antiglomerular basement membrane antibodies. Transplantation 2000;69:679–683.

40. Cochat P. Primary hyperoxaluria type I. Kidney Int 1999;55:2533–2547.

41. Shayakul C, Breton S, Brown D, Alper SL. Gene therapy of inherited renal tubular disease. Am J Kidney Dis 1999;34:374–377.

42. Fraser FC. Genetic counselling. Am J Hum Genet 1974;26:636–661.

43. Clarke A. Is non-directive genetic counseling possible? Lancet 1991;338:998–1001.

44. Bernhardt BA. Empirical evidence that genetic counseling is directive: where do we go from here? Am J Hum Genet 1997;60:17–20.

17 | Renal malformations and renal involvement in syndromes

Bronwyn Kerr and Nicholas J.A. Webb

Introduction

A significant malformation is present in approximately 3% of newborns and approximately 1% have multiple malformations [1]. A congenital anomaly is observed in 5% of liveborn infants, with around one half of these having single-gene, multifactorial, or chromosomal causation [2].

Renal malformations occur in less than 1% of newborns, but when they do occur, the incidence of both multiple renal malformations and other congenital anomalies is high [3]. Despite the clinical assessment of 60% of a series of live and stillborn infants with renal anomalies as being 'syndromic', the cause of the renal malformation remained unknown in more than 90% [3].

The morbidity associated with congenital renal abnormalities is high, with renal malformations, obstructive conditions, and hereditary disorders accounting for 67% of cases of childhood chronic renal failure in the United Kingdom [4].

Comprehensive lists of syndromes associated with particular renal malformations are available from a number of excellent sources [3,5]. The purpose of this chapter is not to duplicate these, but to provide an approach to evaluating the child with a renal abnormality and to summarize renal involvement in common sequences and associations, chromosomal abnormalities, and selected single-gene disorders.

Description of congenital anomalies

The term 'dysmorphology' was coined by Dr David Smith in the 1960s to describe the study of human congenital malformations. Literally, it means 'the study of abnormal form'. A number of terms are used in the literature to describe birth defects in terms of the underlying pathogenesis [6]:

A *congenital anomaly* is an abnormality present at birth, whether it be a malformation, deformation, disruption, or dysplasia. Congenital anomalies are classified as major or minor, single or multiple. A *major anomaly* is defined as one producing significant long-term disability or death. *Minor anomalies*, e.g. ear pits, skin tags, single palmar creases, are unusual morphological features that are of no serious medical or cosmetic consequence in themselves. Their importance is that they may provide a clue to a specific multiple anomaly syndrome or indicate a more generalized error in morphogenesis.

A *malformation* is a morphological defect of an organ, part of an organ, or a larger area of the body that results from an intrinsically abnormal developmental process [1].

A *deformation* is an anomaly produced by aberrant mechanical forces that distort otherwise normal structures. Deformation is commonly associated with abnormal fetal posture and with reduced liquor volume of any cause (Fig. 17.1).

A *disruption* results from destruction of previously normal tissue. Amniotic bands may produce skin constriction and complete or partial amputations or more extensive destruction of normal tissue. Both deformations and disruptions imply that there was no intrinsic abnormality of the involved tissue [1,6].

A *dysplasia* results from abnormal cellular organization or function within a specific tissue type throughout the body. Unlike malformations, disruptions, or deformations, the process that produced the tissue change is ongoing throughout life.

Associations (e.g. VATER, CHARGE) describe a number of birth defects that occur together more frequently than one would expect by chance.

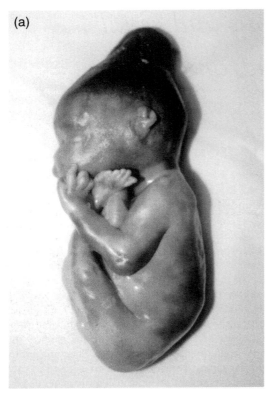
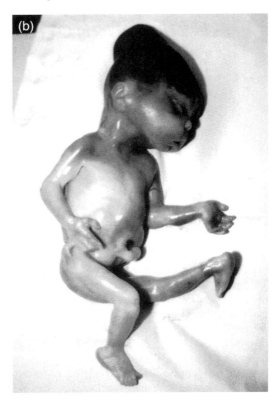

Fig. 17.1   Fetal deformation simulating encephalocele and joint abnormalities (a) post-delivery; (b) presumed *in utero* posture. Photograph courtesy of Professor Dian Donnai.

A *malformation sequence* is a pattern of multiple defects derived from a single known or presumed structural defect. A lumbar myelomeningocele may result in paralysis of the lower limbs, talipes, incontinence, dilatation of the urinary tract, and hydrocephalus, a sequence of malformation wholly derived from the myelomeningocele.

A *syndrome* refers to a particular set of anomalies that occur in a consistent pattern with a single underlying cause.

Clinical evaluation: single or multiple?

The evaluation of an infant with any congenital anomaly begins with determining whether or not the anomaly is a single isolated defect or part of a more generalized disturbance in development. In the history, factors of particular importance are pregnancy history (liquor volume, movements, maternal illness and medication, investigations) and family history (renal disease, congenital anomaly, neonatal death or stillbirth, miscarriages, intellectual disability). On examination, birth weight, head circumference, and facial features should be documented and particular attention paid to the presence or absence of minor anomalies.

Minor anomalies are present in 14% of newborn infants [7]. Only 0.8% of infants have two minor anomalies, and these infants have a rate of congenital anomaly that is five times higher than the background rate. Three or more minor anomalies are found in only 0.5% of newborn infants and 90% of these have one or more significant birth defects [7]. A number of guides to frequency, definition, and interpretation of minor anomalies are available [6,8].

The presence of abnormalities of growth or behaviour or minor anomalies increases the likelihood of a more generalized disturbance in development. Depending on the clinical findings, helpful investigations may include echocardiography, skeletal survey, formal eye examination, cerebral imaging, and karyotype. A normal antenatal karyotype does not necessarily exclude the presence of subtle chromosome abnormality, since, due to the quality of the cell culture, antenatal testing may only reliably exclude major structural arrangements and abnormalities of chromosome number.

Key point

- The presence of minor anomalies can be a clue to a generalized disturbance in development.

Fetal renal abnormality

Increasingly, renal malformations are being diagnosed before birth. The use of ultrasound has become part of routine obstetric practice. One-stage screening has been recommended in the United Kingdom with most pregnancies screened at around 18 weeks' gestation. Evaluation of the efficacy of ultrasound in pregnancy has demonstrated a number of factors that influence its accuracy. The sensitivity and specificity of ultrasound in diagnosing fetal abnormality varies with the timing of ultrasound

examination, the level of expertise of the operator and centre performing the study, the prior risk of the population being studied, fetal factors, the presence or absence of maternal obesity, and the type of abnormality [9,10]. The sensitivity is greatest for central nervous system abnormalities, neck anomalies, and urogenital abnormalities [10].

Case 1

The unrelated parents of this child were first seen in the ultrasound department at 20 weeks' gestation in their first pregnancy because their baby had been found to have unilateral hydronephrosis and agenesis of the corpus callosum. The difficulty of interpreting these findings was discussed; the couple were committed to the pregnancy. At delivery, he was small and microcephalic (birth weight 2.21 kg, head circumference 29.2 cm), with turricephaly, unusual facial features, and round protuberant ear lobes (Fig. 17.2a). On day 3, short-segment Hirschsprung disease was diagnosed and surgically treated. Renal ultrasound confirmed persistent dilatation of the right pelvicalyceal system; a micturating cystourethrogram was normal. A small patent ductus arteriosus (PDA) was found on echocardiography. Other baseline investigations, including chromosomes, were normal. With time, he was found to have severe developmental delay, although a very pleasant and easy personality. Despite

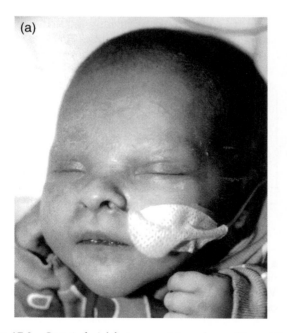 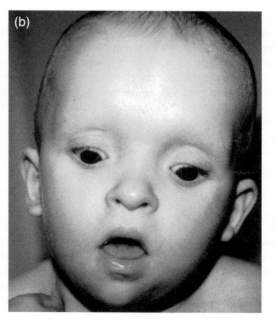

Fig. 17.2   Case 1: facial features as (a) newborn; (b) aged 3 years.

a number of syndromes featuring developmental delay and Hirschsprung disease, no syndrome diagnosis could be made until recognition of a new syndrome [11], thought to be due to a microdeletion or contiguous gene syndrome on chromosome 2q. By this time, he was aged 5 years.

For some antenatally diagnosed renal or urogenital abnormalities, the outlook is known [12–14]. For others, the outlook is not certain. Even with an apparently isolated renal anomaly diagnosed *in utero*, it is not possible to determine antenatally whether or not a given malformation is truly isolated. Even in tertiary centres and with third-trimester ultrasound, the rate of undetected abnormality with ultrasound is high [15]. Additionally, the presence or absence of minor anomalies, on which a syndrome diagnosis is often based, can only be determined post-delivery. Even in fetuses with more than one abnormality visible on ultrasound, definitive diagnosis is often not possible prior to delivery.

Key point

- Accurate diagnosis of an antenatally diagnosed abnormality requires careful examination post-delivery.

When a pregnancy is terminated because of a diagnosis of abnormality, thorough fetal examination is essential after delivery. External assessment and targeted investigation, with or without post-mortem, has been found to modify the pre-termination diagnosis in a way significant for genetic counselling in 40% [16]. For those interested, the literature relevant to fetal dysmorphology has been summarized [17].

Associations and renal abnormalities

The principal anomalies seen in the *CHARGE* association are summarized in the mnemonic: C = coloboma, H = heart defects, A = atresia of the choanae, R = retarded growth and development, G = genital anomalies, E = ear anomalies or deafness. Other frequent anomalies include facial palsy, renal abnormalities, orofacial clefts and tracheo-oesophageal fistula [18]. The cause of the CHARGE association is unknown and the diagnosis is a clinical one. It has been suggested that four of the defining criteria should be present for the diagnosis to be made, and that these should include coloboma or choanal atresia or both. Facial palsy and renal abnormalities are both so common that they can provide confirmatory evidence. Renal ultrasound should be undertaken in all children in whom the diagnosis of the CHARGE association is suspected.

Commonly associated renal abnormalities include duplex renal systems, horseshoe kidney, crossed renal ectopia, abnormal rotation of kidneys, and renal dysplasia with vesico-ureteric reflux. Recurrent urinary tract infections in the presence of a normal urinary tract are also frequent [18].

It is possibly because of this common association that there is a widespread belief that ear abnormalities correlate with the presence of renal abnormalities. In fact the ear shape seen in the CHARGE association is characteristic, the external ear being short and wide with a simple configuration and often protruding, lop, or cup-shaped. Apart from the branchio-oto-renal syndrome (see below), there are few syndromes that combine abnormalities of the external ear and renal abnormalities, namely autosomal dominant dysmorphic pinnae–polysystic kidneys syndrome, autosomal dominant dysmorphic pinnae–hypospadias–renal dysplasia syndrome, and autosomal recessive oto–renal–genital syndrome. In contrast, there are many syndromes that combine hearing loss and renal abnormalities [19].

Key points

- Many syndromes combine hearing loss and renal abnormalities.

- There are only a small number of syndromes combining external ear and renal abnormalities.

The *VATER* or *VACTERL* association describes a combination of anomalies that occur together more often than one would expect by chance: V = vertebral or vascular, A = anal, TE = tracheo-oesophageal fistula or oesophageal atresia, R = radial limb or renal anomalies. The expanded association includes C = cardiovascular, L = limb malformations.

Renal anomalies occur in approximately two-thirds, with 40% having unilateral renal aplasia. Other abnormalities include pelvi-ureteric junction obstruction, crossed renal ectopia, pelvic kidney, or horseshoe kidney [20]. Most cases have been sporadic. It is very important, however, to consider the autosomal recessive *Fanconi anaemia* in the differential diagnosis, because of the implications for general health and the recurrence risk. This condition is most often associated with abnormalities of the radius, thumb, and renal tract, but can have multiple effects in other organ systems, and should be especially considered in the presence of symmetrical upper limb abnormalities. Determining chromosome Mitomycin C sensitivity can make the diagnosis of Fanconi anaemia. The VACTERL association has been reported with the A–G transition mutation at nucleotide position 3243 of mitochondrial DNA and, although this may have been coincidental, a mitochondrially mediated cause should be considered in the presence of a suggestive family history [21].

Major chromosomal abnormalities and renal malformations

Renal malformations are common in children with abnormal chromosomes (Table 17.1). *Trisomy 21* is the most common chromosome abnormality seen in live-born infants. Renal hypoplasia, hydroureteronephrosis, vesico-ureteric and pelvi-ureteric obstruction, vesico-ureteric reflux, and posterior urethral valves have all been reported to occur in association with Down syndrome, and there are a number of reports describing the management of end stage renal failure in this population. The literature has been well reviewed [22] and it has been recommended that all children with Down syndrome undergo ultrasound examination of the urinary tract in the newborn period. *Trisomy 13* is commonly associated with dysplastic renal anomalies and genital anomalies: dysplastic renal anomalies may occur in *trisomy 18*, but are less common. Of particular importance is *7q+*; this anomaly has a greater than chance association with bilateral renal agenesis (Potter syndrome) and is frequently due to a parental translocation [20]. As this would mean a high chance of recurrence, advice about recurrence of bilateral renal agenesis cannot be given without knowledge of the infant or parental karyotype.

Table 17.1 Renal abnormalities associated with chromosomal abnormalities

Karyotype	Frequency of renal abnormality
3q+	60–70%
4p−	Common and variable
4q+	50%
7q+	Potter syndrome
Trisomy 8, often mosaic	40%
10p+	Variable
10q−	Variable
Trisomy 13	Common
Trisomy 18	Less common
Trisomy 21	3.5–16.6%
Marker 22 (cat-eye)	20%
X0	24–60%

Key point

- All children with Down syndrome should undergo ultrasound examination of the urinary tract in the newborn period.

Cat-eye syndrome (CES), the association of coloboma with anal atresia and renal and cardiac malformation, is due to the presence of an extra chromosome fragment (marker) derived from the long arm of chromosome 22. However, the relationship between the presence of a 22 marker and an abnormal phenotype is not a simple one, since even markers known to contain proximal 22q euchromatin (i.e. genetically active material) are not always associated with CES or even an abnormal phenotype [23].

Turner syndrome occurs with an incidence of 1 in 2500 live female births. Girls with Turner syndrome display characteristic major and minor malformations, including structural renal abnormalities. These include horseshoe kidney, duplex collecting systems, renal agenesis, and simple cysts. Studies have estimated the prevalence of renal abnormality at between 24 and 60%, these occurring predominantly in those with pure monosomy compared with a significantly lower incidence in those with mosaicism [24].

Chromosomal microdeletions and renal malformations

Recently, the study of chromosomes has improved due to both higher-resolution banding techniques and the development of new techniques, particularly fluorescence *in situ* hybridization (FISH). Many syndromes are now known to be due to chromosomal microdeletions; deletions below the resolution of conventional cytogenetics. FISH involves the use of a DNA sequence, labelled with a fluorescent tag. When this is hybridized to a glass slide containing patient chromosomes, a signal in the region of interest will only be seen on one chromosome in the presence of a deletion. FISH is a specific technique and can only be performed on specific request when a microdeletion syndrome is suspected on clinical grounds.

Williams syndrome is characterized by mental retardation with a friendly, outgoing personality, typical facies, supravalvular aortic stenosis, peripheral pulmonary artery stenosis, and, sometimes, idiopathic hypercalcaemia in infancy. The cause is a microdeletion on the long arm of chromosome 7, the deletion encompassing the elastin gene. Deletions of, or mutations in, the elastin gene alone cause isolated autosomal dominant supravalvular aortic stenosis. The nature of the other genes involved in the microdeletion seen in Williams syndrome is currently the subject of active research. Hypertension occurs in around one-third of patients. Renal artery stenosis has been reported, and both structural and functional urological abnormalities have an increased frequency. Nephrocalcinosis may occur secondary to hypercalcaemia and hypercalciuria, and renal function may decline with age. Blood pressure monitoring and periodic re-evaluation of the structure and function of the kidney and urinary tract are warranted [25].

A *deletion 22q11* in the DiGeorge syndrome locus has a wide range of phenotypic manifestations, including DiGeorge syndrome, velocardiofacial syndrome, and conotruncal heart defects with characteristic facies [26,27]. In a large European series, renal abnormalities were found in 36% of the 136 who had undergone renal ultrasound [28]. Absent, dysplastic, or multicystic kidneys, obstructive abnormalities, vesico-ureteric reflux, nephrocalcinosis, and duplex kidney were all described. This diagnosis should therefore be considered in children presenting with these renal anomalies and congenital heart disease, cleft palate or velopharyngeal insufficiency, or hypocalcaemia. As deletions visible on standard cytogenetic analysis are uncommon at this locus, the diagnosis will be missed if the specific FISH test is not requested. Conversely, renal ultrasound should be undertaken in children in whom the diagnosis of a 22q11 deletion is made. It should be remembered

that the deletion is inherited in close to one-third of cases, and therefore testing parental chromosomes with appropriate FISH is mandatory once the diagnosis is made.

Smith–Magenis syndrome is a rare chromosome microdeletion syndrome, associated with a deletion of chromosome 17p11.2 [29]. In some children, this will be visible on standard cytogenetic analysis, although in others it will not be recognized unless the specific FISH test is requested. The estimated incidence is 1 in 25 000. Individuals with Smith–Magenis syndrome have a characteristic face (Fig. 17.3), speech delay, growth and mental retardation, a hoarse voice, and a characteristic behavioural phenotype. A variety of congenital heart abnormalities have been described, including septal defects, atrial valve abnormalities, sub- and supravalvular aortic stenosis, and tetralogy of Fallot. Renal abnormalities in one series occurred in 35%, with duplication of the urinary tract being the most common and unilateral agenesis of the kidney and an ectopic kidney also detected. Renal ultrasound is therefore recommended in all patients. Other less common manifestations that have emerged since the first description are a high incidence of ocular anomalies, hearing loss, and peripheral neuropathy, with hypothyroidism and hypogammaglobulinaemia also being seen with increased frequency [30].

Common single-gene diseases in which renal abnormality is a cardinal feature

Meckel–Grüber syndrome is characterized classically by occipital encephalocele, bilateral cystic dysplastic kidneys, and post-axial polydactyly (Fig. 17.4). However, the range of manifestations is broad and not always constant, even in affected siblings. Microcephaly, cleft lip and palate, short limbs, genital anomalies, microcephaly, and microphthalmia have all been described [31]. A nationwide study in Finland concluded that cystic dysplasia of the kidneys, with fibrotic changes of the liver and occipital encephalocele, or some other central nervous system abnormality, are minimal diagnostic criteria, but the validity of this is lessened by findings in some families. The diagnosis should therefore be considered in infants with any combination of the reported

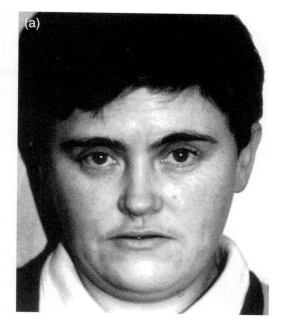

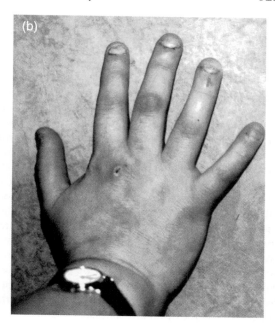

Fig. 17.3   Adult with Smith–Magenis syndrome: (a) facial features; (b) small hands.

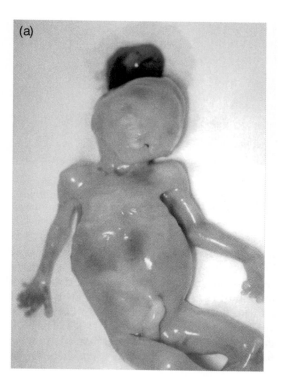

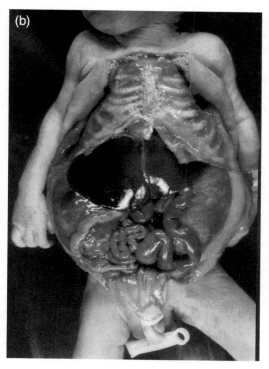

Fig. 17.4   Fetus with Meckel-Grüber syndrome: (a) encephalocele, polydactyly, and distended abdomen; (b) renal enlargement. Photograph courtesy of Professor Dian Donnai.

features. Meckel–Grüber syndrome is an autosomal recessive disorder, with the responsible gene localized in some, but not all families, to 17q21–24 [32]. Detailed fetal ultrasound remains the only antenatal diagnosis in most families.

Jeunes syndrome (asphyxiating thoracic dystrophy or *thoracic–pelvic–phalangeal dystrophy)* usually presents in the newborn period with a long narrow chest, associated with a varying degree of respiratory distress [33]. Affected infants have limb shortening affecting the middle segment of the limbs, hands, and feet, and occasionally polydactyly and nail dysplasia. Skeletal manifestations are milder than in the short-rib polydactyly syndromes. On X-ray, the ribs are variably short and broad with widening of the anterior ends (Fig. 17.5). The pelvis is characteristic, with square iliac wings, and a horizontal acetabular roof, with its medial portion deformed by a rounded protuberance, limited on each side by a spur-shaped projection. The metaphyseal ends may be irregular with a small spine on the distal metaphysis of the humerus or the proximal tibia [20]. The inheritance is autosomal recessive. Identical X-ray findings and polydactyly are seen in *Ellis–Van-Creveld syndrome.* The two conditions may be differentiated by the high frequency of congenital heart disease in Ellis–Van-Creveld syndrome in association with nail dysplasia and abnormalities of the upper lip, typically partial upper lip clefting connected to the alveolar ridge by multiple frenulae. The natural history of the respiratory complications of Jeunes syndrome is improvement with advancing age in those who survive the newborn period. The risk of chronic renal failure secondary to nephronophthisis is high [33]. Symptomatic liver disease has been described [34] and regular monitoring of both renal and hepatic function is important.

Joubert syndrome is a rare autosomal recessive disorder characterized by cerebellar vermis hypoplasia, hypotonia, developmental delay, episodic hyperpnoea, and abnormal eye movements. The diagnostic criteria suggested are the first three manifestations, and at least one of the other two [35]. Post-axial polydactyly and retinal coloboma may be present. Retinal dystrophy occurs in some patients and is consistent within sibships. The group of patients with retinal dystrophy may also have renal involvement, with multiple small cortical cysts and/or interstitial chronic inflammation and fibrosis [35]. Linkage analysis has suggested a locus on 9q in some, but not all, families [36].

Bardet–Biedl syndrome was first reported by Bardet in 1920, and Biedl in 1922. Bardet reported

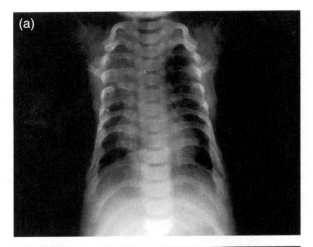

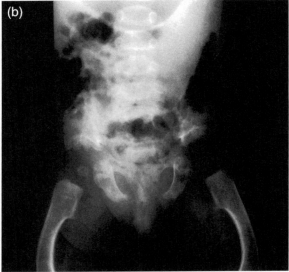

Fig. 17.5 X-ray findings in Jeune syndrome: (a) bell-shaped chest with short ribs with broad anterior ends; (b) pelvis. Photograph courtesy of Dr Maurice Super.

a single patient with congenital obesity, polydactyly, and retinitis pigmentosa and Biedl added mental retardation, hypogenitalism, anal atresia, and skull deformity to the clinical description with a second patient. It is a different condition to *Lawrence-Moon* syndrome, first described in 1866. The original description of Lawrence Moon was of a family with four members affected with a spinocerebellar degeneration, short stature, hypogenitalism, nystagmus, and mental retardation [37]. The original diagnostic criteria proposed that four of five cardinal features needed to be present to make the diagnosis of Bardet–Biedl syndrome; tapetoretinal degeneration, mental retardation, obesity, polydactyly, and hypogenitalism. The frequency of renal manifestations has only been appreciated more recently, with some abnormality of renal structure or function or both being present in all of a series of adult patients [38], although renal failure was present in only 15%. Defects of urinary concentrating ability and acidification and calyceal blunting and clubbing were all common.

A nationwide questionnaire survey of Bardet–Biedl syndrome in the United Kingdom found a lower prevalence of renal abnormalities (present in 26 of 109 patients), although only 57 had undergone renal investigation. Six patients, four of them children, had chronic renal failure, and four, including two children, had undergone renal transplantation. The average age at diagnosis in this group was 9 years; revised diagnostic criteria that may facilitate earlier diagnosis have been proposed [39]. A rod–cone dystrophy had been diagnosed in 93% of patients, all of those aged more than eight years. The mean age at noticing night blindness was 8.5 years, with a mean age of registering as blind of 15.5 years. Learning difficulties were reported in 62%.

Bardet–Biedl is an autosomal recessive condition, where linkage analysis has established five different gene localizations, with some families exhibiting linkage to none of these. A sixth locus has recently been established with the discovery of mutations in the *MKKS* gene in some patients [40]. Different mutations in this gene cause McKusick–Kaufman syndrome, an autosomal recessive disorder which includes congenital heart disease, hydrometrocolpos, and post-axial polydactyly, most commonly in the Amish population. Identification of this gene may facilitate identification of the other genes that can cause Bardet–Biedl syndrome. For the foreseeable future, however, the diagnosis of Bardet–Biedl syndrome remains a clinical one. This may be difficult in early childhood when the recurrence risk to siblings may be most relevant.

In 1951, Fanconi described familial juvenile nephronophthisis. Ten years later, Senior described a family where 6 of 13 siblings had familial juvenile nephronopthisis and a early onset retinopathy [41]. Many similar clinical reports have followed [42]. This combination of juvenile nephronophthisis and early onset retinopathy is referred to in the literature as *Senior–Loken syndrome*. Linkage analysis has established that familial juvenile nephronophthisis is heterogeneous, with one locus on 2q13. This locus has been excluded for Senior–Loken syndrome.

Branchio–oto–renal (BOR) syndrome is an autosomal dominant condition associated with hearing loss, branchial arch defects, ear pits, and renal anomalies. All manifestations are variable. The hearing loss can be conductive, sensorineural, or mixed, and ranges from mild to profound. Renal anomalies include aplasia, hypoplasia, and dysplasia as well as abnormalities of the collecting system. Branchial defects include fistulas and cysts. External ear anomalies may be seen in addition to ear pits and absence of the lacrimal ducts may be seen. The penetrance is high, although the condition is highly variable (i.e. variable expressivity). Around 6% of affected individuals are said to have severe renal involvement, with or without renal failure [19].

BOR syndrome is due to mutations in the *EYA1* gene, located on chromosome 8q13.3. Mutations can be demonstrated in the majority of families with classical BOR syndrome and mutation testing can be used to confirm the diagnosis; however, as there is no correlation between the mutation found and the manifestations, severity cannot be predicted.

The *nail–patella syndrome* is an autosomal dominant condition in which the patellae and nails are small or absent. When nails are present, they are small and the ulnar half may be absent and not reaching the fingertips. The changes are most marked in the thumb, with the severity diminishing across the hand to the little finger. Fingernails are more severely affected than toe nails. Contractures may be present in the fingers and at the elbows. A variety of other skeletal and eye abnormalities have been reported. Of these glaucoma is particularly important. A nephropathy resembling congenital nephrosis or glomerulonephritis has been observed in some families but not others, with the risk of renal disease in an affected person being estimated at 10%. Mutations in the *LMX1B* gene on 9q34 cause nail–patella syndrome, but no correlation has been found between specific mutations and phenotypic features.

Tuberous sclerosis (TS) is a very variable autosomal dominant condition, in which the neurological manifestations dominate the clinical picture. However, renal causes of death are second only to CNS causes [43]. Renal manifestations include angiomyolipoma, cystic disease (isolated cysts and polycystic disease), and, rarely, renal carcinoma. Macroscopically and radiologically, cystic disease in TS, when it occurs, may be indistinguishable from autosomal dominant polycystic kidney disease (ADPKD).

Mutations in two genes cause TS: *TSC1* on 9q34 and *TSC2* on 16p13.3. The *TSC2* gene lies immediately adjacent to *PKD1*, the major disease gene for ADPKD. In 22 of 27 TS patients with renal cystic disease, deletions of both the *TSC1* and ADPKD genes were found. Most patients had constitutional mutations and severe disease. Mosaicism and mild cystic disease were demonstrated in some of their parents [43].

Clinical guidelines and a care pathway for patients with TS have been published recently [44]. These recommend that patients with TS should have a renal ultrasound at diagnosis, at age 5 years and at 5-yearly intervals. If the scan is abnormal, it should be repeated 2–3-yearly, with blood pressure and creatinine measurement. In the presence of an angiomyolipoma that is over 4 cm in size or rapidly growing, scans should be repeated annually. Patients and their families should be aware of the importance of warning signs such as flank pain, unexplained fevers or urinary tract infection, and anaemia and should seek urgent medical advice in the presence of haematuria. Referral to a paediatric nephrologist is recommended when pathology is found and where there is raised blood pressure, elevated plasma creatinine, or any of the warning signs.

Key points: Tuberous sclerosis

- Children with TS should have a renal ultrasound at diagnosis, at age 5 years and at 5-yearly intervals.

- Abnormal scans should be repeated 2–3 yearly with blood pressure and creatinine measurement.

- In the presence of an angiomyolipoma that is over 4 cm in size or rapidly growing, scans should be repeated annually.

- Referral to a paediatric nephrologist is recommended when pathology is found and where there is raised blood pressure, elevated plasma creatinine, or significant symptoms.

Common genetic conditions in which renal abnormality may be found

Neurofibromatosis is an autosomal dominant condition with an estimated incidence of 1 in 2500. While the most obvious signs occur in the skin, complications can occur in many organ systems. Renal artery stenosis occurs in 2.1% and endocrine tumours in 3.1% [45]. Patients with neurofibromatosis should have their blood pressure measured annually as part of routine surveillance for complications and both of these complications considered in those who are persistently hypertensive.

Noonan syndrome is a common disorder. Although dominant inheritance is well established in at least 30% of cases, with maternal transmission being more likely, the cause remains unknown, with a single gene mutation or a microdeletion both possible. The cardinal features of Noonan syndrome are well known: short stature, congenital heart disease, particularly pulmonary stenosis, broad or webbed neck, chest deformity with pectus carinatum superiorly and excavatum inferiorly, and a distinctive facies that changes with age. Renal abnormalities occur in 11% and include cystic dysplasia, duplication, and hydronephrosis [46].

Osteogenesis imperfecta (OI) is a connective tissue disorder associated with osteopenia, skeletal deformity, and fragility, and in some forms, dentinogenesis imperfecta. The clinical classification used is that of Sillence [47]. Types I and IV are autosomal dominant and relatively mild, with the major morbidity in type I often being presenile deafness. Type I is associated with blue sclera. Type III is a more severe disorder, which may occur as a new dominant mutation or as an autosomal recessive condition. Type II is usually lethal in the perinatal period. All variants of OI are due to either qualitative or quantitative mutations in the two genes that are responsible for production of the chains of type I collagen. Renal stones, papillary calcification, and benign renal cysts have been reported in a small number of children with type I, III, and one unclassified [48] associated with unexplained recurrent urinary tract infection. The cause of this is unknown.

Conclusion

The available population surveys of congenital renal abnormality suggest that the majority of infants with a structural renal abnormality will have associated abnormalities. For each child therefore, a careful history and examination with targeted investigation is mandatory for the cause to be determined as accurately as possible, prognosis and recurrence risk derived, and for management to be both appropriate and comprehensive.

References

1. Cohen MM. The child with multiple birth defects. 1982; New York: Raven Press.
2. Baird PA, Anderson TW, Newcombe HB, Lowry RB. Genetic disorders in childen and young adults: a population study. Am J Hum Genet. 1988; 42:677–693.
3. Limwongse C, Clarren SK, Cassidy SB. Syndromes and malformations of the urinary tract. In: Barratt TM, Avner ED, Harmon WE, ed. Pediatric Nephrology. Baltimore: Lippicott Williams and Wilkins, 1998; pp. 427–452.
4. Second Annual Report of the UK Renal Registry. UK Renal Association.
5. Winter RM, Baraitser M. London dysmorphology data base. 2000; Oxford Electronic Publishing.
6. Aase JM. Diagnostic dysmorphology. New York: Plenum Medical Book Company, 1990; pp. 9–13.
7. Marden PM, Smith DW, McDonald MJ. Congenital anomalies in the newborn infant, including minor variations. J Pediatr 1964; 3:357–361.
8. Hall JG, Froster-Iskenius UG, Allanson JE. Handbook of normal physical measurements. 1989; New York: Oxford University Press.
9. Whittle MJ. Screening for fetal anomalies. Curr Obstet Gynaecol 1992; 2:72–76.
10. Levi S, Hyjazi Y, Schaaps J-P, Defoort P, Coulon R, Buekens P. Sensitivity and specificity of routine antenatal screening for congenital anomalies by ultrasound: the Belgian multicentre study. Ultrasound Obstet Gynaecol 1991; 1:102–110.
11. Mowat DR, Croaker GDH, Cass DT *et al.* Hirschprung disease, microcephaly, mental retardation, and characteristic facial features: delineation of a new syndrome and identification of a new locus at chromosome 2q22–q23. J Med Genet 1998; 35:617–623.
12. al-Khaldi N, Watson AR, Zuccollo J, Twining P, Rose DH. Outcome of antenatally detected cystic dysplastic kidney disease. Arch Dis Child 1994; 70: 520–522.
13. Lazebnik N, Bellinger MF, Ferguson JE 2nd, Hogge JS, Hogge WA. Insights into the pathogenesis and natural history of fetuses with multicystic dysplastic kidney disease. Prenat Diagn 1999; 19: 418–423.
14. Slovis TL, Bernstein J, Gruskin A. Hyperechoic kidneys in the newborn and young infant. Pediatr Nephrol 1993; 7:294–302.
15. Manchester DK, Pretorius DH, Avery C *et al.* Accuracy of ultrasound diagnoses in pregnancies complicated by suspected fetal anomalies. Prenat Diagn 1988; 8:109–117.
16. Medeira A, Norman A, Haslam J, Clayton-Smith J, Donnai D. Examination of fetuses after induced abortion for fetal abnormality—a follow-up study. Prenat Diagn 1994; 14:381–385.
17. Kerr B, Donnai D. Fetal dysmorphology. Fetal Mat Med Rev. 1995; 7:31–46.
18. Oley CA, Baraitser M, Grant DB. A reappraisal of the CHARGE association. J Med Genet. 1988; 25: 147–156.
19. Gorlin RJ, Toriello HV, Cohen MM. Hereditary hearing loss and its syndromes. New York: Oxford University Press, 1995; pp. 234–256.
20. Goodman RM, Gorlin RJ. The malformed infant and child; an illustrated guide. New York: Oxford University Press, 1983; pp. 84, 100 and 330.
21. Damian MS, Seibel P, Schachenmayr W, Reichmann H, Dorndorf W. VACTERL with the mitochondrial np3243 point mutation. Am J Med Genet. 1996; 62:398–403.
22. Kupferman JC, Stewart CL, Kaskel FJ, Fine RN. Posterior urethral valves in patients with Down syndrome. Pediatr Nephrol. 1996; 10:143–146.
23. Crolla JA, Howard P, Mitchell C, Long FL, Dennis NR. A molecular and FISH approach to determining karyotype and phenotype correlations in six patients with supernumary marker (22) chromosomes. Am J Med Genet 1997; 72:440–447.
24. Flynn MT, Ekstrom L, De Arce M, Costigan C, Hoey HM. Prevalence of renal malformation in Turner syndrome. Pediatr Nephrol. 1996; 10:498–500.
25. Metcalfe K. Williams syndrome: an update on clinical and molecular aspects. (1999) Arch Dis Child 81: 198–200.
26. Driscoll DA, Salvin J, Sellinger B *et al.* Prevalence of 22q.11 microdeletions in DiGeorge and velocardiofacial syndromes: implications for genetic counselling and prenatal diagnosis. J Med Genet. 1993; 30:813–817.
27. Goldmuntz E, Driscoll D, Budarf ML *et al.* Microdeletions of chromosomal region 22q11 in patients with conotruncal cardiac defects. J Med Genet. 1993; 30:807–812.
28. Ryan AK, Goodship JA, Wilson DI *et al.* Spectrum of clinical features associated with interstitial chromosome 22q11 deletions: a European collaborative study. J Med Genet. 1997; 34:798–804.
29. Smith ACM, McGavran L, Robinson J *et al.* Interstitial deletion of (17) (p11.2p11.2) in nine patients. Am J Med Genet. 1986; 24:393–414.
30. Greenberg F, Lewis RA, Potocki L *et al.* Multidisciplinary clinical study of Smith–Magenis syndrome (deletion 17p11.2). Am J Med Genet. 1996; 62: 247–254.
31. Salonen R, Paavola P. Meckel syndrome. J Med Genet; 1998; 35:497–501.
32. Paavola P, Salonen R, Weissenbach J, Peltonen L. The locus for Meckel syndrome with multiple congenital anomalies maps to chromosome 17q21–24. Nat Genet. 1995; 11:213–215.
33. Oberklaid F, Danks DM, Mayne V, Campbell P. Asphyxiating thoracic dystrophy. Clinical, radiological and pathological information on 10 patients. Arch Dis Child. 1977; 52:758–765.
34. Labrune P, Fabre M, Trioche P *et al.* Jeune syndrome and liver disease; report of three cases treated with ursodeoxycholic acid. Am J Med Genet. 1999; 87:324–328.

35. Saraiva JM, Baraitser M. Joubert syndrome: a review. Am J Med Genet. 1992; 43:726–731.

36. Saar K, Al-Gazali L, Sztriha L *et al*. Homozygosity mapping in families with Joubert syndrome identifies a locus on chromosome 9q34.3 and evidence for genetic heterogeneity. Am J Hum Genet. 1999; 65: 1666–1671.

37. Schachat AP, Maumenee IH. Bardet–Biedl syndrome and related disorders. Arch Ophthalmol. 1982; 100: 285–288.

38. Harnett JD, Green JS, Cramer BC *et al*. The spectrum of renal disease in Laurence–Moon–Biedl syndrome. New Engl J Med. 1988; 319:615–618.

39. Beales PL, Elcioglu N, Woolf AS, Parker D, Flinter FA. New criteria for improved diagnosis of Bardet–Biedl syndrome: results of a population survey. J Med Genet. 1999; 36:437–446.

40. Slavotinek AM, Stone EM, Mykytyn K *et al*. Mutations in MKKS cause Bardet–Biedl syndrome. Nat Genet. 2000; 26:15–16.

41. Senior B, Friedmann AI, Braudo JL. Juvenile familial nephropathy with tapetoretinal degeneration. Am J Ophthalmol. 1961; 52:625–663.

42. Cantani A, Bamonte G, Ceccoli D, Biribicchi G, Farinella F. Familial juvenile nephronopthisis. A review and differential diagnosis. Clinical Pediatr. 1986; 25: 90–95.

43. Sampson JR, Maheshwar MM, Aspinwall R *et al*. Renal cystic disease in tuberous sclerosis: Role of the polycystic kidney disease gene. Am J Hum Genet. 1997; 61:843–851.

44. Bradshaw N, Brewer C, FitzPatrick D *et al*. National guidelines and care pathways for genetic diseases: the Scottish collaborative project on Tuberous sclerosis. 1998; Eur J Hum Genet 6:445–458.

45. Huson SM. Recent developments in the diagnosis and management of neurofibromatosis. Arch Dis Child. 1989; 64:745–749.

46. Sharland M, Burch M, McKenna WM, Paton MA. A clinical study of Noonan syndrome. Arch Dis Child. 1992; 67:178–183.

47. Sillence DO, Senn A, Danks DM Genetic heterogeneity in osteogenesis imperfecta. J Med Genet. 1979; 16: 101–116.

48. Vetter U, Maierhofer B, Muller M *et al*. Osteogenesis imperfecta in childhood: cardiac and renal manifestations. 1989; Eur J Pediatr 149:184–187.

18 | Clinical presentation and evaluation of cystic disease

Katherine MacRae Dell and Ellis D. Avner

Introduction

Renal cystic disorders represent a heterogeneous group of diseases which may present *in utero* or be clinically silent well into adulthood. The age of presentation, family history, and other clinical signs and symptoms are essential in delineating specific disease entities. With the increased utilization of ultrasound (both antenatal as well as postnatal), cystic disease is being detected more frequently and at an earlier age. Accurate diagnosis is essential both in the management of patients found to have cystic kidneys and in counselling their families.

Cystic disorders include autosomal recessive polycystic kidney disease (ARPKD), autosomal dominant polycystic kidney disease (ADPKD), glomerulocystic kidney disease (GCKD), diffuse cystic dysplasia, simple cysts, medullary cystic disease/juvenile nephronophthisis, and acquired cystic kidney disease (ACKD) [1]. Cystic kidneys are an important component of several congenital syndromes, such as tuberous sclerosis and Meckel-Grüber syndrome [2,3]. This chapter will focus on the clinical presentations and management of each of these cystic disorders.

Autosomal recessive polycystic kidney disease

Case 1

Antenatal ultrasound examination in a 25-year-old female at 26 weeks' gestation detected oligohydramnios and a fetus with bilaterally enlarged kidneys with a bright echo pattern suggestive of diffuse parenchymal microcysts. Similar renal changes had been noted with a previous pregnancy, which resulted in a spontaneous abortion at 28 weeks' gestation. At 35 weeks' gestation a 2.8 kg female infant was born with respiratory distress, requiring resuscitation and mechanical ventilation. Bilateral flank masses were palpable on examination. Abdominal ultrasonography showed large, echogenic kidneys with a few small 1–2 mm cysts, and marked loss of corticomedullary differentiation. Liver ultrasound was normal. The infant developed hypertension on day 2 of life and required multiple antihypertensive medications to maintain blood pressure control. Plasma creatinine was 70 μmol/l on day 7 of life but slowly rose over the first few months of life. Though weaned from the ventilator at 4 days of age, the patient had severe feeding difficulties and repeated respiratory exacerbations. She eventually underwent bilateral nephrectomies and was placed on chronic peritoneal dialysis at 8 months of age.

This presentation of a neonate with oligohydramnios, respiratory distress, and large echogenic kidneys is typical of autosomal recessive polycystic kidney disease (ARPKD). The clinical features include large bilateral flank masses, some degree of pulmonary hypoplasia, and hypertension [4]. Renal function is often normal in the neonatal period, although severely affected infants may be azotaemic and anuric [5]. Over 75% of neonates will have hyponatraemia [6]. Severe oliguria, often with hyponatraemia, is frequently present in the newborn period in the presence of apparently well-preserved renal function. The mechanism for this is not clear, but it usually responds to diuretics and salt and water restriction. This oliguria may not be indicative of severe renal failure. Renal ultrasound (Fig. 18.1) typically shows bilaterally enlarged echogenic kidneys with 1–2 mm microcysts, although larger cysts have been reported [7]. Hepatic fibrosis is invariably present histologically, but may not be evident radiographically or clinically at birth [8]. In contrast to the systemic nature of ADPKD, abnormalities in ARPKD are classically restricted to the liver and kidney. However, a recent report noted the occurrence of multiple intracranial aneurysms in an adult with ARPKD [9].

ARPKD occurs with an incidence of 1:20 000 to 1:40 000, although these numbers may underestimate the true incidence since children may die in the neonatal period without a definitive diagnosis [10]. Females and males are affected equally. At present, the gene for ARPKD has not been identified, although a candidate locus has been mapped to chromosome 6p21.1–p12 [11]. To date, no genetic heterogeneity has been identified in affected families with classic ARPKD. However, a recent report described a kindred with ARPKD in association with skeletal and facial anomalies in which linkage to the 6p locus was excluded [12]. The renal pathology of ARPKD is confined to the collecting tubules, following a transient phase of proximal tubular involvement, and is characterized by fusiform dilatations of these nephron segments. The hepatic pathology is that of a characteristic 'ductal plate abnormality' with bile duct proliferation and ectasia with hepatic fibrosis [8].

The differential diagnosis of a neonate presenting with large echogenic kidneys includes ARPKD, early onset autosomal dominant polycystic kidney disease (ADPKD), glomerulocystic kidney disease, and diffuse cystic dysplasia [7,13]. Features that may help to distinguish these diseases presenting in the newborn period are shown in Table 18.1. As noted previously, the hepatic lesion of ARPKD may not be evident by ultrasonography in the newborn period, although if intrahepatic bile duct dilatation is seen, it supports the diagnosis of ARPKD. Liver biopsies are generally not performed for diagnostic purposes in this age group.

Congenital syndromes with polycystic kidneys or diffuse cystic dysplasia as a major feature are listed in Table 18.2. Less common causes of large echogenic kidneys in the newborn period include renal vein thrombosis, congenital nephrotic syndrome, contrast nephropathy, transient nephromegaly, renal candidiasis, glycogen storage disease, and leukaemia [7].

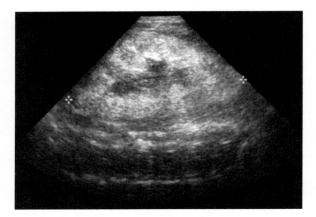

Fig. 18.1 Autosomal recessive polycystic kidney disease. Renal ultrasound (left kidney) in a newborn with ARPKD demonstrates increased kidney size (6.56 cm, mean length for age ± 2SD is 4.48 ± 0.62 cm) and marked echogenicity. A few very small cysts are noted within the renal parenchyma. Findings were identical for the contralateral kidney.

Table 18.1 Clinical features of cystic diseases presenting in the newborn period

Disease	Inheritance	Renal ultrasound	Pathology	Associated anomalies
Autosomal recessive polycystic kidney disease (ARPKD)	AR	Large echogenic kidneys, microcysts[a], occasional macrocysts[b]	Fusiform dilatation of the collecting duct	Hepatic fibrosis/biliary dysgenesis in all cases
Autosomal dominant polycystic kidney disease (ADPKD)	AD	Large echogenic kidneys, occasional macrocysts[b] (infants), multiple macrocysts[b] (older child)	Cysts originating from any portion of the nephron	Mitral valve prolapse, cerebral aneurysm*, AV malformation*, hepatic cysts*, pancreatic cysts*
Glomerulocystic kidney disease (GCKD)	AD, sporadic	Large echogenic kidneys, occasional macrocysts	Cystic dilatations of the glomeruli	May be syndromic. Hepatic fibrosis in up to 10% of non-syndromic
Diffuse cystic dysplasia	Sporadic	Large echogenic kidneys, microcysts or macrocysts[b]	Immature nephron development, dysplastic features (e.g. cartilage)	Usually syndromic

* Rare features in childhood.
AR, autosomal recessive; AD, autosomal dominant.
[a] Microcysts (usually 1–2 mm).
[b] Macrocysts (usually >1–2 cm).

Table 18.2   Congenital syndromes with polycystic kidneys and/or diffuse cystic dysplasia as a frequent feature

Syndrome	Associated features
Tuberous sclerosis	Depigmented ('ash-leaf') macules, adenoma sebaceum, cardiac rhabdomyoma, renal angiomyolipomas, CNS lesions, seizures
Meckel–Grüber syndrome	Microcephaly, occipital encephalocele, cleft palate, polydactyly, hepatic fibrosis
Jeune syndrome (asphyxiating thoracic dystrophy)	Small, short ribs, hypoplastic lungs, cystic lesions in liver and pancreas, hepatic fibrosis
Serpentine fibula–polycystic kidney syndrome	Elongated, serpentine fibulas, short stature, deafness
Short rib–polydactyly syndromes	Dwarfism, short ribs, intestinal atresia, polydactyly
Polycystic kidney disease with microbrachycephaly, hypertelorism, and brachymelia	Microbrachycephaly, hypertelorism, large ears, cardiac defects, brachymelia
Polycystic kidney, cataract, and congenital blindness	Blindness, cataracts, retinal abnormalities
Glutaricaciduria type 2	Abnormal odour, dysmorphic facial features, hepatomegaly, pulmonary hypoplasia, coma
Ivemark syndrome (asplenia with cystic liver, kidney and pancreas)	Asplenia, cardiac defects, cystic liver and/or pancreas, hepatic fibrosis
Orofaciodigital syndrome	Cleft jaw, facial dysmorphisms, syndactyly or other hand malformations
Zellweger syndrome	Abnormal skull and facial features, growth failure
Trisomy 13	Microphthalmia, cleft lip or palate, polydactyly, cardiac defects
Brachymesomelia–renal syndrome	Short limbs, cloudy corneas, cardiac defects
Goldston syndrome	Hepatic dysplasia, pancreatic dysplasia, Dandy–Walker cyst

Source: Online Mendelian Inheritance in Man (http://www3.ncbi.nlm.nih.gov/Omim)

Evaluation of a neonate with suspected ARPKD includes a complete physical examination with attention to the identification of congenital anomalies. As noted previously, features of the oligohydramnios (Potter's) sequence, including pulmonary hypoplasia, flat facies, limb deformities, and arthrogryposis may be present [14]. The family history in ARPKD is often unrevealing; however, consanguinity raises the possibility of an autosomal recessive disorder. Ultrasonography of the parents demonstrates no evidence of renal cystic disease. If renal cysts are identified in either parent, then the diagnosis of ADPKD or dominantly inherited glomerulocystic kidney disease should be considered.

Central to the management of neonates with echogenic large kidneys is assessment and stabilization of respiratory status. It may be clinically difficult to differentiate pulmonary hypoplasia from limitation of diaphragmatic excursion by massively enlarged kidneys, respiratory distress syndrome, or other reversible respiratory insults. An initial period of mechanical ventilation may be indicated until the pulmonary prognosis can be determined. Unilateral or bilateral nephrectomies have been reported in newborns with enlarged kidneys and severe respiratory distress [15,16] but these approaches have not

Key points: Neonatal large echogenic kidneys

- The differential diagnosis of large echogenic kidneys in the newborn period includes ARPKD, ADPKD, glomerulocystic disease, and diffuse cystic dysplasia, as well as a number of non-congenital causes such as contrast nephropathy and renal vein thrombosis.

- Renal ultrasound alone may not be helpful in distinguishing ARPKD, ADPKD, glomerulocystic kidney disease, and diffuse cystic dysplasia in a neonate with large echogenic kidneys. Detailed family history, ultrasonography of the parents, and the presence of associated anomalies are more helpful in establishing the diagnosis.

been studied systematically. Hypertension is often present in the newborn period and treatment with several antihypertensive medications may be necessary [5]. Angiotensin converting enzyme inhibitors and angiotensin II (ATII) receptor antagonists are first agents of choice, although the latter have not been well-studied in infants. Due to the significant collecting tubule involvement, patients with ARPKD have defects in urinary concentration and may be prone to dehydration, particularly with intercurrent childhood illnesses. For additional discussion of the management of neonates with renal disease, see Chapter 15. At present there is no specific treatment for ARPKD. However, an experimental therapy aimed at inhibiting cystic epithelial proliferation has shown encouraging results in an animal model of ARPKD [17].

Because of the complexity of issues involved in managing these patients, including the potential need for renal replacement therapy in infancy, consultation with a paediatric nephrologist in the immediate newborn period is essential. In families with a history of a previously affected infant, prenatal counselling is recommended. In these 'at-risk' families, prenatal genetic diagnosis using linkage analysis can be considered [18].

The prognosis of children with ARPKD has improved with neonatal intensive care, aggressive ventilatory and renal support, and blood pressure control. Currently, approximately 30% of severely affected infants will die in the neonatal period, primarily due to respiratory failure [6,19,20]. Such estimates are based on fragmentary data and the authors' clinical experience, since most published series are based on retrospective analyses of cases from the 1950s through the 1980s. For children who survive the neonatal period, 1-year survival is estimated to be 75–90% and 5-year survival 70–88% [5,6,20,21]. Progression to end stage renal disease (ESRD) occurs in over 50% of patients, especially those who present in the neonatal period. However, the time to reach ESRD may vary from months to years [5,20]. With dialysis and transplantation, death due to renal failure is rare. Commonly encountered clinical problems include feeding problems, growth failure, urinary tract infection, hepatic fibrosis, and complications of dialysis or transplantation [21]. Portal hypertension, with varices and resultant gastrointestinal bleeding, is not uncommon. In fact, a subset of patients with less severe renal involvement will not be diagnosed until later in childhood when they present with stigmata of hepatic involvement. Patients with ARPKD are at significant risk for ascending bacterial cholangitis, which may present as recurrent bacteraemia, without classic clinical features [22]. With improved renal survival and blood pressure control, the liver complications of ARPKD are likely to be of even greater clinical significance in the future.

Autosomal dominant polycystic kidney disease

Case 2

A 14-year-old girl presented to an outpatient clinic with a several-week history of left lower quadrant and abdominal pain. On physical examination she was normotensive with no abnormal findings. Urinalysis revealed 3+ microscopic haematuria with 25–50 red blood cells/high-power field, although no protein or other abnormalities. Screening biochemical tests revealed a normal serum creatinine of 53 μmol/l. Abdominal/pelvic ultrasonography demonstrated multiple small renal cysts (<1 cm) bilaterally, and one large cyst (5.7 cm) in the right kidney. Family history revealed a father with polycystic kidney disease and several paternal relatives who had died of cerebral vascular accidents. In the 2 years following her initial presentation, she had intermittent flank pain and a urinary tract infection. Subsequent urinalyses showed resolution of the haematuria. A follow-up ultrasound showed persistence of renal cysts as well as the appearance of a hepatic cyst. Cerebral magnetic resonance angiography (MRA), performed because of complaints of recurrent headache and the family history of cerebral vascular accidents, showed no evidence of aneurysms.

This case is typical for the initial presentation of ADPKD in the older child or adolescent. Although the majority of ADPKD patients do not become symptomatic until adulthood, children and even neonates may be symptomatic. As noted previously, the presentation of very early onset ADPKD may be indistinguishable from that of ARPKD in the neonatal period [13]. Symptoms include haematuria, hypertension, flank pain (from expanding cysts), and urinary tract infection [23,24]. Sterile pyuria is common. Renal ultrasound (Fig. 18.2) typically demonstrates one or more macroscopic cysts, which may be unilateral early in the disease, but are more typically bilateral. Unlike ARPKD, in which disease is restricted to the kidney and liver, ADPKD is a systemic disease, with multiorgan system involvement [25]. Intracranial aneurysms and other vascular malformations are an important cause of mortality in adults, but are only rarely reported in children [26]. Mitral valve prolapse is common, occurring in about 12% of children [27]. Liver and pancreatic cysts are unusual in children and the former rarely cause hepatic failure [25]. Ovarian cysts,

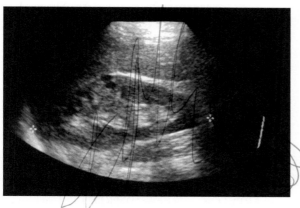

Fig. 18.2 Autosomal dominant polycystic kidney disease. Renal ultrasound (left kidney) in an adolescent with ADPKD shows an enlarged kidney (12.0 cm, mean length for age ± 2SD is 10.04 ± 1.72 cm) with multiple small (<1 cm) cysts throughout the kidney, predominantly in the cortex. The contralateral kidney demonstrated similar findings, as well as a large (5.7 cm) cyst in the upper pole.

intestinal diverticuli, and hernias may also develop. Congenital hepatic fibrosis, an invariable component of ARPKD, has been reported in ADPKD [28].

ADPKD has an incidence of 1/500 to 1/1000 and is caused by mutations in one of at least two identified disease genes, *PKD1* and *PKD2*. The complex genetics of this disease are addressed in recent reviews [29,30]. ADPKD is responsible for 8–10% of cases of end stage renal failure in Europe. *PKD1* accounts for about 85% of cases, maps to chromosome 16, and is a large gene, which encodes polycystin-1. Although polycystin-1 was first described over 5 years ago and is known to be an integral membrane protein, its precise function has not yet been determined. Current studies suggest that it may participate in cell–cell interactions or intracellular signalling. *PKD2* accounts for 10–15% of ADPKD and maps to chromosome 4. *PKD2* encodes a membrane protein, polycystin-2, that putatively functions as a voltage-gated ion channel. Current data support the hypothesis that *PKD1* and *PKD2* interact and that disruption of either can impair the 'polycystin complex'. Genetic diagnosis is possible, and is performed primarily by linkage analysis, since specific mutational analysis is difficult due to gene size and complexity. Approximately 5–10% of patients with ADPKD carry a new mutation. A broad spectrum of clinical severity is present between, and even within, families. Because of this heterogeneity, a family history may not be evident. Affected parents may be identified only after presentation and diagnosis of an affected child [31], as illustrated by the following case.

Case 3

A 2-week-old male infant was admitted to the hospital for evaluation of fever and noted to have persistent hypertension. Family history was unremarkable. Urinalysis and renal function studies were normal. A renal ultrasound showed normal-sized kidneys with several 1–2 cm cysts in each kidney. On repeat questioning, the patient's mother reported that she was once told she had 'a cyst on her kidney' but that it 'wasn't a problem'. Renal ultrasound studies of the patient's mother and maternal grandmother (both of whom had normal blood pressure and renal function) documented enlarged kidneys with diffuse bilateral cystic disease.

Key point: Autosomal dominant polycystic kidney disease

- In a child with renal cysts, a negative family history does not exclude the possibility of ADPKD, since the parent may have clinically silent disease.

The differential diagnosis of the older child with macroscopic renal cysts includes ADPKD, simple cysts, simple cysts associated with tuberous sclerosis (see Chapter 17) or acquired cystic kidney disease [1,32]. Multicystic dysplastic kidney, usually unilateral, is a common cause of palpable mass and macrocysts in the newborn period and is discussed elsewhere in this text. Obstructive cystic dysplasia can present as large kidneys with macrocysts. However, in the face of obvious signs of obstruction (such as severe hydronephrosis), this rarely confounds the differential diagnosis.

Evaluation of an older child with renal cysts includes a careful physical examination, with measurement of blood pressure and particular attention being paid to the presence of congenital abnormalities (such as 'ash-leaf' spots suggestive of tuberous sclerosis). Screening laboratory tests include plasma biochemistries and a urinalysis. Additional laboratory studies are indicated if the patient is found to have abnormal renal function. Ultrasound of the abdomen, including kidney, liver, and pancreas, and echocardiogram complete the initial evaluation.

Ultrasound of the parents can be very helpful in confirming the diagnosis of ADPKD. However, the use of renal ultrasound to screen asymptomatic pae-diatric patients in families with ADPKD is controversial. The psychological implications of carrying a genetic diagnosis for several asymptomatic decades are concerning. With no specific therapies currently available for ADPKD, a presymptomatic diagnosis may adversely affect insurability and employment. A negative ultrasound in an 'at-risk' younger child may be falsely reassuring. The false-negative rate in patients under 18 years of age approaches 20% [33]. The presence of two or more renal cysts is considered diagnostic in a patient under 30 years of age with a positive family history, and even one cyst in an 'at-risk' child is suggestive [33,34].

Screening radiographic studies to detect intracranial aneurysms are currently not recommended, although this remains controversial [35]. The exception is an ADPKD child with a strong family history of cerebral vascular accidents, who appears to have a fourfold increased risk of asymptomatic aneurysm [36]. Of course, patients who are symptomatic (e.g. with headaches or neurological deficits) merit prompt evaluation. Magnetic resonance angiography (MRA) is the study of choice, although small aneurysms may not be detected by this technique [36–38].

Treatment for neonates with ADPKD is identical to that for previously discussed neonates with ARPKD. This includes ventilatory support, close attention to fluid status and metabolic balance, and management of hypertension. In the older child or adolescent, management of hypertension, pain, and urinary tract infection is the mainstay of therapy. Hypertension control has been identified as a major factor influencing progression of disease as well as cardiovascular morbidity and mortality [39]. Based largely on studies in animal experimental models, other factors that may modulate disease progression include protein restriction, flax seed, fish oil, lipid-lowering agents, and angiotensin converting enzyme inhibitors. Pain due to cyst enlargement may require opiate analgesia when severe. In some instances, laparoscopic decortication or surgical decompression may relieve symptoms in selected cases. Infected cysts can be particularly difficult to manage, since standard therapies for urinary tract infections, such as ampicillin and aminoglycosides, are often ineffective in clearing cyst infections [40,41]. Ciprofloxacin has been shown to be effective in eliminating resistant infection [42].

The outcome of paediatric patients with ADPKD is variable. Those presenting in the first year of life generally have a poorer outcome, with about 20%

progressing to ESRD in the first decade of life [5,31]. Patients who present as older children and adolescents generally maintain normal renal function throughout childhood [25], although progression to end stage renal disease in later decades of life is likely.

Glomerulocystic kidney disease

Glomerulocystic kidney disease (GCKD) is an uncommon disorder, which typically presents in the neonatal period with large echogenic kidneys and microscopic glomerular cysts. It may be clinically indistinguishable from ARPKD or early onset ADPKD [13]. Later onset disease has been described in a few kindreds [43]. GCKD can be familial or sporadic. The inherited form is transmitted as an autosomal dominant trait, and in some instances is a distinct morphological subtype of ADPKD. However, a recent study confirmed that, in at least one large kindred, disease linkage to either ADPKD locus was excluded [43]. In the sporadic form, GCKD usually occurs as a major component of certain congenital syndromes, such as trisomy 13, Zellweger syndrome, tuberous sclerosis, orofacialdigital syndrome type I, and brachymesomelia–renal syndrome [2,44].

Kidneys of patients with GCKD demonstrate dilated Bowman's capsules, and dysplasia with abnormal medullary differentiation. Abnormalities of the intrahepatic bile ducts may be present in 10% of patients. The pathology of these liver lesions is similar to that seen in ARPKD [44]. Renal ultrasound findings usually demonstrate diffusely enlarged echogenic kidneys with occasional macrocysts. However, normal-sized kidneys with chronic renal failure have been reported in a father after his daughter was noted to have cystic kidneys [45].

As with other cystic diseases, evaluation includes a complete physical examination, screening chemistry tests, urinalysis, and careful family history. Additional evaluations include renal ultrasonography of the parents. Management of the infant with GCKD is identical to that of ARPKD, outlined previously. Patients with this disorder typically progress to chronic renal insufficiency. Hypertension is a common finding and should be treated aggressively.

Simple cysts

Simple cysts are typically diagnosed as an incidental finding in patients undergoing radiographic studies of the abdomen (ultrasound or CT scan). The incidence of renal cysts increases with increasing age. Although common in adults, the incidence of simple renal cysts is low in children, occurring in less than 1% of patients [46,47]. An increased rate of simple renal cysts (8%) has been reported in paediatric patients with AIDS [48].

The pathogenesis of simple renal cyst formation is not known, although theories include dilated calyces, focal ischaemia, sterilized resolved abscesses, or liquified haematomas [48]. The condition is considered sporadic. Clinically, it is important to differentiate a simple cyst from the early stages of ADPKD. Patients with simple cysts should have blood pressures monitored yearly and a repeat ultrasound examination 3–5 years later to ensure that the cyst is not changing in size or morphology, and that no other new cysts have developed. As noted above, ADPKD in younger children may be evident as only a single cyst and parents with ADPKD may be asymptomatic. The vast majority of simple cysts are asymptomatic and do not require therapy. However, in rare cases where cysts are extremely large or associated with hypertension, cyst decompression may be indicated.

Diffuse cystic dysplasia

Diffuse cystic dysplasia occurs primarily as a sporadic condition, or as part of multiple malformation syndromes. One kindred with autosomal recessive inheritance of non-syndromic cystic dysplasia has been reported [49]. Congenital syndromes for which diffuse cystic dysplasia or polycystic kidneys are a major component are summarized in Table 18.2. Dysplasia with or without cystic changes is a common feature of congenital obstructive uropathies; however, clinical features such as hydronephrosis or bladder abnormalities are usually present. Histological examination of dysplastic kidneys shows disorganized, poorly differentiated nephron segments with primitive elements such as cartilage [50].

Evaluation of a patient with suspected diffuse cystic dysplasia is directed primarily at determining the presence of an underlying congenital syndrome and the extent of other organ system involvement. Renal biopsies are generally not performed for diagnostic purposes. One exception may be patients with non-syndromic cystic dysplasia in whom the diagnosis of ARPKD is a possibility and an accurate diagnosis is

necessary for genetic counselling purposes. In addition to the specific syndromes outlined in Table 18.2, a variety of other congenital syndromes have diffuse cystic kidneys or polycystic kidneys as an infrequent component of the disease [14]. A regularly updated source describing these associations is the Online Mendelian Inheritance in Man (OMIM) registry (http://www3.ncbi.nlm.nih.gov/Omim).

The course of sporadic disease and renal functional prognosis in patients with diffuse cystic dysplasia is dictated by the degree of renal dysplasia relative to the presence of normal renal parenchyma. Involvement of a geneticist is recommended for establishing the diagnosis in syndromic cases, as well as determining the ultimate prognosis. The clinical course of patients with this heterogeneous set of syndromic diseases is based primarily on the course of the underlying disease.

Juvenile nephronophthisis/ medullary cystic disease

Case 4

A 13-year-old boy presented with severe vomiting for several days and increasing fatigue, anorexia and an 11 kg weight loss over the previous 6 months. He also had a history of polyuria and polydipsia since infancy. His family history was unremarkable. He appeared pale and clinically dehydrated. Serum creatinine was markedly elevated at 795 μmol/l and urinalysis showed a low specific gravity with microscopic haematuria and glycosuria. Renal ultrasound showed small echogenic kidneys with marked loss of corticomedullary differentiation and multiple small corticomedullary cysts.

This case illustrates the typical presentation of juvenile nephronophthisis (JN). Patients usually present in late childhood with progressive polyuria, polydipsia, enuresis, and pallor [51]. Because the disease develops slowly over many years, patients often do not come to medical attention until significant renal insufficiency has developed. Anaemia is usually present. Associated features may include eye abnormalities (Senior–Loken syndrome) or skeletal abnormalities. Unlike the large echogenic kidneys of recessive and dominant polycystic kidney disease, JN kidneys are normal-sized or small by ultrasound evaluation. Clearly defined corticomedullary cysts are not always detectable on ultrasound examination.

JN is an autosomal recessive disorder with an incidence of 1 in 50 000 to 1 in 1 000 000. The higher incidences are noted in Europe, whereas the incidence in the United States is very low. Several genetic loci have been identified through linkage analysis, on chromosomes 2, 3, and 9 [52–54]. The gene for the most common form on chromosome 2, *NPH1*, was recently identified [55]. The putative protein, nephrocystin, has an unknown function, but may be involved in cell–cell interactions. Although the pathogenesis remains largely unknown, the disease is characterized by a progressive chronic interstitial nephritis with relative sparing of the glomeruli until late in the disease course. Inflammatory cell infiltrates with interstitial fibrosis and tubular atrophy are characteristic of the disease (Fig. 18.3). Microscopic cysts, usually 1–2 mm diameter, are localized to the corticomedullary region [51]. JN shares many clinical and histological features with an even rarer adult disorder, autosomal dominant medullary cystic kidney disease. These similarities have led some to consider them diseases along a spectrum termed the 'juvenile nephronophthisis/medullary cystic disease complex'.

The differential diagnosis of a patient presenting with small cystic echogenic kidneys includes JN, acquired cystic kidney disease, renal dysplasia, and

familial hypoplastic GCKD [56]. Evaluation of a patient with suspected JN includes a careful physical examination to determine the presence of other syndromic features, including eye or extremity abnormalities. Initial laboratory evaluation should include measurement of serum chemistries, complete blood count, and urinalysis. Additional evaluation should include an ophthalmological evaluation.

Key point: Small echogenic cystic kidneys

- The differential diagnosis of small echogenic cystic kidneys usually does not include polycystic kidney diseases, since PKD kidneys are invariably enlarged.

There is no specific treatment for JN. Current therapy is standard care of progressive renal insufficiency. Patients with JN inevitably progress to ESRD, usually in early adolescence. JN constitutes 3% of paediatric ESRD patients in the USA and 10–20% in Europe.

Acquired cystic kidney disease

Acquired cystic kidney disease (ACKD) is a condition that occurs in patients with chronic renal failure or end stage renal disease. In one longitudinal study in children on chronic peritoneal dialysis, almost 30% had evidence of four or more cysts [57]. Development and severity of ACKD is directly related to duration of dialysis: up to 80% of children receiving dialysis more than 10 years have ACKD [57]. Most patients are asymptomatic and require no treatment. However, flank pain or haematuria may develop in some patients when cysts haemorrhage. Large perinephric haematomas have been reported in patients with haemorrhagic cysts that rupture [58]. Ultrasound or CT scan typically shows macrocysts of varying sizes. Occasionally marked kidney enlargement is seen, which may mimic ADPKD [59]. Patients with ACKD are at increased risk of malignancy, although neoplasms are reported only rarely in children with ESRD [60,61]. Although widespread screening of dialysis patients for the presence of renal masses is not currently recommended, it has been suggested

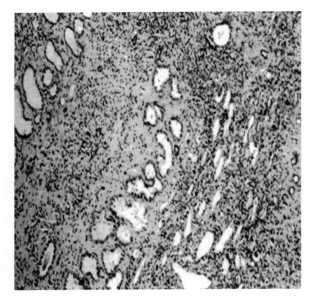

Fig. 18.3 Juvenile nephronophthisis. Renal biopsy specimen of a patient with juvenile nephronophthisis shows a tubulo-interstitial inflammatory cell infiltrate with fibrosis, tubular atrophy, and thickening of the tubular basement membranes. Scattered microscopic cysts are present in the medullary and corticomedullary regions. (Magnification ×570.)

that such a screening programme might be of benefit in younger patients [62].

Conclusions

As these cases and discussions illustrate, cystic diseases in childhood present as a spectrum of diseases in all age groups, ranging from critically ill neonates to totally asymptomatic adolescents. Arriving at a diagnosis can be challenging, but is essential to appropriate patient management and family counselling. In most cases, consultation with a paediatric nephrologist and, in some instances, a geneticist will assist in establishing diagnoses and developing comprehensive treatment plans for these patients.

Acknowledgements

Dr Avner is the director, and Dr Dell a member, of the NIH-supported Rainbow Center for Childhood PKD (#P50-DK27306), Rainbow Babies and Children's Hospital and Case Western Reserve University. Dr Avner is also supported in part by grants from the Polycystic Kidney Disease Foundation and Wyeth–Ayerst Research.

Footnote

After this chapter went to press, two independent groups reported the identification of the ARPKD gene, *PKHD1* (Ward CJ, *et al.* Nat Genet 2002;30:259–269 and Onuchic LF, *et al.* Am J Hum Genet 2002;70:1305–1317). This gene encodes a novel protein, fibrocystin (alternatively called polyductin), which is predicted to be a large membrane-bound protein that may function as a receptor.

References

1. Kissane JM. Renal cysts in pediatric patients: A classification and overview. Pediatr Nephrol 1990;4:69–77.
2. Bernstein J. Renal cystic disease in the tuberous sclerosis complex. Pediatr Nephrol 1993;7:490–495.
3. Salonen R, Paavola P. Meckel syndrome. J Med Genet 1998;35:497–501.
4. Dell KM, Avner ED. Autosomal Recessive Polycystic Kidney Disease (July 2001) In: GeneClinics: Clinical Genetic Information Resource [database online]. Copyright, University of Washington, Seattle. Available at http://www.geneclinics.org.
5. Cole BR, Conley SB, Stapleton FB. Polycystic kidney disease in the first year of life. J Pediatr 1987;111:693–699.
6. Kaplan BS, Fay J, Shah V, Dillon MJ, Barratt TM. Autosomal recessive polycystic kidney disease. Pediatr Nephrol 1989;3:43–49.
7. Slovis TL, Bernstein J, Gruskin A. Hyperechoic kidneys in the newborn and young infant. Pediatr Nephrol 1993;7:294–302.
8. Lieberman E, Salinas-Madrigal L, Gwinn J, Brennan LP, Fine R, Landing B. Infantile polycystic disease of the kidneys and liver: clinical, pathological and radiological correlations and comparison with congenital hepatic fibrosis. Medicine 1971;50:277–318.
9. Neumann HP, Krumme B, van Velthoven V, Orszagh M, Zerrers K. Multiple intracranial aneurysms in a patient with autosomal recessive polycystic kidney disease. Nephrol Dial Tranplant 1999;14:936–939.
10. McDonald R, Watkins SL, Avner ED. Polycystic kidney disease. In: Barratt TM, Avner ED, Harmon WE, editors. Pediatric Nephrology. 4th ed. Baltimore: Lippincott Williams & Wilkins; 1999. p. 459–480.
11. Park JH, Dixit MP, Onuchic LF, Wu G, Goncharuk AN, Kneitz S, et al. A 1 Mb BAC/PAC-based physicial map of the autosomal recessive polycystic kidney disease gene (PKHD1) region on chromosome 6. Genomics 1999;57:249–255.
12. Hallermann C, Mucher G, Kohlschmidt N, Wellek B, Schumacher R, Bahlmann F, et al. Syndrome of autosomal recessive polycystic kidneys with skeletal and facial anomalies is not linked to the ARPKD gene locus on chromosome 6p. Am J Med Genet 2000;90:115–119.
13. Guay-Woodford LM, Galliani CA, Musulman-Mroczek E, Spear GS, Guillot AP, Bernstein J. Diffuse renal cystic disease in children: morphologic and genetic correlations. Pediatr Nephrol 1998;12:173–182.
14. Limwongse C, Clarren SK, Cassidy SB. Syndromes and malformations of the urinary tract. In: Barratt TM, Avner ED, Harmon WE, editors. Pediatric Nephrology. 4th ed. Baltimore: Lippincott Williams & Wilkins; 1999. p. 427–452.
15. Bean SA, Bednarek FJ, Primack WA. Aggressive respiratory support and unilateral nephrectomy for infants with severe perinatal autosomal recessive polycystic kidney disease. J Pediatr 1995;127:311–313.
16. Munding M, Al-Uzri A, Gralneck D, Riden D. Prentally diagnosed autosomal recessive polycystic kidney disease: initial postnatal management. Urology 1999;54:1097.
17. Sweeney WE, Chen Y, Nakanishi K, Frost P, Avner ED. Treatment of polycystic kidney disease with a novel tyrosine kinase inhibitor. Kidney Int 2000;57:33–40.
18. Zerres K, Mücher G, Becker J, Steinkamm C, Rudnik-Schöneborn S, Heikkilä P, et al. Prenatal diagnosis of autosomal recessive polycystic kidney disease (ARPKD): Molecular genetics, clinical experience, and fetal morphology. Am J Med Genet 1998;76:137–144.
19. Kaariainen H, Koskimies O, Norio R. Dominant and recessive polycystic kidney disease in children: evaluation of clinical features and laboratory data. Pediatr Nephrol 1988;2:296–302.
20. Roy S, Dillon MJ, Trompeter RS, Barratt TM. Autosomal recessive polycystic kidney disease:

long-term outcome of neonatal survivors. Pediatr Nephrol 1997;11:302–306.

21. Zerres K, Rudnik-Schoneborn S, Deget F, Holtkamp U, Brodehl J, Geistert J, et al. Autosomal recessive polycystic kidney disease in 115 children: clinical presentation, course and influence of gender. Acta Paediatr 1996;85:437–445.

22. Kashtan CE, Primack WA, Kainer G, Rosenberg AR, McDonald RA, Warady BA. Recurrent bacteremia with enteric pathogens in recessive polycystic kidney disease. Pediatr Nephrol 1999;13:678–682.

23. Fick GM, Gabow PA. Hereditary and acquired cystic disease of the kidney. Kidney Int 1994;46:951–964.

24. Kaplan BS, Rabin I, Nogrady MB, Drummond KN. Autosomal dominant polycystic renal disease in children. J Pediatr 1977;90:782–783.

25. Fick GM, Duley IT, Johnson AM, Strain JD, Manco-Johnson ML, Gabow PA. The spectrum of autosomal dominant polycystic kidney disease in children. J Am Soc Nephrol 1994;4:1654–1660.

26. Proesmans W, Van Damme B, Casaer P, Marchal G. Autosomal dominant polycystic kidney disease in the neonatal period: association with cerebral arteriovenous malformation. Pediatrics 1982;70:971–975.

27. Ivy DD, Shaffer EM, Johnson AM, Kimberling WJ, Dobin A, Gabow PA. Cardiovascular abnormalities in children with autosomal dominant polycystic kidney disease. J Am Soc Nephrol 1995;5:2032–2036.

28. Cobben JM, Breuning MH, Schoots C, Ten Kate LP, Zerres K. Congenital hepatic fibrosis in autosomal-dominant polycystic kidney disease. Kidney Int 1990; 38:880–885.

29. Harris PC. Autosomal dominant polycystic kidney disease: clues to pathogenesis. Hum Mol Genet 1999;8:1861–1866.

30. Watnick T, Germino GG. Molecular basis of autosomal dominant polycystic kidney disease. Semin Nephrol 1999;19:327–343.

31. Fick GM, Johnson AM, Strain JD, Kimberling WJ, Kumar S, Manco-Johnson ML, et al. Characteristics of very early onset autosomal dominant polycystic kidney disease. J Am Soc Nephrol 1993;3:1863–1870.

32. Ewalt DH, Sheffield E, Sparagana SP, Delgado MR, Roach ES. Renal lesion growth in children with tuberous sclerosis complex. J Urol 1998;160:141–145.

33. Sedman A, Bell P, Manco-Johnson M, Schrier R, Warady BA, Heard EO, et al. Autosomal dominant polycystic kidney disease in childhood: a longitudinal study. Kidney Int 1987;31:1000–1005.

34. Ravine D, Gibson RN, Walker RG, Sheffield LJ, Kincaid-Smith P, Danks DM. Evaluation of ultrasonographic diagnostic criteria for autosomal dominant polycystic kidney disease 1. Lancet 1994;343:824–827.

35. Butler WE, Barker 2nd FG, Crowell RM. Patients with polycystic kidney disease would benefit from routine magnetic resonance angiographic screening for intracerebral aneurysms: a decision analysis. Neurosurgery 1996;38:506–515.

36. Huston 3rd J, Torres VE, Sulivan PP, Offord KP, Wiebers DO. Value of magnetic resonance angiography for the detection of intracranial aneurysms in autosomal dominant polycystic kidney disease. J Am Soc Nephrol 1993;3:1871–1877.

37. Huston 3rd J, Torres VE, Wiebers DO, Schievink WI. Follow-up of intracranial aneurysms in autosomal dominant polycystic kidney disease by magnetic resonance angiography. J Am Soc Nephrol 1996;7:2135–2141.

38. Nakajima F, Shibahara N, Arai M, Ueda H, Katsuoka Y. Ruptured cerebral aneurysm not detected by magnetic resonance angiography in juvenile autosomal dominant polycystic kidney. Int J Urol 2000;7:153–156.

39. Gabow PA, Johnson AM, Kaehny WD, Kimberling WJ, Lezotte DC, Duley IT, et al. Factors affecting the progression of renal disease in autosomal-dominant polycystic kidney disease. Kidney Int 1992; 41:1311–1319.

40. Schwab SJ, Bander SJ, Klahr S. Renal infection in autosomal dominant polycystic kidney disease. Am J Med 1987;82:714–718.

41. Gibson P, Watson ML. Cyst infection in polycystic kidney disease: a clinical challenge. Nephrol Dial Transplant 1998;13:2455–2457.

42. Rossi SJ, Healy DP, Savani DV, Deepe G. High-dose ciprofloxacin in the treatment of a renal cyst infection. Ann Pharmacother 1993;27:38–39.

43. Sharp CK, Bergman SM, Stockwin JM, Robbin ML, Galliani C, Guay-Woodford LM. Dominantly transmitted glomerulocystic kidney disease: a distinct genetic entity. J Am Soc Nephrol 1997;8:77–84.

44. Bernstein J. Glomerulocystic kidney disease—nosological considerations. Pediatr Nephrol 1993;7:464–470.

45. Melnick SC, Brewer DB, Oldham JS. Cortical microcystic disease of the kidney with dominant inheritance: a previously undescribed syndrome. J Clin Pathol 1984;37:494–499.

46. Ravine D, Gibson RN, Donlan J, Sheffield LJ. An ultrasound renal cyst prevalence survey: specificity data for inherited renal cystic diseases. Am J Kidney Dis 1993;22:803–807.

47. McHugh K, Stringer DA, Hebert D, Babiak CA. Simple renal cysts in children: diagnosis and follow-up with US. Radiology 1991;178:383–385.

48. Zinn HL, Rosberger ST, Haller JO, Schlesinger AE. Simple renal cysts in children with AIDS. Pediatr Radiol 1997;27:827–828.

49. Sase M, Tsukahara M, Oga A, Kaneko N, Nakata M, Saito T, et al. Diffuse cystic renal dysplasia: nonsyndromal familial case. Am J Med Genet 1996;17: 332–334.

50. Watkins SL, McDonald RA, Avner ED. Renal dysplasia, hypoplasia and miscellaneous cystic disorders. In: Barratt TM, Avner ED, Harmon WE, editors. Pediatric Nephrology. 4th ed. Baltimore: Lippincott Williams & Wilkins; 1999. p. 415–425.

51. Avner ED. Medullary cystic disease. In: Greenberg A, editor. Primer on Kidney Diseases. San Diego: Academic Press; 2001 (in press). p. 320–322.

52. Antignac C, Arduy CH, Beckmann JS, Benessy F, Gros F, Medhioub M, et al. A gene for familial juvenile nephronophthisis (recessive medullary cystic kidney disease) maps to chromosome 2p. Nat Genet 1993;3:342–345.

53. Haider NB, Carmi R, Shalev H, Sheffield VC, Landau D. A Bedouin kindred with infantile nephronophthisis demonstrates linkage to chromosome 9 by homozygosity mapping. Am J Hum Genet 1998;63(5):1404–1410.

54. Konrad M, Saunier S, Calado J, Gubler MC, Broyer M, Antignac C. Familial juvenile nephronophthisis. J Mol Med 1998;76(5):310–316.

55. Hildebrandt F, Otto E, Rensing C, Nothwang HG, Vollmer M, Adolphs J, *et al*. A novel gene encoding an SH3 domain protein is mutated in nephronophthisis type 1. Nat Genet 1997;17:149–153.

56. Kaplan BS, Gordon I, Pincott J, Barratt TM. Familial hypoplastic glomerulocystic kidney disease: a definite entity with dominant inheritance. Am J Med Genet 1989;34:569–573.

57. Anonymous. Acquired cystic kidney disease in children undergoing continuous ambulatory peritoneal dialysis. Kyushu Pediatric Nephrology Study Group. Am J Kidney Dis 1999;34(2):242–246.

58. Levine E, Hartman DS, Meilstrup JW, Van Slyke MA, Edgar KA, Barth JC. Current concepts and controversies in imaging of renal cystic diseases. Urol Clin North Am 1997;24(3):523–543.

59. Gagnon RF, Kintzen GM, Kaye M. Acquired cystic kidney disease: rapid progression from small to enlarged kidneys simulating adult polycystic kidney disease. Clin Nephrol 2000;53(4):307–311.

60. Truong LD, Krishnan B, Cao JT, Barrios R, Suki WN. Renal neoplasm in acquired cystic kidney disease. Am J Kidney Dis 1995;26(1):1–12.

61. Gentle DL, Mandell J, Jennings T. Renal cortical neoplasm in a child with dialysis-acquired cystic kidney disease. Urology 1996;47(2):254–255.

62. Sarasin FP, Wong JB, Levey AS, Meyer KB. Screening for acquired cystic kidney disease: a decision analytic perspective. Kidney Int 1995;48(1):207–219.

19 | *The child with idiopathic nephrotic syndrome*

George Haycock

Introduction

The nephrotic syndrome is defined as the combination of heavy proteinuria, hypoproteinaemia, and oedema. Hyperlipidaemia is invariably present. The nephrotic syndrome is part of the clinical spectrum of proteinuric states and it is neither possible nor desirable to make a sharp distinction between nephrotic and non-nephrotic proteinuria. Two children may have the same disease according to histopathological criteria, one being clinically nephrotic and the other not. A third may have the nephrotic syndrome at some times and not others as a result of the interaction of various renal and non-renal factors; these include spontaneous changes in the amount of proteinuria, dietary energy and protein intake, and the effects of drug and other treatment. In physiological terms, the nephrotic syndrome exists when the rate of urinary protein loss exceeds the rate at which the liver can replace it, leading to depletion of the extracellular albumin pool and a fall in the plasma albumin concentration below the normal range. Because of the influence of non-renal factors, the correlation between the magnitude of proteinuria and the severity of the resulting hypoalbuminaemia is rather weak, though present. Roughly speaking, proteinuria greater than about 50 mg/kg/day (approximately equivalent to $100 mg/m^2/h$ or a urine protein:creatinine ratio of >600 mg/mmol) for a few days or more is likely to cause hypoalbuminaemia. This corresponds to a value of about 3–5 g/day for an adult–sized patient and proportionally less for smaller individuals. The normal range for plasma albumin concentration in well-nourished children is 36–44 g/l, but fluid retention and oedema are unusual until it has fallen below 25–30 g/l, and in some children very much lower levels are seen. Depending on the nature of the underlying glomerular lesion, the urinary protein may be almost entirely albumin (selective proteinuria) or a mixture of albumin and higher molecular weight proteins (non-selective proteinuria). In either case, the salt and water retention leading to nephrotic oedema is determined by the effect on the plasma albumin concentration, although losses of other proteins may be linked to some of the other events which may complicate the syndrome, such as infection and vascular thrombosis.

Causes of the nephrotic syndrome

As stated above, any disease that alters glomerular function so as to cause a large albumin leak from the plasma into Bowman's space may lead to the nephrotic syndrome. Causes include primary glomerulopathies, in which the disease is apparently confined to the glomeruli, and multi-system diseases with a renal component such as Henoch–Schönlein purpura and systemic lupus erythematosus. A comprehensive list of causes, including the rarest entities and single case reports, is very long indeed, but a relatively small number of diseases account for at least 99% of childhood cases, and these are listed in Table 19.1. The mix of causes varies with age; the relative frequency of the most common causes at different ages from 1 to 15 years is shown in Figure 19.1. Note that infants are excluded from this analysis—the nephrotic syndrome in the first year of life, and especially in the first 6 months, is dominated by congenital (usually hereditary) diseases with an almost uniformly bad prognosis (discussed later in this chapter). In adult populations the same primary and secondary diseases that affect children are seen, but their relative importance is different, with membranous nephropathy being the most common and minimal change disease (MCD) being lower down the list. The remainder of this chapter will be confined to a discussion of the primary, idiopathic nephrotic syndrome of childhood, i.e. disease that appears to be confined to the kidney and for which no cause can be demonstrated. In histopathological terms, this means MCD, focal segmental glomerulosclerosis (FSGS), and occasional cases of membranoproliferative (mesangiocapillary) glomerulonephritis and membranous nephropathy. In practice, the large majority of children do not undergo renal biopsy at presentation, but are treated empirically with oral corticosteroids. Those who respond to such therapy rarely have a histological diagnosis made and are referred to as having steroid-sensitive nephrotic syndrome (SSNS).

Table 19.1 Main causes of nephrotic syndrome in children aged 1–15 years

---

Primary glomerular disease
  Minimal change disease (MCD)
    'Pure' MCD
    MCD with mesangial proliferation
  Focal segmental glomerulosclerosis
  Membranoproliferative glomerulonephritis[a]
    type 1
    type 2
    ? type 3
  Membranous nephropathy
Multisystem diseases
  Henoch–Schönlein purpura
  Systemic lupus erythematosus

---

[a] Membranoproliferative glomerulonephritis is also known as mesangiocapillary glomerulonephritis.

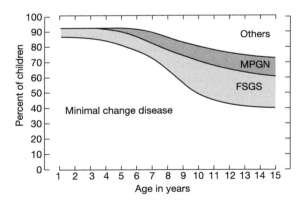

Fig. 19.1 'Smoothed' representation of the distribution of the major causes of childhood nephrotic syndrome by age. MPGN, membranoproliferative (mesangiocapillary) glomerulonephritis; FSGS, focal and segmental glomerulosclerosis. Based on pooled data from the International Study of Kidney Disease in Childhood and patients investigated at Guy's Hospital, London (*n* = 566). From *Clinical Paediatric Nephrology* 2/e by R.J. Postlethwaite. Reprinted by permission of Elsevier Science Ltd.

The mechanism of proteinuria in the nephrotic syndrome

The concepts of glomerular and tubular proteinuria have been discussed in Chapter 1. The proteinuria of the nephrotic syndrome is predominantly glomerular in type. In MCD, and steroid-sensitive patients generally, the proteinuria is usually purely glomerular, but in patients with nephrotic syndrome and progressive loss of renal function it is often mixed with tubular proteinuria superimposed on the underlying glomerular pattern. This is most typical of FSGS of steroid-resistant, progressive type. Even in this subgroup, however, the glomerular albuminuria is responsible for the hypoalbuminaemia and the other, contingent features of the nephrotic syndrome.

Glomerular filtrate is formed by *ultrafiltration* of plasma across the glomerular capillary wall. This structure has three layers: an inner, fenestrated *endothelium*, a *basement membrane* consisting of a hydrated gel rich in proteoglycans, and an outer *epithelium* consisting of highly specialized cells called *podocytes*. The podocyte possesses a cell body from which arise several tentacle-like arms, each of which gives rise to numerous lateral *foot processes (pedicels)* which interdigitate with those of adjacent podocytes to invest the outer surface of the basement membrane, like complex, jigsaw puzzle pieces (Fig. 19.2). The podocytes are separated by a *slit diaphragm*, a critically important part of the ultrafilter that is believed to be limiting for the filtration of albumin. Podocytes have recently been shown to express a membrane protein, nephrin [1], coded by a gene located at 19q13.1. Nephrin is essential for the proper organization and function of the slit diaphragm; mutations in it are responsible for the massive albuminuria of the Finnish type of congenital nephrotic syndrome. However, nephrin is present in normal amounts in the glomeruli in all acquired glomerular diseases studied to date, including MCD [2]. So far there is no evidence that nephrin is involved in the pathogenesis of idiopathic childhood nephrotic syndrome. All three layers of the capillary wall are negatively charged due to the presence of sialic acid residues on the 'glycocalyx' covering both epithelial and endothelial cells, and of sulphated glycosaminoglycans throughout the basement membrane. Plasma albumin is negatively charged at physiological pH, and there is evidence for both a *size-specific* barrier (a sieve) and a *charge-specific* barrier (an electric fence) to the passage of albumin molecules from capillary lumen to Bowman's space.

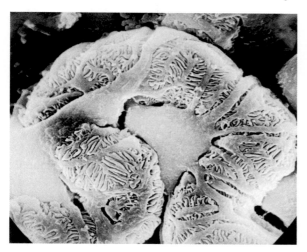

Fig. 19.2 Scanning electron micrograph of a normal rat glomerular capillary loop, showing interdigitation of foot processes (pedicels) from adjacent epithelial cells (podocytes). From Arakawa M (1970). Scanning electron microscopy of the glomerulus in normal and nephrotic rats. *Lab Invest* 23:480–496, by permission; original print kindly supplied by Dr Arakawa.

Most patients with SSNS have MCD on renal biopsy, with no structural changes to the glomerular capillary wall except an appearance usually described as 'fusion' of the epithelial foot processes. This is actually a misnomer: considered in three dimensions, the epithelial cells have altered their shape, with loss of foot processes, so that they now abut one another like simple squames or paving stones. This results in the appearance of a single thin epithelial sheet in the two dimensions of a thin section examined by electron microscopy, instead of the numerous little 'islands' of adjacent foot processes. The nature of the functional change in the properties of the glomerular filter has been the subject of intensive physiological study over more than three decades. The consensus view at present is that the albuminuria is due, mainly or entirely, to loss of the negative electrical charge on the basement membrane and perhaps the epithelium, impairing the charge-specific component of the filtration barrier. The evidence is complex and based on clinical and experimental physiological work as well as ultrastructural studies. It will not be reviewed here, the reader is referred to more specialized articles on the subject [3,4].

The proximate cause of the glomerular lesion

The central, unsolved problem concerning the idiopathic nephrotic syndrome is: what causes the change in glomerular permeability to albumin that underlies the disease? It is widely assumed (though on circumstantial evidence only) that the condition has an immunological basis. Various observations support this hypothesis. All the drugs known to be effective in at least some cases (steroids, alkylating agents, ciclosporin/tacrolimus, levamisole) have effects on the immune system. There is an increased incidence of atopy in affected children and their families. Children with nephrotic syndrome are notoriously susceptible to bacterial peritonitis and sepsis, especially due to *Streptococcus pneumoniae*. A form of minimal change nephrotic syndrome is associated with Hodgkin's disease and other lymphomas, themselves T-cell proliferative disorders. Certain infections (measles and malaria) that depress T-cell function are capable of inducing remissions of the disease. Serum IgG levels are low, and IgM levels frequently raised, in relapses of nephrotic syndrome and do not always normalize in remission. These and other considerations led Shalhoub [5] to propose that MCNS is the consequence of a primary, generalized disorder of T-cell function, a hypothesis that is still under investigation by several groups. The disease has been associated with various class 1 and class 2 HLA antigens in different populations: the known genetic linkage between the HLA system and the immune system makes this a promising area for research using the techniques of modern immunogenetics and molecular biology. The current state of knowledge of the immune system in MCNS is well reviewed by Schnaper [6].

Many workers have pursued the rather obvious possibility that the alteration in charge and permeability of the glomerular capillary wall might be due to the presence of a circulating factor. This is entirely compatible with the immunological hypothesis in that the factor(s) might be produced by cells of the immune system, either as the result of immunological reaction to antigen exposure or due to a primary abnormality of the immune system itself. Candidates for the role of the proposed factor include lymphokines such as *vascular permeability factor* and *soluble immune response suppressor*, and other circulating substances such as *platelet activating factor*, a kallikrein-like substance labelled *100-KF* and various crude, poorly characterized plasma fractions. This aspect of research is being actively followed in several laboratories at the time of writing; although promising, no one factor yet fulfils the equivalent of Koch's postulates as the cause of the disease. The subject has been reviewed by Bakker and van Luijk

[7]. Two women with FSGS have now been described who, between them, gave birth to three babies, all of whom had nephrotic range proteinuria in the neonatal period with rapid spontaneous resolution [8,9]. This experiment of nature is hard to explain other than by the transplacental passage of a chemical that affects glomerular permeability.

Pathophysiology of nephrotic oedema

Oedema is the cardinal clinical feature of the nephrotic syndrome. At least two hypotheses have been advanced in explanation of the renal salt and water retention involved; they are not mutually exclusive. Both involve an alteration in the balance of physical (Starling) forces that govern the movement of water and small solutes between the intravascular (plasma) and extravascular (interstitial) compartments of the extracellular fluid, but the postulated sequence of events in the two is different.

The Starling equilibrium

The interface between the plasma and the interstitial fluid is the capillary wall. This is a semi-permeable membrane that allows free movement of water and small (crystalloid) solutes across it but severely restricts the passage of macromolecules, notably albumin and other proteins. The plasma in the capillary bed differs from the adjacent interstitial fluid in two important respects. First, it is at a higher hydrostatic pressure, being in continuity with the arterial tree; secondly, the albumin concentration is much higher because only very little of it escapes from the circulation by diffusion across the capillary wall. There are therefore two physical pressure gradients acting across the capillary: a *hydrostatic* gradient, favouring filtration of fluid from the plasma into the interstitium, and an *osmotic* gradient, favouring reabsorption of fluid in the reverse direction. Because of the special permeability characteristics of the capillary wall, only those molecules that are too large to cross it contribute to the osmotic gradient. For all practical purposes, this means the plasma proteins, mainly albumin. The relevant quantity is therefore known as the *colloid osmotic* or *oncotic* pressure; in physical terms it is quite small, about 30 mmHg,

compared with the enormous total osmotic pressure of the body fluids (5600 mmHg).

It is conventional to represent hydrostatic pressure in this system as P, and oncotic pressure as Π. If the subscripts C and I refer to capillary lumen and interstitial fluid, respectively, the ultrafiltration pressure (P_{UF}) favouring filtration of fluid from capillary to interstitium can be calculated from the Starling equation:

$$P_{UF} = (P_C - P_I) - \sigma(\Pi_C - \Pi_I)$$

The σ term is the reflection coefficient for albumin, i.e. the reciprocal of the ease with which it crosses the capillary wall, where water has a value of 0 and a substance that does not cross at all has a value of 1. For practical purposes, σ is close enough to 1 to be ignored and both P_I and Π_I are near zero. The equation can therefore be simplified to:

$$P_{UF} = P_C - \Pi_C$$

Increased filtration of fluid from plasma to interstitium, leading eventually to oedema, can therefore result either from an increase in P_C or a decrease in Π_C. Each of the two hypotheses to explain salt and water retention in nephrotic syndrome depends on one of these possibilities.

The underfill theory of oedema formation

The 'traditional' model proposes that the primary change in the Starling equilibrium in the nephrotic syndrome is a fall in Π_C. This leads to a shift of fluid from plasma to interstitium, resulting in an initially small expansion of the latter but also, crucially, a contraction of the former. Contraction of the circulating blood volume, however caused, elicits powerful physiological responses that result in maximal renal salt and water retention. Assuming that the patient continues to eat and drink, a continuously positive salt and water balance ensues, leading to progressive extracellular fluid expansion. Because the Starling imbalance caused by hypoalbuminaemia persists, most of the retained fluid escapes from the circulation into the interstitial space, leading to the progressive and sometimes massive oedema that is characteristic of untreated nephrotic syndrome. This is an example of the *underfill* theory of hypoproteinaemic oedema, and the same argument can be applied to other oedematous conditions, such as cirrhosis of the liver and the oedema of protein–calorie malnutrition (kwashiorkor). A scheme of the genesis of nephrotic oedema according to the underfill theory is given in Fig. 19.3.

The overflow theory of oedema formation

The underfill hypothesis is intuitively attractive on theoretical grounds. However, there are clinical and experimental observations that cast serious doubt on it as the sole and sufficient explanation for nephrotic oedema. Careful measurements in (mainly adult) patients with steroid-responsive, minimal change nephrotic syndrome have shown that circulating blood and plasma volumes are typically *increased* during stable relapse, falling to normal in steroid-induced remission [10]. Indirect measures of blood volume (plasma renin and aldosterone levels and their response to saline volume expansion) suggest that MCD approximates better to the underfill hypothesis, while patients with nephrotic syndrome resulting from structural glomerular disease are more

likely to be volume expanded [11]. These and other observations indicate that, in at least some nephrotic subjects, the proximate cause of oedema may be a primary alteration in renal function causing salt and water retention, circulating volume expansion and an increase in P_C leading to transudation into the interstitial space, as represented in Fig. 19.4. This model is referred to as the *overflow* hypothesis of oedema formation, usually invoked to account for the oedema of the *acute nephritic syndrome*. The consensus of modern opinion, however, favours the hypovolaemic (underfilling) model in MCD in children [12,13].

The question has practical implications as well as theoretical interest. Infusion of plasma or hyperoncotic albumin is logical therapy in a hypovolaemic child but may be dangerous in one who is volume replete or even expanded. There is no doubt that some children present in acute nephrotic relapse with gross clinical evidence of hypovolaemia supported by laboratory evaluation; equally, others are clinically

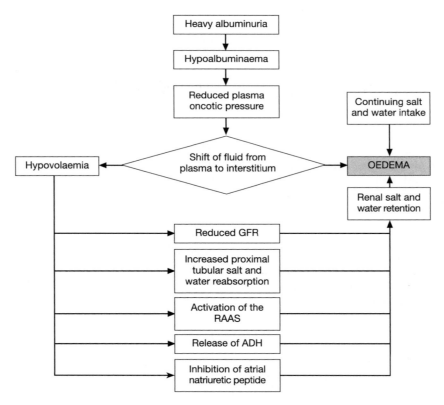

Fig. 19.3 Schematic representation of the pathophysiology of the oedema of the nephrotic syndrome according to the 'underfill hypothesis'. RAAS, renin–angiotension–aldosterone system; ADH, antidiuretic hormone. See text for further details.

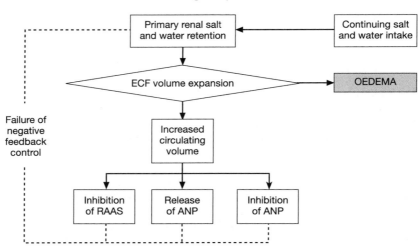

Fig. 19.4 Schematic representation of the pathophysiology of the oedema of the nephrotic syndrome according to the 'overflow hypothesis'. RAAS, renin–angiotension–aldosterone system; ANP, atrial natriuretic peptide; AVP, arginine vasopressin. See text for further details.

euvolaemic. Volume must be carefully assessed and treatment tailored to each patient's individual requirements, as described below under Clinical features and Laboratory findings.

Clinical features

Epidemiology

The disease occurs in both sexes, in all races, and at all ages, but is more common in males, in some races, and at some ages rather than others. It is found in all parts of the world; geographical factors have not convincingly been implicated in its causation.

Sex

There is a consistent male predominance, the male:female risk ratio being in the range 1.5–2:1. The reasons for this are unknown.

Race

Idiopathic nephrotic syndrome is more common in Arabs and the peoples of the Indian subcontinent than in white Europeans and their descendants in North America and Australasia: the per capita risk ratio is about 7:1 if Asian immigrants to the United Kingdom are compared with white children living in

the same cities [14]. It is less common in Africans and African Americans than in Whites. The incidence in Oriental children is probably intermediate between that in Europeans and that in southern Asians. Beyond indicating a probable genetic predisposition to the disease in some populations, the significance of this distribution is not known.

Age

MCD and FSGS are uncommon in the first year of life, and very rare under 6 months. The highest incidence is in the age range 2–5 years, with a smaller peak in later childhood. These two lesions become progressively less common with advancing age thereafter, both in absolute terms and as a proportion of all causes of the nephrotic syndrome, but occasional new cases present even into old age. Membranoproliferative glomerulonephritis is very rare under the age of 10 and occasional cases are seen in the second decade. Its incidence and prevalence in the United Kingdom has declined markedly since the 1960s, for unknown reasons. Membranous nephropathy is rare in childhood, except for cases associated with hepatitis B infection in places where this is common.

Genetic factors

Idiopathic nephrotic syndrome is clearly not inherited as a single gene disorder, but indirect evidence strongly implicates a genetic component in its causation. Several human leucocyte (HLA) antigens, singly and in combination, have been found to be over-represented in different populations of patients as compared with matched controls. HLA-DR7 is the single antigen most commonly identified, while the extended haplotype HLA-B8, -DR3, -DR7 predicted a relative risk of 21.5 in one recent report. The differing prevalence of the disease in different racial subgroups, referred to above, also favours the view that some individuals are genetically more predisposed to the disease than others. So does the slight but definite increased risk to siblings of affected children, especially within consanguineous marriages, and the association with atopy, itself partially a genetically determined trait. The molecular nature of this genetic predisposition is not understood, and it has no implications for practical management. A few families have been described in which a pattern consistent with autosomal recessive inheritance of SSNS is seen, but linkage has not so far been established with any genetic locus [15].

Key points: Idiopathic nephrotic syndrome

- More common in boys.

- More common in Arabs and peoples of the Indian subcontinent.

- Peak incidence is in the age range 2–5 years.

- Minimal change disease is the most common histological lesion.

- Indirect evidence strongly implicates a genetic component in its causation.

Symptoms and signs

The usual presenting feature is oedema. This is generalized and distributed by gravity: thus the face, particularly the periorbital regions, tends to be swollen in the morning and the ankles later in the day. Serous effusions (transudates) are commonly present and ascites without gross oedema is sometimes seen, particularly in very young children and infants, whose tissues are more resistant to the formation of interstitial oedema than those of older patients. Pleural effusions are often present, although seldom clinically significant. Children who are untreated or who fail to respond to treatment may progress to massive anasarca, and gross scrotal or vulval oedema can be particularly distressing. When oedema is severe, minor trauma may breach the continuity of the skin, leading to oozing of fluid from the exposed oedematous tissues.

Blood pressure is usually normal or low, but may be paradoxically raised in up to 21% of patients [16], patricularly in severely volume-contracted patients, probably due to excessive secretion of renin, aldosterone and perhaps other vasoconstrictor hormones in response to hypovolaemia. Persistent, stable hypertension is unusual in MCD and FSGS at presentation, and should raise the suspicion that some other form of glomerular disease, most commonly membranoproliferative glomerulonephritis, may be present. Circulating volume should be carefully assessed before treatment is given (see below). The child is usually miserable but not acutely ill, unless a complication such as infection or severe hypovolaemia is present.

Clinical assessment of circulating volume

The purpose of the circulation is to supply the tissues with blood. In normal conditions, this means that even the most peripheral parts of the body are well perfused, and therefore warm due to the transfer of heat from the centre of the body by the circulating blood. In a warm room, a person with a normal circulation is warm all over and the temperature of the great toe, under thermoneutral conditions, is an excellent indicator of this. If the patient is in bed with the feet covered, the toes should be warm to the touch: if the toe temperature is formally measured, it should be no more than 2 °C less than the core temperature, i.e. not less than 35 °C in an apyrexial patient. The palms, soles, finger, and toe pulps should be pink with prompt capillary return (less than 2 seconds) after being blanched by pressure. Signs of functionally significant hypovolaemia therefore include cold periphery and diminished or delayed capillary return: venous pressure is reduced, although it is often difficult or impossible to assess the jugular venous pressure in an oedematous child. Abdominal pain is common in hypovolaemia, probably due to underperfusion of the splanchnic circulation; it may also be due to peritonitis, which must be excluded in any nephrotic patient presenting with this symptom.

Laboratory findings

Urine

Formed elements. Microscopic *haematuria* is observed in up to 23% of children with steroid-sensitive MCD [16]. Microscopic haematuria is more likely to be continuous in FSGS, but this is only a weak discriminator between the two. Macroscopic haematuria is a pointer to a more serious form of glomerulonephritis, as is the presence of cellular or granular *casts*.

Protein. The urine contains large amounts of *albumin*, typically more than 50 mg/kg/day (100 mg/m^2/h) but sometimes much more, up to 20–30 g/day. The proteinuria may be *selective*, consisting mainly of albumin, or *non-selective*, containing significant amounts of higher molecular weight proteins. This may be quantified by measuring the urine (U) and plasma (P) concentrations of two representative proteins such as transferrin (small) and IgG (large), from which the ratio of their renal clearances can be simply calculated as (U:P transferrin/U:P albumin): a value of less than 0.1 is conventionally described as *highly selective*, greater than 0.2 as *poorly selective* or *non-selective*, and 0.1–0.2 as *moderately selective*. The higher the degree of selectivity, the greater the probability that the patient has MCD; conversely, poorly selective proteinuria predicts some other form of glomerulonephritis (see Table 19.1). However, the correlation between selectivity and diagnosis, though significant, is weak. It is not helpful in the management of individual cases and most paediatric nephrologists have abandoned it as a clinically useful investigation. A recent report [17] suggests that combining measurement of selectivity of proteinuria with the fractional excretion rate of low molecular weight proteins (e.g. β_2-microglobulin) greatly increases both the sensitivity and specificity of prediction of steroid sensitivity. It would be reassuring to see the results of further studies of this novel approach before recommending a change in currently accepted practice.

Lipid. *Lipiduria* is also present, and fat globules and fat-laden macrophages ('oval fat bodies') may be seen on microscopy.

Electrolytes, urea, and creatinine. Measurement of the urinary *sodium* concentration (U_{Na}) is valuable in the diagnosis of suspected hypovolaemia, which is a powerful stimulus to renal sodium retention. In the appropriate clinical setting, U_{Na} less than 10 mmol/l is diagnostic of reduction of effective circulating volume, while a value above 20 mmol/l makes it unlikely. *This rule is invalidated if the patient has received a diuretic*, particularly a powerful loop diuretic such as frusemide. Urinary *potassium* excretion varies in response to dietary intake, as in normal subjects, and measuring it yields no useful information. The urine is usually concentrated with respect to *urea* and *creatinine*, reflecting the reduced urine flow rate that underlies the fluid retention. Fractional sodium excretion (the fraction of filtered sodium excreted in the urine, calculated as U:P sodium/U:P creatinine) is low (<0.0 1) as in all salt-retaining states with normal or near-normal glomerular filtration rate. It will be very low indeed if hypovolaemia is present but clinically this test is no more discriminating than simple measurement of U_{Na}.

Blood

Proteins. *Hypoalbuminaemia* is necessary for the diagnosis of nephrotic syndrome (plasma albumin concentration <25 g/l, often much lower). As would be expected, there is a rough inverse correlation between the plasma albumin and the severity of the clinical manifestations of the disease. *IgG* levels are also reduced, but to a lesser extent than albumin; plasma *IgM* is usually raised. There are no consistent abnormalities of the plasma *complement* proteins C3 and C4, a point which helps to differentiate SSNS from certain forms of glomerulonephritis in which the C3 may be reduced, either transiently (acute post-streptococcal glomerulonephritis) or over a sustained period (membranoproliferative glomerulonephritis, lupus, and the nephritis of bacterial endocarditis or an infected ventriculo-atrial shunt). Of these, only membranoproliferative glomerulonephritis is likely to be confused with the steroid-sensitive disease. The plasma concentration of antithrombin III is reduced due to urinary loss; this accounts in part for the hypercoagulability seen in some nephrotic children. The plasma concentration of several proteins of the coagulation cascade is increased, further increasing the risk of thrombosis.

Lipid. The plasma concentrations of total *cholesterol, low-density* and *very-low-density lipoproteins* are increased, often grossly, while those of *high-density lipoproteins* are usually normal. The plasma may be frankly lipaemic to the naked eye.

Urea, creatinine, and electrolytes. Plasma *urea* and *creatinine* concentrations are usually normal at first presentation of MCD and FSGS, but may be slightly to moderately raised in some cases due to hypovolaemia and renal underperfusion (*prerenal azotaemia*). Plasma *electrolyte* levels are normal in most cases, although *hyponatraemia* is occasionally seen. This is a complication of hypovolaemia: if plasma volume is contracted by more than a few per cent of normal, antidiuretic hormone (ADH) is secreted in response to baroreceptor stimulation even if plasma osmolality, the usual stimulus to ADH release, is normal. Since the normal diet contains proportionately more water than salt, the consequent impairment of water excretion leads to dilutional hyponatraemia. Hyponatraemia may be severe if a diuretic is used, inappropriately, in a hypovolaemic patient. A different form of hyponatraemia, often called *pseudohyponatraemia*, may be seen if the serum is lipaemic. This is because electrolytes are dissolved in the aqueous phase of plasma, and extreme hyperlipidaemia may reduce the fraction of a given volume of serum or plasma which is water. This applies if sodium is measured by flame photometry. Increasingly, cations in plasma are estimated using ion-selective electrodes, which measure *activity* rather than *concentration*, and activity is not affected by changes in plasma lipids or other non-aqueous solids.

Membranoproliferative glomerulonephritis usually presents with a more mixed, 'nephritic–nephrotic' picture than MCD and FSGS. This may include an element of renal impairment due to glomerular inflammation and damage rather than hypovolaemia alone (indeed, patients with this disease are usually

volume expanded). Elevation of the plasma creatinine and urea early in the disease, not responsive to adjustment of volume status, therefore suggests this diagnosis or some other (rare) form of structural glomerular disease. A few cases of membranoproliferative glomerulonephritis follow a rapidly progressive course with deterioration to end stage renal failure in weeks or months, which will obviously be reflected by progressive increase in the plasma creatinine as the glomerular filtration rate (GFR) deteriorates.

Calcium. The total plasma *calcium* concentration is reduced in parallel with the albumin, since it is partly albumin bound. The *ionized calcium* is normal, and it is not necessary to treat the low total concentration of the ion, which normalizes when the hypoalbuminaemia is corrected.

Key points: Initial laboratory investigations in childhood nephrotic syndrome

- Urine:
  - urinalysis and urine microscopy;
  - quantification of proteinuria (early morning protein:creatinine ratio);
  - urinary sodium where hypovolaemia is suspected.

- Plasma:
  - creatinine, urea, and electrolytes;
  - albumin, total protein, calcium, and phosphate;
  - C3, C4, antistreptolysin-O titre (ASOT), antinuclear antibody (ANA);
  - hepatitis B serology;
  - varicella IgG antibody status;

- Full blood count (FBC).

Haematology. The *haemoglobin* concentration and *haematocrit* are increased or decreased in inverse proportion to changes in plasma volume. The absolute values of these variables at presentation are, of course, influenced by other factors, such as pre-existing anaemia, but acute *changes* in them are a reliable guide to changes in volume. Children with MCD or FSGS and severe volume contraction may have marked elevation of these indices, and this should be taken into account as an adjunct to the clinical assessment of circulating volume. Platelet numbers and aggregability

Table 19.2 Major complications of the steroid-sensitive nephrotic syndrome

Infection
Hypovolaemia
Thrombosis
Acute renal failure
Hyperlipidaemia
Malnutrition
Side-effects of treatment:
    Corticosteroids
    Alkylating agents
    Cyclosporin A
    Levamisole

may both be increased. There are no other specific or characteristic changes in the blood count.

Complications

The major complications of the nephrotic syndrome are listed in Table 19.2.

Infection

In modern (post-corticosteroid) times, the steroid-sensitive nephrotic syndrome has come to be regarded as a fairly benign condition, but before steroid therapy was available as many as 30% of affected children died of their illness and before the introduction of antibiotics the proportion was even higher. As this historical note suggests, infection was the major cause of mortality, commonly with *Streptococcus pneumoniae*, which was, and is, prone to cause fulminating peritonitis and septicaemia. This reflects the fact that nephrotic patients are immunocompromised in a number of ways, involving not only humoral factors but also probably lymphocyte function (Table 19.3). In nephrotic children, as in the population generally, the proportion of individuals with preformed antipneumococcal antibody rises with age, which probably accounts for the decreased incidence of serious pneumococcal infection in older patients—it is rarely

Table 19.3 Causes of susceptibility to infection in children with steroid-sensitive nephrotic syndrome

Low plasma IgG
Low serum factor B (C3 proactivator)
Impaired opsonization
Impaired lymphocyte transformation
Drug-induced immunosuppression

seen in adult nephrotics. Low levels of serum factor B (C3 proactivator), probably due to urinary loss, may be of particular importance in this respect, since this substance is necessary for the efficient opsonization and killing of capsulated bacteria in the absence of specific antibody. The significance of the circulating inhibitor of lymphocyte transformation, which has been found in the sera of nephrotic patients in relapse but not in remission, is less certain. Infection remains a serious threat to nephrotic patients during relapse and fever or other clinical evidence of infection should be treated as a medical emergency. It is important to remember that a significant proportion of serious infections in nephrotic children are caused by Gram-negative bacteria and, until an organism has been identified in a particular case, a broad-spectrum antibiotic combination should be prescribed. It is routine practice in many centres for prophylactic penicillin to be commenced in the oedematous child with ascites during disease relapse. Needless to say, nephrotic children receiving treatment with immunosuppressive drugs may be even more susceptible to infections; chickenpox is a life-threatening illness in immunocompromised patients who have not previously had the disease, and parents of such at-risk children should be warned to report any contact with chickenpox or shingles as a matter of urgency, so that protective measures can be taken.

Thrombosis

Both arterial and venous thromboses are prone to occur in patients with the nephrotic syndrome. This is predominantly a problem complicating MCD and FSGS, rather than membranoproliferative disease. Affected sites include the deep veins of the legs and pelvis, the renal veins, mesenteric veins, the pulmonary vasculature, and the arterial supply to the lower limbs. Cerebral thrombosis has been described, fortunately rarely.

Renal vein thrombosis has been recognized as a feature of the nephrotic syndrome for many years; it is particularly associated with membranous nephropathy and used to be considered a *cause* of the syndrome, although it is now thought rather to be a *complication*. Membranous nephropathy is uncommon in childhood, which may account for the relative rarity of renal vein thrombosis in this age group.

The tendency to thrombosis is probably due to a combination of haemodynamic factors and hypercoagulability (Table 19.4). Hypovolaemia, when present,

Table 19.4 Factors predisposing to thrombosis in steroid sensitive nephrotic syndrome

Thrombocytosis
Increased platelet aggregability
Increased plasma concentrations of clotting factors:
   Factor V
   Factor VII
   Factor VIII
   Factor X
   Fibrinogen
Accelerated thromboplastin generation
Reduced plasma concentration of antithrombin III
Hypovolaemia
   Circulatory sluggishness
   Increased blood viscosity
Corticosteroid therapy

probably affects both: the former by causing circulatory sluggishness and the latter by producing haemoconcentration and hyperviscosity. The increased plasma concentrations of clotting factors may be the consequence of a general drive to increased protein synthesis secondary to hypoalbuminaemia; accelerated synthesis and turnover of fibrin have been directly demonstrated. The reduced plasma antithrombin III levels are probably due to increased urinary loss, as suggested by clearance studies and by the close correlation between the plasma concentrations of albumin and antithrombin III. The increased platelet aggregability may also be caused by the urinary loss of albumin, or some substance bound to albumin, since it has been shown to be reversible by the *in vitro* addition or the *in vivo* infusion of albumin, and by the addition of concentrated protein from nephrotic urine although, interestingly, not by aspirin.

Acute renal failure

Prerenal uraemia, usually of mild degree, is quite commonly seen in nephrotic patients in association with hypovolaemia, as discussed above. Much less commonly, acute renal failure unresponsive to volume replacement is seen. The cause of this is not completely understood. It is usually precipitated by hypovolaemia, especially if complicated by sepsis, and the histological appearances are those of acute tubular necrosis (ATN). However, most hypovolaemic episodes and infections do not lead to ATN, and why it should occur in a few cases remains a mystery. Very rarely, SSNS presents with ATN as the initial manifestation [18]. Complete recovery is the rule, although dialysis may be necessary if the renal failure persists for more than a few days.

Hyperlipidaemia

The abnormality of plasma lipids characteristic of the nephrotic syndrome is elevation of total cholesterol, low-density and very-low-density lipoproteins, with high-density lipoproteins remaining relatively normal. Despite several decades of research, the mechanism underlying these changes is poorly understood, but the cause seems to be directly related to hypoalbuminaemia. Whether the hyperlipidaemia of the nephrotic syndrome predisposes to atherosclerosis is an important but unanswered question: fortunately, few children are exposed to it for sustained periods due to the intermittent nature of the disease in most cases.

Malnutrition

Children with unremitting nephrotic syndrome for a long period may develop severe muscle wasting. This may be masked by oedema, and only becomes manifest when this is abolished. This is particularly likely to occur in small children with FSGS, in whom urinary protein loss is often very heavy and sometimes refractory to all forms of treatment. Such patients are at high risk of sudden overwhelming sepsis and the prognosis is poor: fortunately, this 'malignant' variety of FSGS is uncommon. In the much more common SSNS, significant wasting can also occur if

---

Key points: Assessment and treatment of hypovolaemia in nephrotic syndrome

- Children with nephrotic syndrome require repeated careful assessment of their circulatory status with prompt treatment of hypovolaemia with colloid-containing solution such as plasma or human albumin where this is detected.

- The administration of albumin is *not* a routine measure to be given to all patients in relapse and may be dangerous in the child who is not volume depleted.

- Intravenous albumin should be administered at a maximum dose of 1 g/kg (5 ml/kg of 20% solution) over 2–4 hours.

relapses are frequent, although in this case it is difficult to determine the respective contributions of frequent episodes of heavy proteinuria and prolonged corticosteroid therapy.

Management

The initial episode

The child should generally be admitted to hospital for initial assessment and treatment as a matter of some urgency. Exceptions may be made for children who are clinically well, not hypovolaemic, and live within reasonable distance of the hospital. These patients can be managed as daily ward-attenders, their parents having been instructed in how to recognize signs of complications such as hypovolaemia and infection. If hypovolaemia is present according to the criteria discussed above, volume repletion should be undertaken with a colloid-containing solution such as plasma or human albumin, in a dose calculated to provide 1 g albumin/kg body weight. This is *not* a routine measure to be given to all nephrotic patients in relapse—plasma or albumin infusion may be dangerous in children who do not show clinical or laboratory signs of volume depletion (see above) [19].

If the patient is febrile or feels systemically unwell, antibiotics should be given. Penicillin alone is usually appropriate but an aminoglycoside may be added, or a broader-spectrum agent, such as a third-generation cephalosporin, substituted if signs of peritonitis or septicaemia are present, until information on antibiotic sensitivities is available. The urine sediment should be examined, and urine and blood specimens sent to the laboratory for basic biochemical estimations (see above).

Enforced bedrest is not necessary in a child who feels well enough to want to be active. Healthy eating should be encouraged with a no-added-salt diet; there is no indication for altering the protein intake. Children with significant oedema may benefit from fluid restriction with or without the addition of oral diuretic therapy, provided there is no evidence of intravascular volume depletion. Commonly used diuretics include frusemide in conjunction with spironolactone. Children receiving diuretics should be regularly assessed to ensure that their volume status remains normal. As stated above, it is routine practice for oedematous children to receive prophylactic penicillin therapy.

Steroid therapy

In the absence of atypical features (persistent hypertension, continuous or macroscopic haematuria, evidence of reduced GFR, low C3 levels), glucocorticoid therapy should be started as soon as the diagnosis is established. The regimen used by most nephrologists over the past 30 years has been that introduced by the International Study of Kidney Disease in Children (ISKDC), or a modification of it. This begins with prednisone or prednisolone in a dose of $60 \, mg/m^2/day$ (or 2 mg/kg/day), given in two or three divided daily doses, for 4 weeks. This is followed by a second month of treatment with the same drug in a single daily dose of $40 \, mg/m^2/day$ (or 1.5 mg/kg/day) given *either* on three consecutive days (e.g. Monday, Tuesday, Wednesday) in each of four consecutive weeks, *or* on alternate mornings for a further 28 days. In the past few years, however, evidence has been accumulating that a longer course of initial steroid therapy may be significantly protective against the future development of frequent relapses and/or steroid dependency. In a large study from Warsaw, Poland, a tapering course of prednisone lasting 6 months was found to increase the proportion of patients in sustained remission 2 years after completing initial therapy from about 25% to 50% compared with courses lasting 2 and 3 months [20]. Very recently, a meta-analysis including this and several other controlled studies was published by an Australian group [21]. This confirmed that the longer the initial course of treatment, the less was the likelihood of early relapse, frequent relapses and steroid dependency in the first year or two of follow-up, with maximum benefit being seen as a result of 6 or 7 months' treatment compared with 2 or 3 months (Fig. 19.5). A universal consensus is still lacking, and further comparative studies are in progress or planned. Until the results of these are available, the author's reading of the available evidence favours a six month initial course of treatment, the first two months of which are according to the ISKDC regime set out above, alternate day therapy being preferred to three-day-a week therapy for the second month. In months 3–6, alternate day treatment is continued, the dose being reduced by 25% every four weeks. A relatively new alternative to prednisone and prednisolone is deflazacort. This steroid has been claimed to be less catabolic than prednisolone and to be less prone to cause osteopenia and negative calcium balance. Early results of trials from France and

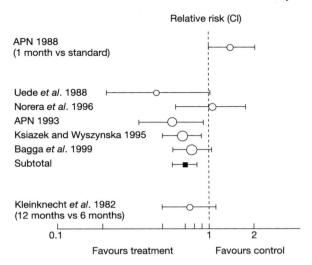

Relative risk (CI)

APN 1988
(1 month vs standard)

Uede *et al.* 1988
Norera *et al.* 1996
APN 1993
Ksiazek and Wyszynska 1995
Bagga *et al.* 1999
Subtotal

Kleinknecht *et al.* 1982
(12 months vs 6 months)

0.1　　　　　　　　1　　　　2

Favours treatment　　　　Favours control

Fig. 19.5　Meta-analysis of controlled studies comparing the effect of courses of prednis(ol)one of varying lengths in the treatment of the initial attack of the nephrotic syndrome on the risk of relapse in the first 21–24 months after treatment. The five studies in the central part of the plot all compared standard (2 months) treatment with 3–7 months in the experimental arm. The entry marked 'subtotal' is the pooled estimate of risk derived from these five studies. (Modified from Hodson *et al.* Arch Dis Child 2000; 83:45–51 with permission from the BMJ Publishing Group.)

elsewhere are modestly encouraging [22], but deflazacort is significantly more expensive than the older glucocorticoids and a general switch to it as the initial steroid of choice in nephrotic syndrome cannot yet be recommended.

STEROID-RESPONSIVE (STEROID-SENSITIVE) NEPHROTIC SYNDROME

The majority (80–90%) of children under the age of 10 presenting with typical nephrotic syndrome respond to steroid treatment within 8 weeks. Response is defined as disappearance of proteinuria and the reversal of all clinical and laboratory features of the syndrome. Failure to respond to steroid is the most generally agreed indication for renal biopsy, and non-responsive children should be referred to a paediatric nephrology centre for evaluation.

Key points: Newly presenting nephrotic syndrome, indications for referral to a paediatric nephrologist and possible renal biopsy

- Age under 12 months (congenital or infantile nephrotic syndrome).

- Age over 16 years (adult disease pattern).

- Persistent hypertension.

- Continuous or macroscopic haematuria.

- Impaired renal function unresponsive to correction of circulatory status.

- Low C3 or C4.

- Failure to respond to initial course of corticosteroid therapy.

Children who do not tolerate steroids well should probably be biopsied earlier, after 4 weeks, because it is inappropriate to continue steroid treatment if the biopsy shows a lesion that is unlikely to respond.

SSNS is most typically a relapsing disease and both morbidity and hospital admission rates can be reduced if relapses are detected early, prior to the child becoming frankly oedematous. To this end, parents need to be trained to perform urinalysis of their child's first morning urine sample (to avoid othostatic proteinuria) and to record the results in a nephrotic syndrome diary, which can also be used to record the administration of drug therapy. They should be instructed to contact the hospital if their child develops evidence of a relapse (defined by the ISKDC as Albustix 2+ proteinuria or more for three consecutive days) or if their child becomes clinically oedematous. Verbal information should be supplemented with written information such as the Nottingham booklet (see Chapter 25). The importance of the continued testing of urine should be stressed, although unfortunately compliance is often not good

In some children who do respond (unfortunately, the minority) no relapse occurs and no further treatment is necessary. After a reasonable period of outpatient observation (12 months) the child can be discharged and told to return if relapse occurs at a later date. No restrictions of any kind should be imposed once treatment has stopped and the child has been released from hospital. The prognosis in this group is excellent in every respect. In most children with SSNS, one or more relapses will occur following the initial episode. The management of these patients ranges from relatively straightforward to extremely difficult, depending mainly on three factors: (1) the frequency of relapses; (2) the dose and duration of steroid therapy necessary to induce remission on each occasion; and (3) the tolerance of the individual to long-term steroid treatment, which varies greatly from patient to patient.

Relapsing nephrotic syndrome

Following the example of the International Study of Kidney Disease in Childhood, it is useful to stratify children with SSNS according to the frequency of their relapses. Four grades of severity are conventionally recognized. They are defined according to carefully specified criteria, and it is important to use the agreed terminology accurately in order that like may be compared with like when the results of therapeutic trials are evaluated:

1. Non-relapsing nephrotic syndrome: children who do not relapse after the first episode of the disease. As indicated above, they need no treatment after the initial attack.

2. Infrequently relapsing nephrotic syndrome: children who relapse after the first attack, but less than twice within the first 6 months and less than four times within any subsequent 12-month period.

3. Frequently relapsing nephrotic syndrome without steroid dependency: this is subsequently referred to simply as frequently relapsing nephrotic syndrome (FRNS). Children who relapse two or more times within the first 6 months after the first attack, or four or more times in any 12-month period.

4. Frequently relapsing nephrotic syndrome with steroid dependency: this is subsequently referred to as steroid-dependent nephrotic syndrome (SDNS). Children fulfilling the criteria for FRNS in whom two consecutive relapses, or two of four relapses in any 6-month period, occurred while a (usually reducing) dose of steroid was still being given, or within 14 days of discontinuing steroid therapy.

Relapses are conventionally treated with an abbreviated corticosteroid regimen, as originally described by the ISKDC. Prednisolone is given at a dose of $60\,mg/m^2$ daily until urinary remission is achieved (3 days of zero or trace proteinuria on Albustix), followed by $40\,mg/m^2$ on alternate days for a total of 28 days (i.e. 14 doses). Treatment should be commenced promptly, to avoid children becoming overtly nephrotic. The median time to remission in more than one study is 11 days from starting high-dose steroid treatment. Using this regimen, children with infrequently relapsing nephrotic syndrome will be receiving corticosteroid therapy considerably less than half the time, allowing recovery from the acute side-effects before the next relapse occurs. It is rarely, if ever, necessary to consider using drugs other than corticosteroids in children in this group. Long-term prognosis is good, with spontaneous resolution after a period of months to years being the rule.

Routine childhood immunizations should be performed, although live vaccines should not be administered when the child is receiving immunosuppressive therapy. Children should additionally be vaccinated against *Streptococcus pneumoniae* and receive influenza vaccine each winter if they are receiving continuous immunosuppressive therapy. A number of centres are now routinely immunizing non-immune patients against varicella zoster virus.

The remainder of this section concentrates on the management of children in the most difficult categories, those with FRNS and SDNS.

Maintenance steroid therapy

Patients with FRNS and SDNS are at risk of severe steroid toxicity, mainly because of the frequency with which they are exposed to continuous, high-dose prednisolone for induction of remission. The main indication for considering treatment other than intermittent steroid therapy as described above is the development of major side-effects. The adverse effects of glucocorticoids are legion and too well known to need listing here, but particular attention should be paid to impairment of statural growth, disfigurement of facial appearance and bodily habitus, and behavioural changes. The last of these is more common than is appreciated by many physicians [23] and may be severe and distressing to patients, parents, and others such as schoolteachers. Because disturbance of mood and conduct is often attributed to the disease or to unrelated factors, rather than to the treatment, it may go unmentioned in the clinic unless specifically asked about by the doctor. An individual clinical judgement must be made in every case as to whether the child's side-effects are acceptable or not (that is, acceptable to him, his family, and his peers). However, many children in the FRNS and most of those in the SDNS categories are best given at least a trial of some treatment other than intermittent, high-dose prednisolone.

If prednisolone is given on alternate days, as a single morning dose, clinical side-effects are milder than if the same total dose is given in single or multiple daily doses—for example, 30 mg every other day is better tolerated than 15 mg daily. Children with FRNS and significant side-effects may therefore be given a trial of alternate-day prednisolone, in the hope of preventing relapses and the consequent exposure to high, toxic doses. By definition, patients with FRNS have not relapsed while still taking steroids and the initial dose should be low, in the range 0.2–0.4 mg/kg (5–15 mg/m^2) per dose. The dose should *not* be divided into two or more doses on treatment days, since the relative freedom from side-effects hoped for from the regimen depends critically on an inter-dose interval of more than 36 h, preferably 48 h. This has been formally documented to be the case with regard to suppression of the hypothalamo-pituitary adrenal axis and to growth, and clinical impression strongly suggests that it is true of other side-effects also. If successful in preventing relapse, this protocol can be followed safely for months or years, and there is usually a gratifying improvement in the patient's appearance and well-being within a few weeks. It is reasonable to attempt gently to withdraw treatment every 6 months or so, to see whether it is still needed, but it is usually extremely well tolerated and the paediatrician should not hesitate to resume the same maintenance regimen if relapse occurs.

Patients with SDNS present a more difficult problem. By definition, they have relapsed while still receiving steroids or within 2 weeks of stopping them, and are likely to need a higher alternate-day prednisolone dose than those with FRNS. The history will reveal the dose at which relapse occurred during the previous few months, and maintenance therapy should be commenced at a level just above this. If this dose is held for 2–3 months it will become apparent whether or not it allows the side-effects to regress to a tolerable level. If so, the dose can be 'fine tuned' by trial and error to establish the minimum amount that will achieve the desired effect—that is, freedom from relapse without unacceptable toxicity. If such a trial is not successful, the use of other drugs must be considered. Particular attention needs to be directed to growth at the time of the expected pubertal growth spurt. Children who have been growing well on alternate-day prednisolone may fall significantly behind in the mid-teens due to steroid-induced pubertal delay.

Alkylating agents

Alkylating agents impair DNA transcription by attaching alkyl chains to purine bases. They are cytotoxic and immunosuppressive. Some members of the group, such as cyclophosphamide, have two alkyl groups and therefore also prevent cell division by cross-linking paired DNA helices. The parent drug, nitrogen mustard (mechlorethamine), was shown to be capable of inducing remission in the nephrotic syndrome in the 1940s. In the past three decades, two orally effective congeners of nitrogen mustard, chlorambucil and cyclophosphamide, have been more widely used. There is no doubt that they work, but their precise role in the management of MCD remains controversial. There are two reasons for this: first, their toxicity, and secondly, the presence of widely conflicting claims in the literature as to their effectiveness in producing sustained remission and allowing the patient to stop taking corticosteroids.

Early reports tended to be optimistic in their conclusions, reporting long-term, relapse-free survival in half or more of treated patients [24]. However, many of these reports are sketchy as to the details of the patients, in particular whether they had FRNS, SDNS, or a mixture of the two, and exactly how much drug was given over what duration. More recent studies have been more consistent, and it is now reasonably clear that patients with FRNS respond well to alkylating agents, with 50–90% long-term remission, while those with SDNS are much more resistant to their action, with only 20–30% long-term remission [25], as shown in Fig. 19.6.

Side-effects of cyclophosphamide (much the most widely used of these drugs in the United Kingdom) can be divided into early, i.e. during or shortly after administration of the agent, and late or long-term. These need to be discussed in detail with parents and the discussion backed-up by additional written information. Early effects include bone marrow suppression, alopecia (always reversible), minor gastrointestinal upsets,

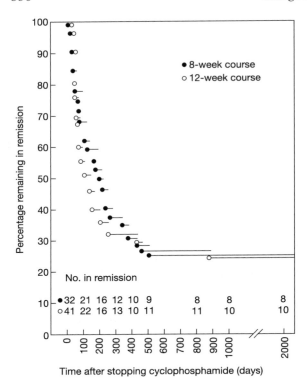

Fig. 19.6 The cumulative probability of sustained remission in children with steroid-dependent nephrotic syndrome following an 8- or 12-week course of cyclophosphamide in a dose of 3 mg/kg/day. Only about 35% were in remission at 1 year, and 25% at 2 years. It is evident from the graph that the longer course conferred no advantage. (From Ueda *et al.* Arch Dis Child 1990; 65:1147–1150 with permission from the BMJ Publishing Group.)

and haemorrhagic cystitis—the latter is rarely seen at the doses usually given in the nephrotic syndrome. Late effects include infertility, especially in males, and malignancy. Although both are obviously serious and worrying possibilities, they are undoubtedly dose related and, in a fairly extensive literature, a cumulative dose of cyclophosphamide of not more than 150–170 mg/kg has not been reported to cause either. Claims that nitrogen mustard and chlorambucil are more effective than cyclophosphamide have been made, but it is not clear whether the drugs were give in equivalent doses as regards both therapeutic and adverse effects. Most of the few malignancies that have been reported after alkylating agent therapy for nephrotic syndrome have followed the use of chlorambucil. However, the cumulative amount of chlorambucil used in these early trials was almost certainly equivalent to several times the amount of cyclophosphamide that is now

conventionally given. It is therefore likely that the ability to cause secondary malignant disease is dose related rather than drug specific.

The only indication for the use of an alkylating agent is failure of intermittent or maintenance prednisolone therapy to achieve stable remission without poisoning the patient with the steroid. Cyclophosphamide should be given at a dose of 3 mg/kg/day for 8 weeks, the calculation being made on ideal weight for height rather than actual (i.e. oedematous or obese) weight. It is usual to start therapy with the patient in a steroid-induced remission but this is not essential: there is some evidence that proteinuria may remit faster if both drugs are given together in relapse than if prednisolone is given alone. Once in remission and on cyclophosphamide, prednisolone should be converted to an alternate-day regimen at 40 mg/m²/day, which is then tapered progressively to stop either just before or just after the cyclophosphamide. Blood counts should be performed weekly during the first 4 weeks of treatment and 2 weekly during the second 4 weeks. Occasionally treatment must be interrupted, usually because of neutropenia, but this is uncommon if the recommended dose is not exceeded. Patients should be advised to report any symptoms of intercurrent infection, or any exposure to infectious disease (especially chickenpox), during treatment so that necessary treatment or protection can be given.

Key points: Side-effects of cyclophosphamide

- Early:
  - bone-marrow suppression (weekly FBCs for 4 weeks then fortnightly);
  - reversible alopecia;
  - gastrointestinal upset;
  - haemorrhagic cystitis.

- Late:
  - impaired fertility;
  - possible malignancy.

At present there is no compelling reason to prefer any other alkylating agent to cyclophosphamide. In one controlled study, a course of eight doses of intravenous nitrogen mustard, 0.1 mg/kg/dose, led to better results than cyclophosphamide, given as described

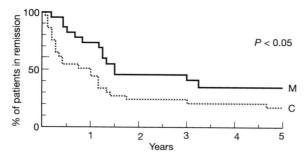

Fig. 19.7 Superiority of intravenous meclorethamine (nitrogen mustard (M)) over oral cyclophosphamide (C) in the induction of prolonged remission in children with frequently relapsing and steroid-dependent nephrotic syndrome. See text for details of dosage. (From Vallo *et al.* Comparative effects of cyclophosphamide and nitrogen mustard in treatment of idiopathic nephrotic syndrome (Abstract) Pediatr Nephrol 1993; 7(suppl):C33 with permission from Springer Verlag.)

in the previous paragraph (Fig. 19.7) [26]. The first four doses were given on each of four consecutive days, the second four being given in the same way after an interval of 4 weeks. It is not clear whether the difference was due to a real difference in the effectiveness of the two drugs, or a difference in patient adherence to the prescribed regimen: the advantage of supervised intravenous infusion is that there is no doubt that the drug enters the patient's bloodstream. If nitrogen mustard is used, a modern anti-emetic such as ondansetron or granisetron should be given to prevent nausea and vomiting, which can be severe. Meticulous attention to intravenous technique is essential, since if nitrogen mustard leaks from a vein it causes tissue necrosis. The recommended method is to set up a fast-running saline infusion through a plastic cannula (not a metal needle) securely placed in a peripheral vein, and to 'piggy-back' the nitrogen mustard into this via a Y-connection. This ensures not only that the intravenous line is free running but also that the drug is infused at high dilution. Any complaint of pain or discomfort at the cannula site must be investigated immediately. Logically, intravenous pulsed cyclophosphamide in eight doses of 20 mg/kg given at 3 week intervals (total dosage 160 mg/kg) should combine the advantage of the intravenous route (compliance) with freedom from the risk of local toxicity if the infusion leaks from the vein but, perhaps oddly, there are no published studies of this regimen in this disease.

Purine analogues

The purine analogues azathioprine, 6-mercaptopurine, and 6-thioguanine have all been used sporadically in the nephrotic syndrome. However, the few controlled trials that have been performed have shown no evidence of a therapeutic effect. These drugs have no place in the modern management of the disease.

Ciclosporin A

Ciclosporin A (CsA) is an immunosuppressive fungal metabolite which acts by modifying T-cell function. Specifically, the drug inhibits the release of interleukin-2 from activated T-helper cells and thus prevents the induction and proliferation of T-effector cells. The previously cited hypothesis of Shalhoub [5], that steroid-responsive nephrotic syndrome is a disorder of T-cell function, led several groups to assess the effect of CsA in the disease. Published reports are fairly consistent in that steroid-responsive patients, including those with FRNS and SDNS, usually respond well to low-dose CsA, and steroids can be withdrawn in most without relapse. However, relapse is almost invariable when the CsA is withdrawn—CsA dependency has been substituted for steroid dependency [27].

Side-effects of CsA include tremor, hypertrichosis, and gum hyperplasia. All of these are dose dependent and can be minimized or prevented by adjusting dosage according to blood levels of the drug. Unfortunately, CsA is also nephrotoxic and it is clear from the experience in transplant patients (especially those in whom the organ transplanted was not the kidney, e.g. recipients of heart, liver, and bone marrow grafts) that permanent kidney damage and even chronic renal failure can result if the drug is given at high dosage for long enough. The matter is made more difficult by the fact that there is also a reversible effect of CsA on renal function, probably due to inhibition of prostaglandin synthesis and consequent constriction of the renal microvasculature. Monitoring renal function by measurement of plasma creatinine or even formal GFR estimation is therefore inadequate to differentiate vasoconstriction from permanent damage.

At Guy's Hospital, we have adopted the following approach to CsA therapy in patients who have failed cyclophosphamide therapy and who remain severely affected by steroid side-effects. First, the drug is introduced at a low dose, typically 4 mg/kg/day in two equal divided doses, and carefully adjusted to keep the measured trough blood level (measured 12–16 h after the last dose) below the upper limit of the target range for transplant patients. This value varies with the assay being used: in our laboratory, using a monoclonal antibody-based radio-immunoassay, it is 150 ng/ml. The lower limit of the target range is defined as the smallest dose that keeps the patient in steroid-free remission. (This is different from the policy in transplant patients, in whom a predetermined lower limit is specified, in our laboratory 70 ng/ml.) Secondly, after 1–2 years of treatment a choice is made: either the drug is withdrawn, or a renal biopsy is performed. The latter alternative is selected if the patient expresses a strong desire to continue taking CsA rather than risk further high-dose steroid exposure. If the biopsy shows no evidence of CsA toxicity, the drug is continued for another year or two and the same choice then repeated. Our experience so far has been encouraging. The drug has not had to be withdrawn from any patient because of clinical or histological evidence of nephrotoxicity. This is probably due to the fact that, in those patients who respond to CsA, the minimum effective dose is very low, often below the range usually considered effective in the prevention of graft rejection. These results encourage us to believe that CsA may have a future in the long-term management of children with FRNS and SDNS.

It must be emphasized that CsA is a potentially toxic drug. At present, it should probably only be used by, or in consultation with, a paediatric nephrologist with experience of its use in transplantation. Control of dosage by regular monitoring of the trough blood level is mandatory. It is very important to emphasize to the patient and parents that the likely effect of CsA is to substitute CsA dependence for steroid dependence, not to cure the disease.

Levamisole

The antihelminthic agent levamisole also alters T-cell function but, in contrast to the immunosuppressive agents discussed above, it stimulates rather than inhibits it. Sporadic reports in the early 1980s suggested that it might be effective in steroid-responsive nephrotic syndrome. Several reports have now confirmed this effect. In one prospective, double-blind, randomized study [28], 61 steroid-dependent patients, 38 of whom had relapsed following treatment with alkylating agents, were treated either with levamisole 2.5 mg/kg on alternate days or with placebo for 112 days. All patients were receiving maintenance alternate-day prednisolone therapy at the beginning of levamisole or placebo treatment; this was tapered and withdrawn over 56 days. At the end of the study, 14 of 31 levamisole-treated patients (45%) and only 4 of 30 placebo-treated patients (13%) were in remission (Fig. 19.8), the difference was highly significant ($P = 0.008$). However, 10 of the 14 children in the levamisole group and 3 of 4 in the placebo group who were in remission at the end of the treatment period relapsed within 3 months of stopping treatment. Thus, like CsA, levamisole can maintain a proportion of steroid-dependent patients in steroid-free remission as long as it is given, but is ineffective as a permanent cure of the disease. On the positive side, levamisole was well tolerated and no important side-effects were reported.

Tacrolimus

Tacrolimus is an immunosuppressive agent similar in its mode of action to CsA but more powerful. Anecdotal evidence suggests that its effect in steroid-dependent nephrotic syndrome is similar to that of the latter. A few patients who have not responded to CsA may respond to tacrolimus, and it may therefore be worthwhile to try it in selected cases. At the time of writing, it should be regarded as an experimental drug in this setting and not used outside centres that are used to prescribing it for transplant recipients. As with CsA, it is necessary to monitor the trough blood level of the drug. The side-effects profile of tacrolimus is also similar to that of CsA.

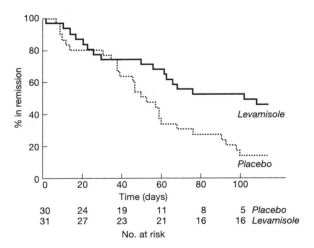

Fig. 19.8 The effect of levamisole compared with placebo on maintenance of remission in a prospective, multi-centre, randomized, double-blind study. For further details see text. (From Anonymous [28]. Reprinted with permission from Elsevier Science.)

Other drugs

There is no evidence that any drugs other than those discussed above have any beneficial effect in the steroid-sensitive nephrotic syndrome. Among those agents tried and found wanting are disodium cromoglycate and intravenous human gammaglobulin. Anecdotal reports of benefit from mizorbine and mycophenolate mofetil await confirmation in larger studies.

It is evident from the foregoing that several options exist for the practical management of children with SSNS in whom steroid therapy alone is proving unsatisfactory. A suggested practical guide to treatment is given in Fig. 19.9. Inevitably, given the 'soft'

nature of most of the evidence for and against the various drugs now available, these proposals reflect the personal experience and prejudices of the author.

STEROID-RESISTANT NEPHROTIC SYNDROME

Steroid-resistant focal segmental glomerulosclerosis and minimal change disease

It is not routine practice, at least in the United Kingdom, to biopsy the kidneys of children with a first attack of nephrotic syndrome, unless atypical 'nephritic' features are present (see Key points, p. 353). Most paediatric nephrologists biopsy children who fail to respond to steroids within 1–2 months. The great majority of these biopsies show either FSGS or MCD. These are probably not distinct clinical and pathological entities. The modern consensus is that they form part of a spectrum ranging from 'pure', highly steroid-sensitive patients with MCD at one end and children with 'malignant' or rapidly progressive FSGS, unresponsive to any form of treatment, at the other. A recent, worrying report from North America [29] suggests that the incidence of FSGS as a cause of idiopathic nephrotic syndrome is rising, from 23% of cases in 1978 to 47% in 1997. No plausible explanation exists for this phenomenon, which appears particularly to affect African–American children. It should be remembered that FSGS is a histological pattern that can occur as the result of several diseases other than the nephrotic syndrome (e.g. advanced reflux nephropathy), and not a disease entity as such. Families have been described with a form of recessively inherited FSGS characterized by nephrotic syndrome resistant to all forms of treatment. This is now known to be due to mutations in a gene mapped to 1q25–31, that codes for a membrane protein, podocin, localized to the podocyte [30]. These familial cases probably form a distinct subgroup, separate from the spectrum of acquired idiopathic nephrotic syndrome. There is some evidence that children showing lesions of FSGS early in the course of the disease are less responsive both to steroids and to other drugs than those with MCD. The matter is further complicated by the fact that some patients with MCD on a first biopsy may have FSGS if a biopsy is done later in the disease, especially if they are persistently steroid resistant or if

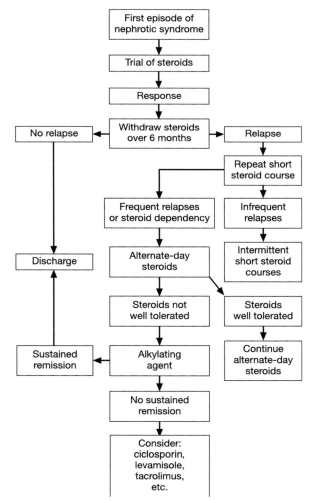

Fig. 19.9 Flow chart summarizing a suggested scheme for managing children with idiopathic nephrotic syndrome who respond to a conventional initial course of corticosteroid.

they have developed secondary steroid resistance, as occasionally happens. Since it is only necessary to identify a single area of focal hyalinosis in a single glomerulus to diagnose FSGS, the question of whether FSGS was present all along but missed on the first biopsy because a representative lesion was not included in the biopsy, or whether 'true' MCD can evolve into FSGS, is unanswerable. There are grounds for believing that the lesions of FSGS arise as a consequence of unremitting heavy proteinuria, rather than being the cause of it. If this is true, it follows that steroid-resistant cases will be more likely to develop FSGS than steroid-responsive patients, in whom proteinuria is, by definition, intermittent. The main reason for performing a biopsy after initial failure to respond to steroids is to exclude one of the rarer causes of nephrotic syndrome, such as membranoproliferative glomerulonephritis, for which a different treatment strategy would be appropriate.

Although treatment for this group of patients is far from satisfactory, an important guiding principle stems from the fact that children whose proteinuria cannot be abolished by one means or another have a very poor prognosis, with a high risk of progression to end stage renal failure, perhaps 50% within 5–10 years. It is therefore justified to try to induce a remission by the empirical use of immunosuppressive drugs of various types, even when (as is usually the case) the evidence for drug effectiveness is weak. Although all these drugs are toxic, if they are used carefully the side-effects can be minimized, and the gain to the patient if treatment is successful is great.

Prolonged steroid treatment

A study by the ISKDC showed that if daily steroid treatment is continued for up to 6 months, a few children will respond after the first 2 months [31]. There are not many of these, however, and it is probably more effective and kinder to the patient to introduce other drugs at this point.

High-dose intravenous methylprednisolone

Methylprednisolone given intravenously daily or on alternate days at a dosage of $1 \, g/1.73 \, m^2$ body surface area to a total of 3–6 doses is effective in the treatment of renal allograft rejection and some forms of rapidly progressive glomerulonephritis. It has succeeded in a small number of cases in inducing remission in children with nephrotic syndrome who have

not responded to a conventional course of oral steroid. This treatment is usually well tolerated, especially if given on alternate days, and some prefer to try this approach before exposing patients to the multiple toxic side-effects of the other drugs discussed below. However, in my opinion these children's long-term exposure to steroids is already so great that I prefer to reserve intravenous methylprednisolone for combination therapy with an alkylating agent at a later stage in children who fail to respond to ciclosporin A (see below).

Ciclosporin A

In a multi-centre study organized by the French Society of Paediatric Nephrology [32], 65 children with primary steroid-resistant nephrotic syndrome were treated with CsA and prednisone for 6 months. CsA was given in a starting dose of $150 \, mg/m^2/day$ in two divided doses, adjusted to achieve a trough plasma CsA concentration of 100–200 ng/ml. Prednisone was given at $30 \, mg/m^2/day$, also in two divided doses, for the first month, followed by 30 mg/m^2 on alternate days for 5 months. Twenty-seven of the 65 patients achieved complete remission and a further four, partial remission. There was no significant difference in the remission rate between children with MCD and those with FSGS. At a mean follow-up interval of 38 months (range 14–60 months) from starting treatment, 17 remained in remission, eight had relapsed and two were clinically nephrotic. It is noteworthy that the eight who had relapsed had become steroid sensitive. Similar findings were obtained in another, smaller multi-centre study from Italy, including both adults and children, treated with CsA alone. These results are superior to those reported for alkylating agents in similar patients, and CsA should now be recommended as the treatment of first choice for steroid-resistant disease with either MCD or FSGS on histology. Because of the nephrotoxicity of the drug, GFR (or plasma creatinine) and the trough blood CsA concentration should be monitored carefully during treatment.

Alkylating agents

Reliable data on the use of alkylating agents in SRNS are scanty, making evidence-based recommendations difficult to construct. There is a suggestion, not solidly based, that steroid-resistant children with MCD are more likely to respond than those with

FSGS. Because of the potentially serious consequences of failure to induce remission of proteinuria, it is worth a trial of a standard course of cyclophosphamide or mustine before abandoning a child to the prospect of renal replacement therapy. Additional force is given to this argument because children with FSGS who receive transplants have a high incidence of early recurrence of their original disease in the graft [33], often leading to loss of the organ. The apparent superiority of CsA over alkylating agents referred to above has led this author to reserve the latter for children in whom a 6-month course of CsA and steroids has failed to induce remission.

One group in California [34] has treated children with SRNS with a prolonged course of intravenous methylprednisolone, combined with chlorambucil or cyclophosphamide if the steroid alone failed to induce a remission after 10 weeks of treatment. Methylprednisolone was given as six alternate-day doses of 30 mg/kg during the first 2 weeks, then weekly in the same dose for a further 8 weeks, then fortnightly for a further 8 weeks, then monthly for a further 32 weeks and finally alternate months for a further 25 weeks (78 weeks in all). After the first 2 weeks of treatment, the children were also given oral prednisone, 2 mg/kg on alternate days until the end of the course. The alkylating agents were given as either cyclophosphamide 2 mg/kg/day or chlorambucil 0.2 mg/kg/day for 8–12 weeks. Of 23 children described in the original report, 12 went into complete, sustained remission, six lost their nephrotic syndrome but remained proteinuric, four remained nephrotic, and one died in chronic renal failure. Fifteen of the 23 had at least one course of an alkylating agent. All patients had FSGS either in the original biopsy or in later biopsies. Although these results are impressive, the regime is potentially very toxic and is perhaps best reserved for those who fail to respond to a 6-month course of CsA and steroids as described above.

Levamisole

There is no evidence that levamisole has any beneficial effect in steroid-resistant nephrotic syndrome.

Tacrolimus

A few cases have been described [35] who were resistant to both steroids and CsA but who entered complete or partial remission when treated with tacrolimus. Controlled data are not available and this drug should be considered experimental at present.

Vincristine

A handful of children with steroid- and alkylating agent-resistant nephrotic syndrome have lost their proteinuria following treatment with the antimitotic alkaloid vincristine [36]. In most cases the drug was given with steroids and a second or third course of an alkylating agent. It is therefore impossible to be certain whether the success of the treatment was due to vincristine or the other simultaneously administered drugs. Vincristine is neurotoxic and must be given intravenously, its effect on tissues being similar to that of mustine if extravasation occurs. It cannot be said to have an established place in the management of steroid-resistant nephrotic syndrome.

Membranoproliferative (mesangiocapillary) glomerulonephritis

This disease is uncommon in children and very rare in the first decade. It typically presents with haematuria (macroscopic or microscopic), non-selective proteinuria which is usually, but not always in the nephrotic range, and frequently hypertension and deteriorating renal function. Hypocomplementaemia (persistently reduced plasma concentration of C3) is present in rather more than half of the cases. Renal histopathologists classify the disease into two subtypes. The commoner is type 1, with mesangial proliferation, narrowing of glomerular capillary lumina due to interposition of mesangial cell cytoplasm between the basement membrane and the capillary endothelial cells, and apparent duplication of the basement membrane ('double contouring'). Subendothelial electron-dense deposits, probably consisting of immunoglobulins and complement, are present. Type 2 is similar except that the narrowing of the capillaries is due to a true thickening of the basement membrane with the deposition of electron-dense deposits, which do not stain positive for immunoglobulins and complement, within the membrane itself (linear dense deposit disease). Some nephrologists and pathologists recognize a type 3, but others regard it as a variant of type 1. Type 2 probably has a rather worse prognosis than type 1, but there is no proven advantage in separating the two variants for the purposes of treatment. As with other types of idiopathic nephrotic syndrome, the cause is unknown. It has been suggested that it may be related in some way to post-infectious glomerulonephritis, or some other exogenous precipitating cause, in that there has been an apparent decline in the incidence of the disease, at least in the United Kingdom, over the past 30 years.

Untreated, the condition has a poor prognosis, with 50% or more of patients progressing to end stage renal disease within 10 years of diagnosis. A few cases present with fulminating, rapidly progressive glomerulonephritis and should be managed as such. The majority exhibit persistent proteinuria of variable degree, and slow loss of renal function. Since the 1960s, West and associates have been treating his patients with long-term (10 years or more), alternate-day prednisone. Although this is an uncontrolled series, the outcome for their patients appears to be superior to that of historical untreated patients in other centres (Fig. 19.10) [37]. However, a controlled study of 5 years' alternate-day prednisone by the ISKDC [38] showed little or no overall advantage of treatment over control, although a small benefit was claimed for patients of types 1 and 3. A recent small series [39] found that children with this disease who never manifested hypertension or the nephrotic syndrome did well without treatment, which should probably be reserved for those with one or both of these. Excellent results were claimed in patients with type 1 membranoproliferative disease for a regimen beginning with six alternate-day high-dose infusions of methylprednisolone followed by alternate-day oral prednisone for 1–5 years [40].

In the absence of good, controlled scientific evidence it seems reasonable to recommend:

(1) that children with persistent urinary abnormalities but normal blood pressure, renal function, and absence of nephrotic syndrome be observed without active treatment; and

(2) that children with persistent nephrotic syndrome, hypertension, or evidence of loss of renal function be treated with six doses of intravenous methylprednisolone, 600 mg/m^2 on alternate days, followed by oral prednis(ol)one 40 mg/m^2 on alternate days for 1 year in the first instance, the dose being adjusted or stopped after that according to response.

Membranous nephropathy

Idiopathic membranous nephropathy is so rare in children that it is impossible to make evidence-based recommendations for treatment. Since there is no good reason to suppose that the disease is significantly different in children from in adults, in the event that a case is encountered, it would be appropriate to consult standard textbooks of renal medicine for guidelines.

A flow diagram summarizing the recommended management of the more common forms of steroid-resistant nephrotic syndrome is depicted in Fig. 19.11.

CONGENITAL AND INFANTILE NEPHROTIC SYNDROMES

As previously mentioned, the nephrotic syndrome presenting in the first year of life usually has different causes from cases presenting after 1 year. *Congenital* nephrotic syndrome (CNS) literally describes disease present at or before birth. Since diagnosis is often

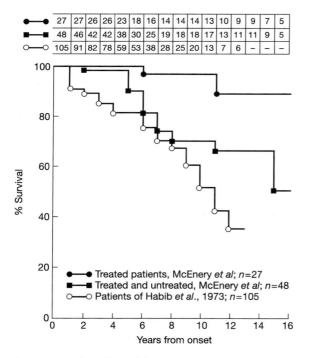

27	27	26	26	23	18	16	14	14	14	13	10	9	9	7	5
48	46	42	42	38	30	25	19	18	18	17	13	11	11	9	5
105	91	82	78	59	53	38	28	25	20	13	7	6	–	–	–

Fig. 19.10 The effect of long-term, alternate-day prednisone treatment on renal survival in a group of children with membranoproliferative glomerulonephritis. Patients from a previous study by Habib *et al.* are included as retrospective controls. (From McEnery *et al.* [37] reproduced with permission from Dustri-Verlag.)

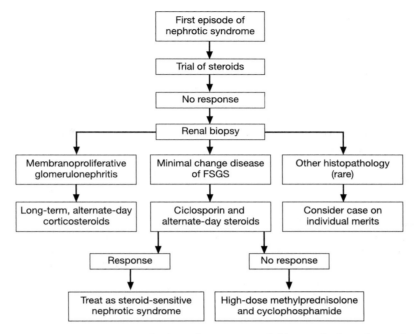

Fig. 19.11 Flow chart summarizing a suggested scheme for managing children with idiopathic nephrotic syndrome who fail to respond to a conventional initial course of corticosteroid. Further details of the included regimes will be found in the text.

delayed for a few days or weeks, partly because of the rarity of the condition in this age group, the term is by convention generally applied to those infants diagnosed within the first 3 months. Cases in whom the first features are seen between the age of 3 months and 1 year are labelled *infantile* nephrotic syndrome (INS). Some cases of CNS and INS are due to congenital infections, some are hereditary, the consequence of mutations in genes that code for essential glomerular components, and others form part of syndromes involving organs other than the kidney (syndromic CNS and INS). The main causes of CNS and INS are listed in Table 19.5.

Congenital nephrotic syndrome

A distinctive form of very early onset nephrotic syndrome has been recognized for many years in the Finnish population and those of Finnish descent. Clinically indistinguishable cases have been found much more rarely in non-Finnish people, including members of most racial and ethnic groups. The clinical features of the 'Finnish' type of CNS include low birth weight, due both to premature delivery and to

Table 19.5 Classification of congenital and infantile nephrotic syndrome (modified from Rapola J. Congenital nephrotic syndrome. Pediatr Nephrol 1987; 1:441–446 with permission from Springer-Verlag.)

Idiopathic
  CNS of Finnish type
  Diffuse mesangial sclerosis
  Other glomerular diseases
Secondary
  Congenital syphilis
  Toxoplasmosis
  Cytomegalovirus
  Rubella
  Hepatitis B
  Malaria
  Other perinatal infections
Syndromic
  Denys–Drash syndrome
  Nail–patella syndrome
  CNS associated with disorders of neuronal migration
  Galloway–Mowat syndrome

CNS, congenital nephrotic syndrome.

intrauterine growth retardation in those born after 34 weeks, placentomegaly (placenta : infant weight ratio > 0.25), heavy albuminuria at birth and, usually, clinically evident oedema within a few days of birth. The cranial fontanelles and sutures are wide, and postural deformities of the hips and knees are common. Proteinuria is massive and unresponsive to steroids or other immunosuppressive drugs. Until it became feasible to offer renal replacement therapy to infants as young as this, the disease was invariably fatal within the first 2 years of life, usually due to infection rather than to progressive renal failure.

It has been clear for a long time that CNS is inherited in an autosomal recessive fashion in Finns, and the recent identification of the gene and its product (nephrin) by molecular methods has confirmed that this is the case in other populations also. Nephrin is a vital component of the slit diaphragm of the glomerular ultrafilter (see above). This important advance in the understanding of the molecular abnormality underlying the condition has not as yet led to any comparable advance in treatment, but these are early days.

Antenatal diagnosis

Finnish CNS is one cause of a raised level of α-fetoprotein (AFP) in maternal blood. This test is widely employed in high-risk populations (Finns and those with a family history of a previously affected child). Measurement of AFP in amniotic fluid is more specific, and is presumed to be a sign of intrauterine proteinuria. Antenatal diagnosis of CNS allows the possibility of termination of pregnancy or, alternatively, of institution of appropriate treatment immediately after birth to promote the best possible outcome if termination is not chosen by the mother.

Histopathology

The most characteristic histological feature of Finnish CNS is dilatation of the tubules, mainly the proximal convoluted tubules, with a typical diameter of 0.1–0.5 mm. The term *microcystic disease* has been applied to this appearance, although this label is best avoided since the appearances are probably non-specific, being the consequence, rather than the cause, of persistent very heavy proteinuria in the immature kidney. Some glomeruli have a primitive, immature appearance with persistence of columnar epithelium, mild mesangial proliferation, and some increase in mesangial matrix. The abnormalities are minimal if tissue is obtained early in the course of the disease, becoming more apparent with time.

Management of Finnish congenital nephrotic syndrome

Treatment is supportive in the first instance, the object being to optimize nutrition and growth and to minimize the amount of time spent in hospital until the child is big enough for renal replacement therapy. Daily, or even twice daily, albumin infusions may be necessary to maintain the plasma albumin and support the circulation, a formidable undertaking in a very small baby. Attempts to reduce the severity of the proteinuria by the use of non-steroidal anti-inflammatory drugs (NSAIDs) and angiotensin converting enzyme (ACE) inhibitors have met with variable success. Paediatric nephrologists in Finland, who have the largest single-centre experience, prefer to perform bilateral nephrectomy at an early stage, and then to dialyse the patient until kidney transplantation is feasible, usually in the second year of life. An alternative approach is to remove only one kidney, which often attenuates the proteinuria to the point at which out–patient management is possible. Unilateral nephrectomy can be combined with NSAID and ACE inhibitor therapy to further reduce proteinuria. As with early onset chronic renal failure of any cause, the definitive treatment is renal transplantation. Surprisingly, the nephrotic syndrome has been observed to recur in some grafts, albeit in a steroid-sensitive form that is quite different from the original Finnish CNS. This may represent an immunological response to nephrin, which is present in the graft but which is presumably seen by the immune system of the recipient as a foreign protein. Whichever of the above strategies is adopted, intensive nutritional support is essential, invariably requiring either nasogastric or gastrostomy tube feeding.

Diffuse mesangial sclerosis

This is another inherited form of nephrotic syndrome. It differs in several important respects from Finnish CNS. There is no association with low birth weight or large placenta. Although proteinuria may be present at birth, its onset may be delayed by weeks or months. The natural history is of progression to end stage renal failure, usually within 2 or 3 years from birth. Proteinuria and the clinical nephrotic syndrome are usually less severe than in the Finnish disease. The histology is distinctive, consisting of uniform, diffuse mesangial sclerosis. It is identical to that seen in the Denys–Drash syndrome (see below), and in at least some cases of diffuse mesangial sclerosis (DMS) mutations have been found in the Wilms' tumour suppressor gene, *WT1*. As with Finnish CNS, management is supportive in the first instance, with renal replacement therapy begun as clinically necessary. Unlike Finnish CNS, it is not usually necessary to perform early unilateral or bilateral nephrectomy to manage the proteinuria.

The Denys–Drash syndrome

This syndrome consists of the combination of male (XY) pseudohermaphroditism, diffuse mesangial sclerosis, and Wilms' tumour. As with isolated DMS, mutations have been identified in the *WT1* gene, although different mutations in different exons of the gene apparently predispose to each of the two conditions. Any infant with apparently isolated DMS who has female or ambiguous genitalia should be karyotyped, since if the Denys–Drash syndrome is confirmed surveillance for the development of Wilms' tumour must be instituted.

Other syndromic forms of congenital nephrotic syndrome

Forms of CNS clinically similar to the Finnish type have been described in several rare syndromes, including the nail–patella syndrome, disorders of neuronal migration, and in a few cases neurological abnormalities with or without arachnodactyly (the Galloway–Mowat syndrome). Management is as for primary CNS and INS, i.e. supportive in the first instance with renal replacement therapy in reserve, if this is thought appropriate in the light of the severe non-renal problems affecting most of these children.

References

1. Holthofer H, Ahola H, Solin ML, Wang S, Palmen T, Luimula P, *et al.* Nephrin localizes at the podocyte filtration slit area and is characteristically spliced in the human kidney. *Am J Pathol* 1999;155:1681–7.
2. Patrakka J, Ruotsalainen V, Ketola I, Holmberg C, Heikinheimo M, Tryggvason K, *et al.* Expression of nephrin in pediatric kidney diseases. *J Am Soc Nephrol* 2001;12:289–96.
3. Carrie BJ, Salyer WR, Myers BD. Minimal change nephropathy: an electrochemical disorder of the basement membrane. *Am J Med* 1981;70:262–8.
4. Taylor GM, Neuhaus TJ, Shah V, Dillon S, Barratt TM. Charge and size selectivity of proteinuria in children with idiopathic nephrotic syndrome. *Pediatr Nephrol* 1997;11:404–10.
5. Shalhoub RJ. Pathogenesis of lipoid nephrosis: a disorder of T-cell function. *Lancet* 1974;2:556–60.
6. Schnaper HW. The immune system in minimal change nephrotic syndrome. *Pediatr Nephrol* 1989;3:101–10.
7. Bakker WW, van Luijk WHJ. Do circulating factors play a role in the pathogenesis of minimal change nephrotic syndrome? *Pediatr Nephrol* 1989;3:341–349.
8. Lagrue G, Branellec A, Niaudet P, Heslan JM, Guillot F, Lang P. Transmission of nephrotic syndrome to two neonates. Spontaneous regression. *Presse Med* 1991;20:255–7.
9. Kemper MJ, Wolf G, Müller-Wiefel DE. Transmission of glomerular permeability factor from a mother to her child [letter]. *New Engl J Med* 2001;344:386–7.
10. Dorhout Mees EJ, Roos JC, *et al.* Observations on edema formation in the nephrotic syndrome in adults with minimal lesions. *Am J Med* 1979;67:378–84.
11. Meltzer JI, Keim HJ, Laragh JH, Sealey JE, Jan KM, Chien S. Nephrotic syndrome: vasoconstriction and hypervolemic types indicated by renin—sodium profiling. *Ann Int Med* 1979;91:688–96.
12. Tulassay T, Rascher W, Schärer K. Intra- and extrarenal factors of oedema formation in the nephrotic syndrome. *Pediatr Nephrol* 1989;3:92–100.
13. Vande Walle JG, Donckerwolcke RAMG, Wimersma Greidanus TB, Joles JA, Koomans HA. Renal sodium handling in children with nephrotic relapse: relation to hypovolaemic symptoms. *Nephrol Dial Transplant* 1996;11:2202–8.
14. Feehally J, Kendell NP, Swift PGF, Walls J. High incidence of minimal change nephrotic syndrome in Asians. *Arch Dis Child* 1985;60:1018–20.
15. Fuchshuber A, Gribouval O, Ronner V, Kroiss S, Karle S, Brandis M, *et al.* Clinical and genetic evaluation of familial steroid-responsive nephrotic syndrome in childhood. *J Am Soc Nephrol* 2001;12:374–8.
16. International Study for Kidney Disease in Children. Nephrotic syndrome in children: Prediction of histopathology from clinical and laboratory characteristics at time of diagnosis. *Kidney Int* 1978;13:159–65
17. Bazzi C, Petrini C, Rizza V, Arrigo G, D'Amico G. A modern approach to selectivity of proteinuria and tubulointerstitial damage in nephrotic syndrome. *Kidney Int* 2000;58:1732–41.
18. Tanaka H, Tateyama T, Waga S. Acute renal failure at the onset of idiopathic nephrotic syndrome in two children. *Clin Exp Nephrol* 2001;5:47–9.
19. Reid CJ, Marsh MJ, Murdoch IM, Clark G. Nephrotic syndrome in childhood complicated by life threatening pulmonary oedema. *BMJ* 1996;312:36–8.
20. Ksiazek J, Wyszynska T. Short versus long initial prednisone treatment in steroid-sensitive nephrotic syndrome in children. *Acta Paediatr* 1995;84:889–93.
21. Hodson EM, Knight JF, Willis NS, Craig JC. Corticosteroid therapy in nephrotic syndrome: a meta-analysis of randomised controlled trials. *Arch Dis Child* 2000;83:45–51.

22. Broyer M, Terzi F, Lehnert A, Gagnadoux MF, Guest G, Niaudet P. A controlled study of deflazacort in the treatment of idiopathic nephrotic syndrome. *Pediatr Nephrol* 1997;11:418–22.

23. Hall AS, Houtman PN. The effects of high dose steroids on behaviour in children with nephrotic syndrome (abstract). *Arch Dis Child* 2001;84 (Suppl 1):A67.

24. Barratt TM, Cameron JS, Chantler C, Ogg CS, Soothill JF. Comparative trial of 2 weeks and 8 weeks cyclophosphamide in steroid-sensitive relapsing nephrotic syndrome of childhood. *Arch Dis Child* 1973;48:286–90.

25. Ueda N, Kuno K, Ito S. Eight and 12 week courses of cyclophosphamide in nephrotic syndrome. *Arch Dis Child* 1990;65:1147–50.

26. Vallo A, Rodríguez-Soriano J, Quintela J. Comparative effects of cyclophosphamide and nitrogen mustard in treatment of idiopathic nephrotic syndrome [abstract]. *Pediatr Nephrol* 1993;7 (Suppl):C33.

27. Hulton S-A, Neuhaus TJ, Dillon MJ, Barratt TM. Long-term cyclosporin A treatment of minimal-change nephrotic syndrome of childhood. *Pediatr Nephrol* 1994;8:401–3.

28. Anonymous. Levamisole for corticosteroid-dependent nephrotic syndrome in childhood. A report of the British Association for Paediatric Nephrology. *Lancet* 1991;337:1555–7.

29. Bonilla-Felix M, Parra C, Dajani T, Ferris M, Swinford RD, Portman RJ, *et al*. Changing patterns in the histopathology of idiopathic nephrotic syndrome in children. *Kidney Int* 1999;55:1885–90.

30. Boute N, Gribouval O, Roselli S, Benessy F, Lee H, Fuchshuber A, *et al*. NPHS2, encoding the glomerular protein podocin, is mutated in autosomal recessive steroid-resistant nephrotic syndrome. *Nat Genet* 2000; 24:349–54.

31. Tarshish P, Tobin JN, Bernstein J, Edelmann CM. Cyclophosphamide does not benefit patients with focal segmental glomerulosclerosis. A report of the International Study of Kidney Disease in Children. *Pediatr Nephrol* 1996;10:590–3.

32. Niaudet P. Treatment of childhood steroid-resistant idiopathic nephrosis with a combination of cyclosporine and prednisone. French Society of Pediatric Nephrology. *J Pediatr* 1994;125:981–6.

33. Senggutuvan P, Cameron JS, Hartley RB, Rigden SPA, Chantler C, Haycock GB, *et al*. Recurrence of focal segmental glomerulosclerosis in transplanted kidneys: analysis of incidence and risk factors in 59 allografts. *Pediatr Nephrol* 1990;4:21–8.

34. Mendoza SA, Reznik VM, Griswold WR, Krensky AM, Yorgin PD, Tune BM. Treatment of steroid-resistant focal segmental glomerulosclerosis with pulse methylprednisolone and alkylating agents. *Pediatr Nephrol* 1990;4:303–7.

35. McCauley J, Shapiro R, Ellis D, Igdal H, Tzakis A, Starzl TE. Pilot trial of FK 506 in the management of steroid-resistant nephrotic syndrome. *Nephrol Dial Transplant* 1993;8:1286–90.

36. Goonasekera CD, Koziell AB, Hulton SA, Dillon MJ. Vincristine and focal segmental sclerosis: do we need a multicentre trial? *Pediatr Nephrol* 1998;12:284–9.

37. McEnery PT, McAdams AJ, West CD. Membranoproliferative glomerulonephritis: improved survival with alternate day prednisone therapy. *Clin Nephrol* 1980;13:117–24.

38. Tarshish P, Bernstein J, Tobin JN, Edelmann CM. Treatment of mesangiocapillary glomerulonephritis with alternate-day prednisone—a report of the International Study of Kidney Disease in Children. *Pediatr Nephrol* 1992;6:123–30.

39. Somers M, Kertesz S, Rosen S, Herrin J, Colvin R, Palacios de Carreta N, *et al*. Non-nephrotic children with membranoproliferative glomerulonephritis: are steroids indicated? *Pediatr Nephrol* 1995;9:140–4.

40. Bergstein JM, Andreoli SP. Response of type I membranoproliferative glomerulonephritis to pulse methylprednisolone and alternate-day prednisone therapy. *Pediatr Nephrol* 1995;9:268–71.

20 | *The child with acute nephritic syndrome*

Jodi M. Smith, M. Khurram Faizan, and Allison A. Eddy

Overview

The acute nephritic syndrome is a constellation of clinical manifestations caused by the abrupt onset of glomerular injury and inflammation that leads to a decline in glomerular filtration rate with sodium and water retention. Urinalysis usually reveals red blood cells, red blood cell casts, and albuminuria. In the paediatric age group the most common cause of the acute nephritic syndrome is acute post-streptococcal glomerulonephritis (APSGN), accounting for approximately 80% of cases. However, it is important to recognize that the acute nephritic syndrome does have multiple causes that must be considered in the differential diagnosis whenever a child has clinical features and/or laboratory findings that would be unusual for classical APSGN. Some of these early warning signs might include: a family history of glomerulonephritis, atypical age (under 4 years and over 15 years), prior history of similar symptoms, presence of extrarenal disease (such as arthritis, rash, or haematological abnormalities), evidence of non-streptococcal infection, and findings suggestive of chronic renal disease (e.g. anaemia, short stature, osteodystrophy, small kidneys, or left ventricular hypertrophy on echocardiography).

Key points: Clinical features suggestive of a pathology other than APSGN in a child with acute nephrotic syndrome

- Family history of glomerular disease
- Age of child (under 4 years or over 15 years)
- Previous history of similar symptoms
- Evidence of extra-renal disease
- Evidence of acute or chronic non-streptococcal infection
- Evidence of chronic renal disease.

Children with acute nephritis most commonly present with gross haematuria, oedema, or symptomatic hypertension. Asymptomatic and self-limiting acute nephritis is thought to be quite common but the true incidence is unknown. The differential diagnosis of children presenting with gross haematuria, oedema, or hypertension is extensive. The algorithms in Figs 20.1, 20.2, and 20.3 suggest a general approach to establishing acute glomerulonephritis as the most likely diagnosis when a child presents with one of these symptoms. The remainder of this chapter will discuss APSGN in some detail, followed by a brief discussion of the other important causes of the acute nephritic syndrome in the paediatric population, and ending with some examples of chronic infections that are associated with glomerulonephritis.

Acute post-streptococcal glomerulonephritis

Epidemiology

APSGN typically follows either a pharyngeal or skin infection with 'nephritogenic' strains of group A beta-haemolytic streptococcus (GAS). There are more than 80 subtypes of GAS as characterized by the M and T proteins found on the outer portion of the streptococcal cell wall. The most common 'nephritogenic' serotypes implicated in pharyngeal and skin infection cases are M-type 1, 3, 4, 12, 25, 49 and M-type 2, 49, 55, 57, 60, respectively. GAS pharyngeal infections occur primarily in the winter and spring, in contrast to GAS skin infections which are more common in the summer and autumn. Regardless of the primary site of infection, the risk of development of APSGN is 10–15%. Within families, the clinical attack rate may be as high as 40%. Although antibiotic treatment of GAS infection does not prevent development of APSGN, treatment is important to prevent further spread of the nephritogenic strain. The simultaneous occurrence of acute rheumatic fever and APSGN has been reported, but is extremely rare [1].

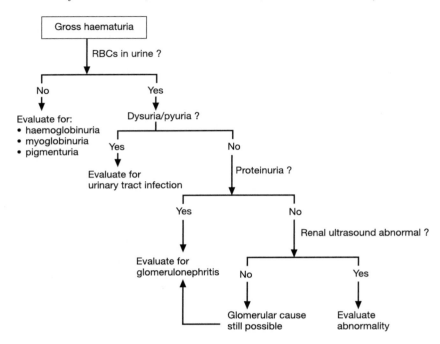

Fig. 20.1   Approach to the investigation of a child with macroscopic haematuria.

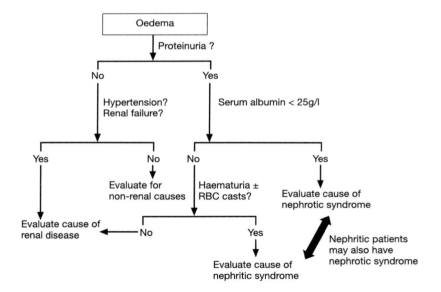

Fig. 20.2   Approach to the investigation of a child with oedema.

APSGN primarily affects school-aged children between 5 and 15 years of age [2]. Children younger than 2 years account for less than 5% of cases. Males are affected more often than females and they are more likely to develop overt nephritis. Children with skin infections tend to be younger than children with pharyngeal infections. The disease may occur sporadically or as an epidemic. Globally, the pattern of disease

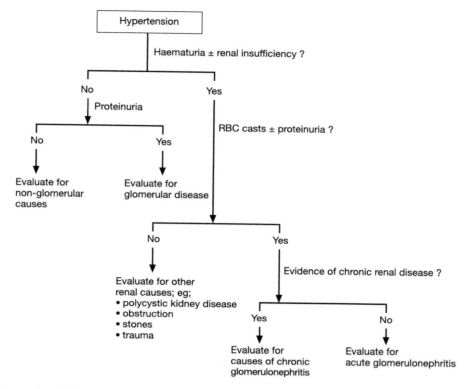

Fig. 20.3   Approach to the investigation of a child with hypertension.

varies; in developed countries, APSGN is usually sporadic and associated with pharyngeal infection, in contrast to the epidemic outbreaks in developing countries that are often attributed to skin infection [3].

Pathogenesis

The exact pathogenic mechanisms underlying APSGN remain unknown. However, considerable knowledge has been gained in recent years, and it is now thought that a number of host- and pathogen-related factors are necessary to produce this syndrome.

Host factors

The fact that only 10–15% of patients infected with nephritogenic strains of GAS develop APSGN is still unexplained, but suggests that certain host factors may be important. APSGN is seen in all age groups but is most common in 5–15-year-olds. It has been reported only rarely in infants [4]. Although throat and skin infections with GAS occur equally amongst both sexes, males are affected approximately twice as often as

females. Such observations suggest that there are risk factors related to the age and sex of the host. The disease is more common in tropical climates and it usually affects individuals from lower socio-economic backgrounds. For example, epidemics have been described in the Australian Aboriginal population, and in parts of Chile, Trinidad, Brazil, and Armenia. Crowded living conditions, poor hygiene, malnutrition, anaemia, and parasitic infestation have all been implicated as risk factors for APSGN. Outbreaks have also occurred in developed countries. Genetic risk factors may also be important. For example, the HLA-DRW4 [5], HLA-DPA1 and HLA-DPB1 alleles [6] are more prevalent in patients than in the general population.

Streptococcal factors

APSGN is initiated when the susceptible host is exposed and develops an antibody to the inciting antigen. The identity of this antigen remains unknown, although several candidates have been investigated, both in animal models and in humans with APSGN. These include streptococcal M protein, endostreptosin (pre-absorbing antigen), cationic proteins, exo-toxin B, nephritis strain associated protein (nephritis plasmin-binding protein), and streptokinase. It is possible that more than one antigen is involved, perhaps at different stages of the renal injury, as suggested for streptokinase and streptococcal M protein.

Streptokinase is a secreted protein that is thought to be involved in the spread of the bacterium through tissue, due to its ability to cleave plasminogen to plasmin. Streptokinase production appears to be a prerequisite for the production of nephritis in APSGN. Streptokinase may also bind to normal glomerular structures, with an affinity that is variable amongst streptococcal strains. It has been suggested that plasmin generated within the glomerulus by streptokinase may activate the complement cascade. Glomerular deposition of C3 is an early histological finding in APSGN (Fig. 20.4).

An association between M protein production by nephritogenic strains of GAS and glomerulonephritis has been known for almost 50 years. M proteins are surface molecules that resist phagocytosis and hence contribute to virulence. They have been isolated from most, but not all, nephritogenic strains. M proteins have been shown to bind both directly to renal antigens such as glomerular basement membrane components and to circulating IgG antibodies. Mice injected with high doses of M protein antigen or M protein immune complexes develop renal lesions [7]. However, since glomerular deposition of C3 often precedes IgG, M proteins may be more important for progression of glomerular injury rather than its initiation.

Initiation and progression of renal injury

A role for the humoral immune system and the complement cascade in the pathogenesis of APSGN is suggested by the characteristic presence of glomerular basement membrane subepithelial deposits of C3 and IgG in affected patients. C3 deposition usually precedes IgG and occasionally may be seen alone, suggesting that complement activation is antibody-independent. Low serum levels of C3 and C5, but normal levels of the classical pathway components (C1q, C2, and C4), indicate activation of the alternate pathway. IgG deposition appears to be a later event and is thought to be secondary to the binding of free antibodies either to intrinsic components of the glomerular capillary and/or its basement membrane or to trapped streptococcal antigens [8]. Whether circulating immune complexes are also deposited within the glomerulus is still unclear (Fig. 20.4).

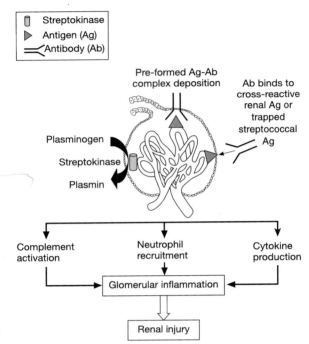

Fig. 20.4 Schematic overview of proposed pathogenic mechanisms of APSGN. The inflammatory cascade that induces renal injury may be triggered by (1) activation of plasminogen to plasmin by streptokinase or similar streptococcal protein and subsequent complement activation; (2) pre-formed antigen–antibody immune complex deposition in the glomerulus, or by (3) binding of pre-formed antibodies against streptococcus, to structurally homologous renal proteins (a process referred to as molecular mimicry).

Glomerular C3 activation leads to recruitment and activation of monocytes and neutrophils. This intense inflammatory infiltrate is obvious histologically and has led to the term 'exudative' glomerulonephritis. Cytokine production by the recruited inflammatory cells propagates glomerular injury. The mesangial hypercellularity that is seen in affected glomeruli is thought to result from resident glomerular cell proliferation, probably induced by locally produced mitogens [9].

An important feature of APSGN is that the inciting event appears to be short lived. With its disappearance, the inflammatory reaction subsides and in most cases the glomerular architecture eventually returns to normal again.

Clinical presentation

The onset of APSGN is usually abrupt, occurring 7–14 days following pharyngitis and 3–6 weeks following skin infection. Patients usually present clinically with acute nephritic syndrome. This term does not refer to a single disease process, but rather a collection of clinical signs, namely acute fluid overload, haematuria (frequently macroscopic), and hypertension. Proteinuria and oliguria may also be present.

Key points: Presenting features of acute nephritic syndrome

- Acute fluid overload
  - Peripheral oedema
  - Pulmonary oedema
  - Congestive cardiac failure
- Hypertension
- Haematuria (microscopic ± macroscopic)
- Proteinuria
- Renal functional impairment
  - Oliguria
  - Elevated plasma creatinine

Acute fluid overload presents early, most commonly as generalised oedema (85%). Less common, but important clinical presentations include acute pulmonary oedema (14%) or signs and symptoms due to congestive heart failure (2%). Microscopic haematuria is seen in virtually all patients. Gross haematuria is usually painless and is classically described as smoky, tea, or coca-cola coloured. Mild to moderate range hypertension is observed in 60–80% of patients and usually develops early in the clinical course. Hypertensive encephalopathy is rare but has been reported even in patients without a significant decline in glomerular filtration rate (GFR). Neurological symptoms secondary to cerebral vasculitis, including headaches and seizures not caused by hypertensive encephalopathy, are rare but may occur [10]. While proteinuria is often present, it is usually in the non-nephrotic range (urinary protein: creatinine ratio <250 mg protein/mmol creatinine). Hypoalbuminaemia is usually not severe and is due

in part to a dilutional effect of intravascular volume expansion. Overt nephrotic syndrome occurs in less than 5% of patients. The degree of renal functional impairment is usually mild with only transient oliguria and/or a mild to moderate rise in plasma creatinine (45%). Anuria, nephrotic-range proteinuria, and more profound renal insufficiency should raise the suspicion of a rapidly progressive glomerulonephritis, which is reported in less than 1% of cases of APSGN. The clinical features of APSGN usually begin to resolve spontaneously within 1–2 weeks. Microscopic abnormalities including haematuria and proteinuria may persist for months to a year, and rarely even longer.

Laboratory investigations

Urinary abnormalities include haematuria, both gross and microscopic, usually associated with proteinuria. Microscopic examination of the urine sediment typically reveals dysmorphic red blood cells and red blood cell casts. Other findings may include pyuria, white blood cell casts, granular and hyaline casts. Although unusual, the urinalysis may be normal. Confirmation of an antecedent streptococcal infection is accomplished through a variety of techniques. A positive throat culture should be interpreted with caution as a 20% carriage rate is reported in otherwise healthy school-aged children. Detection of serum antibodies to streptococcal antigens is a superior measure. Most commonly, the antistreptolysin O titre (ASOT) is used. Antibodies to antistreptolysin O are detected in 80–90% of children with antecedent pharyngitic infections. However, this test is also positive in 16–18% of healthy children. The ASOT is less reliable (<50% positive) for patients with APSGN secondary to skin infections, due to the binding of streptolysin O to lipids in the skin. Use of the streptozyme assay, which detects antibodies to a panel of five different streptococcal antigens (streptolysin O, streptokinase, hyaluronidase, DNAse B, and NADase), increases the likelihood of obtaining a positive test to greater than 95% in cases of antecedent pharyngitic infections and up to 80% in cases of antecedent skin infections. If serological testing for GAS infection is negative, the possibility of acute nephritis due to other infectious agents should be considered. Some of the best-documented examples are summarized in Table 20.1. With recent advances in molecular genetic diagnostic tools it is likely that acute non-GAS post-infectious glomerulonephritis will become increasingly recognized in the future.

Table 20.1 Non-streptococcal causes of acute post-infectious glomerulonephritis

	Examples
Bacteria	*Staphylococcus aureus, Streptococcus pneumoniae, Haemophilus influenzae, Mycoplasma pnemoniae, Escherichia coli, Yersinia, Campylobacter, Salmonella, Syphilis, Mycobacterium tuberculosis*
Viruses	Herpesviruses (EBV, CMV, HSV, varicella zoster), Parvovirus B-19
Rickettsia	Rocky Mountain spotted fever, Q fever (*Coxiella burnetti*), *Legionella pneumophilia*
Fungi	*Candida, Aspergillus,* histoplasmosis, *Cryptococcus, Pneumocystis carinii, Nocardia*
Parasites	Malaria (*Plasmodium vivax, P. falciparum, P. ovale, P. malariae*), schistosomiasis, leishmaniasis, trypanosomiasis, filariasis, trichinosis, echinococcus, toxoplasmosis

EBV, Epstein–Barr virus; CMV, cytomegalovirus; HSV, herpes simplex virus.

Measurement of complement levels is an essential part of the diagnosis of APSGN. C3 levels are almost universally depressed in the acute phase of the illness (often to levels less than 50% of normal). The C3 level typically normalizes within 6–8 weeks. In contrast, C4 levels are usually normal; a small number of cases presenting early in the clinical course of the disease may have very transiently depressed C4 levels, representing early involvement of the classical complement pathway. This pattern distinguishes APSGN from the other types of hypocomplementaemic glomerulonephritis such as bacterial endocarditis, systemic lupus erythematosus, shunt nephritis, and idiopathic membranoproliferative glomerulonephritis, where C4 levels are frequently persistently depressed (Fig. 20.5 and see later).

Metabolic abnormalities reflecting renal functional impairment may be present, such as an elevated plasma urea and creatinine, hyperkalaemia, hyperphosphataemia, and acidosis. Transient hyporeninaemic hypoaldosteronism may contribute to hyperkalaemia. Haematological abnormalities include a mild anaemia due to haemodilution and low-grade haemolysis. A decrease in mean platelet survival time rarely causes thrombocytopenia. Renal biopsy is not required to make the diagnosis of APSGN and is rarely indicated. However, a biopsy may be appropriate for patients with atypical or severe renal disease: indications for renal biopsy are shown in Table 20.2.

Key points: Initial tests to perform in a child presenting with acute nephritic syndrome

- Urinalysis:
  - urine microscopy to confirm the presence of RBCs and to determine whether dysmorphic;
  - urine microscopy to detect casts;
  - quantification of proteinuria (early morning protein:creatinine ratio).

- Bacteriology:
  - throat swab;
  - ASOT;
  - streptozyme assay (antibodies to streptolysin O, streptokinase, hyaluronidase, DNAse B, and NADase).

- Immunology:
  - C3 and C4;
  - anti-neutrophil cytoplasmic antibody (ANCA)*;
  - ANA and anti-double-stranded DNA antibodies*;
  - anti-glomerular basement membrane (GBM) antibodies*.

- Renal function:
  - creatinine, urea, and electrolytes;
  - acid-base status;
  - plasma proteins;
  - calcium and phosphate.

- Haematology:
  - full blood count;
  - peripheral blood film*.

* To exclude alternative diagnoses when indicated.

Management

The management of patients with APSGN consists of eradication of the organism and treatment of the sequelae of acute renal failure. Antibiotic therapy for the antecedent streptococcal throat or skin infection has not been shown to alter the course or severity of the disease. However, antibiotic treatment does prevent the spread of the nephritogenic strains in the community and may help decrease the incidence of glomerulonephritis or prevent outbreaks. Unlike cases of rheumatic fever, antibiotic treatment does not prevent

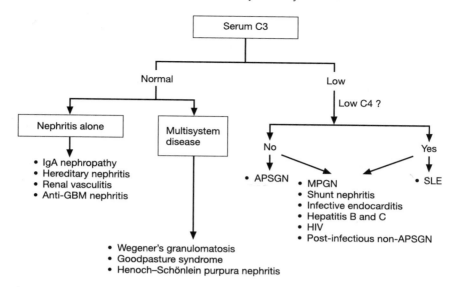

Fig. 20.5 Use of serum C3 levels in the approach to the differential diagnosis of a child with acute glomerulonephritis.
* A small number of cases of APSGN presenting early in the clinical course may have transiently depressed C4 levels.
MPGN = membranoproliferative glomerulonephritis.

Table 20.2 Possible indications for renal biopsy in the child presenting with acute nephritic syndrome

Features suggestive of a diagnosis other than APSGN at presentation***
    family history of glomerular disease
    age under 4 years or over 15 years
    previous history of similar symptoms
    evidence of extrarenal disease
    evidence of acute or chronic non-streptococcal infection
    evidence of chronic renal disease
    atypical investigations, e.g. low C4, positive ANCA,
      ANA, anti-dsDNA, anti-GBM antibodies
GFR <50% of normal for age***
Nephrotic proportion proteinuria***
Macroscopic haematuria persisting for >3 months**
Microscopic haematuria persisting for >12 months*
C3 depressed for greater than 3 months***
Moderate proteinuria persisting >6 months**
Incomplete information*

*** Strong indication; ** moderate indication; * optional.

future recurrences. Subsequent episodes of APSGN after a confirmed case are, however, extremely rare.

The spectrum of renal involvement amongst patients with APSGN ranges from mild asymptomatic haematuria to acute renal failure with oligo-anuria, rarely necessitating dialysis. There is no specific medical therapy for APSGN and treatment remains supportive. Immunosuppressive or corticosteroid

---

Key points: Indications for in-patient management of APSGN

- Hypertension

- Oedema

- Oliguria

- Elevated plasma creatinine

- Electrolyte abnormalities.

---

therapy is not indicated, although there is limited anecdotal evidence that such therapy may be beneficial in the unusual patients with rapidly progressive glomerulonephritis [11,12].

The severity and duration of the acute renal failure varies widely amongst patients. Once the diagnosis is established, it is important to monitor the patient closely and provide supportive therapy. Patients should be admitted to hospital for observation and treatment of complications such as hypertension, oedema, and/or electrolyte abnormalities.

Patients need close observation and supportive medical care until the glomerular injury resolves spontaneously. A general guide to management is outlined in Fig. 20.6. It is advisable to consult with a paediatric

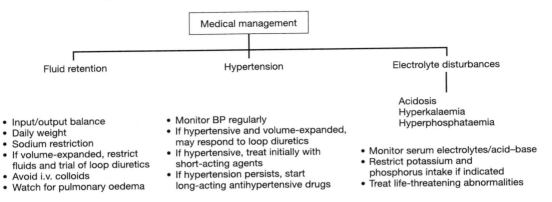

Fig. 20.6   Principles of medical management of a child with acute glomerulonephritis.

nephrologist for assistance with the management of complicated or atypical patients, including those with hypertension, oliguria, oedema, electrolyte abnormalities, impaired renal function, and significant proteinuria.

Key points: When to consult paediatric nephrology regarding a child with APSGN

- All indications for renal biopsy as in Table 20.2

- Hypertension

- Oliguria/oedema

- Electrolyte abnormalities

- Impaired renal function

- Nephrotic proportion proteinuria.

Total fluid intake should be limited to urine output plus insensible losses in patients with oliguria. Further fluid restriction may be indicated in volume overloaded patients. Since these patients may respond to loop diuretics, a trial of frusemide (1–2 mg/kg/dose) may be warranted if the patient is severely fluid overloaded and oedematous. Urine output usually increases spontaneously within 5–10 days. Patients need to be monitored for the development of hyperkalaemia, acidosis, hyponatraemia or hypernatraemia, hyperphosphataemia, and hypocalcaemia. A diet restricted in sodium, potassium, and

phosphorus is usually recommended for patients with significant renal functional impairment. Hypertension is caused primarily by intravascular volume expansion and may respond to salt and water restriction and diuretics. However, in more severe cases, antihypertensive therapy is often indicated in order to avoid serious complications, including congestive heart failure, pulmonary oedema, and cerebrovascular accidents. Anuria lasting more than 2–3 days is unusual and may require dialysis to manage fluid overload and electrolyte disturbances and to optimize nutritional support. Anuria beyond 2 weeks is extremely rare and should be an indication to question the diagnosis; such a clinical course may indicate a bad prognosis for full recovery of renal function.

Clinical course and long-term prognosis

Most of the clinical symptoms of APSGN, including gross haematuria, oliguria, and oedema, usually subside spontaneously by 2–3 weeks after their onset. C3 levels usually normalize within 8–12 weeks. Persistently low C3 levels in a patient thought initially to have APSGN should alert the physician to the possibility of an alternative diagnosis (Fig. 20.5). Microscopic haematuria with or without low-grade proteinuria may persist for 1–2 years after a diagnosed case of APSGN (Fig. 20.7).

The long-term prognosis is excellent in children. In one large prospective study of almost 700 children, who were followed for 2–6 years after diagnosis, less than 2% of patients were found to have persistent urinary abnormalities or hypertension. The prevalence of these abnormalities was directly related to age at diagnosis and decreased over time [13]. Roy and

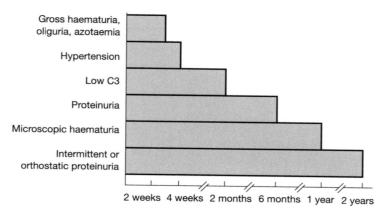

Fig. 20.7   Natural history of APSGN. (Reproduced from *Clinical Paediatric Nephrology*, 2nd edn by RJ Postlethwaite. Reprinted by permission of Elsevier Science Ltd.)

colleagues reported long-term follow-of 35 children (up to 12 years) with APSGN. Follow-up renal biopsies on 34 children (97%) showed complete resolution. Only one patient remained hypertensive [14]. More recent paediatric studies have reconfirmed this excellent outcome, with persistent clinical abnormalities (hypertension, proteinuria, microhaematuria) reported in less than 5% of patients after a follow-up period of 10–17 years [15,16]. The incidence of chronic renal insufficiency after APSGN remains less than 1%. Prompt recognition and aggressive treatment of the small number of patients who remain hypertensive and/or proteinuric after diagnosis, can further delay the onset of end stage renal disease. Persistence of clinical abnormalities is related to the severity of disease on renal biopsy (crescentic glomerulonephritis in particular), the length of the acute phase of renal failure, and older age at the time of diagnosis. Whether 'clinically healed' patients continue to have permanent renal histological abnormalities is debated but remains unknown, as follow-up renal biopsies are rarely performed. The long-term prognosis appears to be less favourable in adults with APSGN [17].

Differential diagnosis: other diseases which may present with acute nephritic syndrome

In addition to APSGN and non-GAS acute post-infectious glomerulonephritis, there are other renal diseases that may present clinically with acute nephritic syndrome. The most common causes in the paediatric population are summarized in Table 20.3.

It is also worth noting that recurrent episodes of gross haematuria during the first decade of life may be observed in children with hereditary nephritis.

IgA nephropathy, a chronic disease, is the most common primary glomerulonephritis world-wide. It often presents in the second or third decade of life but may be seen in younger patients [18]. The development of gross haematuria associated with a respiratory infection is a common clinical presentation. However, a careful history may distinguish between IgA nephropathy and APSGN as gross haematuria usually occurs *at the time* of the respiratory infection in IgA nephropathy (synpharyngitic), while respiratory symptoms have typically resolved at the time of onset of APSGN. Other clinical presentations of IgA nephropathy include asymptomatic microscopic haematuria that may be associated with proteinuria, nephrotic syndrome, renal insufficiency, hypertension, and, rarely, crescentic glomerulonephritis. Routine serological tests are not helpful in confirming the diagnosis of IgA nephropathy. Definitive diagnosis currently requires a renal biopsy. Patients with suspected IgA nephropathy should be referred to a paediatric nephrologist. The disease is discussed in more detail in Chapter 1.

Membranoproliferative glomerulonephritis (MPGN) (also known as mesangiocapillary glomerulonephritis) is a chronic glomerular disease that shares many clinical and laboratory features with APSGN. Like APSGN, most patients present in childhood with microscopic haematuria, proteinuria, and hypertension. C3 levels are low in more than 50% of patients but they fail to return to normal values within 8 weeks [19]. In

Table 20.3 Presenting clinical features of paediatric glomerular diseases that may mimic APSGN

	APSGN	Henoch–Schönlein purpura	IgA nephropathy	MPGN	SLE	ANCA-positive vasculitis
Mean age (years)	5–15	4–14	10–20	8–20	15–20	12–20
Antecedent infection	Yes	35%	Concurrent common	Common	Rare	Flu-like prodrome common
Gross haematuria	30%	20%	50–80%	20–50%	<10%	30%
Nephrotic syndrome*	5%	5–10%	<10%	30–50%	0–50%**	<10%
Serum C3	Low	Normal	Normal	Low	Low	Normal
Serum C4	Normal***	Normal	Normal	Normal/low	Low	Normal
Diagnostic serology	ASOT; streptozyme	No	No	No	ANA, anti-dsDNA	ANCA
Extrarenal disease	Rare	Yes	Rare	Rare	Common	Common

* Some of these values are estimates, as good epidemiological data are not published.
** Incidence depends upon the histological class of lupus nephritis.
*** A small number of cases presenting early in the clinical course of the disease may have very transiently depressed C4 levels.
APSGN, acute post-streptococcal glomerulonephritis; MPGN, membranoproliferative (mesangiocapillary) glomerulonephritis; SLE, systemic lupus erythematosus; ANCA, anti-neutrophil cytoplasmic antibody; ASOT, antistreptolysin-O titre; ANA, antinuclear antibody; anti-dsDNA, anti-double-stranded DNA.

a subset of patients with MPGN, C4 values are also low, serving to further differentiate it from APSGN. Nephrotic syndrome is common, present in 30–50% of MPGN patients at initial presentation. MPGN is discussed in further detail in Chapter 19.

Lupus nephritis, Henoch–Schönlein purpura (HSP) nephritis, and anti-neutrophil cytoplasmic antibody (ANCA) positive vasculitis and other diseases that may present clinically with an acute nephritic syndrome are discussed in further detail in Chapter 21.

Chronic infections associated with potentially reversible glomerulonephritis

While most infection–associated acute glomerular diseases present clinically during the resolution phase of the infection, it is important to remember that glomerulonephritis has also been associated with certain chronic and persistent infections. The best-characterized examples are reviewed below in order to emphasize two points. First, early recognition and treatment of the infection (when effective therapy is available) offers the best chance for reversal of the glomerular disease. Second, is the fact that many of

these glomerular diseases have clinical presentations that are quite distinct from the acute nephritic syndrome. Therefore routine serological testing for these infections is not recommended for patients presenting with typical findings of post-infectious acute nephritic syndrome.

Shunt nephritis

Shunt nephritis occurs in approximately 4% of individuals with infected shunts. Historically, this association was most common amongst patients with hydrocephalus treated with ventriculo-atrial shunts. With the introduction of ventriculo-peritoneal shunts, this association has disappeared. However, another susceptible population is patients with infected vascular access devices. Coagulase-negative *Staphylococcus* is the most commonly isolated organism. Patients typically present with an indolent course of fever, lethargy, arthralgias, hepatosplenomegaly, purpura, adenopathy, and weight loss. Renal manifestations include haematuria (microscopic or gross), proteinuria (nephrotic range in 30%), azotaemia, and hypertension. Laboratory investigations reveal anaemia, leucocytosis, and an elevated erythrocyte sedimentation rate (ESR). C3 and C4 are both depressed in 90% of patients. Blood cultures may be negative but the organism can usually be isolated from the graft itself. Renal pathology typically reveals diffuse proliferative changes resembling idiopathic membranoproliferative glomerulonephritis type I. Treatment includes antimicrobial therapy directed at the underlying pathogen. Removal of the infected shunt is usually required for complete eradication of the organism. Symptoms are typically slow to resolve despite shunt removal, and residual renal abnormalities, including haematuria, proteinuria, and/or renal dysfunction, are reported in up to half of patients.

Infective endocarditis

With the declining incidence of rheumatic fever, subacute bacterial endocarditis is rarely encountered. Acute bacterial endocarditis, most frequently caused by *Staphylococcus aureus*, is now more prevalent, especially among intravenous drug users. Renal manifestations may include haematuria (microscopic or gross), proteinuria, hypertension, and mild renal dysfunction. The spectrum of renal involvement parallels the histological findings, which can range from focal segmental glomerulonephritis to diffuse proliferative glomerulonephritis to a rapidly progressive form with crescents. Hypocomplementaemia with depressed C3 and C4 levels is seen in 60–90% of patients. The degree of complement activation correlates with the severity of renal involvement, with the levels normalizing with successful treatment of the infection. Renal abnormalities such as microscopic haematuria and proteinuria may persist for months to years.

Hepatitis B

An association between hepatitis B virus (HBV) infection and membranous nephropathy (MN) was first reported by Combes *et al.* in 1971 [20]. Other types of glomerulonephritis associated with HBV infection are less common. These include MPGN, minimal change disease, IgA nephropathy, focal glomerulosclerosis, diffuse proliferative glomerulonephritis, and crescentic glomerulonephritis.

The prevalence of HBV-MN varies geographically with the prevalence of the hepatitis B surface antigen (HBsAg) carrier state. The prevalence of HBsAg carriers is 0.3–1% in North America, 1% in western Europe, 7% in Africa, and up to 10% in South-East Asia where it is endemic. One of the most important factors affecting prevalence is the age of the patient when infected. Infection during infancy and early childhood carries

the highest probability of development of a chronic carrier state. The typical age of presentation with nephropathy is between 2 and 12 years, with a male predominance (75–80%). The virus may be transmitted vertically from infected mothers or horizontally from infected siblings. Children present with proteinuria that may be asymptomatic or associated with nephrotic syndrome. Oedema is the usual symptom that brings patients to medical attention. Some patients report a flu-like prodrome with low-grade fever, nausea, and vomiting, but jaundice is typically absent. Hypertension occurs in less than 25% of cases. Microscopic and, rarely, gross haematuria may be seen. Renal insufficiency is unusual.

More than 90% of patients with HBV-MN have evidence of active hepatitis B infection with antigenaemia (positive HBsAg and HBeAg) and absence of antibodies, with the exception that anti-HB core antibodies may be present. C3 and C4 levels have been reported as depressed in 15–64% of cases. Most patients demonstrate little evidence of ongoing liver disease, with only a mild elevation of serum transaminases. Liver biopsy typically reveals chronic persistent hepatitis or minimal pathology. As serum levels of HBV decline, proteinuria improves, suggesting that the renal injury may be related to actual viral replication and is likely to be immunologically mediated. HBV antigens have been identified in the glomerular subepithelial immune complexes. Remission usually coincides with the disappearance of HBe antigenaemia and the appearance of HBV antibodies. Uncontrolled studies suggest that children with HBV-MN have spontaneous recovery rates similar to those reported for children with the idiopathic form of MN. One study reported that two-thirds of the children with HBV-MN were in remission 3 years after diagnosis.

Immunosuppression has not been an effective treatment, due to the importance of cell-mediated immunity in the elimination of the hepatitis B virus. The use of corticosteroids has not improved the course of renal disease and has actually contributed to the progression to chronic active hepatitis. Use of α-interferon to treat HBV hepatitis has not proven efficacious [21]. Newer antiviral therapy is currently under investigation.

Hepatitis C

Hepatitis C infection may present with glomerular disease as the only clinical manifestation. This association was first reported in a group of adults with

MPGN in 1993 [22]. In the paediatric population, hepatitis C is rarely associated with MPGN. The incidence of hepatitis C varies globally, with chronic hepatitis C infection affecting 0.3% of Canada and northern Europe, 0.6% of United States and central Europe, 1.2–1.5% of Japan and southern Europe, and 3.5–6.4% in some regions of Africa. Routes of transmission include intravenous drug use, blood products, and body fluid exposure. Vertical transmission is infrequent. Presenting symptoms include non-nephrotic proteinuria or nephrotic syndrome associated with mild to moderate renal insufficiency. C3 and C4 levels are depressed in hepatitis C associated MPGN. As with HBV-related glomerular disease, signs of clinical liver disease are rare, with the exception of elevated liver enzymes. Liver biopsy usually reveals evidence of chronic active hepatitis. Cryoglobulinaemia is common, seen in 60–70% of patients, associated with symptoms such as arthritis, purpura, or neuropathy in up to 50% of patients. Renal biopsies performed in patients with hepatitis C glomerular disease have shown MPGN, acute proliferative glomerulonephritis, and, rarely, membranous nephropathy. Treatment strategies remain controversial. α-interferon has been shown to decrease proteinuria, but this effect was not sustained after therapy was discontinued [23]. The potential role of antiviral drugs such as ribavarin remains undetermined. Immunosuppressive regimens have been used to treat the associated cryoglobulinaemic states, with encouraging results.

Human immunodeficiency virus associated nephropathy

Initially described in 1984, human immunodeficiency virus nephropathy (HIVN) is a distinct entity seen in human immunodeficiency virus (HIV)-infected adults and children. An estimated 10 million children globally have HIV, many (1–16%) exposed perinatally to HIV-infected mothers. HIVN is more frequently observed in the Black population with an equal sex distribution. The most characteristic presentation is proteinuria with progression to nephrotic syndrome. HIVN should be considered in the differential diagnosis of nephrotic syndrome and, conversely, children with HIV infection should have routine urinalysis screening. Children with HIVN are typically normotensive and they do not have significant haematuria. Serological abnormalities include depressed C3 and C4 levels, elevated immunoglobulins, and positive ANA, ANCA, and anti-dsDNA. The most characteristic pathological

lesion is focal and segmental sclerosis associated with capillary tuft collapse, tubuloreticular inclusions suggestive of viral particles, and interstitial inflammation. Other histopathological lesions have been reported, such as minimal change nephropathy, IgA nephropathy, and microangiopathy resembling the lesions of haemolytic uraemic syndrome. The clinical course of HIVN in children is less fulminant than in the adult population, where rapid progression to ESRD is common (average 9 months; range 1–27 months after diagnosis). Prospective screening of known HIV-positive children has shown that asymptomatic, intermittent proteinuria may be the only presenting symptom. Treatment of HIVN includes the usual antiretroviral therapy. Angiotensin I converting-enzyme inhibitors have been used to decrease protein excretion. There are several case reports of clinical improvement after treatment using steroids and ciclosporin but the concern of infectious complications remains.

References

1. Said R, Hussein M, Hassan A. Simultaneous occurrence of acute poststreptococcal glomerulonephritis and acute rheumatic fever. Am J Nephrol. 1986; 6: 146–48.
2. Nissenson AR, Baraff LF, Fine RF, Knutson DW. Poststreptococcal acute glomerulonephritis: fact and controversy. Ann Int Med. 1991; 91:76–86.
3. Kaplan EL, Anthony BF, Chapman S, Wannamaker WL. Epidemic acute glomerulonephritis associated with type 49 streptococcal pyoderma. I. Clinical and laboratory findings. Am J Med. 1970; 48:9–27.
4. LiVolti S, Furnari MS, Garozzo R, Santangelo G, Mollica F. Acute post-streptococcal glomerulonephritis in an 8-month-old girl. Pediatr Nephrol. 1993; 7: 737–38.
5. Layrisse Z, Rodriguez-Iturbe B, Garcia-Ramirez R, Rodriguez A, Tiwari J. Family studies of the HLA system in acute post-streptococcal glomerulonephritis. Hum Immunol. 1983; 7:177–85.
6. Mori K, Sasazuki T, Kimura A, Ito Y. HLA-DP antigens and post-streptococcal acute glomerulonephritis. Acta Pediatr. 1996; 8:916–18.
7. Humair L, Potter EV, Kwaan HC. The role of fibrinogen in renal disease. I. Production of experimental lesions in mice. J Lab Clin Med. 1969; 74:60–71.
8. Kefalides NA, Pegg MT, Ohno N, Poon-King T, Zabriskie J, Fillit H. Antibodies to basement membrane collagen and to laminin are present in sera from patients with poststreptococcal glomerulonephritis. J Exp Med. 1986; 163:588–60.
9. Oda T, Yoshizawa N, Takeuchi A, et al. Glomerular proliferating cell kinetics in acute post-streptococcal

glomerulonephritis (APSGN). J Pathol. 1997; 183: 359–68.

10. Kaplan RA, Zwick DL, Hellerstein S, Warady BA, Alon U. Cerebral vasculitis in acute post-streptococcal glomerulonephritis. Pediatr Nephrol. 1993; 7:194–5.

11. Dilima MG, Adhikari M, Coovadia HM. Rapidly progressive glomerulonephritis in black children. A report of four cases. S Afr Med J. 1981; 60:829–32.

12. Erwig LP, Rees AJ. Rapidly progressive glomerulonephritis. J Nephrol. 1999; 12: S111–19.

13. Potter EV, Abidh S, Sharrett AR, *et al.* Clinical healing 2 to 6 years after post-streptococcal glomerulonephritis in Trinidad. N Engl J Med. 1978; 298:767–72.

14. Roy SI, Pitcock JA, Etteldorf JN. Prognosis of acute poststreptococcal glomerulonephritis in childhood: Prospective study and review of the literature. Adv Pediatr. 1976; 23:35–69.

15. Popovic-Rolovic M, Kostic M, Antic-Peco A, Jovanovic O, Popovic D. Medium and long term prognosis of patients with acute poststreptococcal glomerulonephritis. Nephron. 1991; 58:393–99.

16. Garcia R, Rubio L, Rodriguez-Iturbe B. Long-term prognosis of epidemic poststreptococcal glomerulonephritis in Maracaibo: follow-up studies 11–12 years after the acute episode. Clin Nephrol. 1981; 15:291–98.

17. Baldwin DS, Schacht RG. Late sequelae of poststreptococcal glomerulonephritis. Annu Rev Med 1976; 27:49–55.

18. Niaudet P, Murcia I, Beaufils H, Broyer M, Habib R. Primary IgA nephropathies in children: prognosis and treatment. Adv Nephrol Necker Hosp. 1993; 22: 121–40.

19. Iitaka K, Igarashi J, Sakai T. Hypocomplimentemia and membranoproliferative glomerulonephritis in school urinary screening in Japan. Pediatr Nephrol. 1994; 8:420–22.

20. Combes B, Shorey J, Barrera A, *et al.* Glomerulonephritis with deposition of Australia antigen–antibody complexes in glomerular basement membrane. Lancet. 1971; 2:234–37.

21. Johnson RJ, Couser WG. Hepatitis B infection and renal disease: Clinical, immunopathogenetic and therapeutic considerations. Kidney Int. 1990; 37:663–76.

22. Johnson RJ, Gretch DR, Couser WG, *et al.* Renal manifestations of hepatitis C virus infection. Kidney Int. 1994; 46:1255–63.

23. Johnson RJ, Gretch DR, Couser WG, *et al.* Hepatitis C virus-associated glomerulonephritis. Effect of alpha-interferon therapy. Kidney Int. 1994; 46:1700–04.

Further reading

1. Couser WG. (1999). Glomerulonephritis. Lancet 353:1509–15.

2. Nordstrand A, Norgren M, Holm SE. (1999). Pathogenic mechanisms of acute post-streptococcal glomerulonephritis. Scand J Infec Dis 31:523–37.

3. Potter EV, Lipschultz SA, Abidh S, Poon-King T, Earle DP. (1982). Twelve to seventeen-year follow-up of patients with poststreptococcal acute glomerulonephritis in Trinidad. N Engl J Med 307:725–29.

4. Lin C-Y. (1991). Clinical features and natural course of HBV-related glomerulopathy in children. Kidney Int 40 Suppl 35:S46–53.

5. D'Amico G. (1998). Renal involvement in hepatitis C infection: cryoglobulinemic glomerulonephritis. Kidney Int 54:650–71.

6. D'Agati V, Appel GB. (1997). HIV infection and the kidney. J Am Soc Nephrol 8:138–52.

7. Zilleruelo G, Strauss J. (1995). HIV nephropathy in children. Pediatr Clin North Am. 42:1469–85.

21 | Renal manifestations of systemic disorders

Nicholas J.A. Webb, Paul A. Brogan, and Eileen M. Baildam

Introduction

Renal disease may be a feature of a number of systemic disorders of childhood. In some of these, e.g. systemic lupus erythematosus (SLE) and Henoch–Schönlein purpura, the renal disease is both common and the major source of morbidity, while in others, e.g. cystic fibrosis, renal disease is relatively rare and of minor importance with regard to overall morbidity. Renal disease may be manifest at disease presentation, or after many years of disease, e.g. in diabetes mellitus.

This chapter will discuss renal manifestations of systemic diseases, focusing on those conditions most commonly encountered in general paediatric practice.

Childhood vasculitis

Introduction

The vasculitides are a group of disorders characterized by the presence of inflammatory infiltrates (which may be predominantly neutrophilic, eosinophilic, or mononuclear) in the walls of blood vessels, with resultant tissue ischaemia and necrosis. Blood vessels of all sizes may be affected. Vasculitis may be the major manifestation of a disease (primary systemic vasculitis, e.g. microscopic polyangiitis) or one aspect of a more widespread disease (secondary vasculitis, e.g. SLE and the other connective tissue diseases).

Classification of the paediatric vasculitic disorders has proved difficult because of the absence of sensitive and specific diagnostic tests, compounded by the fact that many children have constellations of symptoms and findings that overlap the clinical features of the various individual diseases that will be discussed below. The Chapel Hill classification of the primary systemic vasculitides, which is widely accepted in adult practice but not validated in the young, is shown in Table 21.1 [1]. This classification system is based upon the smallest blood vessel involved in the disease process: Wegener's granulomatosis, for instance, is classified as a small vessel disease, but vasculitis may be detected in small and medium-sized arteries, and larger vessels, including the renal artery and aorta, are occasionally involved.

Causes of secondary vasculitis include the connective tissue diseases (e.g. SLE, the juvenile idiopathic arthritides, Behçet's disease) and infection (e.g. hepatitis B and C, Epstein–Barr virus (EBV), and cytomegalovirus (CMV)).

Good-quality epidemiological data regarding the incidence and mortality of the childhood vasculitides are not available, and these data have not, in the main, been included in this chapter. Similarly, the large majority of the treatment regimens discussed have not been ratified by properly conducted randomized controlled trials. Many of the disorders are very rare in paediatric practice. This section will focus deliberately on the more common diseases of importance to the general paediatrician, giving less coverage to those that are only occasionally seen in tertiary centres.

Table 21.1 Chapel Hill Consensus Nomenclature of primary systemic vasculitis

Large vessel
  Takayasu arteritis
  Giant cell (temporal) arteritis
Medium vessel
  Polyarteritis nodosa
  Kawasaki disease
Small vessel
  Wegener's granulomatosis
  Microscopic polyangiitis
  Churg–Strauss syndrome
  Henoch–Schönlein purpura
  Leucocytoclastic vasculitis
  Essential cryoglobulinaemic
   vasculitis

When to consider a diagnosis of vasculitis

The vasculitides are disorders often associated with significant morbidity and mortality. Appropriate treatment, particularly when commenced early in the disease course, can dramatically improve outcome. Prompt recognition is therefore important. Treatment should aim to induce rapid disease remission, which should then be maintained with the use of less potent therapy to limit drug side-effects.

A diagnosis of vasculitis should be considered in children presenting with systemic symptoms (malaise, fever, weight loss) in association with evidence of multiple organ dysfunction. The presence of a palpable purpuric skin rash, an active urinary sediment with red cells and red cell casts with or without evidence of renal dysfunction, arthropathy, serositis, unexplained cardiac or pulmonary disease, and combinations of symptoms suggestive of specific disorders, as discussed below, should raise the paediatrician's suspicion further.

A number of non-specific laboratory abnormalities are common to all of the vasculitides. These include anaemia, neutrophil leucocytosis, thrombocytosis and a raised erythrocyte sedimentation rate (ESR) and C-reactive protein (CRP). Hyperglobulinaemia and immune complexes are frequently detected. Complement studies are generally normal (with the notable exception of the very rare hypocomplementaemic urticarial vasculitis). Where renal involvement is present, there is usually proteinuria, haematuria, and red cell casts on urine microscopy, and the presence of renal impairment and/or hypertension.

Antineutrophil cytoplasmic antibodies (ANCA) are antibodies directed against antigens present in the neutrophil cytoplasm and are detected in a number of the vasculitides. There is emerging evidence that they may be of primary importance in the disease pathogenesis of some, but not all, of the vasculitic syndromes, rather than epiphenomena. cANCA is directed against proteinase 3 and is detected in a high proportion of patients with Wegener's granulomatosis. pANCA is directed against myeloperoxidase and is frequently detected in microscopic polyangiitis. Reports of the detection of ANCA in the other vasculitides are variable and may not be different from rates detected in the other febrile illnesses of childhood or, indeed, the general population.

Key points: When to consider a diagnosis of vasculitis

- Systemic symptoms (malaise, fever, weight loss) in conjunction with evidence of multiple organ dysfunction:
  - purpuric skin rash;
  - active urinary sediment with red cells and red cell casts;
  - arthropathy;
  - serositis;
  - unexplained cardiac or pulmonary disease.

- Laboratory abnormalities:
  - anaemia;
  - neutrophil leucocytosis;
  - thrombocytosis;
  - raised ESR or CRP;
  - positive ANCA titre.

Henoch–Schönlein purpura

Introduction

Henoch–Schönlein purpura (anaphylactoid purpura) is a multi-system small vessel systemic vasculitis with a prominent cutaneous component. It is the most common vasculitis in the paediatric population, with an incidence of around 14 per 100 000 child population [2], and has the most favourable outcome, with the large majority of children requiring no treatment. Younger children are most frequently affected, the peak incidence occurring at around 4–5 years of age. The disease is more prevalent in boys. North American series report a higher incidence of Henoch–Schönlein purpura in White compared with Black children [3]. The disease appears to follow a seasonal pattern, with a higher incidence during winter and the early spring.

Presentation often follows an upper respiratory tract infection. A number of early reports implicated β-haemolytic streptococcus as a significant specific cause, though subsequent publications have failed to confirm this. Allergic reactions to both foods and drugs have also previously been implicated, although again, definitive evidence to support these theories is lacking.

Clinical manifestations

Henoch–Schönlein purpura is a multi-system disease most frequently affecting the skin, joints, gastrointestinal tract, and the kidney. Other organs less frequently involved include the central nervous system, gonads, and the lungs. Many cases follow an upper respiratory tract infection and the onset of the disorder may be accompanied by systemic symptoms including malaise and mild pyrexia. Multiple organ involvement may be present from the outset of the disease, or alternatively an evolving pattern may develop, with different organs becoming involved at different time points over the course of several days to several weeks.

Around one-third of children have symptoms for less that 14 days; one-third, 2–4 weeks; and one-third, more than 4 weeks [3]. Recurrence of symptoms occurs in around one-third of cases, generally within 4 months of resolution of the original symptoms. Recurrences, which tend to be less severe than the initial presenting episode, are more frequent in those with renal involvement.

Skin changes in Henoch–Schönlein purpura are a uniform finding. The skin lesion is typically that of a purpuric rash (Fig. 21.1) which is generally symmetrical, affecting the lower limbs and buttocks in the majority of cases, the upper extremities being involved less frequently. The abdomen, chest, and face are generally unaffected. The rash has a predilection for the extensor surfaces. The earliest skin changes may be those of urticaria with associated oedema, which evolve into non-blanching purpuric lesions. Lesions at different stages of evolution often are present at the same time. New crops of purpura may develop for several months after the disease onset, although they generally fade with time. Lesions can be induced by mild trauma.

Around two-thirds of children have joint manifestations at presentation. The knees and ankles are most frequently involved. Symptoms, which take the form of pain, swelling, and decreased range of movement, tend to be fleeting and resolve without the development of permanent damage.

Around three-quarters of children develop abdominal symptoms. The extent of gastrointestinal involvement is highly variable, ranging from mild colicky abdominal pain to severe pain with associated ileus and vomiting, and gastrointestinal bleeding manifest by haematemesis and melaena. Other complications include intestinal perforation and intussusception.

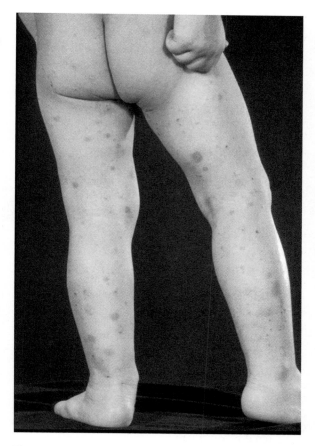

Fig. 21.1 Typical rash in Henoch–Schönlein purpura.

The latter may be difficult to distinguish from abdominal colic, although the incidence of intussusception is significant enough to warrant exclusion by ultrasound where suspected.

Central nervous system involvement may present as headache, behavioural change, seizure, hemiparesis, or coma. Testicular swelling is well recognized in males. Lung involvement presents as pulmonary haemorrhage.

The reported incidence of renal involvement in Henoch–Schönlein purpura (Henoch–Schönlein nephritis) varies according to the intensity with which evidence of renal involvement is sought. Overall, studies report an incidence of between 20 and 100%, although in studies where careful routine in-patient urinalysis was performed, the reported incidence of renal involvement was

20–61% [2,4,5]. Renal involvement is normally manifested between a few days and a few weeks after clinical presentation, but can occur up to 2 months or (rarely) more from presentation. There appears to be an increased risk of renal disease in those with bloody stools.

Renal involvement may present with isolated microscopic haematuria, proteinuria with microscopic or macroscopic haematuria, acute nephritic syndrome (haematuria with at least two of hypertension, raised plasma creatinine, and oliguria), nephrotic syndrome (usually with microscopic haematuria) or a mixed nephritic–nephrotic picture.

Key points: Henoch–Schönlein purpura

- Around one-third of children have symptoms for less than 14 days, one-third 2–4 weeks, and one-third more than 4 weeks.

- Recurrence of symptoms occurs in around one-third of cases, generally within 4 months of resolution of the original symptoms.

- Recurrences are more frequent in those with renal involvement.

Diagnosis and investigation

The diagnosis of Henoch–Schönlein purpura is usually straightforward and made clinically: no single laboratory test has been shown to be helpful. Immunological investigations, including complement levels and antinuclear antibodies, are normal, but IgA is elevated in around one-half of children and a small number exhibit ANCA positivity. Coagulation studies are normal and platelet numbers are normal or occasionally increased. Where significant nephritis is present at presentation, renal function and electrolytes may be correspondingly abnormal.

The differential diagnosis includes sepsis and other systemic vasculitides (SLE, polyarteritis nodosa, Wegener's granulomatosis, and hypersensitivity vasculitis), all of which can present with similar clinical manifestations.

Table 21.2 Henoch–Schönlein purpura: indications for referral to a paediatric nephrologist

Presentation with nephritic and or nephrotic syndrome
Impaired renal function (GFR <80 ml/min/1.73 m²)*
Nephrotic proportion proteinuria (protein : creatinine ratio >250 mg/mmol)
Significant hypertension
Plasma albumin <25 g/l
Persistently abnormal urinalysis after 1 year

* Estimated by the Haycoch–Schwartz formula (see Chapter 28)

It is important to document the extent of renal involvement, and routine daily urinalysis should be performed in all patients: in those where this is initially normal we recommend that urinalysis should continue for 2 months after resolution of the rash, to ensure renal involvement is not overlooked. In most cases this will necessitate issuing the parents with urinalysis sticks and instructions about their use. Quantification of proteinuria (early morning protein : creatinine ratio) and measurement of plasma creatinine, albumin, and total protein should be performed where abnormal urinalysis is detected. The large majority of children can be managed in a district hospital setting; indications for referral to a paediatric nephrologist and possible renal biopsy are shown in Table 21.2.

Pathology

The skin lesion of Henoch–Schönlein purpura is that of a leucocytoclastic vasculitis with perivascular accumulation of neutrophils and mononuclear cells. Immunofluorescence studies reveal vascular deposition of IgA and C3 in affected skin, although similar changes may be observed in skin unaffected by the rash.

The renal lesion of Henoch–Schönlein nephritis is characteristically a focal and segmental proliferative glomerulonephritis. The International Study of Kidney Disease in Children (ISKDC) classification of Henoch–Schönlein nephritis was originally devised by Meadow *et al.* [6] and adopted in a modified form by the ISKDC (Table 21.3) [7].

A broad correlation exists between the clinical presentation and the histological changes on renal biopsy. Those with haematuria alone without significant proteinuria have generally less severe histological changes, which are highly likely to undergo spontaneous resolution, whereas those with heavy

Table 21.3 ISKDC histological classification of Henoch–Schönlein purpura nephritis [7]

I	Minimal alterations
II	Mesangial proliferation
IIIa	Focal proliferation or sclerosis with <50% crescents
IIIb	Diffuse proliferation or sclerosis with <50% crescents
IVa	Focal mesangial proliferation or sclerosis with 50–75% crescents
IVb	Diffuse mesangial proliferation or sclerosis with 50–75% crescents
Va	Focal mesangial proliferation or sclerosis with >75% crescents
Vb	Diffuse mesangial proliferation or sclerosis with >75% crescents
VI	Membranoproliferative-like lesion

proteinuria, a persisting nephritic syndrome or nephrotic syndrome are likely to have more severe changes, which are less likely to resolve.

The renal lesion bears many similarities to that observed in IgA nephropathy (see Chapter 1), and the two diseases are considered by many to share a common pathogenesis and perhaps represent different spectra of one disease. Patients with IgA nephropathy do not, however, have clinical evidence of extrarenal disease.

Treatment

Immunosuppressive therapy. The large majority of cases of Henoch–Schönlein purpura are mild and are associated with a good prognosis: immunosuppressive treatment is therefore not justified. Children should receive symptomatic treatment only.

The skin lesion requires no treatment and the arthropathy should be treated with rest and simple analgesia. While never subjected to a controlled clinical trial, there is some evidence to suggest that the more severe gastrointestinal symptoms, particularly abdominal pain and gastrointestinal bleeding, respond well to corticosteroid therapy [8], which has also been used for the treatment of testicular involvement and pulmonary haemorrhage.

Few prospective randomized controlled studies have been completed relating to the treatment of renal disease associated with Henoch–Schönlein purpura. Mollica *et al.* [9] have reported the results of a prospective study where 168 children with no evidence of renal involvement at disease presentation were alternately assigned to 2 weeks of daily prednisolone (1 mg/kg) or no therapy. No children treated with steroids developed renal involvement, compared with 10 of the 84 control patients. To investigate this further, a randomized prospective study has recently commenced in the United Kingdom to determine whether the administration of corticosteroids in all patients at disease presentation results in an overall reduction in the subsequent incidence of significant renal involvement. Studies investigating antiplatelet therapy have failed to show any benefit in terms of modifying the course of the disease or preventing the development of nephropathy [10].

There is no evidence based on randomized controlled trials to support the use of any of the more potent immunosuppressive therapies in the treatment of more severe grades of Henoch–Schönlein nephritis. A number of uncontrolled studies have reported improvement following therapy with azathioprine, cyclophosphamide, and chlorambucil, anticoagulants, and antiplatelet drugs, often in association with oral corticosteroid therapy. Others, however, have failed to show any benefit. The presence of a large number of crescents may warrant more aggressive additional therapy with intravenous methylprednisolone and plasma exchange, and there are a number of uncontrolled studies reporting good outcomes with these therapies [11–13].

In Manchester, when severe histological changes are detected (Meadow grade IIIb or worse), we use an 8-week course of oral cyclophosphamide in conjunction with daily oral prednisolone, converting to alternate-day prednisolone in combination with azathioprine for a total of 12 months. Where crescentic changes are present, we and others have reported good outcomes following 5–10 days of plasma exchange in addition to steroids and cyclophosphamide, as in other forms of crescentic nephritis. It is important to stress that there are no controlled trial data to support either of these regimens.

Management of hypertension. In addition to specific immunosuppressive therapies, hypertension associated with the acute nephritic syndrome should be treated with salt and water restriction in combination with a loop diuretic, progressing to other antihypertensive agents if this does not settle. The nephrotic state should also be treated cautiously with fluid restriction and/or diuretics, taking care to avoid hypovolaemia.

Key points: Treatment of Henoch–Schönlein purpura

- The skin lesion requires no specific treatment.

- The arthropathy should be treated with rest and simple analgesia.

- Some reports have suggested that the abdominal pain and gastrointestinal bleeding may respond to corticosteroids.

- Severe nephritis may respond to therapy with a variety of immunosuppressive agents.

Henoch–Schönlein purpura: long-term outcome

The overwhelming majority of the long-term morbidity associated with Henoch–Schönlein purpura relates to the associated nephritis. All published data indicate that the great majority of children with the disease make a full and uneventful recovery with no evidence of ongoing significant renal disease. However, Henoch–Schönlein nephritis is reported to be the cause of end stage renal failure in 1.6–3% of children in the United Kingdom [14] and Europe [13].

There is significant reported variability in the relative incidence of the various clinical presentations of Henoch–Schönlein nephritis and the long-term outlook associated with these. Series from tertiary referral institutions report a markedly higher incidence of long-term renal morbidity than unselected series.

The two largest unselected series of children with Henoch–Schönlein purpura are from Finland and Northern Ireland [2,15]. Koskimies *et al.* [15] found 39 of 141 (28%) children to have an abnormal urinary sediment for more than 1 month after presentation. Twenty-nine of these children were followed up, and at an average of 7.2 years after diagnosis, only one child had developed end stage renal failure and died, and two had developed chronic glomerular disease, the overall incidence of chronic renal disease being 2.1%. Stewart *et al.* [2] reported 270 patients presenting over a 13-year period. Fifty-five (20%) were found to have initial evidence of renal involvement. One child died during the acute phase of the illness. At an average of 8.3 years' follow-up, only 3 (1.1%) had evidence of persistent urinary

abnormality with normal renal function. In both of these studies, the large majority of children had relatively minor changes in urinary sediment.

In contrast, series of highly selected patients from tertiary renal centres report significantly higher rates of long-term renal impairment. A 23-year follow-up study from Guys and Birmingham Children's Hospitals found the incidence of long-term renal failure to be 19.2% in a cohort of 78 patients who underwent renal biopsy early in the course of their illness [16]. It must be stressed that the fact that these children were referred into a tertiary centre and underwent renal biopsy is indicative of the relative severity of their renal disease at presentation. A broad correlation was detected between clinical presentation and outcome: 44% of children who presented with a nephritic, nephrotic, or mixed nephritic/nephrotic developed hypertension or renal failure on follow-up, whereas of those with microscopic haematuria with or without proteinuria, 82% were entirely normal at follow-up, with 7.7% developing hypertension or renal failure. A small number of patients showed clinical improvement at 5-year follow-up, only to deteriorate in the longer term, and 16 of 44 successful subsequent pregnancies were complicated by hypertension or proteinuria, including 12 where the mother had made an apparent complete clinical recovery.

The severity of the histology on the initial biopsy correlated well with long-term outcome: 42% of those with WHO grade IV or V changes developed renal failure or died, compared with 7.4% of those with grade I or II changes.

The long-term outcome of the various clinical presentations of Henoch–Schönlein nephritis is illustrated in Fig. 21.2.

From these studies and others, a number of conclusions can be drawn:

1. In unselected populations, the overall risk of significant long-term renal impairment is less than 2%.

2. Children with isolated haematuria with no proteinuria have a negligible incidence of long-term renal morbidity.

3. Patients who present with isolated microscopic and or macroscopic haematuria may have microscopic haematuria that persists for many months and years. Recurrence of episodes of macroscopic haematuria may occur following upper respiratory tract infections. The prognosis

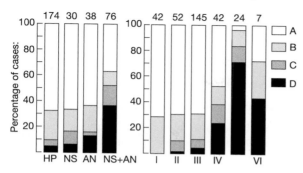

Fig. 21.2 Comparison of (a) clinical and (b) histological features at presentation with eventual outcome. HP, haematuria and/or proteinuria; NS, nephrotic syndrome; AN, acute nephritic syndrome. Histological categories I–VI as in Table 21.3. Outcomes: A, Normal: normal physical examination, no urinary abnormality, normal renal function; B, Minor urinary abnormality: normal physical examination, haematuria (microscopic ± macroscopic) and/or proteinuria <1 g/24 h, normal renal function; C: Active renal disease: proteinuria >1 g/24 h ± hypertension, normal renal function; D: Renal insufficiency: GFR <60 ml/min/1.73 m², actual or renal death (dialysis or transplantation). From Oxford Textbook of Clinical Nephrology 1/e by Cameron JS *et al.* Reprinted by permission of Oxford University Press.

generally remains good here unless there is evidence of significant proteinuria.

4. Where isolated haematuria is associated with proteinuria, the risk of long-term renal impairment is around 5%.

5. Children presenting with the acute nephritic syndrome have a less favourable outcome, with a risk of long-term renal impairment of 10–20%. Those with a mixed nephritic–nephrotic presentation have the worst long-term outlook, with up to 33% developing long-term renal impairment.

6. Those with more aggressive renal biopsy changes are more likely to have a poorer long-term outlook.

7. Children with significant renal impairment at presentation should remain under long-term follow-up.

8. Some instances of hypertension have been reported many years after normalization of renal function and urinalysis: hence the need for long-term follow-up. Most would advocate monitoring of blood pressure for at least 2 years after normalization of urinary sediment, with some recommending that this continue indefinitely through the general practitioner.

Key points: Henoch–Schönlein nephritis

- In unselected patients, the risk of chronic renal impairment is less than 2%.

- In patients referred to specialist paediatric nephrology centres, the risk of chronic renal impairment is greater than 10%.

- The highest risk of developing renal impairment is in those children with a nephritic, nephrotic, or mixed nephritic/nephrotic picture, and those with crescentic changes on renal biopsy.

- Late deterioration in renal function is well recognized, and all children with significant renal disease at presentation should remain under long-term follow-up.

Follow-up

Children with no evidence of nephritis should be followed up for at least 6 months after resolution of their rash, to ensure that they remain well and that there is no evidence of recurrence or other problems. Those with isolated haematuria, or haematuria associated with mild proteinuria, should be followed for a total of at least 2 years after urinalysis becomes normal, in view of the small number of reported cases of late hypertension. Some have recommended lifelong follow-up of this population. Children with evidence of more significant nephritis at presentation, particularly those with a nephrotic, nephritic, or mixed nephritic–nephrotic presentations should undoubtedly remain under lifelong follow-up, although in less severe cases this might be carried out in conjunction with their general practitioner.

Disease recurrence after transplantation

In the small number of children who progress to end stage renal failure necessitating renal transplantation, there are a number of reports of recurrent Henoch–Schönlein purpura in the transplanted kidney [17]. This is complicated by the fact that mesangial IgA deposits have been reported in allografts where the original cause of renal failure was neither Henoch–Schönlein purpura nor IgA nephropathy [18]. There is some suggestion that the rate of clinically significant recurrence is higher with the use of organs from living donors [19]. In

> ## Key points: Recommended follow-up for children with Henoch–Schönlein purpura
>
> - No evidence of nephritis: follow up until 6 months after resolution of rash.
>
> - Isolated haematuria or haematuria and mild proteinuria: follow up for at least 2 years after urinalysis becomes normal (?lifelong follow-up).
>
> - Haematuria and moderate proteinuria: keep under lifelong follow-up, this could be in conjunction with the general practitioner.
>
> - Nephrotic, nephritic, or mixed nephrotic–nephritic picture: need to remain under lifelong hospital follow-up in view of significant risk of renal impairment in the long term.

this publication, where clinical and histological recurrence occurred in five out of 12 living donor transplants compared with none of five cadaveric transplants, transplantation was performed at 27–101 months (mean 46) after presentation with their primary disease. There therefore seems little point in deferring transplantation until 1 year after resolution of the acute illness, as has been suggested by some [20].

Kawasaki disease

First described in Japan, this is the second most common vasculitic disorder of childhood. The disease predominantly affects younger children, boys more frequently than girls, and there is great world-wide variation in incidence. Recent data have demonstrated an increase in the reported incidence of the disease in the United Kingdom to 8.1 per 100 000 child population under 5 years of age in 1999/2000, the corresponding incidence in Japan being significantly higher at 134 per 100 000. The precise aetiology remains unknown: infection has been proposed by many as the cause, though no single organism has clearly been identified. It is likely that the disease represents a final common pathway of immune-mediated vascular inflammation following a variety of infective triggers, and there is ongoing debate regarding a superantigenic versus conventional antigenic trigger.

The acute phase of the disease is manifested by a significant fever lasting from 5 to 28 days, associated with:

(1) a polymorphic generalized rash;

(2) cervical lymphadenopathy;

(3) bilateral non-exudative conjunctival injection;

(4) oral mucous membrane changes, including injected or fissured lips, injected pharynx, or strawberry tongue; and

(5) changes of the peripheral extremities, including erythema of the palms and soles and oedema of the hands and feet (acute phase) and desquamation (convalescent phase).

Desquamation characteristically starts from nail margins proximally and can sometimes involve a whole glove distribution. This is often a late feature and treatment should not be delayed awaiting the presence of peeling for confirmation of the diagnosis. Perineal desquamation is also seen. The diagnostic criteria for Kawasaki disease are shown in Table 21.4 [21].

Arthritis of large joints occurs in around 25% of children. Respiratory (cough, coryza, hoarseness, and pulmonary infiltrates) and gastrointestinal involvement (diarrhoea, jaundice, hydrops of gall bladder) may occur. The most serious and life-threatening feature of Kawasaki disease, however, is the associated cardiac involvement. Coronary artery aneurysms occur in around 20–25% of untreated patients, which may result in myocardial ischaemia, infarction, and sudden death, Kawasaki disease being the most common cause of myocardial infarction in childhood. Furthermore, myocarditis, pericarditis, and arrhythmias can all also occur early in the acute phase of the disease.

Table 21.4 Kawasaki disease: diagnostic criteria

1. Fever for 5 days or more
2. Rash
3. Cervical lymphadenopathy
4. Conjunctivitis
5. Changes of lips/oral mucosa
6. Changes of extremities (erythema of soles, oedema of hands and feet, desquamation of skin from fingertips)

Five of these six symptoms are required for a diagnosis of Kawasaki disease to be made, though four will suffice if there is evidence of coronary artery aneurysms. As with all diagnostic criteria, these are not 100% sensitive and specific. Children who do not have the requisite number of criteria may have incomplete or atypical Kawasaki disease.

Renal disease is uncommon, the most frequent renal manifestation of Kawasaki disease being renal vascular disease. This predominantly affects the larger extraparenchymal and hilar renal arteries, although post-mortem series have shown smaller vessels to be involved [22]. This may present as acute renal impairment during the acute phase of the disease and may result in permanent renal artery stenosis with associated hypertension [23]. Urinalysis may reveal the presence of haematuria and proteinuria, and sterile pyuria may be detected on microscopy. Acute renal insufficiency has also been reported secondary to acute interstitial nephritis [24], and renal biopsy has also detected the presence of immune complex deposition [25] and haemolytic uraemic syndrome [26].

No laboratory investigations are included in the diagnostic criteria for Kawasaki disease. There is commonly a raised ESR and white cell count (neutrophilia). The platelet count may be initially depressed in the acute phase, although it rises in the second week of the illness and thus should not be relied upon diagnostically. Normochromic, normocytic anaemia may occur. Liver enzymes may be moderately raised. Both ANCA and anti-endothelial cell antibodies have been inconsistently detected in the acute phase, but the significance of this observation is unclear.

Children should be admitted to hospital and all should undergo echocardiography early in the acute phase of the illness. Both mortality and chronic sequelae have been greatly reduced by the routine early use of aspirin and high-dose intravenous immunoglobulin [27]. Aspirin is effective in reducing the fever and arthritis, although it was not until the introduction of intravenous immunoglobulin that the incidence of coronary artery aneurysm was reduced to 8% at 14 days and 4% at seven weeks post-diagnosis [28], with a resultant reduction in mortality to less than 1%. There is significant controversy surrounding the use of corticosteroids in this condition.

Takayasu's arteritis

World-wide, this is the third most common vasculitic disorder after Henoch–Schönlein purpura and Kawasaki disease. Segmental vasculitis occurs, leading to stenosis and aneurysms of the large arteries, particularly the aorta and its main branches, including the renal arteries. Presenting clinical features include headache, dyspnoea, palpitations, arthralgia or arthritis, myalgia, fever, night sweats, weight loss, and anorexia. Hypertension in the absence of peripheral pulses ('pulseless disease') should suggest the diagnosis, which is confirmed by aortography.

Glomerular disease does not occur, the major renal manifestations being hypertension and/or renal impairment secondary to reduced renal blood flow.

Children should be treated with corticosteroids and cyclophosphamide in the acute phase, with aortic reconstructive surgery or angioplasty/stenting being performed once the disease is quiescent. Antihypertensive therapy may be necessary while awaiting surgery. Angiotensin converting enzyme (ACE) inhibitors should be withheld unless other therapies have failed to control hypertension because these drugs may diminish renal function further.

Classical polyarteritis nodosa

Polyarteritis nodosa (PAN) is a necrotizing vasculitis of medium-sized muscular arteries with associated aneurysm formation. It is predominantly a disease of middle-aged men and is rare in childhood, although it is observed more commonly in childhood than microscopic polyangiitis (MPA), unlike in adults where MPA is more common than PAN. The vascular lesions are segmental and occur especially at arterial bifurcations. Many organ systems are involved in the disease process, the kidneys being affected most frequently (50–60% of cases). Other organs that are involved include the gastrointestinal tract and liver, heart, lungs, and central and peripheral nervous systems.

The clinical features include an insidious onset of unexplained fever, weight loss, abdominal pain, arthralgia, myalgia, and skin lesions, including livedo reticularis, nodular vasculitis, purpura, peripheral gangrene, and oedema. Renal involvement is manifested as loin pain and haematuria due to renal infarction or renal functional impairment secondary to ischaemia. Hypertension is common and both proteinuria and haematuria are frequently observed. Neurological features include organic psychosis, seizures, hemiparesis, mononeuritis multiplex, and focal neurological defects.

Investigation reveals non-specific changes in common with most of the vasculitides including anaemia, leucocytosis, an elevated platelet count, and raised inflammatory markers. Unlike microscopic polyangiitis, classical polyarteritis nodosa is not generally associated with positive ANCA titres, although these have been reported [29]. Diagnosis is made by the demonstration of aneurysm formation and peripheral vascular pruning in hepatic, mesenteric, and renal vessels on angiography (Fig. 21.3). Renal biopsy is generally avoided as there is a significant risk of inducing major bleeding or arteriovenous malformation production. Other organs, such as skin or muscle, may be biopsied to detect the histopathological changes of fibrinoid necrosis of small and medium-sized arterial walls.

The mainstay of therapy for polyarteritis nodosa is with corticosteroids and cyclophosphamide in combination with antiplatelet agents to induce rapid control of the disease, followed by maintenance therapy with prednisolone and (most commonly) azathioprine. The current mortality of the disease is dependent on the extent of organ involvement, but is around 10% in the United Kingdom [30].

Microscopic polyangiitis

This is a small-vessel vasculitis with focal segmental necrotizing glomerulonephritis, occasionally associated with pulmonary capillaritis, but without granulomatous disease of the upper respiratory tract. Despite its name, the disease is most closely linked to Wegener's granulomatosis, in that the renal lesion is similar and

that ANCA are typically present. Microscopic polyangiitis is a rare disorder in childhood.

The clinical features vary according to the extent of the small-vessel vasculitis. Renal symptoms predominate, with haematuria, proteinuria, hypertension, and acute renal failure which may be rapidly progressive, with a significant proportion of children requiring the early commencement of dialysis. Constitutional features may be present, including a vasculitic skin rash, fever, arthropathy, anorexia, and weight loss. Pulmonary haemorrhage, presenting as dyspnoea, haemoptysis, and anaemia, is an infrequent, though potentially life-threatening disease manifestation.

Similar to other vasculitides, anaemia, leucocytosis, and a raised ESR are frequently present. ANCA directed against myeloperoxidase (pANCA) are present in a high proportion of children. Urine microscopy will detect the presence of red cells and red cell casts. Demonstration of the presence of a small-vessel vasculitis is best performed by renal biopsy, which reveals a pauci-immune segmental necrotizing glomerulonephritis, which when viewed in isolation may be indistinguishable from those changes seen in Wegener's granulomatosis.

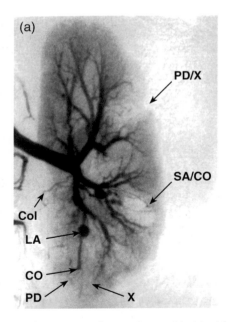 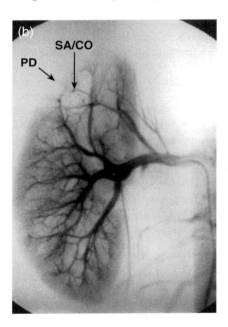

Fig. 21.3 (a) Renal angiogram from a 6-year-old girl with PAN, demonstrating florid aneurysmal and non-aneurysmal changes. Large aneurysms (LA), small aneurysms (SA), perfusion defect (PD), arterial cut-off (CO), lack of crossing of peripheral renal arteries (X), collateral artery (Col). (b) Renal angiogram from an 8-year-old boy with PAN, demonstrating less florid aneurysmal and non-aneurysmal changes. Perfusion defect (PD), small aneurysm (SA) in association with arterial cut-off (CO). For the differentiation of small aneurysms from artefact, it is critical that the arterial swelling is in both antero-posterior and oblique views. From Brogan PA *et al.* Renal angiography in children with polyarteritis nodosa. Pediatr Nephrol 2002;17:277–283 with permission from Springer-Verlag.

As with macroscopic polyarteritis nodosa, high-dose corticosteroids and cyclophosphamide remain the mainstay of therapy. The incidence of permanent renal failure is possibly as high as 50% and in light of this, many advocate the additional use of plasma exchange (even if dialysis independent) at presentation.

A number of authors have proposed that idiopathic focal necrotizing and crescentic glomerulonephritis, where antiglomerular basement membrane antibodies are not detected, is a form of small-vessel vasculitis restricted to the kidney (so-called 'renal limited vasculitis' [31]).

Wegener's granulomatosis

Wegener's granulomatosis is a necrotizing vasculitis with granuloma formation affecting the upper and lower respiratory tract. Although the disease may be limited to the respiratory tract in some, other organs may be involved, with a small-vessel vasculitis affecting the kidneys, eyes, skin, heart, central nervous system, gastrointestinal tract, and joints.

Upper respiratory tract involvement presents with oral and nasal ulceration (leading in some to nasal septum destruction), upper airway obstruction, sinusitis, and otitis media, whereas lower respiratory tract disease presents with cough, haemoptysis, and chest pain. Children are frequently systemically unwell in association with their respiratory disease, with fever, malaise, weight loss, and other constitutional symptoms. Clinical manifestations of renal disease vary from asymptomatic haematuria and proteinuria detected only on routine urinalysis to rapidly progressive renal failure.

Routine laboratory tests are often non-specific. Leucocytosis, thrombocytosis, normocytic normochromic anaemia, and an elevated ESR are frequently observed. Children are frequently, but not universally, cANCA positive with antibodies directed against proteinase-3 detectable by ELISA. Biopsy of affected areas of the upper respiratory tract may be helpful diagnostically if granulomatous change is detected, although such histological changes may be patchy and therefore missed. Renal biopsy should be performed if there is evidence of significant renal disease. Histology classically reveals a segmental necrotizing glomerulonephritis which is pauci-immune, meaning there is little or no immunoglobulin deposition detected on immunofluorescence.

Wegener's granulomatosis is treated with combinations of cyclophosphamide, corticosteroids, and antiplatelet agents. As with microscopic polyangiitis, plasma exchange may be indicated if there is rapidly progressive renal failure. This is most successful when commenced early in the disease course. Mortality approaches 15% [32] and a proportion of children will progress to end stage renal failure necessitating dialysis and transplantation. In those where the disease can be controlled with immunosuppressive therapy, relapse may occur. Unlike polyarteritis nodosa or microscopic polyangiitis in the young, which has a propensity to 'burn out' after several years, Wegener's granulomatosis is a lifelong disease with a chronic relapsing and remitting course.

Systemic lupus erythematosus

Systemic lupus erythematosus (SLE) is a chronic inflammatory multi-system autoimmune disease characterized by widespread inflammation of the blood vessels and connective tissue. The primary pathology is of persistent polyclonal B-cell stimulation resulting in autoantibody production, with the widespread tissue deposition of immune complexes. In the kidney, these are deposited in the glomerular capillary endothelium, with resultant complement-mediated inflammation. Circulating antinuclear antibodies are almost always present, with antibodies to native (double-stranded) deoxyribonucleic acid (dsDNA) being a sensitive and specific test for the disease. The clinical manifestations are diverse and the disease course often unpredictable. There is a significant mortality rate, and in potentially life-threatening cases aggressive treatment needs to be started rapidly.

The incidence of SLE in childhood has been estimated at between 0.5 and 0.6 per 100 000 child population, with most paediatric cases presenting in the teenage years, lupus being a rare disease in the under-fives. SLE affects females more frequently than males (sex ratio 5–10 : 1 for older children), and the disease is much more prevalent in the Black population.

Clinical presentation

The clinical features of SLE are protean, as the disease can affect a wide range of organ systems. Generalized symptoms such as fever, weight loss, and malaise are common. These diverse clinical presentations are shown in Table 21.5, the more common presenting features being highlighted in bold font. The relative frequencies with which different organ systems are involved are shown in

Table 21.5 Clinical features of SLE (more common presentations are highlighted in **bold** font)

General	Tiredness
	Fever and malaise
	Weight loss
	Lymphadenopathy
Skin	**Butterfly rash with photosensitivity**
	Alopecia
	Discoid lesions
	Nail lesions
	Lupus tumidus
	Subacute cutaneous lupus
	Vasculitic purpura
Musculoskeletal	**Non-erosive arthritis/arthralgia**
	Tenosynovitis
	Myopathy
	Avascular necrosis
Gastrointestinal tract	**Oral and nasal ulceration**
	Anorexia, weight loss, diffuse abdominal pain
	Oesophageal dysmotility
	Colitis
	Hepatosplenomegaly
	Pancreatitis
	Protein losing enteropathy/ malabsorption syndromes
Cardiovascular	**Raynaud's phenomenon**
	Pericarditis
	Valvular lesions
	Vasculitic lesions
	Thrombophlebitis
	Conduction abnormalities
	Myocarditis
	Libman–Sacks endocarditis
	Accelerated coronary artery disease
	Peripheral gangrene
Pulmonary	**Pleuritis**, pleural effusions
	Subclinical (abnormal pulmonary function tests only)
	Pneumonitis, pulmonary infiltrates, atelectasis
	Haemorrhage
	Shrinking lung (diaphragmatic dysfunction)
	Pneumothorax
Neurological	**Migraine**
	Depression/anxiety
	Organic psychosis
	Seizures
	Cranial nerve and peripheral neuropathies
	Chorea
	Cerebrovascular accidents
Ocular	Retinopathy, cotton wool spots
	Papilloedema
Renal	**Glomerulonephritis**
	Hypertension
	Renal failure
Haematological	Coomb's positive haemolytic anaemia
	Thrombocytopenia
	Antiphospholipid syndrome
Endocrine	Hypo/hyperthyroidism

Table 21.6, which is based on data from 672 children from a total of 27 publications [33].

Whereas the diagnosis of lupus is often clear-cut in severely ill children with 'full-blown' SLE, milder cases present a diagnostic challenge to the clinician. Many use the American College of Rheumatology (ACR)

Table 21.6 Clinical manifestations at presentation in childhood lupus-data from 672 children. From Cameron J.S. Lupus nephritis in childhood and adolescence. Pediatr Nephrol 1994;8:230–249 with permission from Springer-Verlag.

Clinical manifestation	Proportion affected	Range
Renal disease	82%	28–100%
Fever	78%	54–94%
Arthralgia	75%	44–100%
Rash	68%	14–94%
Weight loss	40%	30–54%
Cardiovascular involvement	40%	19–56%
Neurological involvement	30%	3–48%
Hypertension	28%	12–61%
Splenomegaly	27%	3–59%
Pleurisy	12%	0–36%
Alopecia	10%	0–55%

Table 21.7 Revised 1997 ACR criteria for the classification of systemic lupus erythematosus

Malar (butterfly) rash
Discoid-lupus rash
Photosensitivity
Oral or nasal mucocutaneous ulceration
Non-erosive arthritis
Nephritis[a]
　Proteinuria >0.5 g/day
　Cellular casts
Encephalopathy[a]
　Seizures
　Psychosis
Pleuritis or pericarditis
Haematological abnormality[a]
　Haemolytic anaemia
　Leucopenia
　Lymphopenia
　Thrombocytopenia
Positive immunoserology[a]
　Antibodies to dsDNA
　Antibodies to Sm nuclear antigen
　Positive finding of antiphospholipid antibodies based on:
　　IgG or IgM anticardiolipin antibodies
　　Lupus anticoagulant, or
　　False-positive serological test for syphilis for at least 6 months
Positive antinuclear antibody test

[a] Any one item satisfies the criterion.

criteria (Table 21.7) which have been validated in adult patients with SLE [34]. The presence of any four of the 11 criteria during any period of observation makes the diagnosis of lupus with a sensitivity of 96% and a specificity of 96%. It is important that these criteria are not applied too rigidly: a number of children who fall short of having sufficient diagnostic criteria may develop further clinical problems with time and therefore warrant close observation and possibly treatment. It must also be remembered that SLE is an episodic disease; it is therefore important that the diagnosis be entertained in illnesses where different organ systems are involved either concurrently or serially over a period of time. For example, photosensitive dermatitis may present in the summer with pleuritis and arthritis developing over the ensuing months. It is our experience that clinical clues are available if specifically looked for, i.e. a history of mouth ulcers is often not volunteered unless specifically asked about, faint malar rashes may be put down to more innocent causes, and mild arthropathy may be ignored by the patient and missed by the paediatrician unless careful systematic joint examination has been performed.

It has been noted that certain features usually associated with increased disease severity, such as nephritis or central nervous dysfunction, are more common in children than in adults with SLE. Children have been reported to have a higher incidence of nephritis at disease presentation and a higher incidence of chorea during the subsequent evolution of the disease [35].

Investigations

Children presenting with lupus frequently have haematological abnormalities (Table 21.8), including anaemia, leucopenia, and thrombocytopenia. Abnormalities of coagulation are also seen due to the presence of antibodies against coagulation factors. Almost all children with lupus will have some detectable immunological abnormality. The C3 and C4 components of complement are frequently reduced, reflecting increased consumption or an inherited deficiency. Antibodies to double-stranded DNA are commonly raised, particularly where lupus nephritis is present. Anti-Sm (Smith) antibodies are entirely specific for lupus and are related to CNS involvement, although as they are positive in only 30% of patients, lack sensitivity as a diagnostic test. The ESR is almost

Table 21.8 The prevalence of certain abnormal laboratory tests at presentation in children with lupus (from Cameron JS. *Pediatr Nephrol* 1994;8:230–249)

	Weighted average	Range in different series
Haematological		
Anaemia	56%	45–80%
Leucopenia	47%	33–66%
Thrombocytopenia	25%	7–33%
Coombs positive	48%	36–65%
Clotting prolonged	27%	16–70%
Immunological		
ANF positive	97%	94–100%
DNA binding raised	75%	69–81%
Lupus cells present	84%	69–100%
C3 low	73%	44–90%
C4 low	70%	65–75%
Immune complexes present	70%	55–100%
CRP raised in absence of infection	5%	0–10%
ESR raised	94%	89–100%
IgG raised	64%	44–67%

invariably raised, although the CRP may be normal: this finding is useful in distinguishing acute bacterial infection from disease activity in the patient with lupus. Importantly, however, flares of lupus can occur in association with sepsis, resulting in active disease and a high CRP.

Anticardiolipin antibodies are detected in up to 50% of children with lupus. Their presence is associated with episodes of arterial and venous thrombosis. These antibodies directed against phospholipids paradoxically cause prolongation of *in vitro* clotting times.

Lupus nephritis

Up to 80% of children with lupus have evidence of renal involvement at some point in their disease course, most frequently at disease presentation. Renal disease may, however, present as late as 10 years after initial diagnosis. Lupus nephritis is the most significant cause of morbidity and mortality in this population. As shown in Table 21.9, the most common mode of presentation is with proteinuria and microscopic haematuria, the two frequently occurring concurrently. The proteinuria is often sufficient to cause nephrotic syndrome. Both hypertension and evidence of impaired renal function are seen in around one-half of children.

Table 21.9 Presentation of renal disease in children with lupus nephritis (From Cameron JS. Lupus nephritis in childhood and adolescence. Pediatr Nephrol 1994;8: 230–249 with permission from Springer-Verlag.)

Nephrotic syndrome	55%
Proteinuria <3 g/day	43%
Haematuria	
Macroscopic	1.4%
Microscopic	79%
Hypertension	40%
Impaired renal function	50%
Acute renal failure	1.4%

As non-nephrotic proportion proteinuria and microscopic haematuria are generally asymptomatic, it is essential that children with lupus undergo regular monitoring of their urine for proteinuria (early morning protein:creatinine ratio) and haematuria, and measurement of plasma creatinine (with calculation of glomerular filtration rate (GFR)) and plasma albumin. The regular measurement of blood pressure is also mandatory.

The basic pathological lesions are an immune-complex-mediated vasculitis and fibrinoid necrosis, inflammatory cellular infiltrate, and sclerosis of collagen. The wide spectrum of renal abnormalities has been classified by the World Health Organization (Table 21.10) [36]. The risk of significant long-term renal impairment relates to both the type and extent of these.

Most would advocate a renal biopsy for children with any evidence of renal disease (abnormal urinalysis, impaired renal function with or without hypertension) to obtain a histological diagnosis which will guide therapy. This is in contrast to adult practice, where some have argued that the patient with impaired renal function, an active urinary sediment, and strongly positive lupus serology will almost certainly have diffuse proliferative changes (WHO type IV) and should be treated accordingly, with biopsy being reserved for those with alternative presenting features.

Around two-thirds of children will have a proliferative glomerulonephritis (WHO types III and IV), with two-thirds of these having diffuse proliferative glomerulonephritis, the most severe form of lupus nephritis. Around one-quarter will have WHO type I or II histology [33].

Children with mesangial lupus nephritis (WHO type II) seldom have clinical evidence of disease, although there may be minimal proteinuria and microscopic haematuria. In focal proliferative glomerulonephritis (WHO type III), proteinuria and mild haematuria may occur, and nephrotic syndrome or renal insufficiency

Table 21.10 WHO classification of lupus nephritis [36]

I Normal glomeruli
 (a) Negative IF and EM
 (b) Normal by LM, deposits by IF or EM
II Mesangial alterations (mesangiopathy)
 (a) Mesangial hypercellularity, mild (+)
 (b) Mesangial hypercellularity, moderate (++)
 Both categories have diffuse mesangial deposits by IF and EM
III Focal proliferative glomerulonephritis
 Diffuse mesangial and focal subendothelial and subepithelial deposits by IF and EM
IV Diffuse proliferative glomerulonephitis
 Mesangial, subendothelial, and subepithelial deposits by IF and EM
V Membranous
 Diffuse subepithelial and a few mesangial and focal subendothelial deposits by IF and EM
VI Glomerular sclerosis

IF = immunofluorescence.
EM = electron microscopy.
LM = light microscopy.

occur in 20%. Diffuse glomerulonephritis (WHO type IV) cases usually have significant proteinuria and haematuria and around 60% have nephrotic syndrome or renal insufficiency. Persistent nephrotic syndrome occurs in membranous lupus glomerulonephritis (WHO type V), often with hypertension. The end stage lesion is glomerular sclerosis (sometimes referred to as WHO type VI) with nephrotic syndrome, renal failure, and hypertension being common.

Treatment and prognosis

Once the diagnosis has been made, it is important to start therapy as soon as possible. As outlined above, there is significant variability in the clinical presentation of lupus, and treatment needs to be tailored accordingly. Scoring systems such as the British Isles Lupus Assessment Group (BILAG) score [37] or the Systemic Lupus Erythematosus Disease Activity Index (SLEDAI) [38] may be useful with regard to this. The somewhat more complex 10-part staging criteria [39] may also be useful in determining levels of treatment, including steroid dosage and timing of immunosuppressive therapy.

Treatment is best managed by a multi-professional team experienced in managing this multisystem disease, including a paediatric rheumatologist, physiotherapist, nurse specialist, and social worker, with consultation with a paediatric nephrologist early in the disease course. The goals of treatment should be to reduce symptoms and disease activity while exposing the child to the minimum of side-effects of immunosuppressive therapy.

Children with mild disease without evidence of renal or other life-threatening organ involvement may be managed with non-steroidal anti-inflammatory agents to control musculoskeletal symptoms and/or hydroxychloroquine sulphate. Hydroxychloroquine is useful for cutaneous disease and is helpful in reducing photosensitivity. It also has some anti-inflammatory action and is often a significant disease modifier/ steroid sparer, although rarely ocular toxicity may limit its use. Some advocate combination therapy, with hydroxychloroquine and mepacrine given on alternate days for skin involvement, which limits the toxicity of these two agents. Almost all children require corticosteroids at some stage of their treatment, however, and initial disease control usually requires daily steroids for several weeks or months. Children with mild disease may require as little as 0.25 mg/kg/day of prednisolone to achieve disease control.

Children with moderate disease activity require higher doses of steroids to control their disease. This often exposes the child to the side-effects of these drugs and necessitates the use of 'steroid-sparing' agents such as azathioprine, methotrexate, or, more recently, mycophenolate mofetil. Although azathioprine has been used for longer than any other second-line agent in childhood lupus, there are few trials that have investigated its efficacy. There is limited experience with the use of methotrexate in childhood lupus, although it has been reported to be useful in controlling resistant skin or joint disease [40].

More significant lupus activity, including diffuse proliferative (WHO type IV) lupus nephritis (see above) and CNS lupus, requires the administration of more potent immunosuppressive therapy. Although the number of randomized prospective clinical trials investigating lupus treatment modalities is small, two have shown a benefit of cyclophosphamide over steroids alone in the treatment of lupus nephritis in adults [41,42]. Most authorities would therefore advocate the use of cyclophosphamide as either continuous oral therapy (8–12 weeks in a dose of 2–3 mg/ kg/day [33]) or intermittent intravenous pulse therapy. In our centres, we use the intravenous route, giving cyclophosphamide 500 mg/m^2 increasing to 1 g/m^2 monthly for 6 months. After this initial 6-month 'induction' phase, the standard National Institutes of Health (NIH) treatment regimen for adults recommends 3-monthly pulses of cyclophosphamide for a total of 2 years. Although some paediatric nephrologists adopt this approach for children and adolescents, others adopt a slightly less aggressive protocol (because of concerns relating to gonadal toxicity and long-term malignancy in the young), with only 2 or 3 'consolidatory' cyclophosphamide pulses given at 3-monthly intervals following the initial 6-month induction phase. Intravenous cyclophosphamide is given in combination with a significant volume of intravenous fluid to ensure a satisfactory diuresis, and intravenous mesna to prevent the development of haemorrhagic cystitis.

The side-effects of cyclophosphamide are outlined in Chapter 19. The aforementioned NIH regimen for lupus would administer approximately two and a half to three times the total amount of cyclophosphamide as would be administered for the treatment of frequently relapsing steroid-sensitive nephrotic syndrome, thus increasing the likelihood of some of the longer-term side-effects, including infertility. The risk of infertility is higher in males, particularly those who are sexually mature at the time of therapy. Methods of preserving gonadal function, including the use of gonadotrophin releasing hormone and gonadotrophin releasing hormone agonists, are currently under investigation [43].

The success in treating severe lupus nephritis and CNS lupus with intravenous cyclophosphamide, particularly the assistance that this therapy gives to the reduction of the dose of corticosteroid required, has led many to consider its use earlier, where lupus is less severe, and even before there is evidence of renal dysfunction [44] to avoid the continuous administration of high-dose steroids. Such a course of action appears to be safe [45,46]. Ilowite [47] has likened the chronic relapsing and life-threatening nature of SLE to that of a malignant condition and has suggested that it should be treated in a similar way, with the aggressive use of therapy in the early stages to initiate disease remission, followed by low-dose maintenance therapy.

Cyclophosphamide is generally given in combination with corticosteroid therapy. In some, high-dose intravenous methylprednisolone is used in the initial treatment of severe cases with advanced nephritis, CNS involvement, pulmonary disease, and/or haemolytic anaemia. Intravenous immunoglobulin or plasma exchange may be helpful in refractory cases of thrombocytopenia, although the benefit may be short-lived. Cyclosporin A may be helpful in steroid-resistant cases, particularly for WHO type V nephritis. Induction therapy with mycophenolate mofetil has been used in individual patients, and trials are ongoing in adult and paediatric patients to compare its efficacy with cyclophosphamide. It should be remembered that in some children with severe lupus nephritis unresponsive to conventional therapy, the risks of dialysis and transplantation may be less than those of a progressively escalating immunosuppressive regimen and the kidneys should be 'sacrificed' to save the child.

The child with lupus nephritis should also receive adequate treatment of hypertension if present, to prevent further deterioration of renal function. Where proteinuria is present, an ACE inhibitor is the most logical choice of agent, as this will additionally reduce urinary protein excretion and possibly slow the rate of decline of renal function; however, captopril can be associated with drug-induced lupus, and this should be borne in mind if considering such therapy.

Following the acute treatment of severe lupus with the more potent immunosuppressive agents described above, long-term maintenance therapy should be continued with corticosteroids in conjunction with 'steroid-sparing' agents such as azathioprine. Again, the goal should be control of disease activity using the smallest possible drug dose (usually 2 mg/kg/day of azathioprine and the smallest amount of prednisolone that keeps the child symptom free). In some children, the disease appears to burn out, and it may be possible to gradually withdraw all therapy after a number of years of treatment, though in the vast majority lifelong therapy is necessary. Late relapse of renal disease following cessation of therapy is well recognized, and children and young adults should remain under long-term follow-up.

A number of general measures need to be taken in children with all levels of lupus activity. These include:

1. *Sunscreens*: exposure to the sun and other sources of ultraviolet light (mainly UV-A but also to a lesser extent UV-B) may precipitate a relapse of lupus (or indeed the first attack). Hats and protective clothing will reduce exposure, and high sun protection factor sunblocks should be recommended and prescribed if necessary.
2. *Immunizations*: on the whole all routine childhood immunizations should be given, with the exception of the live vaccines to those on immunosuppressive therapy. Pneumococcal vaccine should additionally be given as there is a risk of functional asplenia and an annual influenza vaccine is recommended, although it has been the observation of some that flaring of the lupus can occur following vaccination, and children and parents may need to be counselled specifically regarding this complication.
3. *Antiplatelet therapy*: children with antiphospholipid syndrome require long-term therapy with antiplatelet agents such as aspirin or dipyridamole, and anticoagulation where there is evidence of thrombosis.
4. *An awareness of the heightened risk of infection*: children with lupus are at increased risk of infection, which remains a major source of mortality in this population, particularly in those who have received the most potent immunosuppressive regimens.

Prior to the availability of modern immunosuppressive therapy, the mortality from renal failure and infection associated with lupus was high. Nowadays, most centres achieve a 5-year survival rate of around 95% [48], although renal failure and sepsis remain the major causes of mortality. Morbidity from the disease and its treatment remain a major problem.

Key points: Lupus nephritis

- Up to 80% of children with SLE will have renal involvement at some point in their disease course.

- Lupus nephritis is the most significant cause of morbidity and mortality in SLE.

- Around two-thirds of children will have a proliferative glomerulonephritis, with two-thirds of these changes being diffuse.

- Most forms of lupus nephritis, particularly those where there are proliferative changes, require treatment with intravenous cyclophosphamide in conjunction with corticosteroids.

- Infection remains a major cause of morbidity and mortality.

Cystic fibrosis

As the prognosis improves for patients with cystic fibrosis, renal complications of the illness may develop. There are several possible mechanisms of renal injury in cystic fibrosis (CF), including complications arising from chronic infection, immunological dysregulation (perhaps as a result of chronic infection or inflammation), and drug therapy. Moreover, the kidney may be inherently involved as part of the underlying defect in the cystic fibrosis transmembrane regulator, since this is widely expressed in the kidney [49].

Cystic fibrosis is associated with an increased risk of nephrocalcinosis and nephrolithiasis. In one autopsy study, 35 of 38 kidneys from cystic fibrosis patients demonstrated microscopic nephrocalcinosis [50]. Notably, nephrocalcinosis was detected in three neonates and three infants, lending support to the hypothesis that such renal calcium deposits reflect the genomic defect and are not due to long-standing pulmonary dysfunction, chronic infection, therapeutic agents, or disease progression. None of the patients with nephrocalcinosis had clinical evidence of renal dysfunction.

There are many reasons other than a primary renal defect for nephrocalcinosis to occur; for example, prolonged periods of immobilization, and the use of steroids or frusemide therapy. Secondary alimentary hyperoxaluria has also been suggested as an additional risk factor [51].

Nephrotoxic drugs

A number of potentially nephrotoxic drugs are routinely used in the management of children with cystic fibrosis, including aminoglycoside antibiotics, cephalosporins, loop diuretics, and non-steroidal anti-inflammatory drugs.

Nephrotoxic acute tubular necrosis (ATN) is a recognized complication of aminoglycosides and differs clinically from ischaemic ATN in that the former is more likely to be associated with a non-oliguric presentation, with gradual onset of renal failure—the so-called 'intermediate syndrome' (i.e. intermediate between pre-renal and renal failure) [52]. Patients with the intermediate syndrome show some characteristics of reversible pre-renal failure, such as a relatively low urinary sodium and a partial response to fluid challenge, but with a shorter maintenance phase of renal failure than associated with ischaemic ATN. It is therefore vital that close monitoring of aminoglycoside levels is undertaken in order to prevent nephrotoxic ATN in cystic fibrosis.

Nephrocalcinosis (mentioned above) is associated with the use of both frusemide (e.g. used to treat right-sided heart failure) and corticosteroids (e.g. used to treat allergic aspergillosis) in cystic fibrosis. NSAIDs are used for the management of cystic

fibrosis-related arthropathy and may be associated with renal vasoconstriction and acute renal dysfunction, especially in the context of the chronic salt depletion associated with the disease [53].

Tubulo-interstitial nephritis

Tubulo-interstitial nephritis may complicate cystic fibrosis as a result of an allergic reaction to antibiotics or infection. Systemic signs of allergy, such as rash, and non-specific symptoms, such as malaise, fever, and vomiting, may be present. Laboratory findings demonstrate elevation of plasma urea and creatinine, occasionally accompanied by hypokalaemia and hypophosphataemia (due to the proximal tubular dysfunction), and sometimes a peripheral blood and/or urinary eosinophilia. Urinary examination may reveal haematuria, proteinuria (positive dipstick for protein, but little urinary albumin, implying tubular rather than glomerular protein leak), and glycosuria. Ultrasonography usually demonstrates large, echobright kidneys, and renal biopsy demonstrates a predominantly T-cell interstitial infiltrate, sometimes with tubular dilatation and areas of tubulo-interstitial fibrosis.

IgA Nephropathy

IgA nephropathy is rare, but has been reported in patients with cystic fibrosis [54]. Since both cystic fibrosis and IgA nephropathy are relatively common, their coexistence may be coincidental, but it is tempting to speculate that there may be a real association due to recurrent respiratory tract infections, with increased circulating IgA and subsequent IgA nephropathy.

Other renal manifestations of cystic fibrosis

Amyloidosis may complicate cystic fibrosis due to the chronic inflammatory nature of the disease. A retrospective autopsy study of 33 patients who were at least 15 years old at the time of death revealed that 11 (33%) had amyloid deposits in multiple organs. The spleen, liver, and kidneys were the principally affected organs, with microscopic deposits mainly restricted to blood vessels. Only one patient had overt clinical renal dysfunction secondary to the presence of amyloid. The prognosis is generally poor, with nearly all dying within a year of clinical onset, although two patients have been treated with colchicine, with some degree of success [55].

Systemic vasculitis occasionally complicates cystic fibrosis, the cause of which is unknown but presumably reflects an aberrant immune response to chronic infection or drug therapy, or both [56]. The vasculitis is predominantly cutaneous, but occasionally is more widespread, with both cerebral and renal involvement (renal failure and focal glomerular sclerosis and capsular adhesions) reported.

Cystic fibrosis may be complicated by diabetes mellitus, and reports of diabetic nephropathy in this context have been documented [57].

Key points: Cystic fibrosis

- As the prognosis for patients with cystic fibrosis improves, renal complications of the illness may develop.

- Reported renal complications include nephrocalcinosis, nephrolithiasis, acute tubular necrosis, tubulo-interstitial nephritis, IgA nephropathy, amyloidosis, systemic vasculitis, and diabetic nephropathy.

Diabetes mellitus

Introduction

Diabetic nephropathy is the most common cause of end stage renal failure in adults in the United States and accounts for 16% of end stage disease in adult patients in the United Kingdom [58]. The natural history in type 1 diabetics includes several stages over 10–15 years, starting with apparent normality in the first few years after diagnosis, followed by incipient nephropathy characterized by the presence of small amounts of albumin in the urine (undetectable on dipstick testing), known as microalbuminuria. This is followed by overt clinical nephropathy with dipstick-positive proteinuria and the associated development of hypertension, with progressive deterioration in renal function leading to end stage renal failure. There is no specific therapy for diabetic nephropathy, and all patient management should be targeted at preventing the onset of renal disease, and slowing its progress once detected.

It has been suggested that 25–45% of patients with type 1 diabetes will develop clinically detectable nephropathy (the minimal criterion for which is a persistently positive urine dipstick for protein)

during their lifetime and a further 20–30% will have subclinical microalbuminuria [59]. There is some evidence that the overall incidence of nephropathy is falling with improved glycaemic control [60]. Patients with nephropathy will almost invariably have other signs of diabetic microvascular disease, such as neuropathy or retinopathy.

Microalbuminuria: definition and measurement

Microalbuminuria refers to levels of albuminuria that are too low to be detected by conventional dipstick analysis and require the use of sensitive radioimmunoassay techniques. Microalbuminuria is defined as an excretion of 30–300 mg/day (20–200 µg/min) of albumin in an adult. In comparison, dipstick-positive albuminuria reflects values greater than 300 mg/day (200 µg/min).

Although a 24-hour urine collection is considered the gold standard for the measurement of microalbuminuria in adult patients, a number of studies have shown that the results of timed urine collections of shorter duration correlate well with those of 24-hour collections. The collection of 24-hour and timed urine samples in children is inherently difficult, and it is now common practice to use early morning spot albumin/creatinine ratios, which are cheap and easy to perform, for the detection of microalbuminuria. There is some debate regarding the albumin:creatinine ratio which best reflects microalbuminuria on a timed urine sample. Shield et al. [61] have shown a level of greater than 2.0 mg/mmol to detect microalbuminuria, based on an overnight timed sample in children, with a sensitivity of 97% and a specificity of 93%. Others have proposed a value in children and adolescents of 2.5 mg/mmol [62], and in adults a value of 3.5 mg/mmol [63]. Further debate centres around whether albumin:creatinine ratios should be used as a screening test to identify those who require a formal timed urine collection performing, or whether the albumin:creatinine ratio itself is a suitable surrogate marker. In light of the fact that there is significant interindividual variation in measured albumin excretion, it is appropriate that repeat samples are collected, and microalbuminuria not diagnosed on the basis of a single elevated value.

The renal excretion of albumin can be elevated by vigorous exercise, acute illness, fever, severe cardiac disease, urinary tract infection, menstrual bleeding, severe hypertension, poor glycaemic control, and ketoacidosis. Sample collection should therefore be avoided when such intercurrent problems are present, and vigorous exercise avoided for 24 hours prior to testing.

The reported incidence of microalbuminuria in the paediatric and adolescent population varies between 7 and 20%: the Microalbuminuria In Diabetic Adolescents and Children (MIDAC) research group, using an albumin:creatinine ratio above 2.0 mg/mmol on at least two out of three early morning urine samples as being diagnostic of microalbuminuria, reported a prevalence of microalbuminuria of 9.7% in a large population of 10–20-year-old diabetics in the United Kingdom. Children with microalbuminuria were more likely to be pubertal, older, female, and have a longer duration of diabetes than those with normal urinary albumin excretion. Puberty itself is regarded by many to be an independent risk factor for the development of, and progression of, microalbuminuria [64]. Importantly, however, the MIDAC study and others [62,65] identified a number of individuals developing microalbuminuria prior to the onset of puberty and during the first 4 years after the development of diabetes.

Key points: Microalbuminuria

- The term 'microalbuminuria' refers to levels of albuminuria that are too low to be detected by conventional dipstick analysis, and is defined as an albumin excretion of 30–300 mg/day in an adult.

- Microalbuminuria is the earliest clinical manifestation of diabetic nephropathy, but not all who develop microalbuminuria progress to overt renal disease.

- Because of difficulties in obtaining timed urine collections in children, it is now common practice to measure albumin excretion by the use of the early morning urine albumin:creatinine ratio.

- Children with diabetes should undergo annual screening for microalbuminuria, commencing 3–5 years after the onset of diabetes, or at the onset of puberty.

- There are a number of causes of false-positive tests for microalbuminuria, and positive tests should be repeated to ensure that the finding is genuine.

Of patients who develop microalbuminuria, the earliest clinical manifestation of diabetic renal disease, less than 50% are at risk of progression to overt clinical nephropathy and renal failure, and there is significant variability in the rate and speed of disease progression. The predictive value of microalbuminuria for the development of later nephropathy is probably weaker in diabetic children and adolescents than in adults. Shield *et al.* [66] followed a population of 81 children, of whom nine had evidence of microalbuminuria: five normalized and the albumin excretion rate fell in a further three with no change in glycaemic control or other therapeutic intervention. Perhaps not suprisingly, microalbuminuria appears more likely to progress where albumin excretion is more pronounced [67]. Other reported adverse risk factors for disease progression include genetic susceptibility (family history of development of nephropathy and possibly the DD ACE genotype), the presence of hypertension, increased GFR early in the disease course, poor glycaemic control, Black, Mexican American, or Pima Indian race, impaired conversion of prorenin to renin, and elevated red cell sodium–lithium countertransport activity. The risk of developing overt nephropathy appears to be less when microalbuminuria occurs late in the course of the disease.

The three major histological changes in the glomeruli in diabetic nephropathy are mesangial expansion, glomerular basement membrane thickening, and glomerular sclerosis, which may have a nodular appearance: the Kimmelstiel–Wilson lesion. There may be associated hyaline deposits in the glomerular arterioles. Renal biopsy in diabetics with microalbuminuria only may reveal normal histology or evidence of glomerulosclerosis or other changes of diabetic nephropathy. Normal histology is more likely where the level of albumin excretion is low and there is no hypertension or impairment of GFR [68,69].

Management of the child with microalbuminuria

The presence of overt diabetic nephropathy in childhood is rare and management should concentrate on the prevention of the development of and screening for the presence of microalbuminuria. Children should undergo annual screening, commencing 3–5 years after the onset of diabetes or at the onset of puberty. Either serial early morning albumin/creatinine ratios (e.g. three consecutive samples) or timed overnight samples are acceptable. The causes of false-positive microalbuminuria should be borne in mind when interpreting results and, if suspected, the investigation should be repeated.

Where microalbuminuria is detected, treatment strategies should be introduced to reduce the degree of albumin excretion, with the aim of postponing the progression to overt nephropathy and renal failure. The clearly emerging consensus opinion is that the optimal management of diabetic renal disease is not based on the administration of a single agent or agents to modify only one adverse factor. All possible risk factors should be targeted, including hyperglycaemia, microalbuminuria, and hypertension.

Glycaemic control

In an attempt to prevent the development of diabetic nephropathy, all efforts should be made to maintain good glycaemic control from the onset of diabetes. There is good evidence from the Diabetes Control and Complications Trial, which included adults and adolescents, that the use of intensive insulin therapy delays the onset and slows the progression of microalbuminuria [70]. Analysis of the adolescent data alone showed intensive therapy to slow the progression of microalbuminuria in those who had evidence of established retinopathy and or microalbuminuria at randomization [71]. Other studies have shown intensive therapy to result in less thickening of the basement membrane and matrix expansion [72]. It needs to be remembered that more intensive insulin regimens are associated with an increased risk of hypoglycaemia, though most believe that the benefits of reducing the incidence of diabetic renal disease outweigh the risks of hypoglycaemia [71].

Where microalbuminuria is detected, an attempt can be made to introduce strict glycaemic control for a period of 6–12 months. This may be very difficult to achieve in the teenage diabetic. If this is not thought to be possible, or if attempted does not result in a reduction in the degree of microalbuminuria, an ACE inhibitor should be commenced, even if the child is normotensive (see below).

ACE inhibition

A large number of studies in adult subjects have investigated the hypothesis that the administration of ACE inhibitors to normotensive diabetics with microalbuminuria reduces both albumin excretion and the rate of decline of GFR in this population. Systematic review of these studies confirms that ACE inhibitor use results in normalization or a significant reduction in albumin excretion rate and a lowering of systemic blood pressure, though to date there is no clear evidence that this reduction in albumin excretion rate is associated with a postponement of end stage renal failure [73]. Studies in adolescents have reported similar findings. It is, at present, difficult to determine whether the reduction in albumin excretion is independent of the reduction in blood pressure induced by ACE inhibition. There are a small number of studies that have shown a slight beneficial effect of ACE inhibitors in the normotensive adult diabetic with normal urinary albumin excretion, but similar paediatric data are not available.

Agents administered once daily such as enalapril and lisinopril are likely to be associated with a greater degree of compliance.

Management of hypertension

The presence of hypertension is a known adverse risk factor for the progression of microalbuminuria to overt clinical nephropathy, and treatment of hypertension will reduce blood pressure and urinary albumin excretion and lessen this risk. ACE inhibitors appear to be the logical drug of first choice as they may have renoprotective effects in addition to their antihypertensive properties [74].

Protein restriction

Systematic review has shown that in adult diabetics, the introduction of a protein-restricted diet (0.3–0.8 g/kg) results in a slowing of the progression of diabetic nephropathy towards renal failure [75]. There are, however, potential problems with such an approach, particularly in young children and adolescents. Compliance is likely to be poor and children may be placed at risk of protein malnutrition because reduction in intake may be associated with enhanced protein breakdown induced by insulin deficiency.

Key points: Management of the child with diabetes and microalbuminuria

- Proven strategies to reduce microalbuminuria include:
  - improved glycaemic control;
  - ACE inhibitors;
  - aggressive management of hypertension.

Non-diabetic renal disease

Whereas the presence of albuminuria in the child with diabetes is most commonly associated with a diagnosis of incipient or overt diabetic nephropathy, it is important to remember that it may occasionally be due to an alternative glomerular disease. Clues pointing to a non-diabetic nephropathy include the early onset of proteinuria (within 5 years of diagnosis), acute onset of disease, heavy proteinuria, the presence of an active urinary sediment (red cells and casts), and absence of diabetic retinopathy or neuropathy.

References

1. Jennette JC, Falk RJ, Andrassy K, Bacon PA, Churg J, Gross WL, Hagen EC, Hoffman GS, Hunder GG, Kallenberg CG *et al.* Nomenclature of systemic vasculitides. Proposal of an international consensus conference. *Arthritis Rheum* 1994;37:187–192.
2. Stewart M, Savage JM, Bell B, McCord B. Long term renal prognosis of Henoch Schonlein purpura in an unselected childhood population. *Eur J Pediatr* 1988; 147:113–115.
3. Allen DM, Diamond LK, Howell DA. Anaphylactoid purpura in children (Schonlein–Henoch syndrome). *Am J Dis Child* 1960;99:833–854.
4. Koskimies O, Rapola J, Savilahti E, Vilska J. Renal involvement in Schönlein–Henoch purpura. *Acta Pediatr Scand* 1974;63:357–363.
5. Kobayashi O, Wada H, Okawa K, Takeyama I. Schönlein–Henoch purpura in children. *Contrib Nephrol* 1977;4:48–71.
6. Meadow SR, Glasgow EF, White RHR, Moncrieff MW, Cameron JS, Ogg CS. Schonlein Henoch nephritis. *QJM* 1972;41:241–258.
7. Counahan R, Winterborn MH, White RHR, Heaton JM, Meadow SR, Bluett NH, Swetschin H, Cameron JS, Chantler C. Prognosis of Henoch–Schonlein nephritis in children. *BMJ* 1977;2:11–14.
8. Rosenblum ND, Winter HS. Steroid effects on the course of abdominal pain in children with Henoch–Schönlein purpura. *Pediatrics* 1987;79:1018–1021.
9. Mollica F, LiVolti S, Garozzo R, Russo G. Effectiveness of early prednisone treatment in preventing the development of nephropathy in anaphylactoid purpura. *Eur J Pediatr* 1992;151:140–144.
10. Peratoner L, Longo F, Lepore L, Freschi P. Prophylaxis and therapy of glomerulonephritis in the course of anaphylactoid purpura. The results of a polycentric clinical trial. *Acta Paediatr Scand* 1990; 79:976–977.
11. Oner A, Tinaztepe K, Erdogan O. The effect of triple therapy on rapidly progressive type of Henoch Schonlein nephritis. *Pediatr Nephrol* 1995;9:6–10.
12. Gianviti A, Trompeter RS, Barratt TM, Lythgoe MF, Dillon MJ. Retrospective study of plasma exchange in patients with idiopathic rapidly progressive glomerulonephritis and vasculitis. *Arch Dis Child* 1996; 75:186–190.
13. Niaudet P, Habib R. Methylprednisolone pulse therapy in the treatment of severe forms of Schonlein–Henoch purpura nephritis. *Pediatr Nephrol* 1998; 12:238–243.
14. Lewis MA. In *UK Renal Registry 1999 Report*, Renal Association, London.
15. Koskimies O, Mir S, Rapola J, Vilska J. Henoch Schönlein nephritis: long term prognosis of unselected patients. *Arch Dis Child* 1981;56:482–484.
16. Goldstein AR, White RHR, Akuse R, Chantler C. Long-term follow-up of childhood Henoch Schönlein nephritis. *Lancet* 1992;339:280–282.
17. Meulders Q, Prison Y, Cosyns J-P, Squifflet J-P, van Ypersele de Strihou C. Course of Henoch Schönlein nephritis after renal transplantation. Report on ten patients and review of the literature. *Transplantation* 1994;58:1179–1186.
18. Durand D, Segords A, Orfila C, Degroc F, Bories P, Giraud P, Suc J. Transplant biopsies and short-term outcome of cadaveric renal allografts. In: Hamburger F, Crosnier J, Grundfeld J, Maxwell M (eds) *Advances in Nephrology*, vol 12. Year Book Medical Publishers, Chicago pp 309–330.
19. Hasegawa A, Kawamura T, Ito H, Hasegawa O, Ogawa O, Honda M, Hajikano H. Fate of grafts with recurrent Henoch Schonlein purpura nephrotis in children. *Transplantation Proceedings* 1989; 21:2130–2133.
20. Bunchman TE, Mauer SM, Sibley RK, Vernier RL. Anaphylactoid purpura: characteristics of 16 patients who progressed to renal failure. *Pediatr Nephrol* 1988;2:393–397.
21. Schulman ST, Inocencio J, Hirsch R. Kawasaki diseaese. *Ped Clin North Am* 1995;42:1205–1222.
22. Ogawa H. Kidney pathology in muco-cutaneous lymphnode syndrome. *Jpn J Nephrol* 1985;27:1229–1237.
23. Foster BJ, Bernard C, Drummond KN. Kawasaki disease complicated by renal artery stenosis. *Arch Dis Child* 2000:83:253–255.
24. Veiga PA, Pieroni D, Baier W, Feld LG. Association of Kawasaki disease and interstitial nephritis. *Pediatr Nephrol* 1992;6:421–423.
25. Salcedo JR, Greenberg L, Kapur S. Renal histology of mucocutaneous lymph node syndrome (Kawasaki disease). *Clin Nephrol* 1988;29:47–51.
26. Ferriero DM, Wolfsdorf JI. Haemolytic uraemic syndrome associated with Kawasaki disease. *Pediatrics* 1981;68:405–406.
27. Curtis N, Levin M. Kawasaki disease thirty years on. *Curr Opin Pediatr* 1998;10:24–33.
28. Newburger JW, Takahashi M, Burns JC, Beiser AS, Chung KJ, Duffy CE, Glode MP, Mason WH, Reddy V, Sanders SP *et al.* The treatment of Kawasaki syndrome with intravenous gammaglobulin. *N Engl J Med* 1986;315: 341–347.
29. Wong S-N, Shah V, Dillon MJ. Anti-neutrophil cytoplasmic antibodies (ANCA) in childhood systemic vasculitis. *J Am Soc Nephrol* 1992;3:668.
30. Brogan PA, Dillon MJ. The use of immunosuppressive and cytotoxic drugs in non-malignant disease. *Arch Dis Child* 2000;83:259–264.

31. Couser WG. Rapidly progressive glomerulonephritis: classification, pathogenetic mechanisms and therapy. *Am J Kidney Dis* 1988;11:449–464.

32. Dillon MJ. Childhood vasculitis. *Lupus* 1998; 7:259–265.

33. Cameron JS Lupus nephritis in childhood and adolescence. *Pediatr Nephrol* 1994;8:230–249.

34. Hochberg MC. Updating the American College of Rheumatology revised criteria for the classification of systemic lupus erythematosus. *Arthritis Rheum* 1997;40:1725.

35. Font J, Cervera R, Espinosa G, Pallares L, Ramos-Casals M, Jiminez S, Garcia-Carrasco M, Seisdedos L, Ingelmo M. Systemic lupus erythematosus (SLE) in childhood: analysis of clinical and immunological findings in 34 patients and comparison with SLE characteristics in adults. *Ann Rheum Dis* 1998;57:456–459.

36. Churg J, Sobin LH. *Renal disease: classification and atlas of glomerular disease*, Tokyo, New York, Igabu Skoin 1982.

37. Symmons DP, Coppock JS, Bacon PA, Bresnihan B, Isenberg DA, Maddison P, McHugh N, Snaith ML, Zoma AS. Development and assessment of a computerized index of clinical disease activity in systemic lupus erythematosis. Members of the British Isles Lupus Assessment Group (BILAG) *QJM* 1988;69:927–937.

38. Bobmardier C, Gladman DD, Urowitz MB, Caron D, Chang CH. Derivation of SLEDAI. A disease activity index for lupus patients. The Committee on Prognosis Studies in SLE. *Arthritis Rheum* 1992;35:630–640.

39. Lehman TJA A practical guide to Systemic Lupus Erythematosis. *Paediatric Clin North America* 1995; 42:1223–1238.

40. Silverman E. What's new in the treatment of paediatric SLE. *J Rheumatol* 1996;23:1657–1660.

41. Boumpas DT, Austin HA III, Vaughn EM, Klippel JH, Steinberg AD, Yarboro CH, Barlow JE. Controlled trial of pulse methylprednisolone versus two regimens of pulse cyclophosphamide in severe lupus nephritis. *Lancet* 1992;340:741–745.

42. Austin HA III, Klippel JH, Balow JE, le Riche NG, Steinberg AD, Plotz PH, Decker JL. Therapy of lupus nephritis. Controlled trial of prednisone and cytotoxic drugs. *N Engl J Med* 1986;314: 614–619.

43. Slater CA, Liang MH, McCune JW, Christman GM, Laufer MR. Preserving gonadal function in patients receiving cyclophosphamide. *Lupus* 1999;8:3–10.

44. Schaller JG. Therapy for childhood rheumatic diseases. Have we been doing enough? *Arthritis Rheum* 1991;36:65–70.

45. Lehman TJ. Long term cyclophophosphamide therapy of childhood systemic lupus erythematosis. *Arthritis Rheum* 1993;36:260.

46. Lehman TJ, Onel K. Intermittent intravenous cyclophosphamide arrests progression of the renal chronicity index in childhood lupus erythematosis. *J Pediatr* 2000;136:243–247.

47. Ilowite NT. Childhood systemic lupus erythematosis, dermatomyositis, scleroderma and systemic vasculitis. *Curr Opin Rheumatol* 1993;5:644–650.

48. Belostotsky VM, Dillon MJ. Systemic lupus erythematosis in children. *Current Paediatrics* 1998;8:252–257.

49. Morales MM, Falkenstein D, Lopes AG. The cystic fibrosis transmembrane regulator (CFTR) in the kidney. *An Acad Bras Cienc* 2000;72:399–406.

50. Katz SM, Krueger LJ, Falkner B. Microscopic nephrocalcinosis in cystic fibrosis. *N Engl J Med* 1988; 319:263–266.

51. Hoppe B, Hesse A, Bromme S, Rietschel E, Michalk D. Urinary excretion substances in patients with cystic fibrosis: risk of urolithiasis? *Pediatr Nephrol* 1998; 12:275–279.

52. Weiss MF. Etiology, pathophysiology, and diagnosis of acute renal failure. In Hrick DE, Sedor JR, Ganz MB, eds. *Nephrology secrets*. Hanley and Belfus, Philadelphia, 1999, pp 29–32.

53. Bennett WM. Drug interactions and consequences of sodium restriction. *Am J Clin Nutr.* 1997; 65: 678S–681S.

54. Stirati G, Antonelli M, Fofi C, Fierimonte S, Pecci G. IgA nephropathy in cystic fibrosis. *J Nephrol* 1999; 12:30–31.

55. Kuwertz-Broking E, Koch HG, Schulze EA, Bulla M, Dworinczak B, Helmchen U, Harms E. Colchicine for secondary nephropathic amyloidosis in cystic fibrosis. *Lancet* 1995;345:1178–1179.

56. Finnegan MJ, Hinchcliffe J, Russell-Jones D, Neill S, Sheffield E, Jayne D, Wise A, Hodson ME. Vasculitis complicating cystic fibrosis. *QJM* 1989; 72:609–621.

57. Magryta CJ, Hennigar R, Weatherly M. Pathological case of the month. Diabetic nephropathy in cystic fibrosis. *Arch Pediatr Adolesc Med* 1999; 153:1307–1308.

58. *Second Annual Report of the United Kingdom Renal Registry*, United Kingdom Renal Association, Dec. 1999.

59. Orchard TJ, Dorman JS, Maser RE, Becker DJ, Drash AL, Ellis D, LaPorte R, Kuller LH. Prevalence of complications in IDDM by sex and duration. Pittsburgh Epidemiology of Diabetes Complications Study I. *Diabetes* 1990:39:1116–1124.

60. Bojestig M, Arnquist H, Hermansson G, Karlberg B, Ludvigsson J. Declining incidence of nephropathy in insulin-dependent diabetes mellitus. *N Engl J Med* 1994;330:15–18.

61. Shield JPH, Hunt LP, Baum JD, Pennock CA. Screening for diabetic microalbuminuria in routine clinical care: which method? *Arch Dis Child* 1995;72:524–525.

62. Jones CA, Leese GP, Kerr S, Bestwisk K, Isherwood DI, Vora JP, Hughes DA, Smith C. Development and progression of microalbuminuria in a clinic sample of patients with insulin dependent diabetes mellitus. *Arch Dis Child* 1998;78:518–523.

63. Marshall SM. Screening for microalbuminuria: which measurement? *Diabet Med* 1991;8:706–711.

64. Barkai L, Vamosi I, Lukacs K. Enhanced progression of urinary albumin excretion in IDDM during puberty. *Diabetes Care* 1998;21:1019–1023.

65. Holl RW, Grabert M, Thon A, Heinze E. Urinary excretion of albumin in adolescents with type 1 diabetes : persistent versus intermittent microalbuminuria and relationship to duration of diabetes, sex, and metabolic control. *Diabetes Care* 1999;22:1555–1560.

66. Shield JPH, Hunt LP, Karachaliou F, Karavanakj K, Baum JD. Is microalbuminuria progressive? *Arch Dis Child* 1995;73:512–514.

67. Rudberg S, Dahlquist G. Determinants of progression of microalbuminuria in adolescents with IDDM. *Diabetes Care* 1996;19:369–371.

68. Fioretto P, Steffes MW, Mauer M. Glomerular structure in nonproteinuric IDDM patients with various levels of albuminuria. *Diabetes* 1994;43:1358–1364.

69. Chavers BM, Bilous RW, Ellis EN, Steffes MW, Mauer SM. Glomerular lesions and urinary albumin excretion in type 1 diabetes without overt proteinuria. *N Engl J Med* 1989;320:759–760.

70. Diabetes Control and Complications Trial Research Group. The effect of intensive treatment of diabetes on the development and progression of long-term complications in insulin-dependent diabetes mellitus. *N Engl J Med* 1993;329:977–986.

71. Diabetes Control and Complications Trial Research Group. Effect of intensive diabetes treatment on the development and progression of long-term complications in adolescents with insulin dependent diabetes mellitus: Diabetes Control and Complications Trial. *J Pediatr* 1994;125:177–188.

72. Bangstad HJ, Osterby R, Dahl-Jorgensen K, Berg KJ, Hartmann A, Hanssen KF. Improvement of blood glucose control in IDDM patients retards the progression of morphological changes in early diabetic nephropathy. *Diabetologia* 1994;37:483–490.

73. Lovell HG. *Angiotensin converting enzyme inhibitors in normotensive diabetic patients with microalbuminuria (Cochrane Review)*. The Cochrane Library, Issue 3, 2001. Update Software, Oxford.

74. Taal MW, Brenner BM. Renoprotective benefits of RAS inhibition: from ACEI to angiotensin antagonists. *Kidney Int* 2000;57:1803–1817.

75. Waugh NR, Robertson AM. *Protein restriction for diabetic renal disease (Cochrane review)*. The Cochrane Library, Issue 3, 2001. Update Software, Oxford.

22 | *The child with acute renal failure*

Margaret M. Fitzpatrick, Steve J. Kerr, and Mark G. Bradbury

Introduction

Acute renal failure is characterized by an abrupt and sustained decline in glomerular filtration rate [1] leading to an increase in the blood concentration of urea and creatinine and the inability of the kidney to regulate fluid and electrolyte balance effectively. While mortality rates in children with acute renal failure in the intensive care setting remain high, full recovery of renal function can be made; this is particularly so for the pre-renal causes, which will often respond promptly to correction of intravascular volume deficit.

The aim of this chapter is to discuss the pathogenesis, diagnosis, and management of the child with acute renal failure. The initial management of the child presenting with acute renal failure to the district hospital is discussed in detail, with particular emphasis on the management of life-threatening emergencies and indications for transfer to a tertiary paediatric nephrology centre. Management of acute renal failure in the tertiary centre is also discussed, including information on the various techniques of renal replacement therapy.

Definitions and pathogenesis

In childhood, acute renal failure may be associated with anuria, oliguria, a normal urine output, or high urine output (polyuric acute renal failure). Oliguria is defined in infants and young children as a urine output of less than 0.5–1 ml/kg/hour and in older children an output of less than 400–500 ml per 24 hours. Anuria is defined as a urine output of less than 1 ml/kg/day. Hyperkalaemia is common and a potentially life-threatening electrolyte abnormality in acute renal failure. True hyperkalaemia (as opposed to pseudohyperkalaemia, see Chapter 2) produces disturbances of cardiac rhythm by its depolarizing effect on the cardiac conduction pathways. The potassium level producing these problems is dependent on the acid–base balance and on other plasma electrolytes. Hypocalcaemia in particular, which also occurs in renal failure, exacerbates the adverse effects of potassium on cardiac conduction. Tall peaked T-waves are the first manifestation of cardiotoxicity. Significant intravascular fluid overload leads to hypertension, cardiac failure, and pulmonary oedema.

Acute renal failure is a multifactorial process involving alterations in renal haemodynamics, specific nephronal susceptibilities, intratubular obstruction, and cellular and metabolic fluxes. Renal vasoconstriction has been considered the dominant renal haemodynamic factor in the pathogenesis of acute renal failure and it has been postulated that an insult to the renal tubular epithelium results in the release of vasoactive compounds that increase cortical vascular resistance, so decreasing renal blood flow and producing injury to the tubule. The release of vasoconstrictive compounds diminishes GFR by constricting the afferent and efferent arterioles, leading to a reduction in urine output. The emphasis has been on identifying and investigating vasoactive compounds that are stimulated or induced by ischaemic or toxic insults, including angiotensin, prostaglandins, endothelin, and nitric oxide. Despite the fact that renal vasoconstriction is well documented as a significant factor initiating acute renal failure, vasodilatation does not consistently result in improvement of renal function, for example the infusion of prostaglandins or dopamine is not associated with a sustained improvement of GFR [2]. Renal haemodynamic factors do undoubtedly play an important role in the initiation of acute renal failure, but alterations in renal vascular resistance and renal perfusion are not the sole determinants of epithelial cell injury.

Cellular and metabolic alterations involving reactive oxygen molecules have been implicated in a variety of renal diseases, including reperfusion injury after ischaemia [3]; the most highly reactive molecules being free radicals, such as the hydroxyl radical or superoxide anion. Reactive oxygen metabolites may contribute to ischaemia by interaction with nitric oxide synthetases, and because of these putative effects the role of reactive oxygen molecules in ischaemia–reperfusion injury has been thoroughly researched, with evidence both for and against their having a dominant role [3,4]. Fluctuations in adenine nucleotide metabolism, associated with energy depletion and restoration, are also believed to play a role in renal cell injury [5] and are both a consequence and a predictor of renal cell injury. A reduction in cellular ATP leads to a disruption of epithelial cell structure and function, with increased intracellular calcium, activation of phospholipases, loss of polarity, and detachment of the cortical cytoskeleton. It is also now appreciated that cell death after an ischaemic or toxic insult occurs by necrosis or apoptosis, a gene-directed process leading to irrevocable DNA damage [6]. Apoptosis is the result of the interaction of promoters such as tumour necrosis factor and inhibitors such as growth factors, and represents an important mechanism of cell death but its role in acute renal failure still remains unclear. It is unlikely that any single mechanism can explain the complexities of acute renal failure that results in the destruction of renal epithelial cells and the acute loss of renal function.

Incidence/prevalence

Two prospective observational studies (total $n = 2576$) in adult practice have found that established acute renal failure affected nearly 5% of patients in hospitals and as many as 15% of critically ill adults, depending on the definitions used [7,8]. In paediatric practice, it is difficult to establish the true incidence of acute renal failure because its definition varies from study to study. It has been reported to be present in between 1 and 3% of admissions to neonatal units, with 50% of cases responding to a fluid challenge [9]. Acute renal failure is particularly prevalent in neonates who survive perinatal asphyxia and shock. The incidence of acute renal failure in older children has been estimated at around 4/100 000 child population. In pre-school children, diarrhoea-associated haemolytic uraemic syndrome remains the most common cause of intrinsic acute renal failure, accounting for more than 50% of all cases in this age group. Glomerulonephritis is a more common cause of acute renal failure in school-age children. There is

concern that an increasing incidence of acute renal failure is occurring in association with multi-organ failure in paediatric intensive care units, following cardiac surgery, and with sepsis/ multi-organ failure in oncology units, although the actual incidence in these areas remains unclear.

Key points: Incidence of acute renal failure in childhood

- The true incidence of acute renal failure is difficult to determine because of variation in its definition from study to study.

- Acute renal failure occurs in between 1 and 3% of admissions to neonatal units.

- There is concern that the incidence of acute renal failure in association with multi-organ failure in paediatric intensive care units, following cardiac surgery, and with sepsis/multi-organ failure in oncology units is increasing.

Classification of acute renal failure

The causes of acute renal failure are classified as pre-renal (Table 22.1), intrinsic renal (Table 22.2), or post-renal (Table 22.3). Pre-renal implies that the cause of the renal failure is reduced blood flow into the kidneys, intrinsic renal that the cause is within the kidney (a renal parenchymal lesion of whatever aetiology),

Table 22.1 Causes of pre-renal failure

Hypovolaemia	Bilateral renal vessel
Gastroenteritis	occlusion
Gastrointestinal drainage	Arterial
Diabetic ketoacidosis	Venous
Hypoproteinaemic states	Drugs
Haemorrhage	Prostaglandin synthetase
Third space losses	inhibitors
Peripheral vasodilatation	Angiotensin-converting
Sepsis	enzyme inhibitors
Antihypertensive	Ciclosporin A
medications, i.e. calcium	Diuretics
channel antagonists	Others
Impaired cardiac output	Increased
Congestive cardiac failure	intraabdominal pressure
Cardiac tamponade	Hepatorenal syndrome

Table 22.2 Causes of intrinsic renal failure

Diseases of kidney or vessels	Tumour infiltrate
Acute glomerulonephritis	Nephrotoxic drugs
Acute tubular necrosis following prolonged	Antimicrobials
pre-renal impairment	Contrast media
Bilateral acute pyelonephritis	Anaesthetics
Haemolytic uraemic syndrome	Heavy metals
Acute interstitial nephritis	
Cortical or medullary necrosis	Organic solvents
Vasculitis, polyarteritis	
Hypercalcaemia, hyperphosphataemia,	Petroleum distillates
Hyperuricaemia	Insecticides
Acute disease in the presence of chronic	Cytotoxic agents
disease	Non-steroidal anti-inflammatory agents
Myoglobinuria, haemoglobinuria	Ciclosporin A
Intratubular obstruction	Diuretics
Sulphonamides	
Uric acid	
Methotrexate	
Iatrogenic factors	
Removal of solitary kidney	
Renal arteriogram	

Table 22.3 Causes of post-renal failure

Obstruction
    Posterior urethral valves
    Blocked bladder catheter
    Neurogenic bladder
    Surgical accident
    Calculi
    Ureterocele
    Tumours
    Trauma

and post-renal that the cause is obstruction to the outflow of urine from the kidney. These groups are not mutually exclusive and the same initial insult may cause both pre-renal and intrinsic renal failure, e.g. shock initially causing pre-renal failure but then progressing to acute tubular or cortical necrosis. The same is true of obstruction such as a severe pelvi-ureteric or vesico-ureteric junction obstruction, which if left untreated may result in permanent renal injury.

All three forms of renal impairment may be associated with a decrease in urine output and rise in plasma creatinine and urea. It is helpful to think about the clinical presentations of acute renal failure in children to alert clinicians to the possible mechanisms of injury. This may provide an opportunity to correct these mechanisms and avoid possible secondary injury due, for example, to the inappropriate restriction of fluids or the prescription of nephrotoxic drugs.

The child with acute renal failure

The aim of this section is to provide a practical guide to the management of acute renal failure with an emphasis on early diagnosis and treatment in the district hospital setting. It is organized to follow the time line of a child admitted to a district hospital and indicates priorities in management.

Clinical history

Given the multiplicity of causes of acute renal failure, a structured approach to the clinical history and examination is important (Table 22.4). Often, the cause of the renal failure is readily apparent from the clinical history: a history of bloody diarrhoea 5–7 days prior to the onset of renal failure points strongly to a diagnosis of haemolytic uraemic syndrome. Other diagnoses, e.g. acute interstitial nephritis, have wide-ranging causes, emphasizing the importance of a comprehensive drug and recent infection history.

Examination will sometimes assist in determining the aetiology of the renal failure. The presence of rash, arthropathy, and fever may indicate a diagnosis of glomerulonephritis, vasculitis, or interstitial nephritis,

Table 22.4 Important aspects of the clinical history and examination in the assessment of the child with acute renal failure

---

A careful history should be taken including the following details:
History of any prodromal illness:
    Diarrhoea ± blood with associated dehydration
    Other events likely to result in volume depletion (see Table 22.1)
    Acute pharyngitis/skin infection
    Other infection
    Fever
    Rash, arthropathy, weight loss
Presence or absence of urinary symptoms
    Haematuria, dysuria, frequency, loin, or abdominal pain
    Poor urinary stream
    Oliguria or anuria
Antenatal history including details of ultrasound scans
Drug history
History of toxin exposure
History of foreign travel
Details of other specific symptoms
Urine output, fluid intake, fluid losses
Recent weight measurements
Previous significant illness, e.g. cardiac or liver disease and previous surgery
Family history of renal disease
A detailed examination should be performed paying particular attention to:
Weight and height
Temperature
State of hydration
    Evidence of dehydration
    Evidence of generalized oedema
Haemodynamic status
    Evidence of intravascular volume depletion (poor capillary refill, hypotension, tachycardia)
    Evidence of intravascular volume overload (hypertension, periorbital or peripheral oedema, tachypnoea)
Respiratory status
    Evidence of tachypnoea secondary to acidosis, fluid overload, or pulmonary interstitial disease
Abdominal examination
    Evidence of renal mass or palpable enlarged bladder
    Evidence of costovertebral tenderness
Neurological examination
    Evidence of confusion, drowsiness
    Manifestations of hypocalcaemia
    Evidence of focal neurological abnormality
Full systems examination for causes or sequelae of renal failure
    Rash, arthropathy

---

and in post-renal renal failure due to renal tract obstruction, flank masses or a palpable bladder may be detectable. Importantly, examination will also help ascertain the degree of fluid overload and other complications that have arisen as a result of the renal failure.

Establishing a diagnosis of acute renal failure

A diagnosis of acute renal failure may be suspected on clinical findings, but requires biochemical confirmation. A comprehensive list of investigations useful in establishing the diagnosis, severity, and likely aetiology of acute renal failure are shown in Tables 22.5 and 22.6. At this early stage, investigations are focused on those necessary to confirm the diagnosis and identify any life-threatening abnormalities (plasma biochemistry, full blood count, urinalysis, urine chemistry, and renal ultrasound scan). Subsequently, further more complex tests may be required (specific immunological investigations, radio-isotope scans, and renal biopsy) to help identify the specific diagnosis.

Table 22.5 Laboratory investigations indicated in acute renal failure

	Indication
Blood	
Electrolytes, creatinine, and urea	Degree of renal impairment and electrolyte disturbance
Glucose	? Hyperglycaemia, e.g. secondary to HUS
Osmolality	? Concentrating abnormality
Calcium and phosphate	Degree of hypocalcaemia/hyperphosphataemia secondary to renal impairment or hypercalcaemia as cause
Albumin and total proteins	? Hypoproteinaemia secondary to proteinuria
Uric acid	? Uric acid nephropathy
Creatinine kinase/LDH	? Intravascular haemolysis, e.g. secondary to HUS
Haptoglobins	? Intravascular haemolysis, e.g. secondary to HUS
Parathyroid hormone	? Evidence of long-standing renal failure
Immunological investigations	? Immunological cause for renal failure
C3, C4, CH50	
ANCA, ASOT	
ANA, anti-double-stranded DNA antibodies	
Anti-glomerular basement membrane antibodies	
Immunoglobulins	
Full blood count and film possibly reticulocyte count	? Evidence of haemolysis, bleeding, long-standing anaemia
Coagulation screen	? Evidence of coagulopathy
Blood culture	? Sepsis related acute renal failure
E. coli antibodies	To determine cause of HUS
Hepatitis B and C serology	To determine cause of renal failure and to determine whether special precautions are necessary if dialysis is commenced
Urine	
Urinalysis – blood, protein, glucose	? Evidence suggesting glomerular/tubular disease
Protein creatinine ratio	? Evidence of glomerular/tubular disease
Microscopy and culture	? Evidence of casts suggesting glomerular disease
	? Evidence of urinary infection
Osmolality	? Evidence of concentrating defect
Sodium, creatinine, and urea	To assist distinguishing renal from pre-renal failure
Myoglobin	? Rhabdomyolysis
Toxicology	? Poisoning as cause of renal failure
Stool	
Culture and sensitivity	Pathogens causing HUS. e.g. E coli O157:H7

Table 22.6 Radiological investigations indicated in acute renal failure

Investigation	Questions to be answered
Chest X-ray	Fluid overload
	Heart size
	Pulmonary infiltrates
Ultrasound kidneys and bladder	Size and structure of kidneys
	Echotexture of kidneys
	Presence of urine in bladder
	Enlarged bladder, thick-walled bladder
	Dilated ureters
	Hydronephrosis
	Cause of obstruction if present
	Nephrocalcinosis
Doppler study	Arterial and venous blood flow
Radionucleotide scans MAG3, DTPA, DMSA	Evidence of renal scarring or renal obstruction
Wrist X-ray (plus other bones)	Renal bone disease
MCUG	Vesico-ureteric reflux
MR or CT scan	Cause of obstruction
	Brain imaging if required

DMSA, dimercaptosuccinic acid; DTPA, diethylenetriaminepentaacetic acid; MAG3, mercaptoacetyltriglycine; MCUG, micturating cystourethrography; MR, magnetic resonance; CT, computed tomography.

Correct life-threatening abnormalities

Life-threatening emergencies in acute renal failure are summarized in Table 22.7.

Hyperkalaemia

Normal values for serum potassium are given in Chapter 28 and pseudohyperkalaemia is discussed in Chapter 2. True hyperkalaemia, particularly when associated with ECG changes, constitutes a medical emergency due to the risk of complex dysrhythmias. The use of a cardiac monitor is therefore mandatory. Where ECG changes are present (see Fig. 2.4), 10% calcium gluconate should be administered to reduce the cardiotoxic effects of potassium (Table 22.8). In this situation, the use of a cardiac monitor is mandatory. Strategies should then be employed to reduce the plasma potassium level (Table 22.8). No studies have compared the relative efficacies of these

treatments, and the choice of potassium-lowering agent remains a matter of personal preference. Many favour the use of nebulized salbutamol as it is rapid in onset of action, safe, and readily available on virtually all paediatric wards. Salbutamol acts by moving potassium from the extracellular into the intracellular space. Other agents with a similar mode of action include sodium bicarbonate and dextrose with or without insulin. The administration of sodium bicarbonate may be complicated by a reduction in the plasma ionized calcium, with possible risk of tetany and, if used repeatedly, the development of hypernatraemia, intravascular volume overload, and hypertension. The administration of dextrose and insulin clearly requires regular monitoring of blood glucose levels.

Ion-exchange resins such as calcium resonium remove potassium from the body by exchanging calcium or sodium for potassium, which is passed from the body in the stool. The onset of action is relatively slow, and these drugs have a very limited role in the management of significant hyperkalaemia associated with acute renal failure.

It is essential that plasma potassium levels are checked regularly once therapy for hyperkalaemia has been commenced. It is important to appreciate that most of the treatments are only stabilizing procedures employed while dialysis is being organized. This is particularly true in the anuric or severely oliguric child, where plasma potassium levels are unlikely to fall spontaneously.

Table 22.7 Life-threatening emergencies in acute renal failure requiring immediate treatment

Hyperkalaemia
Metabolic acidosis
Shock
Hypertension
Fluid overload
Hyponatraemia and hypernatraemia
Hypocalcaemia

Table 22.8 Treatment of hyperkalaemia

1. *Stabilization of the myocardium*	
10% Calcium gluconate	0.5–1 ml/kg i.v. over 5–10 minutes
2. *Shift of potassium from extracellular to intracellular compartment*	
Salbutamol	2.5 mg if <25 kg and 5 mg if >25 kg via nebulizer
	4 µg/kg infused i.v. over 10 minutes
Sodium bicarbonate	1–2 mmol/kg i.v. (=1–2 ml/kg of 8.4% solution)
Dextrose and/or insulin	0.5–1 g/kg/h dextrose (2.5–5 ml/kg/h of 20% dextrose) with insulin 0.2 units for every gram of glucose administered. Aim to maintain blood glucose at 10–15 mmol/l
3. *Removal of potassium from the body*	
Dialysis (see section in text)	
Haemodialysis	
Peritoneal dialysis	
Haemofiltration	
Ion exchange resins	
Calcium resonium	1 g/kg p.o. or p.r.
Sodium resonium	1 g/kg p.o. or p.r.

Key points: Hyperkalaemia

- Hyperkalaemia, particularly when associated with ECG changes, is a medical emergency.

- The use of a cardiac monitor is mandatory.

- The myocardium should be stabilized by the administration of intravenous calcium.

- Salbutamol is effective at rapidly reducing plasma potassium levels, is safe, and is widely available on paediatric wards.

- Repeat blood tests should be performed to ensure that the potassium levels respond to therapy.

- Potassium-lowering agents such as salbutamol act by moving potassium from the extracellular into the intracellular space. Dialysis reduces total body potassium, and should be considered wherever potassium levels are very high or where hyperkalaemia or renal failure are likely to persist.

Metabolic acidosis

In acute renal failure, the inability to excrete hydrogen ions and an increased rate of production result in acidosis (see Chapter 3). Intravenous 8.4% sodium bicarbonate (1–2 ml/kg, equivalent to 1–2 mmol/ kg of bicarbonate or a dose calculated on base-deficit: see Chapter 3) should be administered where blood pH values are less than 7.25. Adequacy of pH correction should be assessed by the regular measurement of blood gases. Side-effects of sodium bicarbonate therapy include hypernatraemia and hypertension. Children with acidosis refractory to intravenous bicarbonate therapy and those who develop side-effects with therapy should be considered for dialysis. Good nutrition reduces the rate of endogenous acid production and is an important aspect of treatment.

Shock

Children with intravascular hypovolaemia require urgent treatment with intravenous fluids: 20 ml/kg of fluid should be given in the first instance and repeated until circulatory insufficiency has been corrected. Where bleeding has occurred, the logical choice of fluid is whole blood, but in the absence of bleeding, there is little to choose between 0.9% saline, 5% albumin, artificial colloids or Ringer's lactate. The child known to have severe hypoalbuminaemia associated with nephrotic syndrome of whatever cause is most logically treated with an albumin-containing solution.

When hypovolaemia is corrected rapidly and adequately and is the sole reason for oliguria (pre-renal failure), the restoration of the circulatory volume should result in an increase in urine output and subsequent correction of the biochemical abnormalities.

Hypertension

Hypertension associated with acute renal failure may be due to volume overload, renal parenchymal or renovascular pathology. Where hypertension is secondary to fluid overload, fluid restriction or diuretic therapy may be helpful. If this proves unsuccessful or the child is oligoanuric and at risk of developing hypertensive encephalopathy, then prompt removal of excess fluid is required using dialysis or haemofiltration. The use of antihypertensive medications may be indicated if the underlying cause is renal parenchymal renovascular disease and if the blood pressure is so elevated that there is a significant risk of neurological sequelae. Bite and swallow nifedipine is simple to use, is effective and generally safe, but may cause headache and palpitation, and has rarely been associated with a rapid fall in blood pressure, which should be avoided. Difficult hypertension or hypertensive encephalopathy are best treated with an intravenous infusion of labetolol, adjusting the rate according to response and aiming to slowly reduce BP to a safe level over 4–6 hours (see Chapter 8).

Fluid overload

The profoundly oliguric child with acute renal failure may present with evidence of intravascular volume overload, manifested by hypertension and congestive cardiac failure. Loop diuretics should be administered in the first instance in an attempt to increase urine output, although if such therapy is unsuccessful, then dialysis is indicated. Some children will require ventilatory support while emergency dialysis is being organized.

Hyponatraemia and hypernatraemia

In oliguric renal failure, losses of sodium are negligible and no additional sodium is generally required unless there are significant losses from the gastro-intestinal tract. These losses can be estimated and appropriate replacement given. In polyuric renal failure, it is necessary to measure the urinary sodium to ensure accurate replacement. Hyponatraemia is the common finding in children with acute renal failure, and is most frequently secondary to water excess rather than sodium loss, unless the history suggests significant gastrointestinal losses. If doubt exists, it is safer to restrict water intake until the cause becomes apparent. Profound hyponatraemia (plasma sodium of less than 120 mmol/l) or hypernatraemia (plasma sodium greater than 160 mmol/l) may cause serious neurological disturbances with seizures, encephalopathy, or intracerebral haemorrhage. Correction of hyponatraemia to a sodium level of around 125 mmol/l with hypertonic saline should be considered, though this may be associated with significant side-effects, particularly if the plasma sodium is corrected too vigorously, and should only be undertaken with extreme caution. The management of hyponatraemia is discussed in detail in Chapter 2.

Hypocalcaemia

Children with acute renal failure may be hypocal-caemic, although they are generally asymptomatic. The administration of sodium bicarbonate for the treatment of either acidosis or hyperkalaemia reduces ionized calcium levels and may induce symptoms including carpopedal spasm and seizures. These should be treated with intravenous 10% calcium gluconate (0.1 mmol/kg/h, which is equivalent to 0.5 ml/kg/h of 10% calcium gluconate), with the infusion rate being titrated according to blood values.

Establish the cause, degree, and complications of renal failure

Identifying an acute presentation of chronic renal disease

Up to 10% of children presenting acutely will have chronic renal disease. A careful clinical and detailed family history are very important in identifying these cases (see Table 23.5). A history of chronic illness, poor growth, and previous recurrent urinary-tract infections is suggestive of reflux nephropathy; poly-dipsia, polyuria, and wetting may be indicative of a concentrating defect, as occurs in many forms of

---

> ## Key points: Acute renal failure emergencies
>
> - Intravenous 8.4% sodium bicarbonate (1–2 ml/kg, equivalent to 1–2 mmol/kg of bicarbonate or a dose calculated on base-deficit: see Chapter 3) should be administered slowly where blood pH values are less than 7.25.
>
> - Children with intravascular hypovolaemia require urgent treatment with intravenous fluids.
>
> - Hypertension associated with acute renal failure may be due to volume overload, renal parenchymal or renovascular pathology.
>
> - The profoundly oliguric child with acute renal failure may present with evidence of intravascular volume overload:
>   - loop diuretics should be administered in the first instance;
>   - if such therapy is unsuccessful, then dialysis is indicated;
>   - some children will require ventilatory support while emergency dialysis is being organized.
>
> - Hyponatraemia is a common finding in children with acute renal failure:
>   - it is most frequently secondary to water excess rather than sodium loss.

---

chronic renal disease including nephronophthisis. Failure to thrive, anaemia, rickets, and signs of end-organ involvement, such as left ventricular hypertrophy and retinopathy, are markers of chronic renal disease, which may be associated with hypertension. Small kidneys on ultrasound, radiological evidence of renal bone disease, and a raised parathyroid hormone all suggest chronic or acute on chronic renal impairment.

Identifying post-renal failure

Post-renal causes of renal failure can be simply and safely identified by performing a renal ultrasound scan looking for the presence of hydronephrosis. This should be done soon after presentation in every child with renal impairment, though is probably best performed when the child is replete of fluids; absence of hydronephrosis in the dry child is not conclusive evidence of the absence of obstruction. Where obstructive lesions, e.g. posterior urethral valves or neuropathic bladder are detected, early referral to a paediatric urologist is essential. Where post-renal causes are not detected, the ultrasound scan will provide additional information. As outlined above, the detection of small kidneys suggests that the child has long-standing renal impairment, and the large majority of children with acute intrinsic renal failure have kidneys which are either enlarged or normal in size and bright ultrasonographically.

Distinguishing pre-renal from intrinsic renal failure

It is important to ascertain whether the newly presenting patient has pre-renal failure or intrinsic renal failure (Table 22.9). The early identification of prerenal failure is important, as restoration of the intravascular circulatory volume may result in an improvement in urine output and plasma biochemistries, whereas failure to do so may result in the development of intrinsic renal failure. It is important in this setting to ascertain the child's urine output accurately; this may necessitate the use of a urinary catheter.

The *fractional excretion of sodium (FE_{Na})* can be a useful tool in delineating pre-renal from intrinsic renal failure. This calculation estimates the amount of sodium that is filtered by the glomeruli but then escapes tubular reabsorption and is excreted in the urine. The use of FE_{Na} is discussed in detail in Chapter 2 with illustrative cases. Others have found calculation of free water clearance to be helpful in

distinguishing pre-renal from intrinsic renal causes. This has not been validated in children and is discussed elsewhere [10].

Determining the precise cause of acute renal failure

Having established that acute renal failure is present and having treated life-threatening abnormalities as outlined above, the next step should be to ascertain the aetiology of the renal failure. Tables 22.5 and 22.6 list those investigations likely to be helpful with regard to this. In conditions such as haemolytic uraemic syndrome, the diagnosis will have been confirmed by the initial investigations as outlined above, though other diagnoses require more comprehensive investigation. This may involve transfer of the child to a tertiary paediatric nephrology centre for consideration for renal biopsy. This is discussed later.

Key points: Investigating specific causes of acute renal failure

- Up to 10% of children presenting acutely will have chronic renal disease.

- Post-renal causes of renal failure can be simply and safely identified by performing a renal ultrasound scan, looking for the presence of hydronephrosis. This should be done soon after presentation.

- The early identification of pre-renal failure is important, as treatment may improve urine output and plasma biochemistries.

Initial management of the child with acute renal failure at the district hospital

Where pre-renal failure is suspected from clinical examination and/or the results of the above investigations, the child should be given a fluid challenge—10 ml/kg 0.9% saline given intravenously over 30 minutes and the urine output reassessed. If there is no improvement and no signs of fluid overload, then this should be repeated. If there is still no improvement, then a clinical decision has to be made regarding the child's intravascular volume status, as further fluid administration could be potentially hazardous in the

---

Table 22.9 Investigations useful in distinguishing pre-renal from intrinsic renal failure

Investigation	Pre-renal renal failure		Intrinsic renal failure	
	Children	Neonates	Children	Neonates
U_{Na} (mmol/l)	<20	<40	>50	>40
U_{osm} (mosm/kg H_2O)	>500	>400	<300	<400
FE_{Na}	<1	<2	>1	>3

U_{Na}, Urinary sodium; U_{osm}, urinary osmolality; FE_{Na}, fractional excretion of sodium (see text).

anuric child who is volume replete. If clinical assessment is for any reason difficult, then more invasive assessment of intravascular volume and cardiac output may be needed. This will nearly always involve transfer to a tertiary paediatric nephrology centre (see below). Where urine output has not improved despite these corrective measures, and the child is felt clinically to be volume replete, many would recommend a trial dose of an intravenous loop diuretic (furosemide up to a maximum of 4 mg/kg/dose) to ascertain whether this induces a diuresis. Non-oliguric acute renal failure is easier to manage than oliguric renal failure. Where diuretic administration results in an improvement in urine output, further doses can be given on a regular basis. There are some problems inherent with such an approach: these are discussed later. At this point, the child's fluid intake should be reduced so that they receive only their insensible losses (300–400 ml/m^2/ day) plus their urine output and other significant losses (e.g. nasogastric or diarrhoeal). Such a fluid regimen will require meticulous measurement of losses and continuous adjustment of input. An indwelling urinary catheter is frequently required, particularly in the child with concomitant diarrhoea. This should be removed at an early stage to reduce the risk of urinary tract infection. The need for regular review of the patient's weight, fluid balance, blood pressure, and general clinical status cannot be overemphasized. Laboratory investigations need to be performed on a regular basis to assist in fluid and electrolyte replacement, and to identify those likely to need dialysis.

A decision has to be made at this point as to whether the child can continue to be managed in the local district hospital, or whether transfer to a tertiary paediatric nephrology centre is necessary (Table 22.10). The cause of the acute renal failure and the severity of the early clinical course is of great importance in making decisions about transfer. Children

Table 22.10 Indications for transfer to a tertiary paediatric nephrology centre

---

Dialysis required or likely to be required (Table 22.11)
Cause of renal failure uncertain
   Need for expert opinion and possible renal biopsy
Need for specialist investigations
   Radiology
   Nuclear medicine
Post-renal failure with urological problem requiring
  paediatric urological opinion
Multiple organ involvement or need for intensive care

---

with pre-renal failure which is fluid responsive, or mild intrinsic renal failure, can safely be managed in the local district hospital and do not require transfer to a tertiary paediatric nephrology centre. In contrast, the child who is early in the course of diarrhoea-associated haemolytic uraemic syndrome and is persistently anuric despite all of the above corrective measures will almost always require early transfer, even if their biochemistry is only mildly abnormal, as the likelihood is that their renal function will continue to deteriorate and dialysis will become necessary. In contrast, the child who is seen late in the course of their illness, where the plasma creatinine and urea are very high, although urine output is increasing and the general clinical status improving, is unlikely to require dialysis, and the child may continue to be managed locally. Early consultation with the tertiary centre should take place where any doubt exists.

Key points: Acute renal failure at the district hospital

- Early management includes fluid challenge where pre-renal failure is suspected, and the use of a loop diuretic once intravascular volume status has been normalized.

- Children with renal failure require regular clinical review, with particular attention being paid to their weight, fluid balance, blood pressure, and biochemistry.

- Children with pre-renal failure which is fluid responsive, or mild intrinsic renal failure, can safely be managed in the district hospital and do not require transfer to a tertiary paediatric nephrology centre.

- Children with persistent anuria will often require dialysis, even if their plasma biochemistry at presentation is not very abnormal. Such children require early transfer to a tertiary centre.

- Early contact with the tertiary centre should be made wherever doubt exists about a child's likely clinical course.

- Medication doses should be adjusted in accordance with the level of renal function, and other further renal insults including dehydration and hypotension avoided.

In all children with established acute renal failure of whatever aetiology, it is important to avoid further nephrotoxic insults that will act as secondary injury mechanisms. Episodes of dehydration, hypoxaemia, and hypotension, the use radiological contrast, and the development of infection in the urinary tract may worsen the renal failure or delay its recovery. Nephrotoxic drugs should be avoided where possible and medication doses should be adjusted according to the level of renal function (Chapter 26).

Further management of the child with acute renal failure at the tertiary centre

If, following fluid challenge at the referring centre, uncertainty about the child's intravascular volume status exists, central venous access should be achieved via the internal jugular or subclavian vein. This is a procedure associated with significant risks, particularly in the awake conscious child, and only experienced practitioners should site these lines. Vascular ultrasonographic aids can significantly improve the rate of successful placement if used regularly [11]. If the child is not under general anaesthesia or sedated in the intensive care unit, or if there is evidence of coagulopathy, many authorities advocate the use of the femoral vein. Central venous pressure measurement via this route approximates to that derived by direct measurement [12], unless there is raised intra-abdominal pressure, in which case direct measurement via the internal jugular or subclavian vein is required. More invasive measurements of intracardiac pressures and of cardiac output using a Swan–Ganz catheter may be useful, but this will require transfer of the child to the intensive care unit. There is, however, no evidence that the information derived from these techniques reduces mortality [13,14] and they are not, therefore, frequently used.

Role of renal biopsy in acute renal failure

When the history, clinical features, laboratory, and radiological investigations have excluded pre-renal and post-renal causes and suggest a diagnosis of intrinsic renal disease other than ischaemic or haemolytic uraemic syndrome-related acute renal failure, a biopsy may establish the diagnosis and guide therapy. Histological diagnosis is particularly important in identifying rapidly progressive glomerulonephritis,

tubulo-interstitial nephritis, and renovascular disease. Management decisions, especially those relating to the use of immunosuppressive agents, depend on an accurate assessment of the histological findings, and specific treatment needs to be started early in the course of these diseases to ensure a successful outcome.

Preventing the development of intrinsic renal failure

A variety of interventions have been investigated in the hope that they may prevent the onset of established acute intrinsic renal failure and the need for renal replacement therapy. These studies have been performed largely in adult patients. *Mannitol* in a dose of 1 g/kg body weight is protective against ischaemia and nephrotoxic renal failure, probably because of its capacity to increase renal perfusion. It can, however, also worsen renal function and induce renal failure, which is recognized by the presence of renal tubular epithelial cells containing vacuoles in the urinary sediment [16]. There is insufficient evidence in both paediatric and adult practice to support the use of *low-dose dopamine* in critically ill patients with acute renal failure [17]. There are no good prospective paediatric studies and recognized adverse effects have been documented. There are two randomized controlled trials in adults which find no evidence that *diuretics* improve mortality, renal recovery, or reduce the number of days on dialysis, although both studies lacked power to rule out the effect [18,19]. Ototoxicity can occur with high-dose loop diuretics; deafness occurred in two patients who received furosemide in one of the trials and the hearing loss was permanent in one of these two [19]. Diuretics may also add pre-renal insult to existing renal injury in acute renal failure, although the frequency of this is uncertain. There is also insufficient evidence on the effects of adding intravenous albumin to diuretic therapy in critically ill people in renal failure. There are no randomized-controlled trials comparing albumin supplementation plus diuretic versus diuretic alone in such cases. The one systematic review of 30 randomized controlled trials [20] found that albumin increased the risk of death in unselected critically ill people (mortality 14% with albumin versus 8% with control; RR, 1.68; confidence interval (CI), 1.26–2.23). However, all of the included trials were small and combined highly heterogeneous populations.

Key points: Preventing the development of intrinsic renal failure

- Mannitol is protective against ischaemia and nephrotoxic renal failure, but can also worsen renal function and induce renal failure, which is recognized by the presence of renal tubular epithelial cells containing vacuoles in the urinary sediment.

- There is, at present, no evidence to support the use of low-dose dopamine to improve renal blood flow in acute renal failure.

Renal replacement therapy

General indications for the commencement of renal replacement therapy (dialysis or haemofiltration) are shown in Table 22.11. As discussed above, information about the cause of the renal failure and the early clinical course are in many ways more important determinants of the need for dialysis than absolute biochemical values, unless these are in themselves life-threatening, e.g. severe hyperkalaemia. Most paediatric nephrologists would start the anuric child with fluid- and diuretic-unresponsive haemolytic uraemic syndrome on dialysis at a very early stage, before the onset of severe acidosis, uraemia or hyperkalaemia. There is some evidence that initiating renal replacement therapy early may reduce the morbidity and mortality of acute renal failure, particularly in the critically ill child on the paediatric intensive care unit. In a retrospective study, Gettings et al. [21]

Table 22.11 Indications for renal replacement therapy

Persistent hyperkalaemia
Diuretic resistant volume overload ± associated
  hypertension and heart failure
Refractory acidosis
Severe uraemia with risk of encephalopathy
  and/or pericarditis
Requirement to create space for the improvement of
  nutritional intake
Resistant hypo- or hypernatraemia
Resistant hypocalcaemia and hyperphosphataemia
Hyperammonaemia with inborn errors of metabolism
Tumour lysis syndrome
Removal of dialysable drug or toxin
Hyperpyrexia/ hypothermia

found that early commencement of renal replacement therapy in post-traumatic acute renal failure improved survival rates. Best et al. [22] and Smith et al. [23] used continuous veno-venous haemofiltration as part of standard treatment for children with severe meningococcal disease. Both reported impressively lower mortality in children so treated when compared with historical controls. However, the number of patients in these studies was small, other novel therapies were used, and there has been no randomized controlled evaluation of this approach.

Choice of renal replacement therapy. The choice of renal replacement therapy in critically ill children is individualized, based upon the availability of various modalities, the patient's requirements for fluid and solute removal, haemodynamic stability, and whether ventilatory support is required. The experience and availablity of relevant expertise in the individual unit is also of considerable importance. The choice is between acute peritoneal dialysis, continuous veno-venous haemofiltration (CVVH), continuous veno-venous haemofiltration and dialysis (CVVHD), and acute haemodialysis. The relative indications for each of these modalities are outlined in Table 22.12. As can be seen, factors determining the choice of replacement therapy include the desired goal of therapy (e.g. the removal of solutes such as potassium and urea, or fluid removal where fluid overload exists) and the clinical stability of the patient.

Acute peritoneal dialysis. The peritoneum has a greater surface area in proportion to body size in children than in adults. It is therefore relatively more efficient at removing fluid and solutes in children. Peritoneal dialysis fluid contains electrolytes, an osmotic agent (glucose or icosodextran), and an acid buffer (lactate or bicarbonate).

Commercially manufactured solutions in the United Kingdom are available in 1.36%, 2.27% and 3.86% glucose concentrations. In North America 0.5%, 1.5%, 2.5% and 4.25% solutions are available. Using higher glucose concentrations in the dialysis fluid will increase the volume of fluid removed from the patient (ultrafiltration). Volumes of 10–50 ml/kg/cycle are used with dwell times varying between 20 and 60 minutes, with 5–10 minutes to drain and fill. Ultrafiltration will also be increased by using a larger volume of fluid. Removal of undesired electrolytes, including potassium, will be increased by increasing the cycle volume or increasing the number of cycles performed in each 24-hour period.

Table 22.12 Relative indications for different renal replacement therapy modalities in acute renal failure

Indication for dialysis	General condition	Modality indicated
Solute removal	Stable	Haemodialysis
	Unstable	CVVH, CVVHD, PD
Fluid removal	Stable	PD, isolated ultrafiltration on HD
	Unstable	CVVH, CVVHD
Solute and fluid removal	Stable	HD, PD, CVVHD
	Unstable	HD, PD, CVVHD
Tumour lysis syndrome or other causes of severe hyperkalaemia	Unstable or stable	HD followed by CVVH or CVVHD
Toxin or drug removal	Stable/unstable	HD or CVVH

CVVH, continuous veno-venous haemofiltration; CVVHD, continuous veno-venous haemofiltration and dialysis; HD, haemodialysis; PD, peritoneal dialysis.

Access to the peritoneal cavity can be achieved using either a permanent or acute Tenchkoff catheter inserted in an operating theatre by a paediatric surgeon under a general anaesthetic or at the bedside by an experienced paediatric nephrologist using a peel away sheath system under sedation and local anaesthesia [24]. Both permanent and acute Tenchkoff catheters have large end and side holes, facilitating good flow and minimizing the complication of catheter blockage. There are neonatal and paediatric acute catheters available which are stiffer than the Tenchkoff catheters and thus easier to insert but are associated with a higher complication rate. Absolute contraindications to peritoneal dialysis include omphalocele or gastroschisis, diaphragmatic hernia, peritonitis or other disease affecting the peritoneal membrane, and bladder exstrophy. Relative contraindications include recent abdominal surgery and high levels of ventilatory support. In haemodynamically unstable patients, peritoneal dialysis may cause hypotension because of a decreased pre-load and increased ventilatory requirements if diaphragmatic splinting occurs. The two major advantages of acute peritoneal dialysis over haemodialysis or CVVH are that central vascular access is not required and anticoagulation is not necessary.

Acute intermittent haemodialysis. Acute haemodialysis has been used for many years for the treatment of acute renal failure in childhood. It has the advantage that metabolic abnormalities and hypervolaemia can be corrected rapidly. The disadvantages include the need to achieve good vascular access, the requirement for anticoagulation, the need for maximally purified water by a reverse osmosis system, and the resource of skilled nursing staff. Relative contraindications include haemodynamic instability and severe coagulopathy. During acute haemodialysis, rapid ultrafiltration may produce hypotension, which may result in additional renal ischaemia, potentially prolonging the episode of acute renal failure. Rapid shifts in the level of blood urea may also result in dialysis dysequilibrium, particularly if the child has a very high urea level at the start of the dialysis session. Dysequilibrium syndrome is complex and the pathogenesis multifactorial; symptoms include restlessness, fatigue, headache, nausea, and vomiting, which may progress to confusion, seizures, and coma. This severe complication can be prevented by attempting to reduce the urea level slowly during haemodialysis.

Continuous veno-venous haemofiltration and continuous veno-venous haemofiltration and dialysis. In continuous veno-venous haemofiltration (CVVH), blood is pumped from the patient via a central vein by a blood pump, through a haemofilter and returned to the patient. The passage of blood through the filter produces an ultrafiltrate containing water and solutes. The amount of filtration achieved is influenced by the filter's surface area and permeability. The hydrostatic pressure gradient, which drives filtration, is increased by increasing the blood flow rate. The removal of a large volume of ultrafiltrate permits convective clearance of solutes and water. The ultrafiltrate, which will contain electrolytes in a concentration equivalent to that in the plasma, is replaced by a replacement fluid (Table 22.13). The rate of replacement will depend on the child's clinical condition: where intravascular volume overload exists, the rate of replacement should be significantly less than the rate of ultrafiltration, resulting in a net loss from the intravascular compartment.

Continuous veno-venous haemofiltration and dialysis (CVVHD) refers to the addition of a counter

Table 22.13   Haemofiltration replacement solution

Electrolyte content of commercially available lactate-based haemofiltration solution (5-litre bags):

Na	142 mmol/l
K	0 mmol/l
Ca	2.0 mmol/l
Mg	0.75 mmol/l
PO_4	0 mmol/l
Lactate	45 mmol/l
Glucose	0 mmol/l

The electrolyte content of the replacement fluid can be altered by the addition of the following:

Additive	Electrolyte content
13.6% potassium acid phosphate	1 mmol/ml of K and 1 mmol/ml of PO_4
21.6% sodium glycerophosphate	2 mmol/ml of Na and 1 mmol/ml of PO_4
15% potassium chloride	2 mmol/ml of K and 2 mmol/ml of Cl
50% dextrose	20 ml/l increases the glucose content by 1%
30% sodium chloride	5 mmol/ml Na and 5 mmol/ml Cl

The addition of:
10 ml 13.6% potassium acid phosphate
2.5 ml 15% potassium chloride
100 ml 50% dextrose
to the 5-litre bag will achieve a replacement fluid with the following electrolyte content:

Na	142 mmol/l
K	3 mmol/l
Ca	2.0 mmol/l
Mg	0.75 mmol/l
PO_4	2 mmol/l
Lactate	45 mmol/l
Glucose	1%

current flow of dialysis fluid across the haemofilter or dialyser. By increasing the diffusion gradient, solute clearance is increased at a rate proportional to the dialysate flow. Both CVVH and CVVHD are significant improvements over the previous technique of continuous arterio-venous haemofiltration (CAVH), in that the need for arterial cannulation is avoided and children with low systemic blood pressures can be maintained on haemofiltration, as the blood pump removes the reliance on arterial blood pressure to maintain adequate blood flow.

A prescription for CVVH/D should include documentation of the venous access achieved, the filter/dialyser size, blood and filtrate pump speeds, anticoagulation and its monitoring, and ultrafiltration rates. Adequate venous access is required to achieve the desired blood flow rates and the size of cannula used will range from 6.5FG in infants weighing less than 10 kg to 11.5FG in children heavier than 20 kg. The filter/dialyser used should be roughly equivalent to the body surface area of the patient and prescriptions also need to take into account the priming volume of the filter and the blood lines, in order to minimize the volume of the extracorporeal circuit. The blood pump speed should be set at 5–10 ml/kg/min with a minimum of 25 ml/min, as below this clearances are poor and clotting almost inevitable. Similar blood flows are required for CVVH and CVVHD and in both situations, if vascular access and cardiovascular stability permit, blood flow can be increased to improve clearances. There are two available filtrate replacement solutions, which are either lactate or bicarbonate based. The lactate-based solution is pre-made and is generally the solution of choice. The bicarbonate-based solution is used in situations of established or expected acidosis and in severely ill children who are unable to convert lactate to bicarbonate in the liver. This solution requires the addition of bicarbonate shortly prior to its use. Potassium and phosphate will need to be replaced if removal lowers plasma levels to below the normal range. This can be achieved by their addition to the haemofiltration replacement fluid in the desired physiological concentrations, i.e. potassium 3–5 mmol/l and phosphate 1–2 mmol/l. The degree of anticoagulation required is dependent upon the coagulation status of the patient, blood flow rates, and the vascular access achieved. More anticoagulation is required in smaller children with smaller lines and lower flow rates. Heparin remains the anticoagulant of choice in most units; a loading dose of 20 units/kg is generally given, followed by an infusion pre-filter of 10–30 units/kg/h to achieve an APTT of 60–90 seconds or an ACT of 130–170 seconds. If citrate is used, then calcium will need to be infused through a separate line to maintain a normal ionized calcium level. Prostacylin is occasionally used when heparin is contraindicated, but is seldom successful unless used with low-dose heparin. Once established on CVVH or CVVH/D and stable, the difference between the amount of ultrafiltrate removed and the fluid replaced each hour can be increased to achieve the desired fluid balance. The child's net fluid balance will depend upon this and all other fluid input (drugs, parenteral nutrition, etc.) and losses (urine, nasogastric, and insensible losses). It is possible to achieve high rates of fluid removal with these modes of treatment, but even in the most extreme states of fluid overload it is unwise to remove more than 10% of the child's body weight in a single 24-hour period.

Key points: Renal replacement therapy

- The peritoneum has a greater surface area in proportion to body size in children than in adults. It is therefore relatively more efficient at removing fluid and solutes in children.

- Haemodialysis has the advantage that metabolic abnormalities and hypervolaemia can be corrected rapidly. Good vascular access and anticoagulation are required, as are skilled nursing staff.

- CVVH and CVVHD allow renal replacement therapy in children with low systemic blood pressure.

Nutrition

Nutrition remains one of the most difficult and important management issues in the child with acute renal failure and needs to be managed by a multiprofessional approach, involving the paediatric nephrologist, dietician, pharmacist, and nursing staff. Children in acute renal failure are in a catabolic state. This is usually multifactorial in origin, reflecting the catabolic nature of the underlying disorder, anorexia, reduced access to food, nutrient losses in drainage fluids or dialysis, increased breakdown and reduced synthesis of muscle protein, and increased hepatic gluconeogenesis. This situation is often compounded by the fact that the infants and children get inadequate nutritional support at this time. The aim of nutritional support is to supply sufficient calories to avoid catabolism and starvation ketoacidosis, while minimizing the production of nitrogenous waste. If the gastrointestinal tract is intact and functioning, then enteral feeding, generally via a nasogastric tube using special formula, should be started as soon as possible. Up to 0.8 g/kg/day of high biological value protein should be given and most of the calories provided as carbohydrate. Protein intake in infants and children may be increased in those who are particularly catabolic, even if this precipitates the need for dialysis. In infants the aim is to provide up to 120 kcal/kg/day. In older children the aim is to provide appropriate maintenance calories or higher if needed. If enteral nutrition via a nasogastric tube using an appropriate formula is not possible, then hyperalimentation should be commenced via a central line, using high-concentration dextrose solution up to 25% and lipids (10–20%). Up to 1–2 g/kg/day of protein should be given. If the child is oliguric or oligoanuric and sufficient calories cannot be achieved with an appropriate fluid balance, then again early dialysis may be required. Indeed, the management of the nutritional state in acute renal failure is often easier after the initiation of dialysis, as ultrafiltration allows adequate volumes of feed to be given. It is believed that adequate nutrition improves survival in acute renal failure [25]; however, consistent benefit has yet to be demonstrated in controlled trials.

Key points: Nutrition in acute renal failure

- Children in acute renal failure are in a catabolic state.

- The aim of nutritional support is to supply sufficient calories to avoid catabolism and starvation ketoacidosis while minimizing the production of nitrogenous waste.

- Input from a dietician with experience in renal disease is essential.

- The oliguric child may need dialysis to be commenced to create fluid space for nutrition to be administered.

Specific causes of acute renal failure

Haemolytic uraemic syndrome

Diarrhoea-associated haemolytic uraemic syndrome (HUS) is the most common cause of acute intrinsic renal failure in children in Europe and North America. It is the most significant complication of infection by verocytotoxin (VT)-producing *Escherichia coli* (VTEC), usually of the serotype O157:H7, but other serotypes are also implicated [26,27].

The annual incidence of VTEC infection, which varies geographically and from year to year, ranges from 1 to 30 cases per 100 000 in industrialized countries and is highest in young children and during the warmer summer months. The reported frequency of developing HUS in outbreaks of VTEC infection is around 8% [28]. The infective dose of *E. coli* is 50–100 organisms, and the incubation period to onset of diarrhoea is 1–8 days. Younger children may continue to excrete the bacteria for more than 3 weeks after the infection, but asymptomatic prolonged carriage of *E. coli* O157 is unusual.

The natural reservoir of VTEC is the intestinal tracts of domestic animals, especially cattle, and foods of bovine origin, such as ground beefburgers and unpasteurized milk, are major sources for human infection. Other foods, including cider and vegetables such as lettuce and radish sprouts, are becoming increasingly recognized as sources, and *E. coli* O157:H7 has been recovered from many retail foods, including fresh seafood, lamb, chicken, pork, venison, and veal. Person to person transmission of VTEC O157, facilitated by the low infectious dose, is a source of human infection.

Clinical features

Affected children are generally healthy before the onset of gastroenteritis. HUS is then characterized by the sudden onset of haemolytic anaemia with fragmentation of red blood cells, thrombocytopenia, and the development of acute renal failure after a prodromal illness of acute gastroenteritis, often with bloody diarrhoea. The gastrointestinal disease may be severe, with haemorrhagic colitis, toxic megacolon, rectal prolapse, and bowel wall necrosis. Hepatomegaly may be common and serum transaminases are often increased. Pancreatic involvement occurs in less than 10% of children and manifests as glucose intolerance and the possible development of insulin-dependent diabetes mellitus, which may be transient or permanent. Oligoanuria occurs in over half of all cases and every child, unless anuric, has microscopic haematuria and proteinuria. The blood pressure may be normal or increased and hypertension may be increased with blood transfusion and may contribute to central nervous system dysfunction. Signs of fluid overload include oedema, hypertension, and cardiac failure. Most children are irritable and they may have behavioural changes, restlessness, ataxia, dizziness, tremors, and twitching. Major neurological dysfunction occurs in a third of patients and is associated with a poor prognosis.

Signs that should alert the paediatrician to the development of HUS in a child with diarrhoea are the presence of bloody diarrhoea, decreasing urine output and the development of oedema when dehydration is being corrected, and the sudden onset of pallor, mild jaundice, and petechiae.

Treatment

Once VTEC-induced HUS has developed, there is no evidence-based specific treatment yet available. It is generally agreed that prompt diagnosis and good supportive care of hydration, electrolyte balance, and nutrition are crucial, as is the management of the critical complications of cerebral oedema, severe ischaemic colitis, myocardial dysfunction, and diabetes mellitus. Inappropriate rehydration in a situation where renal function is compromised may produce significant morbidity, with hyponatraemia and pulmonary oedema. Early dialysis should be commenced to prevent such complications if the child is oligoanuric. The haemoglobin should be maintained above 7–8 g/dl and the institution of early dialysis allows blood transfusions to be given with less risk of volume overload and hyperkalaemia.

Studies are in progress to identify novel treatments that may halt the development of HUS in patients with VTEC, such as the use of a synthetic oligosaccharide receptor for the verotoxin [29], but as yet there is no effective therapy. Antibiotics are not indicated, and might theoretically worsen the renal failure.

Key points: Diarrhoea-associated haemolytic uraemic syndrome

- Commonest cause of acute intrinsic renal failure in children in the United Kingdom and USA.

- Most commonly associated with verocytotoxin-producing *Escherichia coli*, usually of the serotype O157:H7.

- No specific therapy exists: antibiotics are not indicated.

- Major neurological dysfunction occurs in a third of patients and is associated with a poor prognosis.

- Less than 10% may develop pancreatic involvement, manifested by hyperglycaemia which may require insulin therapy. Blood glucose levels should be monitored.

- Mortality is as high as 8.5%, and up to 30% of survivors may develop mild impairment of GFR or albuminuria.

Tumour lysis syndrome

This syndrome is seen most commonly in children with acute lymphoblastic leukaemia and B-cell lymphoma. It is due to the precipitation of uric acid crystals in the renal tubules or the microvasculature, leading to obstruction of urine flow or renal blood flow. Tumour lysis occurs most commonly at the initiation of chemotherapy and can be reduced by aggressive hydration with high urine flow rates, bicarbonate infusion to alkalinize the urine, and the use of allopurinol. This syndrome results in a very rapid increase in serum potassium, urea, and phosphate, and a reciprocal decrease in calcium as tumour cells are lysed. It is generally transient and the child will recover function once tumour lysis is complete. Prolonged haemodialysis is often necessary to control the metabolic imbalance, in particular the hyperkalaemia and hyperphosphataemia, which result from the rapid lysis of tumour cells.

Acute interstitial nephritis

Acute interstitial nephritis may be idiopathic in nature or secondary to drugs, the important ones being the penicillins/cephalosporins, sulphonamides, and non-steroidal anti inflammatory drugs. This form of nephritis often presents with a non-specific prodromal illness and the child may have an erythematous rash, fever, and arthralgia. There is often an associated blood eosinophilia, with white blood cells and occasionally eosinophils detected in the urine. Treatment of acute interstitial nephritis involves withdrawal of the suspected implicating agent(s) and good supportive management. There is no good clinical evidence that steroids are of benefit in this situation.

Acute glomerulonephritis

Acute glomerulonephritis may follow a number of different infections but post-streptococcal glomerulonephritis remains the most important cause. This is discussed in detail in Chapter 20. Rapidly progressive glomerulonephritis (RPGN) is, by definition, a severe form of nephritis and is a rare cause of acute renal failure in children. The clinical features include hypertension, oedema, and haematuria that is often gross. Plasma biochemistries are generally severely deranged, with a significantly elevated urea and creatinine, and the diagnosis is confirmed histologically following a renal biopsy. The characteristic pathological finding is extensive crescent formation. RPGN can occur as a result of post-infectious disease, mesangiocapillary glomerulonephritis, Henoch–Schönlein disease, and systemic lupus erythematosis. In practice, it is more commonly seen in adults presenting with ANCA-associated glomerulonephritis, Goodpasture's disease, or idiopathic rapidly progressive glomerulonephritis. Serological markers are of diagnostic importance and the following should be checked in all suspected cases: ANA, anti-DNA antibodies, ANCA, anti-GBM antibody, complement levels and C3 nephritic factor. A previously healthy child can become dialysis-dependent with irreversible renal failure in a matter of weeks, and specific treatment, to be effective, should be started early once the diagnosis has been confirmed. A variety of treatments have been tried, including steroids, cytotoxic agents, anticoagulants, and plasma exchange, either alone or in combination [30]. The lack of controlled trials, together with a spontaneous remission rate, makes an evidence-based choice of treatment difficult. High-dose intravenous methylprednisolone (20 mg/kg) was found to be beneficial in the treatment of RPGN after Henoch–Schönlein nephritis but not following mesangiocapillary glomerulonephritis [31]. More aggressive treatment regimens have combined pulsed methylprednisolone with cyclophosphamide and dipyridamole. Plasma exchange or filtration have been used, particularly when a measurable antibody can be cleared from the plasma, such as against double-stranded DNA in lupus nephritis or against glomerular basement membrane in Goodpasture's disease. Plasma exchange is, however, a technically difficult technique in small children, it requires very close attention to fluid balance and is itself immunosuppressive.

Renovascular thrombotic disease

Acute renal failure only occurs in large-vessel disease if it is bilateral or if the child has a solitary kidney. Microvascular renal disease occurs most commonly in childhood haemolytic uraemic syndrome. Renal venous thrombosis leading to acute renal failure occurs most commonly in the neonatal period and is associated clinically with the presence of swollen kidneys, haematuria, and thrombocytopenia. It is important that in all cases of renal venous thrombosis a thrombophilia screen is performed to exclude any haematological abnormalities, such as factor V Leiden deficiency. Treatment can be problematic and the risk of therapy needs to be carefully weighed against potential benefit. It is aimed at limiting the extension of clot, and anticoagulation with low molecular weight subcutaneous or intravenous heparin or fibrinolytic therapy should be considered, particularly if the clot is large [32].

Renal cortical necrosis

Cortical necrosis in childhood leads to severe and often irreversible renal failure. It occurs more commonly in the neonatal period and is often associated with multi-system failure. It is commonly associated with a severe hypoxic–ischaemic insult. The infant presents with gross haematuria, oliguria, and hypertension. There is biochemical evidence of severe renal failure and also thrombocytopenia. The ultrasound scan is initially normal but follow-up scans show that the kidney fails to increase in size or, indeed, undergoes atrophy such that follow-up scans show a reduction in the size of the kidneys. Cortical necrosis is associated with a poor prognosis and even those infants who have a partial recovery often develop renal impairment and hypertension later in life.

Acute tubular necrosis

Acute tubular necrosis may follow on from pre-renal failure if the insult is sufficiently severe, and may also result from toxic injury to tubular cells from drugs. It is often reversible, and avoiding secondary mechanisms of injury will improve outcome.

Drug-induced acute renal failure

The most commonly implicated drugs in paediatric practice are the aminoglycoside antibiotics, ifosfamide, cis-platinum, non-steroidal anti-inflammatory drugs, ACE inhibitors, and amphotericin B. Aminoglycoside-associated nephrotoxic renal failure may be non-oliguric. It is generally associated with minimal urinary abnormalities, and the incidence is related primarily to the dose and duration of treatment and any pre-existing renal impairment. The damage is thought to be reversible once the aminoglcoside antibiotics have been discontinued. Other medications, such as amphotericin B and the cytotoxic agents ifosfamide and cis-platinum, together with aciclovir and intravascular contrast media, are thought to induce renal failure in part because of toxic tubular injury.

Causes of acute renal failure in the intensive care unit

Children are not usually admitted to the intensive care unit with acute renal failure alone and tend to have dysfunction of other organ systems, which undoubtedly accounts for the high reported mortality rates.

The disease states most commonly present are infectious diseases, congenital heart disease, complications associated with malignancy and trauma, and only occasionally would a child be admitted with intrinsic renal disease such as HUS or following renal transplantation.

In the United Kingdom, meningococcal septicaemia is the most common infective cause of acute renal failure in the intensive care unit population. All septicaemic illnesses can cause a reduction in intravascular volume and an initial fall in systemic vascular resistance, followed by a fall in cardiac output in the following days. For reasons that are still not fully elucidated, meningococcal disease is particularly adept at causing massive intravascular volume depletion, such that children with severe disease not uncommonly require fluid replacement of twice their blood volume to be administered in the first 24 hours of illness [33].

Children with congenital heart disease are most at risk of developing acute renal failure following cardiac surgery that has involved cardiopulmonary bypass. In past decades, appreciation of the benefits of early repair of congenital defects and the evolution of new surgical procedures have meant more children having surgery in the first weeks or months of life. These patients are particularly at risk of acute renal failure. The mortality associated with this combination may exceed 50% [34]. Some lesions predispose to acute renal failure even before surgery, particularly if the diagnosis is delayed, e.g. severe coarctation of the aorta, severe aortic stenosis, hypoplastic left heart syndrome, and complex cyanotic heart disease.

Severe trauma, including road traffic accidents and burns, can be complicated by acute renal failure, usually as a complication of a reduction in the intravascular volume and occasionally from direct renal injury. It is interesting, though, that a reduction in the incidence of acute renal failure and mortality following penetrating torso wounds was demonstrated when fluid resuscitation was delayed until operative intervention [35].

Key points: Acute renal failure in the ICU

- Meningococcal septicaemia is the commonest infective cause of acute renal failure in the intensive care unit.

- Children with congenital heart disease are at significant risk of developing acute renal failure following surgery that has involved cardiopulmonary bypass.

- Severe trauma, including road traffic accidents and burns, may be complicated by acute renal failure.

Knowing the disease states likely to be associated with ARF should enable clinicians to use a variety of severity of illness scores to alert them to the likelihood of a child developing this complication [36,37]. Those scores whose data are derived at first contact with hospital or ICU staff are most likely to be useful. The Glasgow meningococcal septicaemia prognostic score relies on six clinical signs and one blood gas result.

Children with scores of greater than 10 have high rates of morbidity and/or mortality and may warrant early use of renal replacement therapy, although evidence to support this is, at present, lacking.

Overall prognosis

The mortality rate associated with acute renal failure in adults and children has changed little over the past three decades; despite significant advances in supportive care and in the intensive care unit setting mortality rates remain unacceptably high.

The prognosis in childhood depends significantly on the underlying cause of the acute renal failure. In isolated renal failure, the immediate results of treatment are good, but where there is evidence of other organ failure, mortality increases [38]. Two-thirds of children who develop acute renal failure following cardiac surgery die during the acute illness; mortality is highest in the neonatal age group and those with cyanotic heart disease have the worst outcome [39]. In verocytotoxin-associated haemolytic uraemic syndrome, in which, in the main, only one organ is significantly involved, up to 90% of the children make a good recovery in the short term. Fifteen (8.5%) of 177 children with diarrhoea-associated haemolytic uraemic syndrome seen between 1966 and 1992 at The Hospital for Sick Children, London, died, usually of neurological or gastrointestinal complications [40]. On more detailed examination, however, the longer-term outcome of diarrhoea-associated haemolytic uraemic syndrome is somewhat concerning. A review of 103 children who had diarrhoea-associated haemolytic uraemic syndrome at least 5 years before, showed that 30% had albuminuria and 18% a GFR of less than $80 \, ml/min/1.73 \, m^2$. These children may be at risk of developing hypertension and deteriorating renal function later in life, and therefore require long-term follow-up. Similarly, children who had cortical necrosis during the neonatal period and recovered some renal function, or children following an episode of severe Henoch–Schönlein nephritis who have residual proteinuria or a reduced glomerular filtration rate, are clearly at risk for the later development of renal complications. It is important to recognize that many of the survivors of acute renal failure in the neonatal and childhood period continue to have some degree of renal functional abnormality, which may not be immediately apparent, and for this reason they, too, should remain under long-term observation with monitoring of urinalysis and measurement of blood pressure.

Key points: Prognosis

- The mortality rate associated with acute renal failure in both adults and children has changed little and remains unacceptably high, particularly in the intensive care setting.

- The prognosis in children depends significantly on the underlying cause of the acute renal failure.

- Survivors of acute renal failure in childhood should remain under long-term observation.

References

1. Nissenson AR. Acute renal failure: Definition and pathogenesis. *Kidney Int Suppl* 1998;53:S7–S10.
2. Paller MS, Anderson RJ. Use of vasoactive agents in the therapy of acute renal failure. In: Brenner BM, Lazarus JM, eds. *Acute Renal Failure*. Philadelphia: WB Saunders; 1983:723.
3. Andreoli SP. Reactive oxygen molecules, oxidant injury and renal disease. *Pediatr Nephrol* 1991;5:733–742.
4. Weinberg JM. The cell biology of ischaemic renal injury. *Kidney Int* 1991;39:476–500.
5. Siegel NJ, Devarajan P, Van Why S. Renal cell injury: metabolic and structural alterations. *Pediatr Res* 1994;36:129–136.
6. Lieberthal W, Levine JS. Mechanisms of apoptosis and its potential role in renal tubular epithelial cell injury. *Am J Physiol* 1996;271:F477–488.
7. Hou SH, Bushinski DA, Wish JB, Cohen JJ, Harrington JT. Hospital-acquired renal insufficiency: a prospective study. *Am J Med* 1983;74:243–248.
8. Brivet FG, Kleinknecht D, Loirat C, Landais PJ. Acute renal failure in intensive care units – causes, outcomes and prognostic factors of hospital mortality: a prospective, multi centre study. *Crit Care Med* 1996;24:192–198.
9. Stapleton FB, Jones DB, Green RS. Acute renal failure in neonates: incidence, aetiology and outcome. *Pediatr Nephrol* 1987;1:314–320.
10. Quigley RP, Alexander SR. Acute Renal Failure. In: Levin DL, Morris FC, eds. *Essentials of Pediatric Intensive Care*. Edinburgh: Churchill Livingstone; 1997:509–523.
11. Verghese ST, McGill WA, Patel RI, Sell JE, Midgley FM, Ruttiman UE. Comparison of three techniques for internal jugular vein cannulation in infants. *Paediatr Anaesth* 2000;10:505–511.
12. Yung M, Butt W. Inferior vena cava pressure as an estimate of central venous pressure. *J Paediatr Child Health* 1995;31:399–402.
13. Dalen JE, Bone RC. Is it time to pull the pulmonary artery catheter? *JAMA* 1996;276:916–918.
14. Bernard GR, Sopko G, Cerra F, Demling R, Edmunds H, Kaplan S, Kessler L, Masur H, Parsons P, Shure D, Webb C, Weidemann H, Weinmann G, Williams D. Pulmonary artery catherisation and clinical outcomes: National Heart, Lung, and Blood Institute and Food and Drug Administration Workshop Report. Consensus Statement. *JAMA* 2000;283:2568–2572.
15. Tataranni G, Malacarne F, Farinelli R, Tarroni G, Gritti G, Guberti A, Tartari S, Zavagli G. Beneficial effects of verapamil in renal-risk surgical patients. *Renal Failure* 1994;16:383–390.
16. Dorman HR, Sondheimer JH, Cadnapaphornchai P. Mannitol-induced acute renal failure. *Medicine* 1990;69:153–159.
17. Kellum JA, M Decker J. Use of dopamine in acute renal failure: a meta-analysis. *Crit Care Med* 2001;29:1638–1639.
18. Kleinknecht D. Epidemiology in acute renal failure in France today. In: Biari D, Neild G, eds. *Acute Renal Failure in Intensive Therapy Unit*. Berlin: Springer-Verlag; 1990:13–21.
19. Brown CB, Ogg CS, Cameron JS. High dose frusemide in acute renal failure: a controlled trial. *Clin Nephrol* 1981;15:90–96.
20. The Albumin Reviewers. Human albumin administration in critically ill patients. In: *The Cochrane Library*, Issue 4, 1999.
21. Gettings LG, Reynolds HN, Scalea T. Outcome in post-traumatic acute renal failure when continuous renal replacement therapy is applied early vs. late. *Intensive Care Med* 1999;25:805–813.
22. Best C, Walsh J, Sinclair J, Beattie J. Early haemodiafiltration in meningococcal septicemia. *Lancet* 1996;347:202.
23. Smith OP, White B, Vaughan D, Rafferty M, Claffey L, Lyons B, Casey W. Use of Protein-C concentrate, heparin and haemodiafiltration in meningococcous-induced purpura fulminans. *Lancet* 1997;350:1590–1593.
24. Lewis MA, Nycyk J. Practical peritoneal dialysis—the Tenckhoff catheter in acute renal failure. *Pediatr Nephrol* 1992;6:470–475.
25. Bullock ML, Umen AJ, Finkelstein M, Keane WF. The assessment of risk factors in 462 patients with acute renal failure. *Am J Kidney Dis* 1985;5:97–103.
26. Milford DV, Taylor CM, Guttridge B, Hall SM, Rowe B, Kleanthous H. Haemolytic uraemic syndrome in the British Isles 1985–1988: association with verocytotoxin producing E. coli. Part 1: Clinical and epidemiological aspects. *Arch Dis Child* 1990;65:716–721.
27. Kleanthous H, Smith HR, Scotland SM, Gross RJ, Rowe B, Taylor CM, Milford DV. Haemolytic uraemic syndrome in the British Isles 1985–1988: association with verocytotoxin producing E. coli. Part 2: Microbiological aspects. *Arch Dis Child* 1990;65:722–727.
28. Rowe PC, Orrbine E, Lior H, Wells GA, Yetisir E, Clulow M, McLaine PN. Risk of hemolytic uremic syndrome after sporadic *Escherichia coli* O157:H7 infection: results of a Canadian collaborative study. *J Pediatr* 1998;132:777–727.
29. Armstrong GD, Rowe PC, Goodyer P, Orrbine E, Klassen TP, Wells G, MacKenzie A, Lior H,

Blanchard C, Auclair F, *et al*. A phase I study of chemically synthesized verotoxin (Shiga-like toxin) Pk-trisaccharide receptors attached to chromosorb for preventing hemolytic-uremic syndrome. *J Infect Dis* 1995;171: 1042–1045.

30. Oner A, Tinaztepe K, Erdogan O. The effect of triple therapy on rapidly progressive type of Henoch–Schonlein nephritis. *Paediatr Nephrol* 1995;9:6–10.

31. Cole BR, Brocklebank JT, Kienstra RA, Kissane JM, Robson AM. 'Pulse' methylprednisolone therapy in the treatment of severe glomerulonephritis. *J Pediatr* 1976;88:307–314.

32. Chevalier RL. What treatment do you advise for bilateral or unilateral renal thrombosis in the newborn with or without thrombosis in the IVC. *Pediatr Nephrol* 1991;5:679.

33. Oragui EE, Nadel S, Kyd P, Levin M. Increased excretion of urinary gycosaminoglycans in meningoccoccal septicaemia and their relationship to proteinurea. *Crit Care Med* 2000;28:3002–3008.

34. Fleming F, Bohn D, Edwards H, Cox P, Geary D, McCrindle BW, Williams WG. Renal replacement therapy after repair of congenital heart disease in children. A comparison of hemofiltration and peritoneal dialysis. *J Thorac Cardiovasc Surg* 1995; 109: 322–331.

35. Bickell WH, Wall MJ, Pepe PE, Martin RR, Ginger VF, Allen MK, Mattox KL. Immediate versus delayed fluid resuscitation for hypotensive patients with penetrating torso injuries. *N Engl J Med* 1994; 331:1105–1109.

36. Sinclair JF, Skeoch CH, Hallworth D. Prognosis of Meningococcal Septicaemia. *Lancet* 1987;ii:38.

37. Shann F, Pearson G, Slater A, Wilkinson K. Paediatric Index of Mortality (PIM): a mortality prediction model for children in intensive care. *Intensive Care Med* 1997;23:201–207.

38. Gallego N, Gallego A, Pasaval J, Liano F, Estepa R, Ortuno J. Prognosis of children with acute renal failure. A study of 138 cases. *Nephron* 1993; 64: 399–404.

39. Shaw NJ, Brocklebank JT, Dickinson DF, Wilson N, Walker DR. Long term outcome for children with acute renal failure following cardiac surgery. *Int J Cardiol* 1991;31:161–165.

40. Fitzpatrick MM, Shah V, Trompeter RS, Dillon MJ, Barratt TM. Long term renal outcome of childhood haemolytic uraemic syndrome. *Br Med J* 1991; 303:489–492.

23 | *The management of chronic and end stage renal failure in children*

Susan P.A. Rigden

Introduction

Renal failure is a continuum extending from mild renal insufficiency to end stage renal failure (ESRF), its severity being proportional to the reduction in functioning renal mass [1] (Table 23.1). For the purposes of this chapter, chronic renal failure (CRF) is arbitrarily defined by a glomerular filtration rate (GFR) of less than $50\,ml/min/1.73\,m^2$ surface area (SA), i.e. to include moderate and severe renal insufficiency, since below this level of renal function metabolic abnormalities such as acidosis and secondary hyperparathyroidism become increasingly apparent, growth may be impaired, and further progressive loss of function is likely to occur. Renal replacement therapy (RRT), either by dialysis or transplantation, does not usually become necessary until the GFR falls below $10\,ml/min/1.73\,m^2$ SA. The initiation of RRT defines the onset of ESRF, and pre-terminal renal failure (pre-TRF) defines those patients with CRF before RRT becomes necessary.

Ideally, the care of children with renal failure should also be a continuum: those with pre-TRF require careful conservative management in order to prevent metabolic abnormalities, optimize their growth, and to preserve their renal function for as long as possible, which for some, will be into adult life. They should be under the supervision of a paediatric nephrologist, though often their care can be shared with their local paediatrician. Children with ESRF should be treated in specialized children's units, where facilities can be concentrated and expertise developed. Their management is complex, requiring the resources of a multi-professional team comprising not only medical and nursing staff trained in paediatric renal medicine and surgeons experienced in paediatric urology and transplantation, but also specialist children's dieticians, social workers, psychiatrists, psychologists, teachers, and play therapists. The main disadvantage of providing children's ESRF services in specialized units is that many families have to travel, sometimes considerable distances, for treatment. For some children the number of visits to the specialized centre can be reduced by co-opting the local paediatrician or nephrologist to the multidisciplinary team to share in the child's care.

Incidence and prevalence

The incidence of ESRF in children is, fortunately, low. In the United Kingdom in 1997–1999 [2], the annual take-on rate for RRT in patients less than 18 years old, was 101, or 7.4 per million age-adjusted population. On 1 August 1999, 725 patients under 18 years of age were receiving RRT, giving a prevalence of 53.4 per million age-adjusted population: 2.4% of these children were less than 2 years old; 6.4%, 2–5 years; 20.5%, 5–10 years; 41.2%, 10–15 years; and 29.5%, 15–18 years. The fall in numbers after 15 years of age

Table 23.1 Stages of renal failure

	Residual functioning renal mass (%)	GFR ($ml/min/1.73\,m^2$ SA)	
Mild renal insufficiency	50–25	80–50	Asymptomatic
Moderate renal insufficiency	25–15	50–30	Metabolic abnormalities, impaired growth, progressive renal failure
Severe renal insufficiency	15–5	30–10	
End-stage renal failure	<5	<10	RRT required

reflects both the direct referral of some older adolescents presenting with renal failure to adult renal units and the variable age at which patients who commence RRT during childhood are transferred to adult units. In keeping with other studies of ESRF in children, there is a predominance of male patients in all age groups, with an overall male to female ratio of 1.76:1.

A Swedish report [3] gives a median annual incidence of ESRF of 6.4 (range 4.4–9.5) per million children less than 16 years old for the period 1986–1994, during which time the prevalence increased significantly from 17.8 to 38 per million age-adjusted population.

The prevalence of pre-TRF is less well defined because of differing definitions of pre-TRF, the use of different age ranges and the under-reporting that occurs when infants or children are not referred to specialized units. In Sweden [3], in the period 1986–1994,

the prevalence of pre-TRF, defined as a GFR of less than $30 \, ml/min/1.73 \, m^2$ SA, in children aged 6 months to 16 years, decreased from 29.3 to 21 per million age-adjusted population, while in the United Kingdom in 1992 [4], in units defining pre-TRF as a GFR of less than $2.5–30 \, ml/min/1.73 \, m^2$ SA, the prevalence of pre-TRF in children less than 15 years old was 44.2 per million age-adjusted population.

Causes of chronic renal failure

The causes of CRF, compiled from three sources [2,3,5], are summarized in Table 23.2. The primary renal diseases of 683 children less than 18 years of age, undergoing RRT on 8 August 1999, in the United Kingdom, are given in column 1 and

Table 23.2 Causes of chronic renal failure

	UK $n = 683$ %	NAPRTCS $n = 6878$ %	Sweden	
			CRF $n = 118$ %	ESRF $n = 97$ %
Congenital abnormalities	55.1	40	40.7	34.1
Aplasia/hypoplasia/dysplasia	25.5	15.8	17.8	15.5
Obstructive uropathy	20.2	16.1	19.5	15.5
Reflux nephropathy	7.2	5.4	0	0
Prune belly syndrome	2.2	2.7	3.4	3.1
Hereditary conditions	17.6	13.3	26.3	35
Juvenile nephronophthisis/medullary cystic disease	5.3	2.8	6.8	10.3
Polycystic kidney disease-autosomal recessive	1.8	2.8	5.1	7.2
Hereditary nephritis with or without nerve deafness	1.2	2.4		
Cystinosis	2	2.1		
Primary oxalosis	0.4	0.6		
Congenital nephrotic syndrome	6.9	2.6	5.1	7.2
Other hereditary conditions			9.3	10.3
Glomerulonephritis	10.3	22	14.4	14.4
Focal segmental glomerulosclerosis	6.4	11.6	2.5	3.1
Other glomerulonephritides	3.9	10.4	11.9	11.3
Multisystem disease	5.6	6.8	3.4	4.1
Lupus erythematosus		1.7		
Henoch–Schönlein purpura	1.6	1.4		
Haemolytic uraemic syndrome	3.2	2.7	3.4	4.1
Other multisystem diseases	0.8	1		
Miscellaneous	9	12.6	15.2	12.4
Renal vascular disease	4.5	1.7	6.8	4.1
Kidney tumour	1.6	0.6		
Drash syndrome		0.6	2.5	3.1
Others	2.9	9.7	5.9	5.2
Chronic renal failure	2	5.4		
Cause unknown	2	5.4		

those of 6878 patients receiving renal transplants before 21 years of age in North America in the period 1987–2000, in column 2; the causes of CRF (GFR <30 ml/min/1.73 m^2 SA) in 118 Swedish children, 97 of whom required RRT in the period 1986–1994, are shown in columns 3 and 4. It is noteworthy that in the Swedish series, no children were identified as having reflux nephropathy as a cause of CRF.

Congenital abnormalities, which occur more frequently in boys and in younger children, account for the largest proportion of cases in all three series and inherited conditions for a further 13.3–35%. The cause of ESRF is, therefore, determined prenatally in more than 50% of children requiring RRT, which has important implications for antenatal diagnosis and intervention, genetic counselling, and future research.

Presentation

Children with CRF present to their paediatricians in a wide variety of ways, which may be related to the primary renal disease or the consequence of impaired renal function. The onset of CRF may be silent and its progression insidious, with symptoms only developing late in its course.

Key points: Modes of presentation of chronic renal failure

- Antenatal ultrasound scanning
- Abdominal mass
- Urinary tract infection
- Enuresis
- Failure to thrive
- Short stature
- Lethargy and pallor
- Haematuria
- Nephrotic syndrome
- Hypertension
- Congestive cardiac failure
- Seizures
- Failure to recover from acute renal failure
- Screening siblings of index cases.

Antenatal ultrasound scanning

Routine antenatal ultrasound screening has resulted in an increased detection of fetal renal tract anomalies [6], some of which will result in post-natal CRF, e.g. obstructive uropathy due to posterior urethral valves, autosomal recessive polycystic kidney disease. Such an *in utero* diagnosis requires close co-operation between the obstetrician, neonatologist, paediatric nephrologist, and urologist to ensure appropriate pre- and post-delivery management and that the parents are given accurate information (see Chapters 13 and 14).

Abdominal mass

The detection of a renal mass or a palpable bladder may be the first clue to underlying CRF. Investigation, initially by renal tract ultrasound examination and assessment of renal function, will lead to the correct diagnosis.

Urinary tract infection

Investigation of the child presenting with urinary tract infection may reveal a serious underlying renal tract abnormality or reflux nephropathy of sufficient severity to cause CRF (Chapter 11).

Enuresis

The large majority of children with enuresis will have no organic cause found (Chapter 9), but CRF may present in this way in a small number of children. Useful clues are a history of urinary tract infection, the presence of daytime wetting, the onset of secondary enuresis, and a history of polydipsia and polyuria. Early morning urine osmolality is a useful screening test and will often avoid the need for renal tract imaging studies.

Failure to thrive

Chronic uraemia frequently results in anorexia, vomiting, and failure to thrive, particularly in infants and young children, making assessment of renal function mandatory in children presenting with these symptoms. Failure to thrive, with dehydration and electrolyte disturbances, is a common presentation in children with renal tubular disorders (see Chapter 5), which are either associated with CRF, e.g. obstructive uropathy, or which will progress to CRF, e.g. Fanconi's syndrome due to cystinosis.

Short stature

Poor height velocity, short stature, and pubertal delay may all be caused by, and be presenting symptoms of, CRF.

Lethargy, pallor

Pallor, due to the normochromic–normocytic anaemia which results from uraemia, and lethargy, are classic symptoms of CRF, though they do not usually develop until late in its course. Occasionally a child with even less-specific symptoms of ill health is found to have CRF.

Haematuria

The causes and investigation of haematuria are discussed in Chapter 1. Rarely haematuria, usually macroscopic, is the first symptom of a condition which will ultimately cause renal failure, e.g. Alport's syndrome, autosomal dominant polycystic kidney disease.

Nephrotic syndrome

The outcome for children with minimal-change nephrotic syndrome is generally excellent, but for those with steroid-resistant disease the outlook is less favourable, with a significant number progressing to chronic and ESRF (Chapter 19). Infants with congenital nephrotic syndrome also have a poor prognosis, either succumbing to infection or eventually developing CRF.

Hypertension

Hypertension, usually symptomatic, is not infrequently the presenting feature of renal parenchymal scarring due, for example, to reflux nephropathy, which may also result in CRF. Assessment of renal function is therefore essential in all children with hypertension (Chapters 7 and 8). Non-renin-dependent hypertension due to salt and water retention also occurs in children with CRF, but is less likely to be a presenting feature unless it results in cardiac failure (see below).

Congestive cardiac failure

Congestive cardiac failure resulting from untreated hypertension and/or salt and water overload does not usually develop until late in the course of CRF, but in some children it may be the presenting symptom, requiring urgent treatment with diuretics or dialysis, and occasionally ventilation.

Seizures

Children with unsuspected CRF may present with seizures secondary to hypertension or fluid and electrolyte disturbances, particularly hypocalcaemia.

Failure to recover from acute renal failure

Occasionally a child with acute renal failure will make no or an incomplete recovery and be left in chronic or ESRF, e.g. as a result of rapidly progressive glomerulonephritis, or there may be a slow but inexorable decline in renal function, usually heralded by hypertension and/or proteinuria, in a child who had apparently made a good recovery from acute renal failure, e.g. haemolytic uraemic syndrome [7] or Henoch–Schönlein purpura.

Asymptomatic: detected by screening

Very rarely an asymptomatic child is found to be hypertensive or to have proteinuria or microscopic haematuria on routine urinalysis, which on investigation is found to be due to serious underlying renal disease.

It is important to screen even the apparently healthy siblings of children with genetically determined CRF, e.g. juvenile nephronophthisis, Alport's syndrome, or reflux nephropathy, while realizing the potentially devastating effect on the family of finding a further affected child.

Investigation of the child with CRF

It may not be clear at presentation whether a child has acute, and therefore potentially reversible renal failure (see Chapter 22), or CRF. However, the priority is to establish whether the child requires urgent referral to a specialized children's unit, based on the criteria listed in Table 23.3.

History and examination may provide valuable pointers to the underlying cause of renal failure, but in some children this will only be revealed by specific investigations (Table 23.4). The features listed in Table 23.5 may help differentiate ARF from CRF, and those in Table 23.6 establish the severity and duration of CRF.

Table 23.3 Indications for transfer to a specialist paediatric nephrology centre

Symptomatic electrolyte abnormalities
   Hyperkalaemia: $K^+ > 6$ mmol/l
   Hypernatraemia, hyponatraemia
   Metabolic acidosis
   Hypocalcaemia, hyperphosphataemia
Severe hypertension
Pulmonary oedema
Anuria/oliguria

Table 23.4 Specific investigations to elucidate the underlying cause of chronic renal failure

Renal tract ultrasound
Micturating cystourethrogram
Radio-isotope scans: DMSA, MAG3, or DTPA
Antegrade pressure flow studies
Intravenous urogram
Urinalysis
Urine microscopy and culture
C3, C4, antinuclear antibody, anti-DNA antibodies, anti-GBM antibodies, ANCA
Renal biopsy
White cell cystine level
Oxalate excretion
Purine excretion

Table 23.5 Features suggestive of acute and chronic renal failure

Acute renal failure	Chronic renal failure
Previously healthy	Family history of renal disease
Normal or slightly enlarged kidneys on ultrasound	Small/asymmetric kidneys, cystic kidneys, abnormal collecting systems, ureters, and bladder on ultrasound
Microangiopathic haemolytic anaemia, thrombocytopenia	Normochromic, normocytic anaemia
	End-organ effects of hypertension, e.g. retinopathy
	Poor growth
	Radiological evidence of rickets or secondary hyperparathyroidism

Table 23.6 Investigations to assess the severity and duration of CRF

Full blood count	
Biochemistry	Blood electrolytes, urea, creatinine, calcium, phosphate, alkaline phosphatase, total protein, albumin, urate
	Blood pH and bicarbonate
	Parathyroid hormone using an intact molecule assay
	Urine creatinine, phosphate, protein, albumin
GFR	Of less value in severe chronic renal failure
Left hand and wrist X-ray	For bone age and evidence of renal osteodystrophy
Chest X-ray	
ECG or echocardiogram	To assess left ventricular hypertrophy

• be *normal*, i.e. to be like his or her friends and have sufficient energy to take a full part in all school and social activities; or, for the pre-school child, to achieve normal motor, social, and intellectual development;

• maintain *normal* growth;

while:

• preserving *normal* family functioning;

• slowing the rate of progression to ESRF;

• preparing the child and family for RRT.

For the child with moderate to severe CRF (GFR < 30 ml/min/1.73 m² SA), these objectives are best met by a multiprofessional team approach in the setting of a dedicated clinic, where ample time can be spent with each child and his or her family [8].

For children with less severe degrees of CRF, it may be appropriate for their care to be shared with their local paediatrician, either in out-reach clinics or by alternating clinic visits with those to the specialist centre.

The frequency of clinic visits is determined by:

• the child's age: babies and infants generally require more intensive input and therefore more frequent clinic visits than older children;

• the level of renal function, e.g. children with GFRs below 20 ml/min/1.73 m² SA usually need to be seen every 4 weeks, whereas those with GFRs above 30 ml/min/1.73 m² SA do not normally need to attend clinic at less than 12-weekly intervals;

Management of pre-terminal renal failure

The aims of conservative management of pre-TRF are, from the child's viewpoint, to:

• feel *normal*, i.e. not to have uraemic symptoms such as nausea or vomiting;

- the rate of progression of renal failure: children with stable CRF require less frequent clinic visits than those with declining renal function;
- the presence of complications of CRF, e.g. the child with poor growth or severe secondary hyperparathyroidism may require more frequent clinic visits while the problem is being brought under control.

Measurements

Regular and reliable measurements of height or length according to the age of the child and weight are essential for the optimal management of CRF.

Weight and blood pressure should be recorded at each clinic visit. Height or, for children less than 18 months of age or unable to stand, supine length, should also be measured, ideally by the same trained observer using suitable equipment, at each visit, unless the child is attending clinic more frequently than every month. Children under 2 years old should also have their head circumference measured and plotted on a suitable chart.

In older children pubertal status should be assessed and recorded using the Tanner classification and in boys, testicular volume measured using an orchidometer.

Laboratory measurements are listed in Table 23.7. A urine sample should be collected under sterile conditions at each visit for urinalysis and, if indicated, microscopy and culture. The urine protein/creatinine ratio should also be measured. Increasing proteinuria often heralds the progression of renal failure.

An annual X-ray of the non-dominant wrist and hand should be obtained for the determination of bone age and for radiological evidence of renal osteodystrophy (see below).

Table 23.7 Laboratory parameters to be monitored in clinic

Full blood count	
Serum ferritin	3 monthly
Biochemistry	Plasma electrolytes, creatinine
	Urea, total protein, albumin
	Calcium, phosphate, alkaline phosphatase
	Urate
	Parathyroid hormone (PTH)— using an intact molecule assay
	pH, bicarbonate
	Urine protein/creatinine ratio

Management points

The following management points need to be considered at each clinic visit.

Nutrition

Untreated, renal failure results in malnutrition and, in children, growth retardation [9]. Nutritional therapy, carefully applied, can ameliorate the effects of renal failure and promote improved well-being and growth [10]; it may also have a role in slowing the rate of progression of renal failure. The services of a skilled paediatric renal dietician are invaluable in the provision of individualized nutritional therapy, without undue disruption to the family's eating pattern.

The recommended intakes of nutrients for children with CRF are given in Table 23.8 [11], but the following points need to be emphasized:

1. The intake of nutrients should be monitored by prospective 3-day dietary assessments performed twice a year, and more often if clinically indicated.

2. Children with CRF tend to be anorexic and frequently have spontaneous energy intakes below the estimated average requirement (EAR) for age. The term EAR refers to the 'estimated average requirement of a group of people for energy or protein or a vitamin or mineral: about half will usually need more than the EAR and half less'. This has superseded recommended daily allowance (RDA), defined as 'sufficient or more than sufficient for the nutritional needs of practically all healthy people in a population'. Energy intakes of less than 80% of the RDA have previously been shown to be associated with growth retardation [12], which can be reversed by increasing energy intake to 100% RDA. Energy intakes in excess of this do not confer any additional benefit, except perhaps in children with low weight-to-height ratios, who may require energy intakes of up to 120% RDA. To achieve EAR for age for energy, most children with CRF require calorie supplements in the form of glucose polymers or fat emulsions, which, for infants and young children, may need to be added to a feed to be delivered by a naso-gastric or gastrostomy tube [13].

3. In order to prevent or treat secondary hyperparathyroidism, plasma phosphate must be maintained between the mean and −2SD for age, by restriction of dietary phosphate and the use of calcium carbonate as a phosphate binder (see below) [14]. As the major dietary sources of phosphate are

dairy products, adequate phosphate restriction can usually be achieved by limiting the intake of cow's milk to less than half a pint a day and by avoiding cheese and yoghurt.

4. In animal models, dietary protein restriction slows the progression of renal failure. However, in patients, the use of low protein diets has proved much more problematic with only marginal benefit in properly controlled trials [15]. In children, who have a higher protein requirement because of the demands of growth, protein restriction has been shown to be of no benefit in retarding progression of renal failure [16] and in a short-term study in infants was associated with inferior growth [17]. Children with CRF should therefore receive a minimum protein intake of EAR for age (Table 23.8). If dairy proteins have been restricted as above to limit phosphate intake, and energy intake ensured to promote anabolism, further protein restriction is seldom necessary. If, despite these measures, a child's blood urea remains above 20 mmol/l, a gentle step-wise protein restriction, using the child's 3-day dietary assessment as the basis for advice, should be introduced to reduce the blood urea to less than 20 mmol/l.

Fluid and electrolyte balance

Clinical assessment of the child's state of hydration using skin turgor, mucous membrane moisture, blood pressure, jugular venous pressure, and weight should be performed at each clinic visit. Many causes of CRF in children are associated with excessive sodium loss, e.g. obstructive uropathy, renal dysplasia, juvenile nephronophthisis. Sodium depletion results in contraction of the extracellular fluid volume and further impairment in renal function: it is also detrimental to growth [18]. Sodium chloride supplements should be gradually increased until an improvement in growth is seen or the child develops peripheral oedema or hypertension, when they should be reduced to the maximum tolerated level. Some infants may require an intake of sodium chloride of 4–6 mmol/kg/day to ensure normal physical and intellectual development.

Water intake is determined by the child and should, therefore, be offered freely to infants, to satisfy thirst.

Children with primary renal diseases resulting in hypertension may benefit from a reduction in sodium intake to 1–2 mmol/kg/day, but it is seldom necessary to restrict fluid intake until ESRF supervenes.

Most children with CRF are able to maintain potassium homeostasis satisfactorily despite fluctuations in intake. If hyperkalaemia occurs, it is important to exclude drugs such as ACE inhibitors, catabolism, and metabolic acidosis as correctable causes, as well as giving individually tailored advice based on the child's dietary assessments.

Table 23.8 Recommended daily energy and nutrient intakes for children with chronic renal failure[a]

Age	Mean weight (kg)	Energy EAR (kcal)	Protein EAR (g)	Protein RNI (g)	Sodium RNI (mmol)	Calcium RNI (mg)	Phosphorus RNI (mg)
0–3 months	5.9	115/kg	–	2.1/kg	9	525	400
4–6 months	7.7	100/kg	1.4/kg	1.6/kg	12	525	400
7–9 months	8.8	95/kg	1.3/kg	1.6/kg	14	525	400
10–12 months	9.7	95/kg	1.2/kg	1.5/kg	15	525	400
1–3 years	12.5	1230	11.7	14.5	22	350	270
4–6 years	17.8	1715	14.8	19.7	30	450	350
7–10 years	28.3	1970	22.8	28.3	52	550	450
11–14 years							
Males	43	2220	33.8	42.1	70	1000	775
Females	43.8	1845	33.1	41.2	70	800	625
15–18 years							
Males	64.5	2755	46.1	55.2	70	1000	775
Females	55.5	2110	37.1	45.4	70	800	625

[a] Based on UK dietary reference values (Department of Health, 1991).
EAR, Estimated average requirement.
RNI, Reference nutrient intake = EAR + 2SD.

Key points: Management points in the child with CRF

- Nutrition

- Fluid and electrolyte balance

- Acid–base status

- Renal osteodystrophy

- Hypertension

- Infection

- Preservation of renal function

- Anaemia

- Growth

- Education and preparation

- Social and psychological support.

Acid–base status

Maintenance of acid–base balance is particularly important in infants and children. Persistent metabolic acidosis is associated with failure to thrive in infancy and contributes to muscle degradation, bone demineralization and hyperkalaemia. The severity of metabolic acidosis may be masked by ECF volume contraction (see above) and only becomes apparent when this is corrected. Although reducing protein intake, and therefore the intake of sulphur-containing amino acids, reduces endogenous acid production, sodium bicarbonate supplements, in a starting dose of 2 mmol/kg/day, are frequently required to correct metabolic acidosis. Treatment should be monitored and dosage adjusted according to venous blood gas determinations of pH and bicarbonate concentration.

Renal osteodystrophy

The optimal management of renal osteodystrophy in children is controversial [14,19], but several important points should be noted:

1. Parathyroid hormone (PTH) levels may be increased and 1,25-dihydroxycholecalciferol levels decreased even with relatively mild renal insufficiency, i.e. with GFRs of 50–80 ml/min/1.73 m² SA. It is therefore essential to monitor PTH levels, using

an intact molecule assay, in all children with renal insufficiency in order to prevent not only the skeletal, but also the non-skeletal consequences, e.g. bone marrow suppression, of secondary hyperparathyroidism.

2. Plasma phosphate concentration is central in the pathogenesis of secondary hyperparathyroidism. There is now convincing evidence that phosphate regulates parathyroid cells independent of its effects on serum calcium and endogenous 1,25-dihydroxycholecalciferol levels [20]. Control of plasma phosphate is therefore the most important factor in the prevention and treatment of secondary hyperparathyroidism, but is also the most difficult to achieve long term, since it requires both compliance with diet to restrict the intake of phosphorus and oral phosphate binding drugs to reduce its absorption. Dietary phosphate intake should be reduced, initially by limiting cow's milk and cow's milk-derived products, to the recommended level for age (Table 23.8): if the plasma phosphate remains above the mean value for age [21], oral phosphate-binding drugs, e.g. calcium carbonate in a starting dose of approximately 100 mg/kg/day, should then be prescribed to be taken with meals or feeds, and the dosage adjusted until the plasma phosphate falls between the mean and −2SD for age [22]. Calcium acetate and, more recently, the non-calcium/non-aluminium containing polymer, sevelamer [23], are also used as phosphate-binding agents.

3. Reduction in plasma phosphate results in increased levels of endogenous 1,25-dihydroxycholecalciferol and ionized calcium, which may be sufficient to normalize PTH levels [24]. If, however, PTH remains elevated and the plasma phosphate normal, additional hydroxylated vitamin D₃ should be prescribed.

4. The type, dose, frequency, and route of administration of vitamin D used in the prevention and treatment of renal osteodystrophy remain controversial. In the author's unit, we have used, almost exclusively, relatively low-dose oral 1α-hydroxycholecalciferol, in a starting dose of 15–30 ng/kg/once daily for children weighing less than 20 kg and 250–500 ng once daily in older children, to increase the plasma calcium to the upper limit of normal: once the PTH has normalized, it is often possible, and indeed is desirable, to discontinue the 1α-hydroxycholecalciferol for a period of time. Intermittent, and particularly intravenous, administration of 1,25-dihydroxycholecalciferol is reported to be more effective in decreasing serum PTH levels, but it may be associated with,

and is perhaps the cause of, adynamic bone, since 1,25-dihydroxycholecalciferol has, at high doses, an antiproliferative effect on osteoblasts [25].

5. Careful monitoring is mandatory to avoid hypercalcaemia and metastatic calcification. Plasma calcium, phosphate, and alkaline phosphatase are measured each time the child is seen. The PTH level should be checked using an intact molecule assay, monthly or at each clinic visit if the child is attending clinic less frequently and therapy adjusted accordingly. If the child is asymptomatic and the biochemical parameters normal, it is only necessary to perform an annual X-ray of the left hand and wrist to assess bone age.

Hypertension

Hypertension may result from the primary renal disease, e.g. reflux nephropathy, autosomal recessive polycystic kidney disease, or, in advanced CRF, from sodium and water retention. If, in the absence of circulatory volume overload, the child's systolic or diastolic blood pressure is repeatedly in excess of the 90th centile for age, specific hypotensive therapy should be instituted to prevent the morbidity and mortality associated with hypertension and to retard the progression of CRF (see below). If there is evidence of circulatory volume overload causing or contributing to hypertension, a diuretic, usually frusemide in a dose of 1–3 mg/kg, should be commenced and sodium restricted as above. (see also Chapters 7 and 8).

Infection

Children with renal tract abnormalities predisposing them to recurrent urinary tract infections must have a urine sample cultured at each clinic visit. They should be maintained on low-dose prophylactic antibiotics, remembering that nitrofurantoin becomes less effective with declining renal function, and practise the general measures to prevent reinfection, as outlined in Chapter 11. Other bacterial infections, e.g. otitis media, should be treated promptly to reverse catabolism.

Preservation of renal function

In the majority of patients with CRF, renal function continues to decline, irrespective of the primary renal disease and whether or not it is still active. Progression of CRF is associated histologically with progressive glomerulosclerosis, interstitial fibrosis, and vascular or arteriolar sclerosis. Numerous hypotheses, which are not necessarily mutually exclusive, have been proposed to explain these scarring processes [26,27].

Various therapeutic interventions have been proposed to slow the progression of CRF, including the control of hypertension, reduction of proteinuria, and modification of dietary protein intake (see above) [28]. In the proteinuric patient, the urine contains numerous toxic/inflammatory factors that promote the progression of renal disease, including complement, inflammatory lipoproteins, and iron species which induce free oxygen-radical formation. There is now compelling evidence that the use of ACE inhibitors to reduce proteinuria is renoprotective, independent of their effect on blood pressure in both diabetic and non-diabetic nephropathies [29,30]. Proteinuria should therefore be monitored at each clinic visit and treated if significant.

Anaemia

CRF is associated with normochromic, normocytic anaemia due to inadequate erythropoietin production by the peritubular interstitial cells of the inner cortex and outer medulla of the kidney. Recombinant human erythropoietin (rHuEPO) is available and now widely used to reverse anaemia in CRF [31]. However, there are other contributory aetiological factors, including reduced red blood cell survival, bone marrow inhibition, particularly by PTH, intestinal blood loss, and, most commonly, iron and folate deficiency.

The majority of children with pre-TRF can maintain satisfactory haemoglobin levels without exogenous rHuEPO therapy, provided that careful attention is paid to nutrition, iron and folate supplements are given if indicated, and secondary hyperparathyroidism is suppressed without the use of aluminium-containing phosphate binders. If, despite these measures, a child's quality of life is being limited by anaemia, rHuEPO should be commenced in a dose of 50 units/kg subcutaneously twice weekly and the dose titrated according to response, to achieve a target haemoglobin of 100–120 g/dl. The serum ferritin level should be maintained above 100 μg/l to ensure adequate iron supplies. In children with pre-TRF, this is usually possible using oral iron supplements, though those treated by dialysis may require intravenous supplementation (see below).

Growth

Growth is the most sensitive indicator of adequacy of CRF treatment. Height or supine length, weight and, for children under 2 years of age, head circumference, should be measured at each clinic visit (see above) and the values obtained plotted for chronological age on appropriate centile charts. Using these data, early fall-off in growth velocity or weight can easily be identified and its cause investigated, with a view to correcting it, rather than simply ascribing the poor growth to 'CRF'. The main factors affecting growth in children with CRF are listed in Table 23.9.

The pattern of growth in any individual child with CRF is influenced by the age of the child, the age at onset of CRF and the treatment given [32]. In normal children, growth velocity is maximal during the first 2 years of life: growth then slows through mid-childhood, only to accelerate again with the pubertal growth spurt. Suboptimal growth during either or both of these two critical periods results in reduction in final height.

During the first 2 years of life, during which growth is mainly driven by nutritional factors, normal infants achieve approximately 50% of their ultimate height potential: it is hardly surprising therefore, that CRF dating from infancy has a disproportionate effect on final height. Infants with CRF may lose as much as 0.6 height SDS (standard deviation score) per month during the first few months of life [12], and many are, as a result, already significantly growth retarded when first seen in a specialist centre, emphasizing the need for early referral. This poor growth can be prevented or arrested and in some infants catch-up growth, induced by scrupulous attention to the provision of adequate nutrition and water and electrolyte balance [13].

Table 23.9 Possible factors contributing to growth retardation in chronic renal failure

Inadequate energy intake
Inappropriate protein intake
Disturbances of water and electrolyte balance, particularly sodium chloride deficiency and metabolic acidosis
Renal osteodystrophy
Hypertension
Infection
Anaemia
Hormonal abnormalities
Corticosteroid therapy
Psychosocial factors

Growth during childhood is under the influence of growth hormone (GH) and with the advent of puberty, sex steroids play a major role. Children with CRF usually maintain a normal or near normal growth velocity during mid-childhood. Catch-up growth occurs less commonly than in infants with pre-TRF. Pre-pubertal children with CRF growing below the 3rd centile for age respond well to supra-physiological doses of recombinant human GH (rhGH) (see below).

The onset of puberty is often delayed in children with CRF, although it occurs at the appropriate bone age. The normal pre-pubertal decrease in growth velocity may be prolonged in children with CRF and followed by a pubertal growth spurt of only 50% of that expected, resulting in further reduction in final height [33].

If, despite optimal management, growth remains poor, i.e. the child's height velocity SDS is below -2 or the height SDS is below -2, a trial of rhGH therapy should be considered. Given in a dose of 30 units/m² SA/week, divided into seven daily doses, by subcutaneous injection or high-pressure gun. Pre-pubertal children with pre-TRF have, in many studies [34], shown a significant increase in growth velocity and, with continued treatment and improvement in final height [35]. Results in pubertal children and in those treated by dialysis or who have received renal transplants have, in general, been less impressive, making it even more important that a child realizes their genetic potential for height before puberty or transplantation.

Potential side-effects of rhGH treatment include exacerbation of pre-existing glucose intolerance due to peripheral insulin resistance in uraemia, although in clinical practice this has not proved a problem. Concern has also been raised that rhGH may have a deleterious effect on renal function as a result of glomerular hyperfiltration, but this has not been borne out in controlled trials, either in children with pre-TRF or after renal transplantation. However, rhGH is an immunomodulatory substance and, in a prospectively controlled study, there was an increase in acute rejection episodes in patients who had experienced more than one rejection episode before the start of rhGH therapy [36]. Benign intracranial hypertension has been recorded more frequently in children with pre-TRF receiving rhGH than in GH-deficient children under treatment and there is a theoretical risk of malignancy.

Synthetic androgens, usually oxandrolone, and testosterone derivatives have been used in boys with constitutional delay of growth and puberty, to induce the onset of puberty without compromising final height, but data on their use in children with CRF are less conclusive.

Key points: Growth in chronic renal failure

- Growth is the most sensitive indicator of adequacy of CRF treatment. Height or supine length, weight and, for children under 2 years of age, head circumference should be measured at each clinic visit and the values obtained plotted for chronological age on appropriate centile charts.

- If, despite optimal management, growth remains poor, i.e. the child's height velocity SDS is below −2 or the height SDS is below −2, a trial of growth hormone therapy should be considered.

Education and preparation

The conservative phase of CRF management is an ideal time for an ongoing programme of education for the child and family. It is very important that the child and their family understand the rationale of pre-TRF therapy and that ultimately RRT will be necessary. It is usually possible to predict with reasonable accuracy, when ESRF will supervene, from a plot of the reciprocal of the plasma creatinine or the calculated GFR. Using this prediction, there should, at an appropriate time, be full discussion of the various RRT options available (see below). It is very helpful for the child and family to meet other children treated by peritoneal and haemodialysis and also those who have been transplanted. They should also meet the various staff involved, including the transplant surgeon, and visit the dialysis unit, so that by the time RRT becomes necessary, they are thoroughly acquainted with all therapeutic options.

In addition to education, there are also important practical preparations for ESRF management to be considered:

1. Immunizations, including BCG, hepatitis B, and, if indicated, varicella zoster, should be completed at least 3 months before RRT is anticipated to be required.

2. If a child with pre-TRF is receiving an enzyme–inducing anti-epileptic drug, this should, if possible, be replaced by a non-enzyme-inducing agent such as sodium valproate or lamotrigine, to facilitate adequate immunosuppression following transplantation.

3. Children with CRF associated with bladder dysfunction require very careful assessment, including urodynamic studies, to ensure that the bladder is safe prior to transplantation. Management with clean intermittent catheterization and/or bladder augmentation surgery, with or without the creation of a Mitrofanoff channel, may be necessary to achieve this.

4. Children who are likely to require dialysis prior to transplantation, but who are not suitable for peritoneal dialysis, should, if appropriate, have an arterio-venous fistula created to provide access for haemodialysis (see below).

Social and psychological support

The management of a child with progressive pre-TRF can be extremely stressful, even to the best-adjusted families. CRF and its treatment may be disruptive to a child's schooling, social life, and family life: siblings may feel excluded and the parents' relationship put under stress; there may be financial difficulties as a result of a parent having to give up work and the expense of travelling, sometimes long distances, to the specialist centre.

Good medical management will minimize illness, and good patient and family education the fear of the unknown. It is important that the child attends a normal school, develops normal peer-group relationships, and takes part in out-of-school activities: liaison between the hospital-based teacher and the child's school can be useful in this respect. The problems of denial and non-compliance with treatment may be helped by encouraging school friends, as well as siblings, to visit the hospital and to become part of the extended team. All families should have easy access to a social worker for help with practical and financial difficulties, as well as for psychological support. Many families derive support from each other, either informally or through a parents' support group. More difficult problems, such as behavioural disorders, feeding problems, and poor family functioning ideally require skilled intervention by a child psychologist or psychiatrist, who should be seen as part of the team (see Chapter 24).

With careful attention to the management points detailed above, it is possible to improve the well-being, activity, and growth of children with pre-TRF and possibly prolong the time until RRT is required. However, even with meticulous management, most children with pre-TRF eventually progress to ESRF, while other children present in ESRF.

Management of end stage renal failure

The aims of ESRF treatment for children are not only to sustain life, but also to permit a worthwhile quality of life, with the ultimate goal of an enjoyable and satisfying adult life.

The treatment of ESRF is much better considered as a potentially repetitive cycle (Fig. 23.1) rather than as a simple progression from pre-TRF to dialysis to transplantation to cure, since for those less fortunate patients, who do not attain a successful transplant, this model exacerbates the sense of failure and disappointment. Children with pre-TRF may enter the cycle at point A for pre-emptive transplantation or at

point B, with those presenting in ESRF, for a period of dialysis prior to transplantation. The ideal exit is with normal renal function, but if this is not achieved and further treatment is appropriate, the cycle continues, and the child returns to dialysis with a view to a further transplant.

Treatment options

Successful renal transplantation is undoubtedly the treatment of choice for all children with ESRF [37].

Some families will have a choice between living-related kidney donation and cadaveric transplantation: they *must* understand the arguments for and against both types of transplantation before making such a decision. Living donor transplantation avoids an unpredictable and sometimes long wait for a suitable cadaveric graft and facilitates pre-emptive transplantation. The results of living donor transplantation are superior to those obtained by cadaveric transplantation, with 6-year graft survival rates of 74% and 58%, respectively [38]. None the less, a quarter of living-related kidney grafts are lost by 5 years post-transplant. The psychological consequences of such loss, particularly if due to rejection, may be profound for donor and recipient.

The advantages to the recipient of living-related kidney transplantation have to be weighed against the risks to the donor. Living-donor organ donation is the only operation with no planned physical benefits to the patient, though there may be psychological benefits. The peri-operative mortality rate for donors in North America has been estimated to be 0.03% [39]. The same authors, in a study of 57 donors over a mean follow-up period of 23.7 years, have observed no progressive rise in plasma creatinine levels and no increased incidence of hypertension or proteinuria, when compared with sibling controls or the general population. They conclude that renal transplant donors are not at increased risk for the development of renal failure. The arguments favouring living-related kidney transplantation appear more persuasive in North America than in Europe: in North America in 2000, more than 60% of transplanted kidneys came from a living-related donor [5], compared with only 30% in the United Kingdom [40].

For some children there will be a choice between entering the treatment cycle at point A (Fig. 23.1) for pre-emptive transplantation or at point B for a period of dialysis prior to transplantation. Pre-emptive transplantation is being performed more frequently,

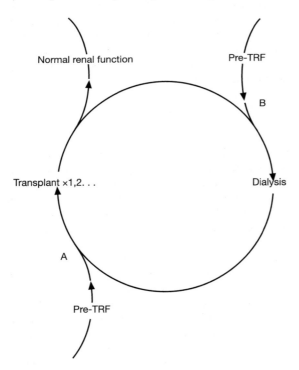

Fig. 23.1   The circular model of ESRF management.

with several recent reports confirming that it is detrimental neither to the patient nor to graft survival [41,42]. Pre-emptive transplantation is obviously easier using a living-related donor but is also possible with a well-organized cadaveric programme. Potential benefits of pre-emptive transplantation before the child develops symptoms and adopts the 'sick' role, include improved growth, nutrition, and neurological outcome, particularly for the younger child; less time lost from school and less disturbance in established social patterns, leading to better rehabilitation; avoidance of access surgery and therefore fewer scars; and reduced financial costs.

Pre-emptive transplantation in adults has been associated with an increase in non-compliance with medications, but this has not been the case in children. Critics have suggested that pre-emptive transplantation leads to decreased involvement and education of the patient and family before transplantation and to greater difficulties in adapting to dialysis if the transplant should fail. However, both of these objections can be overcome by improving patient and family education during the conservative phase of CRF management.

Dialysis should be seen as a complement to transplantation, which may be needed before or between transplants, but ideally not as an alternative to transplantation. When dialysis options are being discussed with the family, there are two basic choices: is the child to be treated by haemodialysis or peritoneal dialysis and is the child to be dialysed at home or in hospital? There may be medical constraints to the first choice (e.g. difficult vascular access may dictate peritoneal dialysis, or intra-abdominal adhesions may preclude peritoneal dialysis), but if not, the child and family should decide which mode of dialysis they prefer. The second decision depends on the family's resources. Home peritoneal dialysis offers advantages in psychosocial adjustment, compared with hospital haemodialysis, but if continued for long periods of time, it may be associated with family 'burn-out'. Nightly peritoneal dialysis, particularly if naso-gastric or gastrostomy feeding, and regular injections of rhGH and rHuEPO are also required, may result in an immense responsibility and burden on the principal care-giver.

The third option, that of no active treatment, is becoming increasingly rare, but remains a valid, if difficult, choice on behalf of some children. The critical questions are whether intervention by dialysis or transplantation will permit the child a worthwhile quality of life and whether the expected medical gain is greater than the harm or risk of harm of treatment. These questions are particularly difficult to answer on behalf of infants and the increasing number of children with severe learning difficulties and ESRF. The results of ESRF treatment in infants without co-morbid conditions are improving [13], but treatment may be arduous, particularly if dialysis access proves difficult. Dialysis is the only active treatment option available for infants with ESRF, since transplantation is not usually undertaken in children weighing less than 10 kg.

The decision to embark on treatment by dialysis and transplantation or to withhold active treatment, should be made for each child individually after full discussion with the family, the child at a level appropriate to their age and maturity, and the multidisciplinary team. A decision to pursue active treatment, particularly for a child who cannot express his or her own views, should be coupled with an agreement to review the child's treatment at regular intervals, to try to ensure that the gain outweighs the pain. If the treatment is proving too arduous for the quality of life obtained, the question of withdrawing treatment must be discussed and agreed by the parents and the whole treatment team. Difficult problems arise if the family and the multidisciplinary team cannot agree on the most appropriate treatment for a child. Second opinions from other clinicians can be helpful, but if agreement still cannot be reached, then it may be necessary to apply to the courts for a decision.

Indications for initiating renal replacement therapy

Ideally children with progressive pre-TRF should be transplanted just before they become symptomatic from their renal failure and require dialysis, i.e. undergo pre-emptive transplantation. For children of families who have opted for cadaveric transplantation resident in the United Kingdom, this is usually possible if the child is registered on the national 'active' waiting list for cadaveric transplantation held at UK Transplant, when their calculated GFR has fallen to approximately 10 ml/min/1.73 m^2 SA. Waiting time is dependent on blood group, tissue type, and the supply of kidneys, but in the United Kingdom with the current kidney allocation scheme, the median waiting time for a kidney, for the 50% of children classified as 'easy to match', is 96 days and 368 days for the 50% of 'hard to match' children.

Not all children are suitable for pre-emptive transplantation, e.g. those with nephrotic-range proteinuria and/or hypertension require bilateral nephrectomy and therefore a period of dialysis before transplantation. Other children present in ESRF and require dialysis before the necessary assessment, education, and preparation for renal transplantation can occur: it is particularly important to give such children and their families adequate time to adjust to their new situation before planning for long-term RRT.

If pre-emptive renal transplantation is not possible, indications for commencing dialysis are:

- uraemic symptoms such as lethargy, anorexia, or vomiting, which interfere with daily life;
- dangerous biochemical abnormalities, e.g. hyperkalaemia, unresponsive to the measures outlined above;
- circulatory overload refractory to diuretic therapy.

Dialysis

The relative merits of peritoneal (PD) and haemodialysis (HD) are summarized in Table 23.10. In the United Kingdom [40], the USA [5], and many other countries, PD is the preferred dialysis modality for children. Of the 135 children less than 15 years old, maintained on dialysis in the United Kingdom in 2000, 111 (82%) were first treated by PD, but only 79 (58.5%) were receiving PD at the time of the cross-sectional survey. The increase in HD was predominantly in the 10–15-year-old band, suggesting that either through choice or necessity, older children or those with ESRF for longer are being treated with HD. If this is because of loss of peritoneal access or function, it will have important implications for their future treatment [40].

Peritoneal dialysis

PD uses the child's peritoneal membrane as an exchange mechanism for small solutes, by diffusion down a concentration gradient, and for water together with larger solutes, by convective mass transfer. Peritoneal membrane transport capacity can be assessed using a standardized peritoneal equilibration test, the results of which can be helpful in determining the child's PD prescription. Adequacy of PD should then be monitored by regular clearance studies.

Successful PD requires a reliable peritoneal catheter: there are multiple types of soft, permanent PD catheters in a variety of configurations, available for surgical placement, although curled Tenckhoff catheters, when combined with an omentectomy, are probably less prone to blockage [43]. Peritoneal catheters pose a risk of infection, either at the exit site, in the subcutaneous tunnel or within the peritoneum, with peritonitis being the single most common complication of PD [44].

PD may be performed either intermittently, usually overnight, using an automated cycling machine to deliver 8–10 exchanges over 8–10 hours, or continuously by CAPD (continuous ambulatory peritoneal dialysis) or by CCPD (continuous cycling peritoneal dialysis). CAPD utilizes the peritoneum 24 h per day, with the child or carer performing four exchanges of dialysate during the day with a long overnight dwell. CCPD combines five or six overnight exchanges delivered by an automated cycling machine with a long daytime dwell. CCPD obviates the need for daytime exchanges and reduces the number of system disconnections to two per day, as well as improving PD adequacy in patients with average peritoneal transport rates. In the United Kingdom, automated cycling dialysis is clearly preferred over CAPD with, in 2000, only 11.6% of children being treated with PD using CAPD [40].

Table 23.10 Relative merits of peritoneal and haemodialysis

Peritoneal dialysis	Haemodialysis
Technically easier to perform	Can provide greater levels of small molecule mass transfer
Avoids sudden shifts of fluid and metabolites	Only available in specialized centres
Preferable for young/small patients	Usually requires greater fluid restriction
Can be performed at home and on holiday	Relieves family of stress and responsibility
Minimizes fluid and dietary restrictions	Usually requires 3 × 3–5 hour sessions/week
Associated with a less severe degree of anaemia	depending on patient size
High level of responsibility for principle care-giver	
Can lead to treatment fatigue/ 'burn-out'	
Less disruptive to daily routine	
Facilitates regular school attendance	

Haemodialysis

Haemodialysis is a technique of removing or 'clearing' small molecular weight solutes from the blood by diffusion through a semi-permeable membrane. As blood is passed over the dialyser membrane, water and small molecular weight solutes pass through the membrane to form the ultrafiltrate. The rate at which ultrafiltrate is formed is controlled by two variables—the ultrafiltration coefficient, which is a characteristic of the membrane, and the pressure gradient across the membrane, which with modern dialysis machines can be varied and controlled.

Haemodialysis requires access to the circulation, which is best provided by an arterio-venous fistula created from the radial or brachial vessels of the non-dominant arm. However, it is more usual [40,45], particularly in young children, to use a surgically placed, double-lumen, central venous catheter to access the circulation, in order to avoid the trauma of placing dialysis needles in a fistula. However, central venous catheters do pose an infection risk and, perhaps more importantly, may result in stenosis or occlusion of large central veins, making further access difficult [46]. The problem of optimal long-term vascular access for children, remains unsolved. In a recent cross-sectional survey in the United Kingdom [40], all children under 10 years old being treated by HD and two-thirds of those aged 10–15 years, had a central venous catheter for vascular access.

Limitations of dialysis

Although HD and PD provide effective RRT, the mortality rate for dialysis is higher than that for transplantation for all age groups of children [47]. Dialysis also imposes physical and psychosocial limitations [48].

Children treated by dialysis require regular review of all of the points listed under 'Management of pre-terminal renal failure' (see above) and in addition will require an individually adjusted fluid restriction, depending on their residual urine output, if any, and their mode of dialysis. Insensible fluid losses should be calculated as 300 ml/m^2 body SA per day. Several points deserve special mention:

- *Growth*: it is, in general, more difficult to achieve normal growth in children treated by dialysis, and rhGH would seem to be less effective [49].

- *Nutrition*: the nutritional strategy for children on dialysis is very similar to that discussed for the child with pre-TRF. An adequate energy intake is of paramount importance. Children on PD may require an increase in protein intake to compensate for losses on dialysis [50].

- *Anaemia*: the availability of rHuEPO therapy has dramatically reduced the need for blood transfusions in children maintained on dialysis [31]. It is important to ensure adequate iron supplies to make optimal usage of rHuEPO. In PD patients, rHuEPO is best administered subcutaneously, which prolongs the half-life of the drug. Intraperitoneal administration is not cost effective and seldom used.

- *Social and psychological support* become even more necessary during periods of dialysis, which increase stress for the child and family [48].

Transplantation

Transplantation is the preferred treatment for children with ESRF since it offers the potential for the best rehabilitation to a near normal life style [37].

Transplantation is performed using a cadaveric kidney or a kidney from a live relative over the age of consent, which for a child usually means a parent. Overall, in Europe, in the period 1984–1993, almost 21% of first grafts in patients under 21 years old, were derived from live donors, although there was wide intercountry variation [51]. In North America, live-donor sources accounted for approximately 50% of grafts performed in children and adolescents aged less than 21 years between 1987 and 2000 [5]; 24% of the 6878 primary transplants performed during this period were pre-emptive, i.e. these patients had never received maintenance dialysis. In the United Kingdom in 2000, 30% of the 83 renal allografts performed were live-donor grafts and 20% were pre-emptive [40].

Immunosuppression

Immunosuppressive agents and regimens continue to proliferate [52], while the quest for immunological tolerance continues. Most children in the United Kingdom are receiving maintenance immunosuppression in the form of triple therapy, with a calcineurin inhibitor (cyclosporin A or tacrolimus), steroids, and either azathioprine or mycophenolate: 97.6% of the 459 patients were receiving a calcineurin inhibitor, 1 in 4 of them tacrolimus, and the remainder cyclosporin A [40].

The following general points can be made:

1. The intensity of immunosuppression required is, in general, inversely related to the degree of human leucocyte antigen (HLA) matching achieved between the donor and the recipient.

2. Immunosuppression needs to be continued indefinitely, a fact not always appreciated by patients, particularly non-compliant teenagers [53].

3. Cyclosporin A and tacrolimus are nephrotoxic and therefore blood levels must be monitored to ensure adequate immunosuppressive effect and avoid nephrotoxicity. Levels taken 2 hours after a dose may prove to be more reliable in this respect than trough levels.

4. Alternate-day steroid regimens are associated with better post-transplant growth than those using daily steroids [54]. Steroid-free regimes are at present unusual, if desirable from the point of view of growth, but some of the newer immunosuppressive agents, e.g. rapamycin, may enable steroids to be discontinued.

5. The incidence of post-transplant malignancy leading to death would appear to be lower in the United Kingdom (UKT data) than in North America, where the use of induction monoclonal or polyclonal antibody is more common.

Graft survival

European Dialysis and Transplant Association data for children and adolescents receiving first transplants before the age of 21 years in the period 1984–1993 show a 1-year graft survival for living-donor grafts of 91%, falling to 74% by 5 years and, for cadaveric grafts, a 1-year survival of 80%, falling to 60% at 5 years [51].

Similar graft survival figures of 90% at 1 year and 74% at 6 years for live-donor grafts and 80% at 1 year and 58% at 6 years for cadaveric grafts have been reported by the North American Pediatric Renal Transplantation Co-operative Study [38].

Key points: Renal transplantation

- Successful renal transplantation is the treatment of choice for children with ESRF.

- Live donors provide kidneys for 21% of European and 50% of US paediatric transplants.

- The survival of living donor grafts are superior to cadaveric grafts (74% versus 58% 6-year graft survival, respectively).

- Most children receive triple immunosuppressive therapy, with cyclosporin A or tacrolimus in combination with azathioprine and corticosteroids.

- Cyclosporin A and tacrolimus are potentially nephrotoxic: blood levels must be monitored to ensure adequate immunosuppression and to avoid nephrotoxicity.

In a study of factors influencing the outcome of paediatric cadaveric transplantation in the United Kingdom and Ireland, performed by UK Transplant, donor and recipient age and HLA matching were identified as the most important determinants of outcome [55]: kidneys from donors under 2 years of age had a 1-year graft survival of only 48%, compared with 80–90% for kidneys from donors more than 5 years old: similarly, graft survival in recipients less than 2 years old was significantly worse than in any other age band. Kidneys with no more than one mismatch at HLA A locus and HLA B locus fared significantly better than those less well matched.

Patient survival and rehabilitation

The survival of children with ESRF continues to improve: of the 1070 children less than 18 years old receiving a cadaveric kidney transplant in the United Kingdom and Ireland in the 10-year period 1986–1995, 91 (9%) were reported to have died by the time of analysis [55]. The principle causes of death were infection (19%), lymphoid malignant disease (4.5%), and uraemia due to graft failure (4.5%). Registry data from North America demonstrates 5-year patient survival following living donor transplantation ranging from 80.8% in those aged less than 1 year at transplant to 97.4% for those aged 6–10 years [56].

Rehabilitation following a successful renal transplant is, in general, good [57]. However, some young adults, particularly young men, who commenced RRT during childhood, still have problems [58]. They were concerned about their physical appearance, particularly their height, and the effect this had on their social life and on forming lasting relationships. The challenge now is to try and ensure that the present generation of children with ESRF, and particularly those commencing RRT in infancy, achieve more complete rehabilitation in adult life.

What to tell families of children with CRF

Hopefully, the information in this chapter will enable paediatricians to give families and children realistic answers to their questions about CRF. It is important that everyone realizes that CRF treatment is lifelong and extends beyond having a successful kidney transplant. It is really very like the little girl in the nursery rhyme, who, when she was good, she was very, very good, but when she was bad, she was horrid! There are now many young adults with successful kidney transplants, who are doing everything that their peers are doing, be that being a professor of dermatology, raising their own families (and some of them bringing their offspring to the paediatric nephrology clinic— remember the relevant genetic advice!), enjoying an exciting 'gap' year in the Antipodes, or residing at Her Majesty's pleasure in a detention centre for young offenders—yes, everything their peers are doing. Only 3 or 4 decades ago these children would have died of renal failure. There are, though, still children who have a difficult time with ESRF treatment and a small minority for whom it is really horrid, e.g. a small infant with difficult dialysis access, who is still a long way from being transplanted: we, the professionals, must not forget that we are not obliged to treat at any cost, but only to care, and sometimes withdrawal of active treatment is appropriate.

The future must lie with research into means of preventing the congenital and genetically determined causes of CRF; into methods of early detection of CRF in order to prevent growth retardation and perhaps progression to ESRF; to improving dialysis access and into more specific methods of immunosuppression, with the ultimate goal of immunological tolerance.

References

1. Kaufman JM, DiMeola HJ, Siegel NJ, Lytton B, Kashgarian M, Hayslett JP. Compensatory adaptation of structure and function following progressive renal ablation. *Kidney Int* 1974; 6: 10–17.
2. Lewis M. Report of the Paediatric Renal Registry. In: Ansell D, Feest T. (eds) *UK Renal Registry Report 1999*. Bristol, UK Renal Registry, 1999: Chapter 15.
3. Esbjorner E, Berg U, Hansson S, writing on behalf of the Swedish Pediatric Nephrology Association. Epidemiology of chronic renal failure in children: a report from Sweden 1986–1994. *Pediatr Nephrol* 1997; 11: 438–442.
4. Report of a Working Party of the British Association for Paediatric Nephrology 1995: The provision of services in the United Kingdom for children and adolescents with renal disease. London: British Paediatric Association.
5. North American Pediatric Renal Transplant Cooperative Study 2001 Annual Report.
6. Scott JES, Renwick M. Antenatal diagnosis of congenital abnormalities of the urinary tract. *Br J Urol* 1991; 62: 295–300.
7. Fitzpatrick MM, Shah V, Trompeter RS, Dillon MJ, Barratt TM. Long term renal outcome of childhood haemolytic uraemic syndrome. *BMJ* 1991; 303: 489–492.
8. Rees L, Rigden SPA, Chantler C, Haycock GB. Growth and methods of improving growth in chronic renal failure managed conservatively. In: Scharer K (ed) *Growth and Endocrine Changes in Children and Adolescents with Chronic Renal Failure. Pediatric and Adolescent Endocrinology*, Vol 20. Basel, Karger, 1989: 15–26.
9. Chantler C. Growth in children with renal disease with particular reference to the effects of calorie malnutrition: a review. *Clin Nephrol* 1973; 1: 230–242.
10. Shaw V. Nutritional management of renal disease. *Paediatric Nursing* 1999; 11(4): 37–42.
11. Department of Health. Dietary reference values for food energy and nutrients for the United Kingdom. *Report on Health and Social Subjects 41*. London, HM Stationary Office, 1991.
12. Rizzoni G, Baso T, Setari M. Growth in children in chronic renal failure. *Kidney Int* 1984; 26: 52–58.
13. Kari JA, Gonzalez C, Ledermann SE, Shaw V, Rees L. Outcome and growth of infants with severe chronic renal failure. *Kidney Int* 2000; 57: 1681–1687.
14. Rigden SPA. The treatment of renal osteodystrophy. *Pediatr Nephrol* 1996; 10: 653–655.
15. Klahr S, Levey AS, Beck GJ *et al.* for the Modification of Diet in Renal Disease Study Group: The effects of dietary protein restriction and blood pressure control on the progression of chronic renal failure. *N Engl J Med* 1994; 330: 877–884.
16. Wingen AM, Fabian-Bach C, Schaefer F, Mehls O and the European Study Group for Nutritional Treatment of Chronic Renal Failure in Childhood: Randomised multicentre study of a low protein diet on the progression of chronic renal failure in children. *Lancet* 1997; 349: 1117–1123.

17. Uauy RD, Hogg RJ, Brewer ED, Reisch JS, Cunningham C, Holliday MA. Dietary protein and growth in infants with chronic renal insufficiency: a report from the Southwest Paediatric Nephrology Study Group and the University of California, San Francisco. *Pediatr Nephrol* 1994; 8: 45–50.

18. Haycock GB. The influence of sodium on growth in infancy. *Pediatr Nephrol* 1993; 7: 871–875.

19. Salusky IB, Goodman WG. The management of renal osteodystrophy. *Pediatr Nephrol* 1996; 10: 651–653.

20. Lopez-Hilker SA, Dusso A, Rapp N, Martin KJ, Slatopolsky E. Phosphorus restriction reverses hyperparathyroidism in uraemia independent of changes in calcium and calcitriol. *Am J Physiol* 1993; 259: F432–F437.

21. Clayton BE, Jenkins P, Round JM. *Paediatric Chemical Pathology*. Oxford, Blackwell, 1980.

22. Tamanaha K, Mak RHK, Rigden SPA, Turner C, Start KM, Haycock GB, Chantler C. Long term suppression of hyperparathyroidism by phosphate binders in uremic children. *Pediatr Nephrol* 1987; 1: 145–149.

23. Slatopolsky EA, Burke SK, Dillon MA, and the Renagel Study Group. RenaGel, a nonabsorbed calcium- and aluminium-free phosphate binder, lowers serum phosphorus and parathyroid hormone. *Kidney Int* 1999; 55: 299–307.

24. Portale AA, Booth BE, Halloran BP, Morris JC Jnr. Effect of dietary phosphorus on circulating concentrations of 1–25 dihydroxy vitamin D and immunoreactive parathyroid hormone in children with moderate renal insufficiency. *J Clin Invest* 1984; 73: 1580–1589.

25. Owen TA, Aronour MS, Barone LM, Bettencourt B, Stein GS, Lian LB. Pleiotropic effects of vitamin D on osteoblast gene expression are related to the proliferative and differentiated state of the bone cell phenotype: dependency upon basal levels of gene expression, duration of exposure, and bone matrix competency in normal rat osteoblast cultures. *Endocrinology* 1991; 128: 1496–1504.

26. Hostetter TH, Oslon JL, Rennke HG, Venkatachalam MA, Brenner BM. Hyperfiltration of remnant nephrons: a potentially adverse response to renal ablation. *Am J Physiol* 1981; 241: F85–93.

27. Johnson RJ. The glomerular response to injury: progression or resolution? *Kidney Int* 1994;45:1769–1782.

28. Hebert LA, Wilmer WA, Falkenhain ME, Ladson-Wofford SE, Naham NS Jr, Rovin BH. Renoprotection: One or many therapies? *Kidney Int* 2001; 59: 1211–1226.

29. Maschio G, Alberti D, Janin G, Locatelli F, Mann JFE, Motolese M, Ponticelli C, Ritz E. Effect of the angio-tensin converting enzyme inhibitor benazepril on the progression of chronic renal insufficiency. ACE inhibition in Progressive Renal Insufficiency Study Group. *N Engl J Med* 1996; 334: 939–945.

30. Taal MW, Brenner BM. Renoprotective benefits of RAS inhibition: From ACEI to angiotensin II antagonists. *Kidney Int* 2000; 57: 1803–1817.

31. Van Damme-Lombaerts R, Herman J. Erythropoietin treatment in children with renal failure. *Pediatr Nephrol* 2000; 13: 148–152.

32. Betts PR, McGrath G. Growth pattern and dietary intake of children with chronic renal insufficiency. *BMJ* 1974; 2:189–193.

33. Schaefer F, Seidel C, Binding A *et al*. Pubertal growth in chronic renal failure. *Pediatr Res* 1990; 28: 5–10.

34. Hokken-Koelega ACS, Stijnen T, de Muinck Keizer-Schrama SMPF, Wit JM, Wolff ED, de Jong MCJW, Donckerwolcke RA, Abbad NCB, Bot A, Blum WF, Drop SLS. Placebo-controlled, double-blind, cross-over trial of growth hormone treatment in prepubertal children with chronic renal failure. *Lancet* 1991; 338: 585–590.

35. Haffner D, Schaefer F, Nissel R, Wuhl E, Tonshoff B, Mehls O. for the German Study Group for Growth Hormone Treatment in Chronic Renal Failure. Effect of growth hormone treatment on the adult height of children with chronic renal failure. *N Engl J Med* 2000; 343: 923–930.

36. Broyer M. Results and side-effects of treating children with growth hormone after kidney transplantation – a preliminary report. Pharmacia & Upjohn Study Group. *Acta Paediatr Suppl* 1996; 417: 76–79.

37. Fine RN. Renal transplantation for children – the only realistic choice. *Kidney Int* 1985; 1: 15–17.

38. Benfield MR, McDonald R, Sullivan EK, Stablein DM, Tejani A. The 1997 Annual Renal Transplantation in Children Report of the North American Pediatric Renal Transplant Cooperative Study. *Pediatr Transplant* 1999; 3: 152–167.

39. Najarian JS, Chavers BM, McHugh LE *et al*. 20 years or more of follow up of living donors. *Lancet* 1992; 340: 807–810.

40. Lewis M, Shaw J. Report of the Paediatric Renal Registry. In: Ansell D, Feest T (eds), *UK Renal Registry Report 2000*. Bristol, UK Renal Registry, 2000: Chapter 15.

41. Rigden SPA. Pre-emptive Kidney Transplantation. *Pediatr Nephrol* 1996; 10: C44.

42. Mahmoud A, Said M-H, Dawahra M, Hadj-Aissa A, Schell M, Faraj G, Long D, Parchoux B, Martin X, Cochat P. Outcome of preemptive transplantation and pretransplantation dialysis in children. *Pediatr Nephrol* 1997; 11: 537–541.

43. Alexander SR, Tank ES, Corneil AT. Five years experience with CAPD/CCPD catheters in infants and children. In: Fine RN, Scharer K, Mehls O (eds), *CAPD in children*. New York, Springer, 1985; 174–189.

44. Warady BA, Campoy SF, Gross SP *et al*. Peritonitis with continuous ambulatory peritoneal dialysis and continuous cycling peritoneal dialysis. *J Pediatr* 1984; 105: 726–730.

45. Lerner GR, Warady BA, Sullivan EK *et al*. Chronic peritoneal and hemodialysis in children, the 1996 annual report of the dialysis arm of the North American Pediatric Renal Transplant Cooperative Study. *Pediatr Nephrol* 1999; 13: 404–417.

46. Harland RC. Placement of permanent vascular access devices: surgical consideration. *Adv Renal Repl Therapy* 1994; 1: 99–106.

47. United States Renal Data System (USRDS). The 1997 Annual Report. Bethesda: National Institutes of

Health, National Institute of Diabetes and Digestive and Kidney Diseases, 1997: 113–128.

48. Fielding D, Brownbridge G. Factors related to psychosocial adjustment in children with end-stage renal failure. *Pediatr Nephrol* 1999; 13:766–770.

49. Wuhl E, Haffner D, Nissl R *et al*. Short children on dialysis treatment respond less to growth hormone than patients with chronic renal failure prior to dialysis. German Study Group for GH Treatment in children with CRF. *Pediatr Nephrol* 1996; 10: 294–298.

50. Quan A, Baum M. Protein losses in children on continuous cycler peritoneal dialysis. *Pediatr Nephrol* 1996; 10: 728–731.

51. Rigden S, Mehls O, Gellert R. Factors influencing second renal allograft survival. *Nephrol Dial Transplant* 1999; 14: 566–569.

52. Suthanthiran M, Strom TB. Immunoregulatory drugs: mechanistic basis for use in organ transplantation. *Pediatr Nephrol* 1997; 11: 651–657.

53. Wolff G, Strecker K, Vester U, Latta K, Ehrich JHH. Non-compliance following renal transplantation in children and adolescents. *Pediatr Nephrol* 1998; 9: 703–708.

54. Broyer M, Guest G, Gagnadoux M-F. Growth rate in children receiving alternate day corticosteroid treatment after kidney transplantation. *J Pediatr* 1992; 120: 721–725.

55. Johnson R, Belger M, Postlethwaite RJ, Rigden SPA, Verrier-Jones K for UKTSSA, Bristol and the British Association for Paediatric Nephrology. UKTSSA Paediatric Task Force report on factors affecting paediatric transplant survival. *Pediatr Nephrol* 1998; 12: C61.

56. U.S. Scientific Registry for Transplant Recipients and the Organ Procurement and Transplant Network. Graft and patient survival rates. In: *The 1997 Annual Report of the U.S. Scientific Registry for Transplant Recipients and the Organ Procurement and Transplant Network: 1988–1996 UNOS and DHHS*, 1997: 101–194.

57. Reynolds JM, Garralda ME, Postlethwaite RJ, Goh D. Changes in psychosocial adjustment after renal transplantation. *Arch Dis Child* 1991; 66: 508–513.

58. Henning P, Tomlinson L, Rigden SPA, Haycock GB, Chantler C. Long term outcome of treatment of end stage renal failure. *Arch Dis Child* 1988; 63: 35–40.

24 | *Psychosocial care of children and their families*

Hilary Lloyd and Mary Eminson

Introduction

It is a truism, familiar to all clinicians, that children can show remarkable emotional resilience in their adjustment to major life-threatening illness. None the less, studies have repeatedly shown that having a chronic illness increases the risk of child psychiatric disorder by approximately twofold, and, if that illness is accompanied by physical disability, or impairment, by a greater degree. Lesser degrees of maladaptation or psychological problems appear to be common [1–3].

The argument throughout this chapter is for good understanding and recognition of psychosocial factors relevant to the management of problems that present to physicians via the renal tract. For the most part, the chapter concentrates upon chronic renal failure, but many of the issues can be generalized to other conditions.

Overall, the management of psychosocial issues is concerned with engendering three things:

(1) a team culture that, by its awareness, sensitivity and ethos, promotes discussion of psychosocial issues generally (e.g. addressing how to provide a ward environment suitable for adolescents as well as children; thinking of ways of minimizing disruption to peer group relationships for sick children; approaches to information giving; addressing the effects of patient deaths on other patients and on staff);

(2) an approach of looking for achievable practical solutions (e.g. early involvement of support from Social Services for disadvantaged and burdened families; liaison with schools);

(3) recognition of cases with more severe mental health problems that may need specialist mental health involvement (e.g. depression is recognized and not rationalized as understandable sadness,

relationship difficulties between parents and children resulting in severe adherence problems being picked up early enough for intervention to be effective).

All team members have a role in psychosocial care. Dieticians, play workers, physiotherapists, hospital teachers, as well as social workers, nurses and doctors, may be the first (or only) recipients of highly important information about the psychological well-being of children and their families, and may be especially well placed to play a part in the management of psychosocial difficulties.

This chapter offers an overview of the relationships between psyche and soma, a discussion of physical illness and the burden of care as factors increasing the risk of psychiatric disorders in children and parents, a review of psychosocial research in paediatric nephrology and a discussion of general issues in psychosocial care, and specific issues and problems in paediatric nephrology, with case examples. Attention is drawn to the importance of early detection and to treatability and evidence-based practice in child and adolescent mental health. Finally, an outline of liaison child and adolescent mental health is discussed, with suggestions of useful and effective models.

Relationships between psyche and soma

Cartesian mind–body dualism is alien to useful understanding in all branches of medicine, and particularly where chronic illness is concerned. Nevertheless, separating the possible interactions of psyche and soma in a structured way is a means of ensuring that all the main mechanisms and possibilities in a given clinical situation are considered. It is worth teasing these out for both children and parents.

Figure 24.1 lists each 'type' of psychosomatic relationship: soma on psyche, psyche on soma, and the interaction with another person's soma and psyche. Any may be presented, alone or in combination, to general and specialist paediatricians through complaints focusing on any body system, including the renal tract.

Soma influences psyche (Fig. 24.1, A1): even minor illnesses have an effect on mental state, albeit subtle. Lethargy and avolition, frustration, and fear are all common reactions to acute illnesses. Lethargy and avolition may be systemic somatic effects. Frustration and fear are more usually understood to be psychological reactions to illness and its limitations and prognosis or uncertainties. Minor degrees of lowering of mood (e.g. dysphoria) seem also to arise by similar mechanisms. There are other systemic illnesses that are commonly associated with low mood, and in which this appears to be a biological response, e.g. systemic lupus erythematosus, Cushing's syndrome.

Brain pathology can, albeit uncommonly, cause symptomatic mental illness in children and adolescents, e.g. schizophreniform illnesses, severe depression, mania. Lesions or deposits in the temporal lobes are particularly potent in this respect. Toxic confusional states (acute, chronic, and subacute) all occur in children. Aetiologies may be infective, metabolic, anoxic, traumatic, adverse drug effects. Steroids regularly produce mild to moderate psychological effects and may cause frank mood disorders and/or disinhibited behaviour (Fig. 24.1, A2).

Indirect effects of soma on psyche (Fig. 24.1, A3): any or all of acute or repeated experience of pain, unpleasant treatments, limitations, disability, disruption to social life, or lifestyle changes may precipitate psychological reactions, including low mood, adjustment reactions including disturbed conduct (oppositionality, defiance, rebellion), anxiety disorders. For adolescents in particular worries may include concern about future prospects including medical prognosis, career, marriageability, and fertility.

Psyche influences soma (Fig. 24.1, B1, B2): psychiatric conditions may have significant effects on the soma. For example, the biological symptoms of depression include changes in sleep, appetite, fitness; anorexia nervosa may result in loss of weight, anergia, cold intolerance, bradycardia, peripheral cyanosis, and lanugo hair in the short term, and infertility and osteoporosis later. In severe anorexia nervosa, we also see the soma's effect on the psyche, with the typical mental state characteristics of starvation.

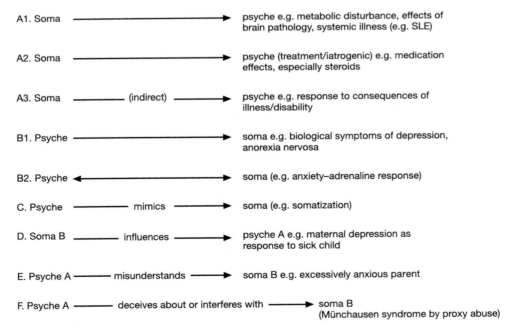

Fig. 24.1 Mutual influences between psyche and soma.

The somatic manifestations of anxiety (Fig. 24.1, B2) and the mechanisms (adrenaline response) are, of course, a prime example of psychosomatic and somatopsychic relationships (psychological provocation results in release of adrenaline causing somatic symptoms of anxiety which in turn increase psychological discomfort). Urinary frequency may be a symptom of anxiety (i.e. psychogenic presentation to paediatrics via urinary tract). Secondary nocturnal enuresis may be symptomatic of an adjustment reaction (see Chapter 9) rather than genitourinary pathology.

Psyche mimics soma (Fig. 24.1, C): members of this group of disorders suggest somatic problems at initial presentation, but are in fact somatizations. Somatoform disorders is the term used to include a range of somatic presentations which have a psychological origin, and includes apparent losses of function, such as incontinence, as well as positive symptoms such as pain. However, somatic complaints may also be the marker for other common psychiatric disorders such as anxiety. Recurrent abdominal pain with loin pain may lead to suspicion of urinary tract or other renal pathology such as stones, but may, in fact, be a presentation of school refusal, or an anxiety disorder. Somatoform pain disorder describes those situations in which the presenting complaint is psychogenic pain without other marked abnormality of mental state or other identifiable psychiatric disorder. Somatization disorder describes the occurrence of multiple somatic symptoms without organic cause. In all these somatoform disorders psychopathology in the patient may be strikingly inapparent. Family dysfunction is variable, but secondary gains of the illness role are common.

Effect of the soma of one on the psyche of another (Fig. 24.1, D): seeing one's own child sick, may contribute to a mood disorder or, indeed, some other psychological reaction of a parent.

Effect of the soma of one on the psyche of another (Fig. 24.1, E): the psyche of one may misperceive or erroneously fear that the soma of another is sick. For example, depressed or anxious mothers may worry excessively about the health or potential sickness of their child.

Finally, *the psyche of one may deceive in order to persuade that the soma of another is diseased* (Fig. 24.1, F). This is seen in Münchausen by proxy abuse, where illness in the child is invented verbally or actively physically induced by a parent. This may present with many different renal symptoms, according to the inventiveness and dangerousness of the abuser. These include blood in the urine (which may be a fictional report, fabricated using blood from another source, or actively induced), GU bleeding (again this may be fabricated or induced), effects of salt poisoning, alleged polyuria, alleged frequency.

Physical illness as a risk factor for child psychiatric disorder

In addition to clinical experience, there is a wealth of evidence in the epidemiological literature supporting the view that chronic physical illness and disability are risk factors for mental health problems in children and adolescents. In the Isle of Wight study [1], psychiatric disorders were found in 17% of chronically ill children, compared with 7% of healthy children. Broadly comparable rates were found by Cadman *et al.* in the Ontario Child Health Study [2] and Pless and Roghman [3].

Cadman *et al.* [2] found that the children with physical illness and disability were more likely to be socially isolated (i.e. to have fewer social contacts with friends), raising the possibility that this may be a contributory mechanism for mental health problems.

There are other risk factors for child psychiatric disorders: many are linked to social disadvantage, poverty, poor housing, educational failure, learning disability, family instability, being looked after by the local authority. Boys are at greater risk of disruptive behaviour disorders, and older girls of emotional disorders. An awareness of these risk factors may assist paediatric teams to identify those children at particularly high risk of developing (or of having pre-existing) mental health problems in the wake of chronic illness and disability. Where physical illness befalls a child with pre-existing mental health problems, these are likely to be exacerbated and treatment may be compromised by them.

General issues for the psychosocial care of children

Breaking bad news

Breaking bad news must be understood to be a process, and not an event. The news may be of renal disease, its treatment and prognosis, plus other problems if there is a syndrome. Breaking bad news taxes the communication skills of the most articulate doctor. The doctor needs to:

- convey information about his or her own area of expertise;
- put it in the context of the rest of the child's development;
- establish which areas are of primary concern to parents;
- listen.

Antenatal diagnosis

Where renal disease is detected antenatally, serious ethical issues may arise. How severe or, indeed, certain should disability or prognosis be for termination of the pregnancy to be allowable? Where the renal problems are part of a wider syndrome, the parents' preoccupation may be about the possibility of mental handicap or associated dysmorphology. Doctors need to be prepared for stark questions such as 'What will the child look like?' or 'What are his chances?' For many parents, the anticipatory joy of expecting the birth of a healthy child will be severely tainted by antenatal diagnosis.

Communication skills

It has become widely accepted that all doctors in all specialities need to give thought to communication skills, and there are books [4,5] and courses, examining and teaching those aspects that can be taught and which provide more detail than is appropriate here. The doctor who is a 'good communicator' probably acknowledges that he or she does not 'get it right' all of the time, and that communication skills are something we continue to develop throughout our professional lives.

Time, respect, and listening skills are arguably the most vital equipment for successful communication with parents and children. Communication skills training often mentions the importance of avoiding jargon. What is really important is that there is a shared, mutual understanding of the language used by clinician and parent/patient.

The process of breaking the news

It is generally recommended that both parents should be seen together when critical news is being imparted, but this may not be possible. A variety of responses should be anticipated. The breaking of some bad news can and should be planned, for example when informing the parents of a substantive diagnosis. In such situations, it is important to take time to ascertain what current knowledge and understanding the parents have reached, what their fears are, and the things about which they have been wondering. This helps the doctor to introduce the difficult areas and issues sensitively. Indeed, the doctor may find that the parents are not as ill-prepared or shocked as he had anticipated. Summarizing, recapitulating, inviting questions, and checking that parents have understood are important elements of the dialogue.

Bad news should be given as early as possible and is such a skilled task that the parents have a right to expect that it will be done by the most senior doctor available. However, there are, of course, many situations where bad news has to be given very promptly (e.g. what has just happened in theatre, the latest blood results). Often, in these instances, it is the more junior members of the medical team who find themselves giving the news or facing the anxious questions of the child or parents. In such circumstances, it may be advisable that junior doctors emphasize the provisional nature of what they are saying until someone more senior arrives.

In communicating emotive issues, the needs of the child and parents must be paramount. It is easy to be seduced into thinking that things that make oneself feel more at ease must be to the good of the parents. For example, addressing parents by their first names without seeking permission, or using touch in an attempt to console may not be well received. Experience allows one to develop confidence in the limits of one's knowledge and expertise. Parents will feel confident with honesty in this respect. Prevarication and anxious fudging in such situations will be picked up by most parents very promptly and recognized for what they are. Those who are breaking the news need to be able to deal sensitively with the emotional reactions that are provoked, and these may involve frank distress and tearfulness, anger (that may be displaced onto the staff), or stunned disbelief.

The presence of another team member may be very helpful by providing joint reflection on the interview, and another point of reference for the family when they have questions or seek reiteration and clarification. Parents should be informed of the opportunities that will be afforded them later (e.g. a follow-up interview or a nominated team member they can approach).

What to tell the child patient

What, how, and when to tell their child may be sources of considerable anxiety to parents and discussion about this with professionals may be very welcome. An approach that is flexible and takes account of the child's developmental stage and previous experiences and the parent's views is recommended.

Key points: Breaking news

- Is a process, not an event.

- Needs a senior, experienced doctor and nurse/ social worker with with plenty of time.

- Necessitates mutually understandable language.

- Should occur in the context of previous open and honest dialogue.

- Should be done with both parents together in most cases, but consult about this.

- Remember to:
  – check parents' understanding before impart-ing new information;
  – offer a named team member to consult with further questions;
  – emphasize positive issues as well as negative (e.g. ability to continue at school);
  – be prepared for emotional responses and acknowledge them;
  – discuss how, what, and when to tell child.

Coping behaviours and psychological defences

Notwithstanding the strong evidence that chronic physical illness and disability increase the risk of psychiatric disorders in children, the majority of children with physical illness and disability do not have substantial mental health problems. Consideration of how such children and parents may cope with their predicaments may assist in both recognizing when others are not coping and in intervention to assist them to develop coping strategies.

Coping is the means of adaptive psychological management of an adverse, stressful situation or predicament such as chronic illness or disability. Models of conscious cognitive and behavioural strategies or 'coping behaviours' have been described by Hamburg and Hamburg [6], as succinctly outlined by Graham *et al.* [7].

In Hamburg and Hamburg's view, children and parents who deal successfully with stress tend to:

- have a 'day to day outlook'—they ration the amount of stress to be coped with at any one time (e.g. think only about the next stage of treatment, such as an operation or starting dialysis, and not further ahead);

- seek information about their condition and treatment;

- rehearse what is going to be difficult (e.g. prepare responses to expected teasing);

- try a variety of ways of dealing with a problem rather than persisting with one unsatisfactory, unsuccessful approach;

- construct buffers against disappointment, e.g. prepare for failure of an operation and not just for its success.

Coping depends upon physical resources (money and employment), social resources (support from friends, family, Social Services), and psychological resources such as beliefs, problem-solving skills, personality. Eiser [8] gives a detailed and comprehensive review of other models of coping.

The other psychological ingredient of adaptation to stress is generally considered to be defence mechanisms. This acknowledges a model of unconscious psychological process. Defence mechanisms relevant to adaptation to physical illness and disability are described by Graham *et al.* [7], and the reader who wishes to know more is referred there. Defence mechanisms are an important and essential aspect of adaptation but can become maladaptive. In addition, it is not uncommon in clinical experience, to find that coping children 'compartmentalize' areas of their lives. That is to say, they do not allow the illness to intrude at all into some arenas in which they operate, and in which they are, to all intents and purposes, healthy and normal. For example, a young person may attend a regular social activity without allowing other participants to know of his or her medical condition. Such compartmentalization was apparent in the Manchester paediatric haemodialysis study, although not described in the publications (R.J. Postlethwaite, personal communication).

Defence mechanisms are also used by professionals in helping them to cope with the emotional stress of dealing with sick, disabled, and dying children. It is not only the defence mechanisms of children and parents that can become maladaptive.

The burden of care: effects on the family

Practical consequences of the care and treatment of children with renal disease may be a major source of strain in families, e.g. dietary restrictions, having to support the subjection of the child to unpleasant and distressing procedures 'for his or her own good', limitations on holidays, time off work for appointments, restrictions on social life and career development. Parents whose young child is on continuous ambulatory peritoneal dialysis (CAPD) need to be sufficiently organized and able to find the time for weighing, measuring blood pressure, caring for the catheter, frequently administering injections and giving nasogastric or gastrostomy feeds by day and night. Younger couples tend to have greater difficulties in mobilizing the support of friends and relatives.

Effects on parents

Despite advances in treatment and survival, one would surely think it very abnormal if parents showed no hint of distress in the face of realization that their child had serious renal disease. The impact on parents depends on various factors, such as the nature and severity of the condition, (especially the amount of physical care the child needs), the child's age at diagnosis, associated handicaps, the parents' personality and previous experience, the temperament of the child, the help available from family and friends, the quality of the available health, social welfare, and educational services.

Adaptation. The adjustment process for parents can be understood as being akin to that seen in bereavement. The stages include: **shock** and **numbing** (a sense of unreality), with difficulty in absorbing information; **denial**, when seriousness is questioned, and perhaps with fantasies that the child will be miraculously (or 'alternatively') cured, and 'doctor shopping'; then **sadness** and **anger**—depressive feelings and sensations of guilt—rage against fate, each other, the child, or the professionals. Healthcare teams need to understand that parental anger may be part of the process of coming to terms. It is unpleasant to be the recipient of such displaced anger, but understanding its origin is likely to assist in dealing with it appropriately and in the way most useful for the family. Parents who emerge from the process of adaptation relatively unscathed reach a stage in which they can reorganize their lives to truly accommodate the sick and disabled child. They become able to see the child and his future in more realistic terms, making plans for his care and education that accord with his real potential.

Not all parents go through these various stages and there is not necessarily anything amiss if they adapt via a different route. The rate of adaptation is hugely variable between individuals. Often the process takes several months but may be longer or shorter. Cultural and religious beliefs may be prominent in the adaptation of some families, and healthcare teams may need to understand these.

Maladaptive responses

Maladaptive parental adjustment to a child's illness may lead to an exaggerated tendency to protect (see Case 1), or, at the other extreme, to neglect emotionally or physically (e.g. administration of medication). These difficulties are likely to occur in those parents most vulnerable prior to the onset of the child's illness: parents in psychosocial adversity, those currently unsupported, those with other risk factors such as anxiety or substance misuse or learning difficulties. Gaining an understanding of these issues, for the sake of the child patient, places demands on the renal team for comprehensive assessments of families early in an illness.

Mothers of children with severe disability as a group show high levels of psychological distress [9]. Paediatric teams must be alert to the real possibility that a parent of a sick child may be clinically depressed.

Effects on marriage

Defining and assessing a concept such as 'marital strain' caused by the burden of care of a sick child is a complicated and imprecise activity. Notwithstanding this, few would challenge the premise that caring for a child with chronic renal failure represents a burden of care, and that such a burden may well pose a marital strain. However, studies suggest that while couples acknowledge such strain, actual divorce rates are, if anything, only slightly increased by this burden of care. It is suggested that in some families the strain of the child's illness may unite the couple and strengthen the marriage [10]. It also seems possible that some are simply deterred from separating by practical issues or a wish to protect the child from overt family breakdown. In individual cases, it may be that the exception proves the rule (see Case 1), but of course, caution must be applied when extrapolating from research to the individual human story of the case confronting one. As in bereavement, parents adjust to their child's condition and treatment at different rates. This may impede the couple in being able to support each other in the way that they would in another predicament.

Case 1: Mother and child's adjustment to illness

Stephen was a vulnerable (premature) child born into a marital relationship characterized by mutual dissatisfaction. His mother had been frustrated in her career by the marriage. She had thought that having a child would be gratifying, enriching her life and compensating for the disappointing marriage.

Stephen was born prematurely (31 weeks), and spent 5 weeks in SCBU. He was a crying, fractious baby.

At 18 months he developed nephrotic syndrome that was subsequently refractory to treatment. His mother became unable to set limits on Stephen's behaviour, because of wanting to indulge him and because of her guilt. She appeared to be frightened of setting limits.

When it was confirmed that peritoneal dialysis was necessary, mother confided that she had been experiencing extreme negativism, oppositionality and clinginess, and demandingness from Stephen since the diagnosis had been made. She had confided this now because of her intense anxiety about how she would gain her child's co-operation with dialysis. Both parents argued with each other about the need for treatment. Stephen's mother decided to divorce her husband while Stephen was on dialysis.

The liaison psychiatrist referred Stephen to his local child mental health service where his mother would be assisted in developing more effective parent management strategies, and where she would receive some psychotherapeutic support, focusing on issues of adjustment to Stephen's illness. The local service was more accessible than the liaison service, especially in view of the frequency of appointments that would be required early on in treatment.

Effects on siblings

Eiser has reviewed the main studies in this area [10]. Individual reactions of healthy children to their chronically sick siblings are many and varied. Siblings may be relatively neglected in families coming to terms or dealing with the illness of another child. The timing of the diagnosis or crisis may be critical for a sibling, for example, coinciding with major examinations or starting school. When the healthy sibling is a toddler and the parent has had to spend time away with the sick child, an increase in separation difficulties, oppositionality, tantrums, or other behaviour problems would not be surprising. Some parents may not recognize this for what it is, and may be assisted by being made aware of the possibility in advance.

Although there is evidence that, overall, chronic physical disease appears to act as a risk factor for emotional and behavioural maladjustment in healthy siblings, for some children it seems possible that the consequences are not all adverse. For example, it has been suggested that such a circumstance may lead to some children becoming more companionable, sensitive, understanding, or mature.

Care of the dying child

The principles of breaking bad news have been outlined above. The various identifiable phases of grief have been written about elsewhere [11,12]. Such general patterns must not be seen as a rigid model and it is to be emphasized that families respond in different ways to the anticipated and actual death of a child [13,14]. Couples do not necessarily progress in their grief at the same rate as each other. Staff may become the target of a parent's anger that is a manifestation of grief. Siblings may also need support.

Parents' views on what to tell the child patient are important. Although it is usually agreed that openness about outcome with reassurance about palliative care are important principles, some children make it clear that they are not ready to confront the fact that they are dying, and therefore flexibility of approach is needed. Children come to understand the finality of death between the ages of 5 and 8 years. The older dying child may try to avoid distressing their obviously upset parents further by expressing their own fears and anxieties. Children may be highly sensitive to their parents' anxieties and anger. The dying child may himself be angry and may direct the anger towards parents or staff.

The support of a key worker from amongst the hospital staff may be very valuable to families. Teams need to think through how and when requests for autopsies or donation of organs should be made. Post-bereavement appointments with the consultant and, sometimes, other staff are now routine in many hospital units. Some hospitals offer post-bereavement counselling or bereavement groups as an option for families.

While grief is an essentially normal human process, atypical and complicated grief reactions occur in both adults and children, and may warrant specialist mental health consultation or intervention.

Hospital staff may be emotionally affected by the anticipated or actual death of a patient, and thought should be given to how staff can be supported. Clinical supervision provides some opportunities for nursing staff. Psychosocial meetings of the team, described in greater detail below, may provide useful opportunities for such support.

Awareness of the likely and actual effects of the death of a patient on other patients, with whom they may have developed a relationship over weeks, months, or even years of meeting in clinic, ward, or dialysis unit settings, is also needed. Again, psychosocial team meetings provide a useful forum in which to discuss such issues and formulate a considered approach.

Psychosocial research in paediatric nephrology: The Manchester Studies

Paediatric nephrology has not been neglected in psychosocial research. Beginning in the mid 1980s, the psychiatric nephrology liaison teams in Manchester have produced perhaps the most substantial series of publications examining the psychological effects and adjustment at various different stages of renal disease and treatment, through into adulthood; a set of studies of the impact of growth hormone in the CRF arena, an audit of psychological risk factors, and a paper examining appropriate psychological research methodologies [15]. The early papers reflect management of renal disease which has undergone radical changes.

Renal teams now work with a group of children facing more severe illness and carrying greater physical and cognitive handicaps, thus limiting the extent to which conclusions from the earlier work can be extrapolated to the present day. Nevertheless these studies still provide substantial information and some merit repeating.

Psychiatric morbidity was increased in children with ESRF, when compared with controls, whatever the stage of illness. Most of these problems were short-lived adjustment disorders or minor symptoms which were not seriously deleterious to the child's emotional state or quality of life. For children in the pre-dialysis stage these minor psychiatric problems were manifested primarily in the school setting and

through mood changes, but there were no deleterious effects on the child's self-concept. Children on haemodialysis (no children were on peritoneal dialysis when these studies were carried out) manifested prominent mood changes, lowered self-esteem, and problems seen primarily at home rather than at school. After transplantation children's moods and self-concept improved, paralleled by parental perceptions of improvements in their physical and psychological health, but psychiatric morbidity was still greater than in healthy controls: a finding likely to be more marked currently because of the inclusion of more children diagnosed *in utero* and with many very severe physical and other problems. Social development measured by having a special friend, showed a clear gradient according to severity of illness.

The young adult survivors of ESRF in the late 1980s did not have increased psychiatric morbidity compared with healthy controls: if there was continuity of findings between child and young adult, it was for those with mood disorders. However, lower self-esteem was found in adults with earlier onset of illness and lower educational attainments: both are more common today. In the young adults there was evidence of more limited and later independence from families, but generally these young people had adjusted their expectations as well as their lifestyle. Parental mental health problems and family stress were closely related to stage of illness, with more problems in the families of severely affected children: this risk factor, too, is likely to have increased proportionally. Parental mental health improved after transplantation but increased behaviour problems were still reported.

Specific issues for psychosocial care of children with renal disease

The following are important, frequently occurring issues, but not mutually exclusive.

Complexity of syndromes

To the practitioner new to paediatric nephrology, be they paediatrician or psychiatrist, the complexity of the syndromes and conditions of children with chronic renal failure may make a striking impact. For those who have been immersed in the field for some time, there may be an understandable tendency for the focus to become very fixed upon the speciality system. But these are not simply children with renal disease, nor children with simple renal disease. Within a CRF population, there is a high proportion of children with multi-system disease or complex syndromes affecting other organs, often including the brain. These complexities may interact as risk factors for emotional and behavioural problems, as well as increasing the burden of care on families and staff. In a review of a case series by North and Eminson [16], 50% had specific or global learning disability and 25% had a dysmorphic syndrome or neurological condition.

Each wave of new treatments brings with it new psychological demands for families and it takes time for these impacts to become familiar to the physician so that he or she can help treatment recipients to adjust and cope. Currently, the morbidity in survivors of the new and powerful treatments for meningococcal septicaemia may have significant impact for renal teams. Not only may the team be confronted by issues regarding the ongoing acute renal failure management following the discharge from ICU of a meningococcal septicaemia survivor, but also with the day to day care, including the emotional care of a young person with multiple digit and/or limb amputations.

Early adjustment

Early adjustment of the child patient to illness, to diagnosis, to prognosis, or to dealing with uncertainty may tax the clinician. A wide variety of responses may be anticipated. There is a wide spectrum of normal responses and adjustment. Severe responses including elements of maladjustment are those in which the reaction gives rise to increased impairments, which may be emotional, behavioural, or social. Such adjustment disorders are described in greater detail below.

Burdens of illness and treatment on the child

In chronic renal failure, the burden of illness and treatment will vary according to 'control' of the disease and response to, or stage of, treatment. In addition, malaise, fatigue, intrusive or painful procedures, growth failure, effects on appearance (such as those caused by other treatments), uncertainty of the course of the illness and response to treatment, ultimate prognosis, and disruption to school may add to the burden. Children with chronic low-grade metabolic disturbance are likely to be irritable and sometimes dysphoric. Some children may be taking *many* tablets every day. Peritoneal dialysis is a vast advance and allows children to miss less schooling but necessitates

$1\frac{1}{2}$–2 hours of treatment per day (CAPD), which must surely be a significant burden. The younger the child, the greater the proportion of the waking day will be taken up with treatment [17].

Stages of illness

Parental morbidity and family stress are related to stage of illness. There are increased problems in more severely affected children. Successful transplants tend to be associated with improved parental mental health and psychosocial adjustment of children.

Non-adherence (medication/diet)

This is a familiar and major problem for renal teams [18–22]. Consequences can be dire, for example the loss of a transplant. The autonomy of adolescence, side-effects (including changes to appearance), depression, desire to be no different from one's peers, risk-taking, or denial may all be relevant. In some cases, non-adherence appears to be a suicidal metaphor. The lack of immediate effects of adherence or non-adherence may be relevant. Even adults do not always do what is good for them. If you are taking many tablets per day, it is unsurprising that the ones which are left out are those which taste bitter or are unpleasant to swallow or are the last few of the day.

Careful education of parents, but more particularly of adolescents, may need to be revisited. In some instances parents may need to take greater control of medication or do more reminding. In other instances the adolescent may respond to being allowed a greater degree of independence and autonomy. While there are those young people who are poorly adherent both before and after transplant, there are others whose adherence improves markedly in apparent response to a transplant.

Young people who are struggling to develop autonomy and take control of their lives may well resent or deny their illness, with implications for their adherence. Non-adherence may become a suicidal metaphor for those who feel helpless and hopeless in their predicament. For others, non-adherence may have the characteristics of risk-taking behaviours that are so common in adolescents, or be a readily accepted new focus for 'acting out' of other conflicts, including issues of autonomy and rebellion against parents.

It may sound a banal and trivial suggestion, but it is strongly recommended that clinicians strive to understand the reasons for non-adherence in each particular case, and plan a response accordingly [21].

Review of whether this is an isolated problem or occurs in the context of more major parenting difficulties is always necessary. If the latter, practical support with some other parenting tasks may release energy to attend to medication adherence. Discussing parents' understanding and beliefs about the relative importance of different components of the regimen may help. It is crucial that problems of adherence are not swept under the carpet until the situation becomes critical, but are tackled early in the child's illness career. One of the responses at an early stage may involve assessment by a child and adolescent psychiatrist, but when problems are severely entrenched little movement can be expected no matter how high the stakes or charismatic the professional.

Non-adherence often evokes strong emotional responses from health professionals. Understanding the dynamics of non-adherence in the individual patient may help the professionals to deal with it non-pejoratively and with compassion. Seeing non-adherence as naughtiness or simple 'defiance' is most unlikely to be helpful (see Cases 2 and 3).

Key points: Non-adherence

- May be:
  - symptomatic of a mood disorder (depressed mood);
  - symptomatic of an adjustment disorder;
  - related to body image concerns or other side-effects;
  - symptomatic of pre-existing general problem with structure and boundaries within family;
  - symptomatic of difficulties in putting boundaries and limits on sick child (reaction to illness);
  - related to over-rigidity by the parents (pre-existing style of reaction to illness);
  - related to beliefs or understanding of child and/or family.

Case 2: Non-adherence in the context of conduct disorder and multiple family psychosocial problems

Danny presented to the renal team at 5 years of age in end stage renal failure. He was being treated with peritoneal dialysis, but contracted recurrent peritonitis. Danny refused medication and was uncooperative with dialysis. His mother was highly distressed at her inability to ensure that her young child received vital treatment.

When ward staff had little time to take bloods, Danny protested vociferously and violently. At home Danny had been generally and intensely oppositional and defiant well before his renal disease declared itself. His treatment was seriously compromised by his emotional and behavioural problems.

The family had multiple, long-standing psychosocial problems. Theirs was a reconstituted family, living on benefits, caring for five children. There was a previous history of marital violence, and Danny's mother had a history of overdosing in response to stress and in the context of her depression. Danny's older sister took an overdose at age 12 years.

Due to the severity of Danny's conduct disorder and the degree to which his treatment was compromised, he was admitted to the child psychiatry day unit, attending 2 days per week, in the same hospital where his renal condition was being treated. Danny attended the Day Unit whether he was on the paediatric ward or at home. The aims of this day unit admission were to assess his emotional status, develop a greater understanding of his non-adherence, assist his mother and ward staff to develop more effective management of his challenging behaviour. The scope for Danny to benefit from direct psychological intervention would also be assessed. The underlying purpose was to attempt to use psychological intervention to minimize risks to Danny's physical health posed by his emotional and behavioural problems.

On the day unit, it became apparent that, although Danny had an undeniable long-standing and severe conduct disorder, his conduct deteriorated when he was physically unwell (e.g. due to a peritoneal infection or high blood pressure). At other times he became more quiescent when he was more acutely ill. It became apparent in play sessions that Danny had a lot of anxieties about his condition. His behaviour could be very challenging on the day unit but over time, he developed positive relationships with the staff. His mother appeared to benefit from attending the parents' group on the unit and her management skills improved with focused parent management skills training. Ward staff developed a better understanding of his multiplicity of problems and needs, and viewed him less negatively.

The day unit attendance was unusually protracted (18 months) because it was seen that this was an effective way of maximizing Danny's compliance with treatment. Gains were modest but significant. Danny subsequently lost his first transplant but not through non-adherence. He was assiduously compliant with treatment after his second transplant, which continues to function well.

It may be expected that this case would tax health economists.

Case 3: Non-adherence successfully treated

John presented with renal failure at age 7 years, necessitating CAPD. While in hospital for the CAPD training and initiation, he was noted to be generally non-adherent with his mother, and would refuse to accept his medication from her. He would accept medication from the nursing staff. His mother became increasingly tense and unconfident when offering John medication. The nursing approach was to nurture and support the mother, offering her the opportunity to discuss her difficulties and fears about John's illness and behaviour, and to devise a programme of handing responsibility for administering John's medication to her in a gradual way, with a positive reinforcement of his adherence. This was highly successful and she had no difficulty in gaining his adherence with CAPD, although the process of handing over responsibility to her by the nurses was done more gradually than usual.

Early detection of mental health problems

As in most other areas of medicine, interventions for mental health problems are more likely to be successful early in the course of the disorder. Awareness of the manifestations of child mental health problems should lead to their early identification with prompt referral or consultation. In addition, identification of high-risk cases (i.e. those with other, pre-existing risk factors such as social disadvantage; impaired parental mental health; previous history of emotional/behavioural difficulties; learning disability) and awareness of high-risk situations (treatment failures, life-threatening complications, aversive procedures) are necessary.

Some specific psychiatric disorders

The whole range of child psychiatric disorders may be seen in children with renal disease, but the following deserve particular mention.

Adjustment disorders

Adjustment disorders are a group of psychiatric disorders that are defined by virtue of their onset being in the period of adaptation to a significant life change or to the consequences of a stressful life event. The life change or consequences of the life event are regarded as the sufficient and necessary cause of the adjustment disorder, although individuals have greater or lesser degrees of predisposition and vulnerability. In renal disease, the precipitating life event may be the diagnosis, understanding (or misunderstanding) of prognosis, the illness itself, or a particular treatment,

Key points: Key issues

- Children and adolescents with chronic illness and disability are at high risk of mental health problems.

- Treatability of child psychiatric disorders: there are effective, evidence-based treatments for many child psychiatric disorders, including those that affect children with chronic illness and disability.

- Dismissing psychiatric disorders as understandable reactions to stress denies children effective treatments.

- Early detection: disorders are more likely to be responsive to treatment the earlier in their course the intervention is offered.

- Non-adherence to treatment of renal conditions may be symptomatic of depression, a severe adjustment disorder, or may be an expression of hopelessness by a disaffected adolescent, or may become a new focus for longstanding autonomy struggles with parents.

- Adolescent conflicts about dependence/independence and freedom/responsibility are common; adolescents may be highly sensitive to body image issues such as drug side-effects (hypertrichosis, weight gain, Cushingoid side-effects), scars, fistulas, stomas; and may become very concerned about sexual attractiveness, short stature, fertility, life expectancy, being different, lifestyle restrictions.

- Families with pre-existing problems (of relationships, mental health, or severe psychosocial stress) are at substantial extra risk of mental health problems (especially adherence).

the consequences of which may be varied and in any one or several of the spheres of physical debility, lifestyle restrictions, treatment regimes, disruption to social relationships, disruption to education, or to family functioning. Adjustment disorders may be predominantly manifest in conduct problems or emotional difficulties, or a mixture of the two. Younger children may regress (e.g. start to speak less maturely, return to sucking thumbs or fingers, return to bedwetting). In addition to the clear onset within a month or so of the adverse life change or event, adjustment disorders virtually all resolve within 6 months, although this will inevitably depend to some degree on what the future holds. It seems likely that adjustment disorders are more likely to occur when circumstances have prevented preparation for the precipitating event (see Case 4).

Depressive adjustment disorders are characterized by persistently low mood (although this may fluctuate in the course of a day) often accompanied, according to severity, by poor concentration, sleep disturbance (early morning wakening that is typical in adult depressive disorders is less common in young people), irritability, reduced appetite, and weight loss. Occasionally appetite and weight may increase in depression. Depressive adjustment disorders may be severe and prolonged and should be referred to child and adolescent psychiatric teams.

Case 4: Adjustment disorder in a pre-school child

Laura, aged 4 years, presented with marked non-adherence and frequent severe tantrums when thwarted. She cut up her previously favourite dresses, smashed a mirror, and threw a framed photograph of herself at her third birthday party at the wall.

These problems started suddenly as she became ambulant after the emergency laparotomy at which her Wilms' tumour had been found. Laura had previously been a healthy and well adjusted, albeit rather indulged, child. Her Wilms' tumour had declared itself suddenly, with abdominal pain and increasing girth. At laparotomy it was found to be unresectable, and a decision was made to start chemotherapy immediately. Laura woke up in ICU and there was little time for psychological preparation before chemotherapy began. She had previously revelled in frilly dresses and fancy hairstyles.

Her single mother was taken aback at and distressed by Laura's non-adherence and tantrums and found it difficult to be firm with her little daughter who was so ill. Nursing staff saw her as a spoiled child.

The child psychiatry team provided an opportunity for Laura's mother to reflect on their predicament and assisted her in understanding and managing Laura's challenging and distressed behaviour and individual play therapy for Laura in which she showed a preoccupation with control, appearance, and pain.

Laura did very well psychologically, and, fortunately, she responded very well to the chemotherapy.

Depression

Depression is not uncommon in adolescents but less so in younger children; bipolar (manic–depressive) illness is increasingly recognized in adolescents. Both are illnesses with a genetic component. The symptoms are, of course, those of depressive adjustment disorders (see above) but may also include intense self-criticism and guilt, with distorted perceptions about the future, the risks of renal illness, or treatment. Severe biological symptoms of depression, including psychomotor retardation, are uncommon in children.

Depressive cognitions may include suicidality and hopelessness (which may not necessarily be apparent and about which enquiries may need to be made) and may be linked to non-adherence. Depression in children and adolescents is easily missed or attributed to normal 'moods' or to an understandable response to the renal disease or treatment. It is responsive to psychiatric treatment (usually antidepressants and cognitive therapy) and carries an increased risk of relapse and recurrence in adulthood. A low threshold for referral to child psychiatrists should be firmly maintained (see Case 5).

Case 5: Eating disorder and depression

Jill developed bulimia nervosa at age 15 years, some 5 years after her successful renal transplant. She had been inducing vomiting in an attempt to lose weight and had recently secretly missed several doses of cyclosporin. Jill had had her transplant as she entered puberty. She had been very distressed by her Cushingoid facies while on high doses of prednisolone.

Her bulimia developed during her GCSE year while she was concerned about her future career prospects and while there were a number of tensions within the family. Her older, healthy sister had recently left home.

On psychiatric assessment, Jill was clinically depressed, but did not want to take psychotropic medication (a selective serotonin re-uptake inhibitor was recommended). Psychiatric intervention was a combination of individual cognitive behaviour therapy and family therapy.

Jill's mood improved substantially over the subsequent 4 months. Her vomiting reduced. The family used the family sessions to reflect on the stress of Jill's acute illness years previously, the continuing psychological burden of care, and anxieties about the future, to good effect. Communication had broken down in the family in the wake of Jill's illness as they each attempted not to burden the others with their worries and other emotions.

Jill retained a sensitivity about her weight and a slightly distorted body image.

Eating disorders

Whether there is any overall increased risk of eating disorders with chronic renal failure is unknown. As only 1% of 18-year-old girls suffer from anorexia nervosa, and as it is still more rare in boys and in younger adolescents, a very large study would need to be done to investigate this possibility. Clinical practice, however, suggests that there may well be a link. The continued focus on the female form and the media's premise that thinness is desirable are powerful societal pressures for vulnerable youngsters. Shunts, catheters, hypertrichosis from medication, fluid retention, Cushingoid facies, dietary restrictions, and frequent weighings of chronic renal failure patients, those dialysed, and those post-transplant, may key into the sensitivities of their adolescence. When a young person begins to control their weight because of an eating disorder (anorexia or bulimia nervosa), the treatment and control of the renal condition, most particularly when dialysis is involved, may be rapidly jeopardized. It is worth thinking about the possibility of an eating disorder in any young person, but particularly in a teenage girl, whose weight is fluctuating unexpectedly and unexplainedly. Again, referral to a child psychiatrist who is able to liaise closely with the paediatric team will be essential and physicians should not be reassured by bland reassurances from the patient that they are not trying to lose weight (see Cases 5 and 6).

Case 6: Anorexia nervosa

Mary presented with all the cardinal features of anorexia nervosa at the age of 17 years. She had had several years on peritoneal dialysis and a failed transplant. Prior to her renal disease becoming manifest, she had been 'a very picky eater' with a restricted range of food preferences. After her transplant, her parents would travel 30 miles to the particular take-away restaurant she preferred to try to tempt her with the one dish she said she wanted. Her body image disturbance was profound and she was highly distressed by her abdominal scarring and A-V shunt. Her anorexia nervosa severely compromised the management of her dialysis.

The psychiatric team offered individual psychotherapy and family therapy, and worked closely with the renal team in respect of dietary advice, weight monitoring, and target weights. Mary's weight loss ceased but she remained underweight and the psychopathology of anorexia nervosa remained.

Her age eventually dictated that she be transferred to adult services, for which careful liaison was needed with both renal and psychiatric teams.

Post-traumatic stress disorder

This is a delayed and/or protracted response to an exceptionally threatening or catastrophic stressful situation. Unfortunately, such situations can, of course, be medical, and can happen either as a direct result of acute illness or as a catastrophic consequence of treatment. Virulent, serious disease and emergency situations may severely constrain, if not completely preclude, the psychological preparation that would otherwise have been offered. Post-traumatic stress disorder (PTSD) should be suspected in children who have enduring intense maladaptive reactions following intrusive medical procedures, or catastrophes or complications, particularly if there is low mood, poor concentration, and sleep disturbance. People with post-traumatic stress disorder are often clinically depressed and have intense anxiety symptoms, nightmares, and intrusive memories of the adverse events ('flashbacks'). PTSD needs skilled psychiatric intervention that may involve psychotherapy, cognitive behaviour therapy, and/or psychotropic medication.

Postoperative, infective, or metabolic confusional states

These may be especially difficult to recognize in younger children. Signs of impaired or fluctuating consciousness may be subtle. Children so affected will not be registering new information. Visual misinterpretations and hallucinations tend to be exacerbated by poor light, and children may need to be nursed with lights on at night.

Fear of procedures

Most doctors learn early in their career not to put questions to children if unprepared for the answer or unable to modify their behaviour in response. One learns to avoid such pitfalls as asking, 'May I take some blood please?' What is surprising is not why some children show extreme fear of procedures, but that so few do. Children who appear to enjoy procedures or are too readily compliant are a source of concern because it is unusual to deny fear, pain, and distress so strongly, and a high cost may be paid later, in psychological terms, for such repression of normal reactions. Most children manage to put up with procedures with proper preparation, attention to pain and discomfort during, and praise afterwards for bravery, but some become frankly phobic. Parents cannot always manage to be supportive to their children in respect of procedures. Finding out the parent's own attitudes, views, and fears may be useful. Children will only be reassured about procedures if they are properly assured in the first place. Developmentally appropriate explanations should be offered where possible. Lies such as 'it won't hurt' are likely to damage the child's fragile trust and are likely to make future compliance waiver. An understanding, calm, patient, and firm attitude is usually the most successful. Clinical team members should let each other know when a child is intensely fearful. It is much easier to deal with a panic-stricken child when one has been forewarned. Dealing with frightened children demands judgement and a mixture of firmness and flexibility that is not contradictory. Play specialists can offer very useful distraction or guided imagery. Child mental health teams may be able to assist in situations where children have become phobic of procedures (most commonly termed 'needle phobia') (see Case 7).

Case 7: Fear of procedures

Joel, aged 16 years, presented with frank and severe anxiety symptoms in relation to the prospect of further surgery. He had had two failed transplants, and a close family acquaintance had recently died from renal failure. Ward, theatre, and anaesthetic staff offered a careful, well-planned graded exposure programme with supported opportunity for familiarization with equipment and theatre. Cognitive behaviour therapy was offered to assist him in managing his anxiety. Short-term anxiolytics would be considered if his anxiety symptoms intensified as further operative procedures became imminent.

Other complications with potential mental health consequences

Separations

Attachment is the infant's predisposition to seek proximity to certain people and to be more secure in their presence. It is a process fundamental to the development of secure, meaningful social relationships. Separation anxiety is the anxiety and distress shown by small children when they are separated from their primary attachment figure(s). Separation anxiety is a normal phenomenon in young children and may be intensified or prolonged in response to stress. Although increased separation anxiety is common as a response of young children to enforced separation and hospitalization, there is little to suggest that serious illness and its consequences have

a significant effect on attachment, especially now that parents are encouraged to room in and admissions are generally short.

As described by Graham *et al.* [7], the short-term effects of hospitalization depend upon: the age of the child (above 1 year, the younger the more severe the distress); the social circumstances of the family (financial and parental relationship); the adequacy of preparation for hospitalization; the child's condition (the greater the degree of discomfort and distress, the greater the degree of disturbance); the frequency of painful procedures [23]; the presence of familiar figures (rooming-in facilities); the previous experience of hospitalization; the parent–child relationship; the temperament or personality of the child; the coping style of the child; the provision of play and education facilities of the ward; the attitudes of hospital staff; the degree to which the ward is child-centred.

Children who have been repeatedly admitted to hospital in early and mid-childhood are slightly more likely to develop behavioural and emotional disturbances in adolescence [24]. The effects are particularly likely if admissions are for long periods and if the children come from disadvantaged homes. Reasons for this are unclear and it is possible that with improvements in hospital practice, this adverse effect may be minimized or may disappear altogether [25].

Parents may be taken aback by the fact that their young child becomes more oppositional on discharge home, but this may be related to the separation experiences or to other aspects of treatment. Preparation for these reactions should be routine (rather than an assumption that everything will be 'plain sailing' once the onerous phase of hospital admission is over) and, if introduced carefully, such explanation will be perceived as useful.

Short stature

Many of the chronic renal conditions or their treatment have an impact on growth, sometimes so severe that comparison with 'normal' short stature seems ridiculous for those who are six or seven standard deviations below it. Nevertheless there is limited literature relating specifically to psychological effects of growth limitation in the context of renal disease, and some generalization from other sources of information, and from clinical studies, is necessary.

In early childhood, the problem demands practical adaptations at home and school and will mostly have an impact on parents and other adults who may be overprotective. This is a good time, however, to prepare parents for the difficulties ahead, with discussions about why overprotectiveness is bad for children (it has demonstrable negative effects on their self-esteem and confidence) and about ways in which parents will need to ensure that their children are included in a range of age- and development-appropriate activities, even though others may think them too small.

In middle childhood, as self-concept develops, the child's own self-image becomes more relevant and peer group issues begin to arise, although not always negatively at this stage. Being treated as a 'baby' in big girls' games is not to everyone's taste, however. Smallness and quickness may be joined in the child's mind, so that they are perceived as useful members sometimes, and being 'cute' or a mascot may convey benefits. For those with learning difficulties, short stature may be protective, signalling greater youth and therefore less demands from the outside world. Parents can help their children problem-solve practical difficulties and become used to demonstrating their true age with a variety of identity cards and passes.

It is in adolescence that, for boys particularly, clear social and peer group advantages are conveyed by early physical development and being the tallest increases popularity with both sexes and signals maturity. Thus short boys are disadvantaged in all these areas. For girls, it seems that being 'average' in development is more important than being first and so short-statured girls may be less severely affected than boys in adolescence, and indeed advantaged by the protectiveness they may attract.

Preparations for the practical difficulties and the problem-solving approach to peer group issues can always be improved, but it is hard to prepare for the intensity of feelings of some adolescents, or the reactions to an unpleasant or bullying peer group. These should obviously be tackled through the school system as well as individually. Interventions depend on the strength and nature of the young person's distress, but brief cognitive and behavioural inputs in relation to teasing, confidence, and 'acting tall' have been demonstrated to be effective [26]. Frank anxiety or depression should receive attention from mental health professionals and not be rationalized as normal reactions to an abnormal predicament. Firm parental approaches to well-meaning infantilization by other adults may be necessary. Where groups are held by the renal and psychosocial team with the young people themselves, peer group talk about the problems and sharing of reactions and solutions may be very supportive.

Other complications of treatment

A number of treatments for renal disease can have noxious effects on mental functioning, whether via a direct effect on the brain or through a psychological reaction to side-effects that affect appearance. Steroids can lead to behavioural problems because of irritability and can cause mood disorders. Children, and particularly adolescents, may be very distressed by their Cushingoid appearance. Similarly, ciclosporin can cause hypertrichosis that can be very distressing, especially for adolescent girls. Operative procedures may cause worrying scarring and disfigurement.

Disruptions to schooling

The consequences here may be to academic achievement, peer group (social) relations, or to self-esteem. The significance of missing GCSE or A level coursework, revision or examinations is obvious. Younger children may miss leaving their primary school and the potential difficulties of joining a new class or school out of step with one's peer group should not be underestimated. Hospital schools and teachers have a crucial function in liaising with the child's usual school and in keeping the child as academically active as possible. Hospital schools may have a very normalizing function when they can educate the children away from the ward environment and in a group.

Other problems with peer group

Although there are those situations in which a group of children become protective to the vulnerable or 'different' member, less altruistic aspects of human nature, group dynamics, and children's inventiveness often result in persecutory, derogatory situations for children with almost any chronic illness or disability. Short stature may give form to the persecution, but 'Steak and kidney', 'You belong in the pie shop', and 'Look it's...—get the gravy' are but a few examples children with CRF have encountered. Young people may even encounter difficulties with situations brought about by the best of misguided intentions. For example, in a PSE (personal and social education) class, the teacher showed a video of transplants and our patient, who had had her transplant some months previously and who was a member of the class, was asked to say something about her experiences. She had not been consulted or forewarned and was mortified.

Key Points: Situations requiring vigilance (high-risk situations)

- Repeated stressful separations.

- Disruption to school and peer-group relationships.

- Social disadvantage (single parents, lack of support, financial worries).

- Teenage girls and adverse effects on appearance and thereby body image (steroids, hypertrichosis, scars, cannulas, weight).

- Boys with poor growth.

- Pre-existing emotional and behavioural difficulties.

- Serial treatment failures.

Liaison child mental health

With good liaison psychiatry/psychology, paediatric teams will develop some expertise in recognition of mental health problems and in managing the less severe of these. Teams will be able to identify those children for whom more specialist mental health input is required. The whole range of assessment and therapeutic resources of specialist CAMHS (Child and Adolescent Mental Health Services) may be needed by renal patients who have significant mental health problems. Those likely to be most frequently needed are: child and adolescent psychiatry; child clinical psychology—behavioural skills (e.g. needle phobias, management of feeding difficulties), elucidation of complex cognitive deficits; play therapy; social work.

We advocate a model that includes all of the following liaison activities:

(1) emergency/urgency: confusional states, severe mood disorders, severe adjustment disorders;

rapid response for serious psychiatric problems in inpatients;

(2) planned non-urgent case assessment/intervention (outpatient);

(3) case by case liaison to care team;

(4) regular psychosocial liaison meetings (some case-related function, but also looking at general issues for team/ward).

Resources and professional relationships may well be limiting factors in the structure of a psychosocial team. We suggest that one identified senior mental health professional be nominated as the key liaison person who can involve other members of CAMHS as appropriate.

As outlined above, psychiatric disorders and less severe psychological problems are many and varied. Effective, evidence-based treatments are increasingly available for mental health problems (e.g. cognitive behaviour therapy, behavioural treatments, parent management training, psychotropic medications). There is a spectrum of treatability from cure through remitting and relapsing conditions to palliation and prevention of deterioration and secondary impairments, but this certainly does not, in our view, compare unfavourably with the medical and surgical treatments of renal failure and its causes.

The advantages of regular psychosocial liaison meetings are that the CAMHS specialist becomes known to and, hopefully, trusted by the renal or paediatric team, the culture of considering and discussing psychosocial issues as a matter of course is promoted, and the appropriateness of referral of cases can be clarified in the meeting. A team that is used to recognizing, rather than denying, and reflecting on and considering sympathetically the psychosocial aspects of illness, is likely to promote enhanced meeting of mental health needs of all of its patients, not just those who have major difficulties.

We would suggest that psychosocial meetings offer a more efficient and effective model of liaison than joint clinics.

Given the number of complex and severe emotional and behavioural difficulties, the potential contribution of medication and the metabolic problems, we suggest that for renal teams, the key liaison CAMHS specialist should be a psychiatrist. Given the complexity of the children, the psychiatrist should also be a port of entry to a range of CAMHS professionals, especially clinical psychology.

Key points: CAMHS referral guidelines

For paediatric services that do not have a close liaison relationship with child mental health services, the following guideline for thinking about and prioritizing referrals to CAMHS is suggested:

- High priority—urgent referral:
  - any symptoms or signs suggestive of psychotic illness (delusions, thought disorder, hallucinations) including schizophrenia, mania, psychotic depression, or organic mental state (other than the most transient febrile confusional state).

- High priority—urgent discussion/early referral:
  - high concern about suicidal risk (suicidal thinking or attempts) or self-harm;
  - where family dynamics are significantly affecting adaptation to illness or medical treatment;
  - symptoms or signs suggestive of moderate to severe depressive illness;
  - symptoms or signs suggestive of eating disorder (anorexia nervosa or bulimia nervosa).

- Less urgent but important—early discussion/planned referral:
  - school refusal;
  - impairing obsessions and compulsions;
  - other emotional disorders, including needle phobias;
  - neuropsychiatric problems;
  - serious non-adherence, where a fuller understanding may be useful or where non-adherence is thought to be symptomatic of other problems;
  - complex presentations where the relative contributions of physical, psychological, and social factors require skilled assessment of each element.

References

1. Rutter, M., Tizard, J. and Whitmore, K. Education, health and behaviour. 1970; Longman Press, London.
2. Cadman, D., Boyle, M., Szatmari, P., and Offord, D.R. 1987. Chronic illness, disability and mental and social well-being: findings of the Ontario Child Health Study. Pediatrics. 1987; 79, 5: 805–813.
3. Pless I.B. and Roghman, K.J. Chronic illness and its consequences: observations based on three epidemiologic surveys. 1971; J Pediatr. 79: 351–359.
4. Lloyd, M. and Bor, R. (eds) Communication skills for medicine. 1996; Churchill Livingstone, Edinburgh.
5. Billings, A. and Stoeckle J.D. The Clinical encounter (a guide to the medical interview and case presentation). 1998; Mosby, St Louis.
6. Hamburg, D. and Hamburg, B. A life-span perspective on adaptation and health. In: Family and Health: Epidemiological Approaches, Kaplan, B and Ibrahim, M (eds). 1980; University of South Carolina Press, Chapel Hill.
7. Graham, P., Turk, J. and Verhulst, F. Child Psychiatry: A developmental approach. 3rd Edition. 1999; Oxford University Press, Oxford.
8. Eiser, C. Growing up with a chronic disease: the impact on children and their families. Jessica Kingsley, 1993; London and Bristol, Pennsylvania.
9. Sloper, P. and Turner, S. Risk and resistance factors in the adaptation of parents of children with severe physical disability. 1993; J Child Psychol Psychiatr. 34 (2): 167–188.
10. Eiser, C. 1990. Chronic Childhood Disease. An Introduction to Psychological Theory and Research. CUP.
11. Lindemann, E. The symptomatology and management of acute grief. Am J Psychiatry. 1994; 101:141.
12. Parkes, C.M. Bereavement: studies of grief in adult life. 1972; Penguin Books, London.
13. Burton, L. Care of the child facing death. 1975; Routledge and Keegan Paul, London.
14. Gyulay, J.E. 1978. The dying child. McGraw-Hill, New York.
15. Postlethwaite, R.J., Garralda, M.E., Eminson, D.M. and Reynolds, J.C. Lessons from psychosocial studies of chronic renal failure. Arch Dis Child. 1996; 75: 455–459.
16. North, C. and Eminson, D.M. A review of a psychiatry-nephrology liaison service. Eur Child Adolesc Psychiatry. 1998; 7: 235–245.
17. Moghal, N.E., Wittich, E. and Milford, D.V. The impact of renal replacement therapy on toddler time. ANNA J. 1999; 26: 331–335.
18. Korsch, B.M., Fine, R.N. and Negete, V.F. Non-compliance in children with renal transplants. Pediatrics. 1978; 61: 872–876.
19. Beck, D.E., Fennell, R.S., Yost, R.L., Robinson, J.D., Geary, D. and Richards, G.A. Evaluation of an educational program on compliance with medication regimens in pediatric patients with renal transplants. J Pediatr. 1980; 96: 1094–1097.
20. Ettenger, R.B., Rosenthal, J.T., Marik, J.L., Malekzadeh, M., Forsythe, S.B., Kamil, E.S., Salusky, I.B. and Fine, R.N. Improved cadaveric renal transplant outcome in children. Pediatr Nephrol. 1991; 5: 137–142.
21. Wolff, G., Strecker, K., Vester, U., Latta, K. and Ehrich, J.H.H. Non-compliance following renal transplantation in children and adolescents. Pediatr Nephrol. 1998; 12: 703–708.

22. Watson, A.R. Non-compliance and transfer from paediatric to adult transplant unit. Pediatr Nephrol.
2000; 14: 469–472.

23. Saylor, C., Pallmeyer, T.P., Finch, A.J., Eason, L.
Treiber, F. and Folger, C. Predictors of psychological
distress in hospitalized pediatric patients. J Am Acad
Child Adolesc Psychiatry 1987; 26, 2: 232–236.

24. Quinton, D. and Rutter, M. Early Admissions and
later disturbances of behaviour: an attempted replication of Douglas' findings. Dev Med Child Neurol.
1976; 18: 447–459.

25. Shannon, F.T., Fergusson, D.M. and Dimond, M.E.
Early hospital admissions and subsequent behaviour
problems in 6 year olds. Arch Dis Child 1984; 59:
815–819.

26. Eminson, D.M., Powell, R.P. and Hollis, S. Cognitive
Behavioural Interventions with Short Statured Boys. In:
Growth, Stature and Adaptation. Stabler, B. &
Underwood, L. (eds). 1994; North Carolina USA.

25 | *Meeting the information needs of children and their families*

Alan R. Watson

Parents bring to a doctor concerns about their child. The doctor's role is to gain as accurate a picture as possible of the child's problems. This information must then be processed to develop a plan for management of the problem. This must be done in collaboration with the parents and child. To enable this to happen there will be a need to explain and discuss what has been found and what investigations and management are planned. In chronic and/or relapsing illness this discussion must include a general review of the likely course of the illness. Thus, giving and receiving of information is an integral part of clinical care and the support offered to families [1–4].

This chapter is concerned with what might be thought of as the routine information needs of parents and children with renal problems. On occasion the information that is being imparted is of such a serious nature, either from the parents' or the professional's perspective, that it is considered to be 'breaking bad news'. The same principles underpin 'breaking bad news' as the more routine communication considered in this chapter, but this more heightened situation is discussed in Chapter 24. The boundary between these two situations is arbitrary and on occasions what had been expected to be a routine communication of information escalates into 'breaking bad news' because of an unanticipated reaction from the parents.

Standard texts describe good practice in communication [5,6]. This chapter aims to place these general recommendations in the context of paediatric renal medicine. Additionally, a number of methods of communication are available to reinforce verbal communication and this chapter will highlight some useful methods of communication or sources of information. The different types of information should be considered to be complementary and should be deployed to maximize the chances of meeting the information needs of children and their families.

Why give information?

The provision of adequate information before operations and procedures has been shown to reduce patient anxiety [7]. It is important that families have an opportunity to plan for both good and bad outcomes. There is evidence that if warned of possible poor outcomes, families are more able to cope if they have had time to prepare their reactions. There is also evidence from studies in adult cancer patients that those who were more satisfied with the information imparted by the staff were more likely to be content with their level of involvement in decision making [8].

> ## Key points: Provision of information to patients and their families
>
> - Reduces anxiety and stress [7].
> - Allows families and child to plan for outcomes.
> - Enables decision making and informed consent.
> - Improves outcomes.
> - Enhances parent and child satisfaction.
> - Improves compliance with treatment.

We are now in an era of evidence-based healthcare and unprecedented access to information technology. Although the evidence base for paediatric renal care is often limited, there is increasing focus on evidence-based patient choice, where patients are offered research-based information and given the opportunity to influence decisions about their treatment and

Table 25.1 Important aspects of a unit's information strategy

Keeping the child and his or her family informed and hopefully enhancing adherence to treatment
Preparing the child for procedures and reducing anxiety [7]
Explaining illness to siblings
Explaining illness to extended family, friends, and family practitioner
Informing school of expected progress [13]

care [9]. This will increase demand for patient-orientated information about medical effectiveness.

There is increasing evidence that the use of education programmes for adult renal patients may delay the onset of renal replacement therapy [10], improve patient knowledge [11], and enhance patient satisfaction [12].

This chapter will review the practical aspects to be considered in developing a unit's 'information strategy' (Table 25.1). This will be achieved through discussion of:

(1) the information needs of patients and their families;

(2) what sources of information are available for providing this information;

(3) the sources of information that patients and parents are using;

(4) where this information should be given;

(5) support for parents of children with renal disease.

The information needs of patients and their families

Research on information needs

Although there has been research investigating patient satisfaction with communication and the ability to retain information [14], little work has been done to ascertain what information parents require. If parents are to participate actively in the care of their children, then the parent's perspective on information needs must be taken into consideration. Few studies have attempted to research this topic [15–17] and there is little information available in the field of paediatric nephrology [1,18].

Research in Nottingham has emphasized the information needs of parents of children with nephrotic syndrome, which remains a chronic illness for many families [19]. We have also assessed the information needs of parents of children with end stage renal failure compared to the parents of children with insulin-dependent diabetes mellitus (IDDM) using questionnaires over a 2-year period [20]. The main findings were that most information needs were for:

• detailed test results;

• new information about the condition;

• their child's future social development.

The questions that achieved the highest ratings were those concerned with the future, such as the child's fertility, their future social and marriage prospects, and the hope for new improved treatments or a possible cure. Other studies have concurred with these findings [21]. These were also the highest scoring questions in parents of children with nephrotic syndrome [19] and cystic fibrosis [22]. In the study, the mean general information need scores from mothers and fathers of children with end stage renal failure tended to decline over the 2-year study period. There was no similar trend for mothers or fathers of children with diabetes. We speculated that the decrease in information needs of the parents of children with end stage renal failure during this time may have been due to the more frequent inpatient/outpatient contact with healthcare professionals that these parents encountered compared to those of children with diabetes. Another important observation was that occupation was significantly associated with the mean general information need scores for parents, with occupations of a lower socio-economic status being associated with higher information need scores. This was similar to findings in a study of parents of children with cystic fibrosis [22] and is an important factor to recognize. Healthcare professionals should not assume that those with occupations of lower socio-economic status have lower information needs.

What sources of information are available?

There are different ways of imparting information. The most important point to recognize is that different families may need different types of information delivered at different intervals and reinforced by different members of the multidisciplinary team in different settings.

We should avoid the paternalistic approach of assuming that the interview between the doctor and the family is the only source that matters. If the news is bad we know that the majority of parents will hear little, whatever the duration of the interview, hence the importance of tailoring the information to the needs of the family and using the members of the multidisciplinary team to support and expand on the information. The different types of methods of transmission of information should be considered as complementary and should be deployed to maximize the information for the child and family.

Verbal information

Verbal information allows direct contact between professionals and the family and remains the mainstay of communication. It provides a flexible communication opportunity with the possibility of immediately correcting misinterpretations and amplifying points. Thus it can be tailored to the parents' as opposed to the professional's information needs. Professional interpreters can be arranged if the patient or their family do not use English as their first language Standard texts should be consulted for a more detailed discussion, but the more important points for the paediatric renal service are summarized in Table 25.2.

Written information

Patients and families can read written information at their leisure and use it as a permanent record of the discussions. The written information should cover all of the points that the family consider important. The requirements for written information are set out in Table 25.3.

In addition to written information specific for individual patients, a number of information booklets about various children's renal conditions and investigations are available. The production of booklets is not without its problems. The production of a quality booklet takes a great deal of time and effort, particularly as all members of the multiprofessional team should have an input. Separate booklets will be required for parents and children of different ages. It is difficult to produce generic booklets for national distribution as practices vary from unit to unit. Booklets

Table 25.2 Important points regarding the provision of verbal information

Setting
  For new or important information, ensure that adequate time without interruptions is scheduled
  Try to ensure that both parents or carers hear the message together
  Arrange for a professional interpreter to be present if appropriate
  Ensure that one other member of the multiprofessional team who is accepted by the family is present. Too many team members inhibit parents and children
Content
  Describe what information you plan to give
  Summarize your understanding of the child's problem
  Explore the parents' (and child's) understanding of the problem
  Outline the rest of the interview
  Give the most important piece of information first
  Use appropriate language
  If relevant, use drawings to supplement the information
  Explore the parents' (and child's) response to the information given
  Negotiate management
  Check the parents' (and child's) understanding of what you have said
  Always ensure that the child's needs are considered and agree with the parents how to attend to these
Afterwards
  For new or important information, follow up with a written or tape-recorded summary
  Feed back what has been said to members of the multi-disciplinary team

Table 25.3 Key requirements for written information

Information should be:
  easy to read using short words and sentences
  expressed in the active rather than the passive voice
  expressed in positive rather than negative sentences
  attractively presented

in several languages will be required to meet the needs of families whose first language is not English.

Suggestions for the production of written information are given in Table 25.4. Desktop publishing may help to produce additional leaflets on certain aspects, which require more explanation. This can be included in booklet updates.

Tape recordings of consultations

The audiotaping of consultations can help to overcome the effect of 'shock block' when information is poorly received by the family and, similar to written

Table 25.4 Suggestions for written information

Each patient and family should have their own
  information folder
National organizations should be used to fund booklets
Generic booklets should be produced in discussion
  with other units
Booklets need to be updated regularly

Examples of booklets are included in Appendix 1 at the end of this
chapter.

Table 25.5 Suggestions for the use of audiotaping as an
aid to consultation

Agree as a unit strategy
Give parents a choice as to whether audiotaping is
  carried out
Discuss with others who may also be using the
  technique [23]

summaries, provides a permanent record of the consultation [23]. The tape can also be played to relatives who were not able to attend the consultation themselves. The use of tape recordings does require a level of organization to have working equipment available at the time of consultation and some feel the presence of a tape recorder could be an impediment to dialogue. Suggestions regarding the use of audiotaping are given in Table 25.5.

Videos

The use of professionally produced video recordings may supplement information given to children and their families. Video recordings tend to be somewhat more realistic than booklets, which often use line drawings or cartoons for illustrations. Hospital or university audiovisual departments are becoming increasingly experienced in their production. They are useful for those with poor literary skills and the technology is widely available, with most households owning a video player. Similar to written and audiotaped material, they are a useful means of reaching the extended family and are a useful teaching tool for trainee nurses and doctors. They may, however, be both costly and time-consuming to produce in a professional manner, the costs of keeping the material up to date will be much greater than, for instance, written material. In light of the relative rarity of renal disease in childhood, these videos will have a relatively small market and hence the cost may be hard to justify unless commercial or other sponsorship is available.

CD-ROMs

These are an attractive alternative medium to video for children with facilities for animation. CD-ROMs are, however, expensive to produce and adults are not always as computer literate as their children. They require a large investment of time and money to be produced well. A CD-ROM may be particularly useful when children have a choice of treatments available to them, e.g. in nocturnal enuresis (see 'Boss of my Bladder', ERIC, 34 Old School House, Britannia Road, Bristol BS15 2DB, UK).

The Internet

The Internet offers children and their families rapid access to a wealth of information produced by a variety of sources. It is an increasingly popular source of knowledge and many children are becoming increasingly adept at Internet navigation. The major downside is that the information available is generally not peer-reviewed, is not always appropriate, and can confuse and sometimes alarm families. To try and circumvent some of these problems, clinicians need to be involved in the production and monitoring of the renal information available on websites. This requires time and effort to produce quality material for websites and to provide regular updates. Clinicians could consider providing their patients with a list of suitable websites specifically for children and families with renal problems (see Appendix 2 at the end of this chapter).

What sources of information are parents using?

We conducted a questionnaire survey of 84 parents of children who attend the outpatient department of our institution with general nephrological problems (UTI, enuresis, nephrotic syndrome, nephritis, hypertension, etc.) and 42 parents of children who attend the chronic renal failure clinic (including dialysis and transplant patients). Parents were asked about the sources that they used to obtain information about their child's medical condition. The results are shown in Fig. 25.1.

This survey was conducted at the end of 2000 and shows that in Nottingham, less than 25% of families of children with renal disease had sought medical

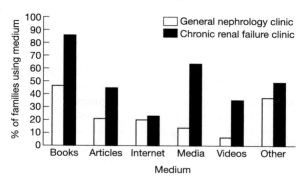

Fig. 25.1 Sources of information used by 84 parents of children attending a general nephrology clinic and 42 parents of children attending a chronic renal failure clinic.

Table 25.6 Provision of information for families and associated professionals

Clinic	Team members
	Parent contact and organized 'linkage'
	Information library
	CD-ROM computer program
	Parent support groups
Ward	Team members
	Parent contact
	Structured visits before procedures
Home	Team members
	Update visits
	Videophone link
School	Visits by team members
	Hospital–schoolteacher liaison
	Schoolteacher visits to unit
GP	Visits by team members
	Regular correspondence

information on the Internet. Between 11 and 12 Internet sites were quoted by the general and chronic renal failure patients as sources of information. Books are seen as a particularly important source of information for chronic renal failure families. These consisted mainly of the chronic renal failure, dialysis, and transplant booklets produced by our unit. The media (predominantly television and newspapers) was referred to more often in the end stage renal failure group, with the parents reporting a lot of interest in programmes dealing with transplantation and medical issues.

These local results emphasize the various information sources used by parents. They have encouraged us to continue to develop and refine our booklets and videos, which are still seen as important information sources. Anecdotally, we all remember parents who arrive in the clinic with an Internet printout, but this source of information appears to be of lesser importance in our population of patients at present.

Where should the information be given?

Although the clinic and ward are the usual venues where information may be given, these are also places where there may be a lack of privacy, and anxiety may reduce information retention. Home visits by team members such as social workers and nurses provide an opportunity for the whole family to discuss their anxieties and worries in their own home environment. As well as obtaining detailed information about family structure and support in a relaxed atmosphere, the

visits allow family members to raise questions which might have been worrying them, but which they felt reluctant to ask the doctor about [24]. Since information needs to be reviewed regularly, we have introduced update visits to the family home for both chronic peritoneal dialysis and transplant patients [25,26].

Since children spend a great deal of their time at school, it is essential that, with the parent's consent, information about the child's condition is imparted to schoolteachers [13]. Compared to asthma and diabetes, renal failure is a rare problem in childhood and very few schools will have encountered the problem of a child requiring dialysis or a kidney transplant. Visiting the school and meeting the teachers directly will provide teachers with some understanding of the child's problems. The hospital schoolteacher can then liaise with the school over issues such as preparation for exams and home tuition [13]. The Internet now allows children to liaise directly with their school if attending for regular haemodialysis.

In the United Kingdom, the general practitioner (GP) is the first port of call for the child and family. Again, the rarity of paediatric renal disease means that any single GP's experience of a particular disorder will be small. Nursing staff can combine a home and school visit with one to the GP to provide information about the child's condition, prognosis and, particularly, medications. As many children have to travel large distances to the unit for treatment, it is important to establish this link, especially as many GPs can arrange blood tests and monitoring locally if requested.

Table 25.6 summarizes where and how information can be given.

Support for parents of children with renal disease

Parent contact

Information is also gained by families from the parents and relatives of other patients. Families are often in close contact on the ward or in the clinic. Although there may be some negative aspects to this contact, with each child's clinical course being different, on balance, parents find the support helpful. It can be a positive move to assess the information needs of a family and suggest, with both families' consent, linking them with another family who have been through the experience, e.g. children who have received cyclophosphamide for nephrotic syndrome or a young child commencing dialysis therapy. In our weekly chronic renal failure clinic we facilitate such meetings by providing a coffee room where parents can meet and mingle. In the coffee room there is also a library of non-specialist medical books appropriate to all developmental levels. These can be borrowed and used by parents to explain bodily parts and functions to children and siblings.

Parent support groups

A logical extension of the parent support strategy is to arrange parent support groups [27]. Here, parents can meet and talk with others in a similar situation or with those who have already passed on to another stage. These are generally organized twice a year by our social worker and psychologist and are held on a weekend day with crèche facilities provided, so that parents can bring all of their children and not be distracted at the group meeting. These groups provide a forum for free discussion of issues for parents with children at different stages of treatment. They have certainly provided feedback on many important qualitative issues for our unit and have resulted in the development of information leaflets and the respite care or home support strategy [1]. Occasionally, meetings have been organized for extended family members such as grandparents, who can be a major source of support for a child with a chronic illness. We know, for instance, that having a child at home on peritoneal dialysis and overnight feeding is very intimidating for grandparents who feel reluctant to babysit [28]. Informing them about the treatments and other issues does help to allay some of their own anxieties and helps them to support the patient and their parents.

Patient support organizations

These can be an important source of information and support for families. The names and contact details of a number of different organizations dealing with a wide range of paediatric renal disease and enuresis are shown in Appendix 3 of this chapter.

Helplines

A recent development in the United Kingdom has been the creation of helplines, both by the National Health Service in general and more notably by the National Kidney Research Fund (helpline 0845 300 1499) and National Kidney Federation (helpline 0845 601 0209). Their stated aims are to provide information on all aspects of kidney disease and dysfunction (including sending out patient information fact sheets); support for those in a traumatized state following a difficult diagnosis; advice on questions to ask the general practitioner or hospital medical team; plus useful contacts to other sources of help. The helplines have only been in operation for around 12 months in the United Kingdom. Many of the queries require answers from a nephrologist and difficulties can arise with confidentiality and liability issues for any advice that is given. However, it will be useful to audit the range of questions that are asked in order to more clearly identify areas where our information sources are deficient.

Internet sources

Although our local survey in Nottingham did not suggest major internet use at present, there is no doubt that there has been a proliferation of websites and an increasing number of families will use this modality [29]. Since there may well be a generation gap between children and adults in the level of computer literacy, the Internet may provide an opportunity for improving children's education and understanding. They could also support each other with 'chatrooms', although caution with general chatrooms has been emphasized recently because of potential contact with paedophiles.

Several large companies active in the renal field appear to have supported the development of websites as well as major research organizations, who have used the opportunity to advertise their needs for research funding. One's impression is that, as with the production of booklets, a great deal of time and effort is required to put good information on the Internet. Only time will tell if the initial effort has been sustained. The hope is also that the world-wide web will improve the information flow to poorer countries, and hence improve health, but this remains a big disappointment at present [30].

Conclusions

The information needs of children and their parents necessitates a strategy involving all members of the multiprofessional team and is an essential component of the treatment partnership. Information has to be individualized for each child and family, taking into account the socio-economic and cultural aspects that impact upon information giving. Information needs to be updated as the child grows, the clinical condition changes, and new information becomes available. As well as the child and family, there is a need to impart information to extended family members, schoolteachers, and other professionals involved in the child's care.

There are a number of modalities which can be employed to impart information, and all require time and effort. The Internet will spread only confusion if the nephrology community does not ensure that quality information is available. Feedback from families about their information needs should be sought and further research conducted into this important aspect of care.

Acknowledgements

I thank Alison Cargill for the parent survey and Judith Hayes for typing this manuscript.

References

1. Watson AR. Strategies to support families of children with end-stage renal failure. *Pediatr Nephrol* 1995, 9; 628–631.
2. Lewis CC, Pantell RH and Sharp L. Increasing patient knowledge, satisfaction and involvement. Randomised trial of a communication intervention. *Pediatrics* 1991, 88(2); 351–358.
3. Van Stuijvenberg, M, Suur MH, de Vos S, Tjiang GCH, Steyerberg EW, Derksen-Lubsen G and Moll HA. Informed consent, parental awareness and reasons for participating in a randomised controlled study. *Arch Dis Child* 1998, 79; 120–125.
4. Sharp MC, Strauss RP and Lorch SC. Communicating medical bad news: Parents' experiences and preferences. *J Pediatr* 1992, 121(4); 539–546.
5. Street RL. Communication styles and adaptations in physician-patient consultations. *Soc Sci Med* 1992, 34(10); 1155–1163.
6. Street RL. Information-giving in medical consultations: The influence of patients' communicative styles and personal characteristics. *Soc Sci Med* 1991, 32(5); 541–548.
7. Collier J, MacKinlay D and Watson AR. Painful procedures: preparation and coping strategies for children. *Matern Child Health* 1993, 18; 282–286.
8. Turner S, Maher EJ, Young T, Young J, Vaughan Hudson G. What are the information priorities for cancer patients involved in treatment decisions? An experienced surrogate study in Hodgkin's disease. *Br J Cancer* 1996, 73; 222–227.
9. Holmes-Rovner M, Llewellyn-Thomas H, Entwistle V, Coulter A, O'Connor A and Rovner DR. Patient choice modules for summaries of clinical effectiveness: a proposal. *BMJ* 2001, 322; 664–667.
10. Binik YM, Devins GM, Barre PE, Guttmann RD, Hollomby DJ, Mandin H, Paul LC, Hons RB and Burgess ED. Live and learn: patient education delays the need to initiate renal replacement therapy in end stage renal disease. *J Nerv Ment Dis* 1993, 181(6); 371–376.
11. Gomez CG, Valido P, Celadilla O, Bernaldo de Quiros AG, and Mojon M. Validity of a standard information protocol provided to end stage renal disease patients and its effect on treatment selection. *PDI* 1999, 19(5); 471–477.
12. Campbell A. Improvement of patient care through a collaborative approach to patient education and triage. *Adv Renal Replacement Therapy* 1999, 6(4); 347–360.
13. Beadles E, Stephenson R and Watson AR. Kidney failure at school. *Family Medicine* 1997, 1(3); 19–20.
14. Ley P. Communicating with patients: improving communication, satisfaction and compliance. Chapman and Hall, London, 1988.
15. Perlman NM, Freedman JL, Abramovitch R, Whyte H, Kirplani H and Perlman M. Information needs of parents with sick neonates. *Pediatrics* 1991, 88(3); 512–517.
16. Weichler NK. Caretakers' informational needs after their children's renal or liver transplant. *ANNA J* 1993, 20(2); 135–146.
17. Weichler NK. Information needs of mothers of children who have had liver transplants. *J Ped Nurs* 1990, 75(2); 88–96.
18. Reynolds JM, Garralda ME, Jameson RA and Postlethwaite RJ. How parents and families cope with chronic renal failure. *Arch Dis Child* 1988, 63; 821–826.
19. Moore EA, Collier J, Evans JHC and Watson AR. The need to know: Information needs of parents with children with nephrotic syndrome. *Child Health* 1994; 2(4); 147–149.
20. Collier J, Pattison H, Watson AR and Sheard C. Parental information needs in chronic renal failure and diabetes mellitus. *Eur J Pediatr* 2001, 160(1); 31–36.
21. Garralda ME, Jameson RA, Reynolds JM and Postlethwaite RJ. Psychiatric adjustment in children with chronic renal failure. *J Child Psychol Psychiatry* 1988, 29; 79–90.

22. Henley LD and Hill ID. Global and specific information needs of cystic fibrosis patients and their families. *Pediatrics* 1990, 85(6); 1015–1021.

23. Rylance G. Should audio recordings of outpatient consultations be presented to patients? *Arch Dis Child* 1992, 67; 622–624.

24. Moore EA, Gartland C and Watson AR. The role of the community paediatric renal nurse (CPRN). *Br J Renal Med* 1996, 1; 8–9.

25. Wright E, Gartland C and Watson AR. An update programme for children on home peritoneal dialysis. *EDTNA/ERCA Journal* 1995, 3; 25–27.

26. Moore EA and Watson AR. Home update programme following renal transplantation. *Dial Transpl* 1999, 28(8); 465–467.

27. Argles J, MacKinlay DRE, Middleton D and Watson AR. The parents' support group: support for families attending a paediatric renal unit. *Mat Child Health* 1994, 19(5); 152–158.

28. Watson AR. Home health and respite care. *Perit Dial Int* 1996, 16; S551–S553.

29. Austin J. Leveraging the internet for better patient education. *Dial Transplant* 2000, 333–341.

30. Editorial. Global information flow. *BMJ* 2000, 321; 776–777.

Appendix 1: Sources for booklets and leaflets (a more comprehensive international list is available from author)

1. Children and Young People's Kidney Unit, City Hospital, Nottingham NG5 1PB, UK

- Childhood Nephrotic Syndrome (also available in Urdu, Arabic, Greek)
- Nephrotic Syndrome Package (including video)
- Painful Procedures Package (including video)
- Your Child and Chronic Renal Failure
- Kidney Transplantation in Childhood
- Children with Recurrent UTI
- Bertie Button (gastrostomy feeding)
- Dietary Advice for Children on Dialysis
- Colin Has Constipation

Other booklets

- Graham has a GFR
- Sharon has a Very Important Test (MCUG)
- Darren has a Very Important Test (MCUG)
- Rebecca has a Renal Biopsy
- Arnold has an Ultrasound
- Arnold goes for a DMSA Scan
- Mary has a MAG 3 Scan
- Why Annie Needs a Blood Test
- Brian has Bladder Pressure Studies

- Reimplantation of Ureters
- Your Child is Having a Nephrectomy
- Your Child is Having a Pyeloplasty
- Haemolytic Uraemic Syndrome
- Multicystic Dysplastic Kidney Disease
- Kidney and Bladder Problems Detected Before Birth by Ultrasound
- Urinary Tract Infection in Children
- A Guide to the Management of Childhood Nephritis

2. Kidney Foundation of Canada, 300–5165 Sherbrooke Street West, Montreal QC, Canada H4A 1T6

Booklets available in English and French

- Your Child and Chronic Renal Failure. An Introductory Guide for Families
- Kidney Transplantation
- Urinary Tract Infections
- Hemodialysis
- Patient Services—Because We Care
- Childhood Nephrotic Syndrome
- Organ Donation—Have You Thought About It?

3. National Kidney Foundation of America, 30 East 33rd Street, New York, NY 10016, USA

- Alport Syndrome Information Package
- Hemolytic Uremic Syndrome—Information Packet

- Childhood Nephrotic Syndrome—Information Packet
- Professional and Patient Education Publications List
- Financing Transplantation: What Every Patient Needs to Know
- Questions and Answers About Organ Transplantation
- Urinary Tract Infections
- When Bedwetting Becomes a Problem

4. American Kidney Fund, 6110 Executive Boulevard, Suite 1010, Rockville, MD 20852, USA

- Children and Kidney Disease
- Kidneys for Kids
- The Kid
- Caring for Children with Primary Vesicoureteral Reflux—A Guide for Parents and Others

5. Renal Resource Centre, 37 Darling Point Road, Darling Point, NSW 2027, Australia

- Urinary Reflux—Information for Parents
- Nephrotic Syndrome in Children

6. Australian Kidney Foundation, 82 Melbourne Street, North Adelaide, South Australia 5006

- Finding Kidney Problems Before your Baby is Born
- Let's Talk About Kidney Problems in Children
- Let's Talk About Blood in the Urine

7. National Kidney Research Fund, Kings Chambers, Priestgate, Peterborough PE1 1FG, UK

- What I Tell Parents About Childhood Nephrotic Syndrome

- What I Tell My Patients About Alport's Syndrome
- What I Tell My Patients About Adult Polycystic Kidney Disease
- What I Tell my Patients About IgA Nephropathy
- What I Tell Parents About UTIs and Reflux in Children
- What I Tell Parents About HUS Syndrome
- What I Tell Families about Kidney and Bladder Problems Detected before Birth
- What I Tell Families about Renal Biopsy in Children

Appendix 2: Internet sites

Internet sites to consider include:

- www.nkrf.org.uk (National Kidney Research Fund, UK)
  - email helpline (helpline@nkrf.org.uk)
  - booklets on 'What I tell my patients about…'
  - books on 'Kidney Failure Explained' and 'Kidney Failure The Facts'
  - includes patient histories
  - the website is also useful for those who are interested in the kidney research that is being sponsored by the charity.

- www.kidney.org (National Kidney Foundation, USA)
  - very good A–Z guide of kidney terms
  - long list of publications including on-line patient fact sheets about a variety of predominantly adult renal diseases.

- www.renal.org (Renal Association, UK)
  - not much practical information for patients
  - good list of nephrology internet sites and resources.

- www.nephronline.org (UK: unrestricted grant from pharmaceutical company)
  - large glossary of terms
  - list of dialysis units and holiday dialysis facilities
  - good diagrams of kidneys but not much explanation as yet.

- www.renalweb.com (commercially sponsored)
  - heavy with adverts
  - lots of links to other sites, chat rooms, discussion groups and fast food tips.

- www.renalnet.org
  - the kidney information clearing house offering valuable information for both professional and consumer
  - wordsearch facility.

- www.healthfinder.gov (US Dept of Health and Human Services)
  - helps consumers find reliable health information that can help them stay healthy, understand diagnoses, explore treatment options, find support and generally become more informed about health and medical topics
  - publishes a list of questions that consumers can ask to decide if a website is trustworthy.

- www.niddk.nih.gov (National Institute of Diabetes and Digestive and Kidney Diseases, US)
  - offers a number of publications on line
  - has a large kidney disease dictionary index.

- www.cochraneconsumer.com (UK)
  - the Cochrane database 'used to help people make well informed decisions about health care'
  - limited nephrology information to date.

- www.kidneydirections.com (US; dialysis company sponsored)
  - there is a 'kids' section with paediatric nephrology input
  - e-mail lists for 'kids' to exchange
  - list of summer camps
  - virtual tours of hospitals
  - links to a number of other websites such as nephrotic parents support group, 'nephrology kids' cyber support group and stories about patients
  - available in Japanese and Spanish.

- www.kidneywise.com (UK; dialysis company sponsored)
  - similar to above with 'wise kids club'
  - little development at time of writing of 'wise kids club', but useful links to other sites.

- http://cnserver0.nkf.med.ualberta.ca/nephkids (Nephkids cyber support group, Canada)
  - interactive email group if parents of children with chronic renal disease of all varieties.

- www.ikidney.com (iKidney corner, US)
  - useful lists of summer camps in USA
  - pen pals.

- www.enuresis.org.uk (Enuresis Resource and Information Centre, UK)
  - much useful information about enuresis
  - information for teenagers
  - literature and products.

Appendix 3: Parent support organizations

- ERIC (Enuresis Resource and Information Centre, 34 Old School House, Britannia Road, Kingswood, Bristol BS15 2DB, UK) is a national organization involved in support for families with incontinence problems, particularly nocturnal enuresis.

- If children have renal failure in association with other syndromes or genetic conditions, national directories or genetic departments will provide information about support groups which often hold national and international meetings, e.g. Cystinosis Foundation, 174 Corwen Road, Tilehurst, Reading RG30 4TA, UK; March of Dimes Birth Defects Foundation, 1275 Mamaroneck Avenue, White Plains, NY 10605, USA.

- Many countries have national kidney patient associations which provide much support to families and nephrology units. As well as responding to numerous enquiries over the years they have also been a major source for the development of information materials.
  - British Kidney Patient Association, Bordon, Hants GU35 9JZ, UK
  - National Kidney Foundation, 30 East 33rd Street, New York, NY 10016, USA
  - Kidney Foundation of Canada, 300–5165 Sherbrooke Street West, Montreal QC, H4 1T6, Canada
  - National Kidney Federation, 6 Stanley Street, Worksop, Notts S81 7HX, UK

26 | Practical guidelines for drug prescribing in children with renal disease: preventing nephrotoxicity and adjusting doses in renal impairment

Imti Choonara and Richard S. Trompeter

Introduction

The use of drugs in patients with renal disease may be a source of some considerable confusion. Nephrotoxic drugs may induce renal dysfunction in the child with normal kidneys and this adverse effect is compounded in the child with pre-existing renal impairment of any degree. The presence of renal impairment will result in the reduced clearance of a number of drugs which rely on the kidney for their excretion. Here, dosage alteration is necessary to protect the child from overexposure to the drug, with the attendant risk of increased renal and non-renal side-effects. The purpose of this chapter is to provide the reader with an introduction to the basic principles of clinical pharmacology and to discuss the use of therapeutic drug monitoring in paediatric patients. The chapter will go on to discuss the prevention of nephrotoxicity in a variety of patient groups and finally discuss prescribing in varying degrees of renal impairment.

Introduction to clinical pharmacology

Pharmacokinetics

Clinical pharmacokinetics is the quantitative study of the relationship between a drug dosage regimen and the concentration profile over time. There are a number of parameters that control these relationships and these need to be understood if one is to understand pharmacokinetics at a basic level. Individuals who wish to have a more detailed understanding of clinical pharmacokinetics should refer to the excellent review by Thomson [1].

Bioavailability

The bioavailability of a drug is the proportion of the dose administered that enters the systemic circulation. Conventionally, this is determined by comparing the area under the concentration–time curve following oral (or other non-parenteral) administration of the drug with the value obtained after intravenous administration. A number of factors influence bioavailability, including individual drug characteristics, local factors including gut motility and blood supply, and the extent of first-pass metabolism in the gastrointestinal mucosa or liver. This may be of great clinical significance. Cyclosporin A, a calcineurin inhibitor used extensively in renal transplantation, undergoes some first-pass metabolism, a process which may be significantly inhibited by the patient drinking or eating grapefruit-containing products or other drugs (see below).

Volume of distribution

The volume of distribution does not represent a physiological volume but an apparent volume into which the drug would have to distribute to achieve the measured concentration. The volume of distribution is therefore determined by the ratio of plasma to tissue binding and by how much of the total amount of drug in the body is outside of the sampling compartment. Lipid and water solubility may be important. Gentamicin, which is water soluble, has a volume of distribution that approximates to the extracellular fluid volume; whereas the volume of distribution of chloroquine, which is widely distributed throughout the body, is much higher.

Knowledge about volume of distribution can be applied to determine the loading dose of a drug required to reach a target concentration. The loading dose can be calculated by multiplying the volume of distribution by the target concentration. For example, the gentamicin dose required to achieve a peak gentamicin concentration of 10 mg/l in a neonate weighing 1 kg would be 10 mg/l × 0.5 l/kg (the volume of distribution of gentamicin in a neonate) × 1 kg. This equals 5 mg [1].

Clearance

Clearance represents the irreversible removal of a drug from the body and is usually expressed in relation to volume divided by time. It can be defined as the volume of fluid (most frequently plasma) that is completely cleared of a drug per unit time. Therefore if the plasma clearance is 10 ml/min, then this means that 10 ml of plasma is completely cleared of the drug in a period of 1 minute. In children, one usually describes plasma clearance in relation to body weight or surface area, i.e. ml/min/kg or ml/min/m². A drug may be cleared by hepatic and/or gut wall metabolism, renal excretion, or a combination of both of these mechanisms.

Elimination half-life

This is the pharmacokinetic parameter most commonly quoted by clinicians. The elimination half-life is the time taken for 50% of the drug to be eliminated. For most drugs, the rate of elimination is proportional to the amount of drug present. This means that the elimination half-life is constant and is not dependent upon the amount of drug in the body, i.e. if the elimination half-life is 4 hours and 100% of the drug is present at time 0, at times 4, 8, and 12 hours, 50%, 25%, and 12.5% of the drug, respectively, will be present. After seven half-lives, 97% of the drug will be eliminated. Similarly, when a new drug is commenced, after five half-lives the concentration of the drug in the body will be 97% of that achieved at steady state. This is assuming that dosing remains constant.

The elimination half-life is dependent upon two parameters, clearance and volume of distribution. Clearance and the elimination half-life are inversely related to each other: as clearance increases, the half-life decreases.

Key points: Clinical pharmacokinetics, definitions

- Volume of distribution: the apparent volume into which the drug has distributed to produce the measured concentration.

- Clearance: volume of fluid (usually plasma) completely cleared of drug per unit time.

- Elimination half-life: the time taken for 50% of the drug to be eliminated.

Pharmacodynamics

The study of pharmacodynamics is the study of the effect of a drug. This may be considerably more difficult to assess in children than in adults. If one wished to study the pharmacodynamic effect of an antihypertensive agent, then this would be relatively easy, assuming one had an appropriately sized blood-pressure cuff. If, however, one wished to study the pharmacodynamic effect of an analgesic drug, then one would need to use a validated pain tool appropriate for the child's age and the type of pain they were experiencing.

Therapeutic drug monitoring

Therapeutic drug monitoring (TDM) can be defined as the use of drug measurements in body fluids as an aid to the management of patients receiving drug therapy for cure, and alleviation or prevention of disease [2]. For certain drugs, the desired or toxic effect cannot always be assessed clinically and is related to the amount of drug in the body and thus controlled only by limiting the quantity of drug administered. This is achieved by defining a standard dose, which will produce a satisfactory response in the majority of patients. However, for many drugs, the primary determinant of clinical response is the correlation which can be achieved at the site of action, i.e. the cell receptor, or site of infection [3].

Frequently, wide variations in drug concentration above a minimum or 'threshold' level will make little difference to clinical effect, but for some drugs the desired, and possibly unwanted, effects may be very sensitive to the drug concentration at any given time. The characteristics of a drug that make it suitable for therapeutic drug monitoring are shown in Table 26.1. The number of drugs which fulfil these criteria is relatively small (Table 26.2), although a number will be of importance for patients with renal disease and their doctors.

Table 26.1   Therapeutic drug monitoring

If therapeutic drug monitoring is to be practical for a
  particular drug:
    Plasma drug concentrations must correlate
      well with effect
    Measurements made must give accurate information
      about the biological effect that is being obtained
    The close concentration–effect relationship requires
      minimal intraindividual pharmacodynamic variability
    No active unmeasured metabolites of the drug should
      contribute to the biological effect
    The drug must have a reversible mode of action
      at the receptor site

Table 26.2   Drugs for which therapeutic drug monitoring is of established value

Aminoglycoside antibiotics
Anticonvulsants: phenytoin, carbamazepine
Immunosuppressants: cyclosporin A, tacrolimus
Digoxin
Lithium
Theophylline
Methotrexate

To make effective use of any laboratory investigation, it is essential to be clear about the question being asked. This is particularly true of TDM, and a failure to define the indications for analysis diminishes the value of TDM (Table 26.3).

A single measurement is insufficient to determine why the plasma concentration is inadequate. A series of measurements will be required at appropriate time intervals or under supervised dosing if non-compliance is suspected. Other indications for TDM would include situations where pharmacokinetic parameters are changing rapidly, i.e. in the neonate and in children with deteriorating renal and/or hepatic dysfunction.

Table 26.3   Questions to which therapeutic drug monitoring can provide effective answers

Patient is not responding to therapy, could this be due to
  inadequate plasma concentration?
Why is the plasma/blood drug concentration inadequate?
    Inappropriate dosage?
    Poor compliance?
    Malabsorption?
    Rapid metabolism?
Could the patient's symptoms be caused by drug toxicity?

Preventing nephrotoxicity

Medication errors

Medication errors are an invariable part of drug prescribing. It is important to recognize that some medicines (e.g. aminoglycosides and cytotoxic agents) are more dangerous than others [4]. Tenfold errors are a particular problem in young children. The risk of such errors is significantly increased where ampoules contain adult amounts of drugs and it is possible to overdose a young infant with a single ampoule. The importance of the meticulous checking of the child's weight and the dose of the drug prescribed cannot be overstated. It is important to recognize that blaming individuals is often unhelpful in preventing medication errors. It is more important to look at the process of drug prescribing in a hospital and see whether safety checks can be introduced.

It is essential that following recognition of a medication error, that the parents and patient (dependent upon age) are informed. Parents and patients recognize that doctors and nurses are human and make mistakes. It is when the medical profession tries to conceal mistakes that relationships with parents break down.

Key points: Medication errors

- Medical and nursing staff should double-check the weight of the child, the dose required, and the medicine whenever any drug is administered.

- Be aware of the danger of tenfold errors in dose calculations.

Nephrotoxic drugs

The list of drugs that can induce nephrotoxicity includes many of the medicines that may be prescribed to children. It is worthwhile recognizing that the aminoglycosides and cytotoxic drugs have a low threshold for causing renal impairment. With the increased use of non-steroidal anti-inflammatory drugs in paediatric patients, particularly for the management of simple pyrexia, the paediatrician needs to recognize that these drugs also have the ability to cause renal impairment [5].

Nephrotoxicity in the sick neonate may be more difficult to detect, and one prospective study, which confirmed that aminoglycosides have a nephrotoxic effect in the newborn infant, failed to show any correlation between the nephrotoxic effect and serum gentamicin concentrations [6]. This is not an argument against therapeutic drug monitoring. It is, however, important to recognize that we do not fully understand the inter-relationships between serum drug concentrations and nephrotoxicity in all age groups.

Key points: Nephrotoxic drugs

- Many drugs have the potential for nephrotoxicity.

- Aminoglycosides and cytotoxic drugs are the drugs most likely to cause nephrotoxicity.

- Be aware of the potential of non-steroidal anti-inflammatory drugs to cause nephrotoxicity.

Patients at risk

The major route for drug excretion in postnatal life is the kidney, supplanting the placenta which performs this function during fetal life. Drug excretion is effected by three mechanisms: glomerular filtration, active tubular secretion, and passive tubular resorption. Factors contributing to the susceptibility of the kidney to drug toxicity are shown in Table 26.4 and the potential mechanisms for drug-induced renal dysfunction are shown in Table 26.5.

Table 26.4 Factors contributing to the susceptibility of the kidney to drug toxicity

Exposure to potentially harmful compounds, reflecting the magnitude of blood flow through glomerular and peritubular vessels
The concentration of toxic substances within the tubular lumen, predisposing to toxic accumulation within the renal tubular cell
Dependence of the tubular cell for function on a high metabolic rate, and transport systems for the concentration of pharmacological agents

Table 26.5 Potential mechanisms for drug-induced renal dysfunction

Alterations in renal perfusion and glomerular filtration
Tubular cell damage
Tubular obstruction

The neonate is at particular risk for drug-induced renal dysfunction, particularly if there has been a history of hypovolaemic or hypoxaemic episodes at any time in the antenatal or immediate postnatal period. Glomerular filtration rate (GFR) and tubular secretory capacity are markedly reduced prior to 34 weeks' gestation, increasing as a function of post-conceptual age. GFR corrected for body surface area reaches near adult values at 1–2 years of age. Alterations in body water compartment sizes will affect the volume of distribution of a drug. At term, the extracellular fluid volume (ECF) approximates to 40% of body weight, decreasing to approximately 25–30% by the age of 1 year. The clinical importance of this gradual reduction in the size of body water compartments with age is clear; when attempting to achieve comparable plasma concentrations of a drug distributing into the ECF, higher doses per kg body weight are prescribed in infants and children compared to adults.

Although the renal function of infants and children admitted to intensive care units may have been normal prior to their presenting illness, any multi-system dysfunction associated with such an illness may result in a degree of renal insufficiency requiring careful assessment and management, particularly when prescribing potentially nephrotoxic drugs. Similarly, renal function should be assessed in children prior to cardiopulmonary bypass surgery for correction of congenital heart anomalies or heart and heart–lung transplant surgery. Again, knowledge of pre-existing renal insufficiency will be helpful when having to prescribe potentially nephrotoxic drugs. It should be remembered that calculated GFRs derived using the Schwartz formula (see Chapter 28) might significantly overestimate the true GFR in the chronically ill child with a reduced muscle mass.

Children with malignant disease may present for management in two circumstances where there may be significant risk of the development of renal dysfunction. The first is that of tumour lysis syndrome, where care of fluid balance, correction of acidosis and hyperuricaemia are essential components of therapy [7]. The second is that associated with the administration of chemotherapeutic agents.

Prescribing in renal failure

The effect of renal failure on pharmacokinetics

Drugs are eliminated by either metabolic processes that occur within the liver or the gut wall or by renal excretion. Renal failure will not have a direct effect on drug metabolism but will significantly reduce the elimination of drugs that are excreted via the kidneys. This will result in a prolongation of the plasma half-life and a reduction in plasma clearance. Renal failure may alter the protein binding of drugs and this may affect the volume of distribution.

It is important to recognize that for some drugs, although renal failure does not affect drug metabolism, it may affect the elimination of metabolites of the parent drug. The importance of this is illustrated by drugs such as morphine, where the metabolite is active but is excreted via the kidneys. Renal failure, therefore, necessitates a reduction in the dose of morphine due to impaired elimination of the metabolites [8].

If a drug is excreted via the kidneys and renal function is impaired, it is logical to increase the interval between doses of the drug. Alternatively, one can reduce the dose. There are certain instances when one of these methods of dose modification may be preferable, e.g. where the action of the drug is dependent on a minimum peak concentration. Practical advice regarding dose and dosage interval modification for specific drugs is given in the section below.

Key points: Prescribing in renal failure

- The plasma half-life of drugs that are excreted via the kidneys will be increased in renal failure.

- Drug metabolism will not be directly affected by renal impairment.

- Dialysis may affect the clearance of the drug.

- Involve your local paediatric clinical pharmacist in discussions regarding individual patients.

Effect of dialysis on pharmacokinetics

Both peritoneal dialysis and haemodialysis may have a significant effect on the clearance of a drug. There are limited data available regarding the effects of either peritoneal dialysis or haemodialysis on the pharmacokinetics of many drugs [9,10]. It is important to recognize that the clearance of a drug by haemodialysis depends upon the properties of the apparatus as well the properties of the drug itself. The elimination of drugs with a large molecular weight may vary depending on the pore size of the membrane. Different dialysis membranes will therefore have different effects on drug concentrations [10].

Studies in adults have shown that patients with end stage renal disease have numerous problems with their medicines. Prospective studies have shown the value of clinical pharmacy input [11]. If your patient has renal impairment, then it would be advisable to contact your paediatric clinical pharmacist and ask for help.

Prescribing specific drugs in renal impairment

The following are provided as examples only. Other review articles are available [12]. Whenever medications are prescribed to children with renal impairment, it is essential that the prescribing doctor consults a specialist paediatric pharmacopoeia, which contains specific information about dose alterations in renal failure (e.g. Medicines for Children, Royal College of Paediatrics and Child Health). Where there is any doubt, expert opinion should be sought.

Aminoglycosides

The aminoglycoside antibiotics, gentamicin, tobramycin, and amikacin are commonly used antimicrobial agents associated with nephrotoxicity. The incidence of toxicity is variable but a significant rise in serum creatinine concentration is seen in approximately 10% of adults receiving a course of such treatment. The neonate is particularly susceptible to renal toxicity with this group of agents. The concomitant administration of another nephrotoxic antimicrobial agent such as amphotericin B and certain cephalosporins, ciclosporin A, and extracellular fluid volume depletion increases the overall risk of nephrotoxicity [13].

Aminoglycosides are primarily excreted by glomerular filtration, partially resorbed by the proximal tubule and then accumulated in lysosymes, which play a role in the development of phospholipid accumulation, thus forming electron-dense myeloid bodies. The initial functional abnormality in aminoglycoside toxicity is manifested as an increased loss of tubular enzymes in the urine followed by polyuria and a defect in urinary concentration. Finally, there is a decrease in GFR often associated with mild proteinuria. The renal failure is usually non-oliguric

in nature and associated with a marked increase in the fractional excretion of sodium.

Strategies for the prevention of aminoglycoside toxicity are shown in Table 26.6. In children with renal dysfunction, aminoglycoside dosing should be adjusted. As the GFR falls to levels between 10 and 50% of normal, the frequency of dosing with aminoglycosides should be reduced to a dose every 12 hours, and further reduced to a dose every 24 hours when GFR is less than 10% of normal.

β-Lactam antibiotics

The β-lactam antibiotics are related to the penicillins and are extracted from renal venous blood by the organic transport system. The original compounds, such as cephaloridine, are no longer used; ceftazidime and cefotaxime appear to cause little nephrotoxicity, with dosing alterations only necessary in patients with more severe renal failure. However, newer drugs such as meropenem, a carbapenem, are nephrotoxic and thus adjustments are necessary at less significant levels of reduced renal function (Table 26.7).

Amphotericin B

Amphotericin B is an antifungal agent and has the potential to cause a variety of renal injuries, primarily related to renal tubular toxicity. Nephrotoxicity is invariably predictable as GFR falls, and is usually reversible. The presence of a metabolic acidosis will indicate distal renal tubular dysfunction associated with salt wasting, hypomagnesaemia, and hypokalaemia. In addition to an ion-transport defect, amphotericin B may cause a vasopressin-resistant urinary concentrating defect. Sodium loading may therefore have a beneficial effect on preventing nephrotoxicity by maintaining intravascular volume expansion and reducing renal vasoconstriction. Dose reduction or

Table 26.6 Prevention of aminoglycoside toxicity

Careful dosing schedules—avoid prolonged and
  repeated courses
Blood level monitoring with target trough level (less than
  4 mg/l for amikacin; less than 2 mg/l for gentamicin)
Recognition of potentiation of nephrotoxicity, i.e.
  Amphotericin B
  Cephalosporins
  Ciclosporin A
  ECF volume contraction, especially with diuretic use
  Hypokalaemia
  Hyperphosphataemia

Table 26.7 Dosing schedule for β-lactam antibiotics with reduced renal function

	Creatinine clearance (ml/min/1.73 m²)				
	>50	25–50	10–25	5–10	<5
Cefotaxime[a]	N	N	N	N	$\frac{1}{2}$ dose same frequency
Ceftazidime[b]	N	N	Normal dose every 24 h	$\frac{1}{2}$ dose every 24 h	$\frac{1}{2}$ dose every 48 h
Meropenem[b]	N	Normal dose every 12 h	Normal dose every 24 h	$\frac{1}{2}$ dose every 24 h	$\frac{1}{2}$ dose every 24 h

N, Normal dose/kg body weight.
[a] Removed by peritoneal and haemodialysis.
[b] Removed by haemodialysis, dose administered immediately post haemodialysis.

liposomal amphotericin or lipid-associated amphotericin B should be used if the drug is suspected of causing deterioration in renal function.

Antiviral agents

Aciclovir and ganciclovir are antiviral agents effective against herpes viruses and cytomegalovirus. Aciclovir is probably excreted by both glomerular filtration and tubular secretion, 30–90% of the drug being excreted unchanged in the urine of healthy individuals. Neither drug is normally associated with causation of renal insufficiency or toxicity, except in the situation where the pre-treatment GFR is already reduced, and in the presence of ECF volume depletion, or with the concomitant administration of nephrotoxic agents. Recommendations for dose reductions in children with varying degrees of renal impairment are shown in Table 26.8.

Non-steroidal anti-inflammatory drugs

This group of drugs inhibits the enzyme fatty acid cyclooxygenase, thus decreasing the synthesis of prostaglandin from arachidonic acid. Synthesized in the kidney, prostaglandins are active in the renal cortex, i.e. modifying regional blood flow, GFR, and renin production; and in the medulla, regulating blood flow, tubular response to vasopressin, and tubular resorption of sodium chloride in the loop of Henle.

In states of normal health, non-steroidal anti-inflammatory drugs (NSAIDs) have little effect on renal function; however, in states of altered physiology such as volume depletion, congestive cardiac failure, and hypoalbuminaemia, acute renal failure may result from excessive vasoconstriction of the afferent arterioles.

NSAIDs may also produce a tubulo-interstitial nephritis characterized by a mononuclear cell infiltrate. Functional disturbances associated with this are usually reversible. Long-term use may cause papillary necrosis as well as chronic renal failure secondary to chronic ischaemia. Children receiving NSAID therapy, e.g. ibuprofen, for febrile illness are potentially at risk of nephrotoxicity in view of coexisting reduced fluid intake and increased insensible losses. NSAIDs should be used with great caution in children with renal impairment.

Chemotherapeutic agents

Cisplatin (*cis*-diaminedichloroplatinum II) is commonly used in the treatment of childhood malignancies, acting by inhibition of DNA synthesis. Its use is complicated by the fact that it is highly nephrotoxic, characterized by both acute and chronic renal failure and tubular dysfunction, i.e. magnesium, sodium, and potassium wasting. Polyuria is a common finding, with a fall in urine osmolality occurring within 24–48 hours of administration. Optimal saline hydration before, during, and after administration reduces the risk of renal toxicity. Dosage modification is essential in patients with reduced levels of GFR determined prior to treatment. A reduced GFR secondary to cisplatin injury may improve with long-term follow-up, although tubular defects may persist.

Ifosfamide is a structural isomer of cyclophosphamide used to treat a wide variety of solid tumours in children. The tumoricidal action is related to alkylation and inhibition of cell replication. Although alkylating agents are associated with haemorrhagic cystitis, myelosuppression, alopecia, and gastrointestinal symptoms, ifosfamide additionally has significant renal toxicity, inducing a tubulopathy with wasting of glucose, protein, amino acids, and phosphate, as well as decreased GFR. The incidence of nephrotoxicity is variable, dependent on cumulative dosing, rapidity of administration, and concomitant therapy, particularly with platinum-based compounds. The clinical pattern in most cases is one of a transient tubular wasting, although reduced GFR may persist. As for the use of all potentially nephrotoxic chemotherapeutic agents, knowledge of GFR pre-treatment is essential.

Table 26.8 Dosing schedule for aciclovir and ganciclovir with reduced renal function

	Creatinine clearance (ml/min/1.73m^2)			
	50–75	25–50	10–25	<10
Aciclovir (oral)	N	N	Normal dose every 8 h	Normal dose every 12 h
Aciclovir (i.v.)	N	Normal dose every 12 h	Normal dose every 24 h	$\frac{1}{2}$ dose every 24 h
Ganciclovir (i.v.)	$\frac{1}{2}$ dose every 12 h	$\frac{1}{2}$ dose every 24 h	$\frac{1}{4}$ dose every 24 h	$\frac{1}{2}$ dose every 24 h

Bladder toxicity results primarily from the metabolite acrolein, and mesna (sodium-2-mercaptoethine sulphonate) has been used to ameliorate both ifosfamide and cyclophosphamide bladder toxicity. Unfortunately this does not afford protection against tubular toxicity.

Ciclosporin A

Ciclosporin A is an immunosuppressive agent designed for use in post-transplant patients, although it is also routinely used for the treatment of idiopathic nephrotic syndrome and a variety of autoimmune diseases. Metabolism is by the hepatic and gut-wall cytochrome P450 system; thus the concomitant administration of compounds stimulating the P450 system results in increased clearance, and those inhibiting cytochrome P450 increase ciclosporin levels, thus potentiating toxicity. Drugs altering ciclosporin metabolism are shown in Table 26.9. It is clearly important that all doctors caring for children with renal and other solid organ transplants, including their general practitioners, are aware of these interactions. Metabolism may be age related, with infants and young children having faster metabolic clearance and a larger volume of distribution. Therefore, dose requirements may be relatively greater than in adults to achieve a comparable blood concentration [13].

Nephrotoxicity can be detected in the form of a proximal tubulopathy with impaired secretion of

urea and uric acid and reduced fractional excretion of sodium, potassium, and phosphate, and reduced bicarbonate reabsorption, leading to a hyperchloraemic metabolic acidosis. Toxicity is dose-related and the functional changes include vasoconstriction of the afferent arteriole with evidence of reducing GFR, rising plasma creatinine concentration, and hypertension. Monitoring ciclosporin A, using a 12-hour post-dose (trough) whole blood level to avoid overdosing and toxicity, is mandatory.

References

1. Thomson AH. Introduction to clinical pharmacokinetics. Paediatric and Perinatal Drug Therapy. 2000; 4:3–11.
2. Marks V. A historical introduction. In: Widdop B (ed). Therapeutic Drug Monitoring. 1985; Edinburgh: Churchill Livingstone: 3–15.
3. Hallworth M and Capps N. Theoretical considerations. In Therapeutic Drug Monitoring. 1993; London ACB Venture Publications: 1–28.
4. Choonara I How to harm children in hospital – A guide for junior doctors. Paediatric and Perinatal Drug Therapy. 1999; 3:34–35.
5. Bhangoo P, Choonara I Transient acute renal insufficiency following an overdose of ibuprofen. Journal of Pediatric Pharmacy Practice. 1998; 3:163–165.
6. Adelman RD, Wirth F, Rubio T A controlled study of the nephrotoxicity of mezlocillin and gentamicin plus ampicillin in the neonate. J Pediatr. 1987; 111: 888–893.
7. Jones DP, Mahmoud H, Chesney RN Tumour lysis syndrome: pathogenesis and management. Pediatr Nephrol. 1995; 9:206–212.
8. Chauvin M, Sandouk P, Scherrmann JM *et al.* Morphine pharmacokinetics in renal failure. Anesthesiology. 1987; 66:327–331.
9. Paton TW, Cornish WR, Manuel MA, Hardy BG Drug therapy in patients undergoing peritoneal dialysis. Clinical pharmacokinetic considerations. Clin Pharmacokinet. 1985; 10:404–425.
10. Reetze-Bonorden P, Bohler J, Keller E Drug dosage in patients during continuous renal replacement therapy. Pharmacokinetic and therapeutic considerations. 1993; Clin Pharmacokinet 24:362–379.
11. Tang I, Vrahnos D, Hatoum H, Lau A Effectiveness of clinical pharmacist interventions in a hemodialysis unit. Clinical Therapeutics. 1993; 15:459–464.
12. Trompeter RS A review of drug prescribing in children with end-stage renal failure. Pediatr Nephrol. 1987; 1:183–194.
13. Mendoza SA Nephrotoxic drugs. Paediatr Nephrol. 1988; 2:466–476.

Table 26.9 Drugs affecting ciclosporin metabolism

Increase ciclosporin level	Decrease ciclosporin level	Increase nephrotoxicity
Chloroquine	Carbamazepine	Acyclovir
Cimetidine	Methylprednisolone	Aminoglycosides
Colchicine	Octriotide	Amphotericin B
Diltiazem	Phenobarbitone	Ciprofloxacin
Doxycycline	Phenytoin	Cotrimoxazole
Erythromycin	Rifampicin	Melphalan
Fluconazole	St John's wort[a]	Methotrexate
Ketoconazole		NSAIDs
Metoclopramide		Trimethoprim
Methyl prednisolone (high dose)		
Nicardipine		
Progestogens		
Verapamil		

[a] Emphasizing the importance of discussing whether the patient is taking herbal and homeopathic medications.

27 | Paediatric nephrology in developing countries

Rasheed Gbadegesin and Rajendra Srivastava

Introduction

Developing countries contain 75% of the world's population, Asia accounting for 57%. Most of these are in different stages of development. Whilst some have made remarkable progress over the past two or three decades, a majority share a low per capita income, rapidly increasing population and high mortality rates. Political instability and natural and man-made calamities are important in many countries. Educational and health facilities are poor, having received a low priority. As a consequence, the majority of the population remains uneducated and has poor access to information. The standards of sanitation and hygiene are low and safe water is largely unavailable. The prevalence of preventable and infectious diseases, which are the major cause of morbidity and mortality, is high. Malnutrition in children is common. National health efforts are mostly utilized on provision of primary healthcare and preventive programmes, although in many countries the governments support medical education and teaching hospitals, which provide free medical care, and research. Vast differences often exist in the availability of medical care between urban and rural areas. Most large cities have modern hospitals, many comparable to those in developed countries, whilst basic medical care may be difficult to obtain in villages. Qualified doctors and specialists chiefly work in cities. Practitioners of indigenous systems of medicine and even quacks attend to large segments of the population.

Although paediatrics as a discipline is well developed in most developing countries, paediatric specialities remain confined to a few tertiary centres. This is in contrast to specialities of internal medicine, which are very well established at medical colleges and a number of excellent hospitals in the private sector. In recent years neonatology has gained wide acceptance. The number of well-trained paediatric nephrologists in developing countries remains very small (none in many small countries) and there are only a few centres that undertake chronic dialysis and renal transplantation. Children with renal disorders are often managed by general paediatricians and adult nephrologists.

Spectrum of renal diseases

Renal registries are well established in developed countries. These registries provide high-quality data on disease patterns in the community, thus allowing planning and allocation of resources. Unfortunately, registries are not available in most developing countries and the nephrologist often has to rely on published data from large hospitals. The disadvantage of this approach is that data from these sources are often incomplete, because not all renal cases are managed in these hospitals. There are, additionally, problems with case ascertainment because of poor diagnostic facilities; thus data from these sources should be interpreted with caution. Furthermore, regional differences also occur within large countries.

The prevalence of renal diseases is much greater, since many are related to preventable conditions, mostly eradicated from developed countries. Thus, post-infectious glomerulonephritis, hepatitis B nephropathy, *Plasmodium malariae* nephropathy, acute renal failure due to acute gastroenteritis, leptospirosis, falciparum malaria, snake-bite and other envenomations, and post-dysenteric haemolytic uraemic syndrome are quite frequent in different countries. Furthermore, the problem is compounded by delayed detection, inadequate initial management, and late referral of patients, which are responsible for a large number of hospital admissions and high mortality. In recent years, neonatal renal disorders have assumed increasing importance since newborn care units have become widely established

Table 27.1 Spectrum of renal diseases in 2266 Nigerian Children [1–4]

Diagnosis	n	%
Nephrotic syndrome	704	31.1
Acute glomerulonephritis	576	25.4
UTI	573	25.3
ARF and CRF	143	6.3
Wilms' tumour	69	3.0
Obstructive uropathies and other malformations	59	2.6
Haemolytic uraemic syndrome	3	0.1
Others	139	6.2
Total	2266	100

UTI, Urinary tract infection; ARF, acute renal failure; CRF, chronic renal failure.

and many of these are managing very sick and low birthweight babies.

Table 27.1 is a summary of the spectrum of renal disease from a study based on four hospitals in different parts of Nigeria [1–4]. Nephrotic syndrome, acute glomerulonephritis (AGN), and urinary tract infection (UTI) constitute more than 75% of cases seen in these series. This pattern is similar to reports from other developing countries [5,6]. In a report from Brazil, UTI, nephrotic syndrome, haematuria, and AGN were reported to be the common renal diseases seen in children, while in black South African children, AGN was reported to be responsible for one-third of all renal cases seen in hospital. When these data are compared with those from developed countries, what stands out prominently is the fact that vesico-ureteric reflux (VUR) and renal dysplasia are not very common. It is difficult to know what the contribution of underdiagnosis is to this, but there are studies from the developed world to suggest that VUR is uncommon in children of African origin. Haemolytic uraemic syndrome was uncommon in these studies, but recently large numbers of cases have been observed in Zimbabwe and South Africa [7]. The high prevalence of infection-related renal disease is a reflection of the general high incidence of infectious disease in the community and prevailing low standard of living. The impact of the HIV epidemic on the incidence and pattern of renal disease in developing countries has not been studied systematically, but limited data from West Africa showed that up to 27% of HIV patients may have renal involvement [8].

The pattern and behaviour of various paediatric renal disorders in Asian countries is by and large similar to that in developed countries. In addition, certain conditions are more prevalent in different regions.

Paediatric nephrology services are better established in Latin America as compared to many other areas of the developing world and the pattern of renal diseases is largely similar to that of developed countries. One exception is *haemolytic uraemic syndrome*, which is particularly common in Argentina, where it is the most important cause of acute renal failure (see later).

Key points: General issues

- Absence of registry data and selective referral to hospital means that the picture is biased and incomplete.

- There are major regional differences even within countries.

- The prevalence of renal disease is much higher because of the incidence of preventable and infectious diseases.

- Vesico-ureteric reflux is uncommon in African black children.

Nephrotic syndrome

Nephrotic syndrome is the most common disease encountered in children in many developing countries. There is variability in the incidence of minimal change disease (MCD) and steroid-sensitive nephrotic syndrome (SSNS), with a low incidence among black Africans [9–12], but an incidence among Asians and Arabs similar to that seen in Western countries. Infectious agents are prominent as trigger factors [10–15]. The incidence of nephrotic syndrome, mostly minimal change, steroid–responsive type, may be higher in the Indian subcontinent. A clinicopathological study of children with nephrotic syndrome carried out in Delhi in the early 1970s disclosed a pattern of renal histological abnormalities that was remarkably similar to that published by the International Study of Kidney Disease in Children (ISKDC) [16]. A wider experience with non-referred cases indicates the proportion of steroid-responsive cases (presumably minimal change type) to be about 90%. Studies from Nigeria have reported a high

Table 27.2 Comparison of histology of childhood nephrotic syndrome from different parts of Africa with the ISKDC data [9–12,16]

Histology	ISKDC (n = 234) (%)	Nigeria (n =521) (%)	South Africa	
			Non-Black (n = 202) (%)	Black (n = 246) (%)
Minimal change disease	76.4	8.9	55.3	13.7
Membranoproliferative glomerulonephritis	7.5	22.8	3.7	5.1
Focal segmental glomerulosclerosis	6.9	2.5	28.0	28.6
Membranous glomerulonephritis	1.5	3.0	5.3	40.2
Mesangioproliferative glomerulonephritis	2.3	2.5	3.7	7.3
Proliferative glomerulonephritis	2.3	10.4	0.0	0.0
Quartan malarial nephropathy	0.0	35.1	0.0	0.0
Others	3.1	14.9	4.0	5.1

incidence of quartan malarial nephropathy (see below and Table 27.2) [9,10,12].

Steroid-sensitive nephrotic syndrome

The proportion of those with frequent relapses and steroid dependence in the Indian subcontinent seems to be high, but the final outcome is satisfactory and most patients are permanently cured. The incidence of serious infections in nephrotic syndrome is high because of delayed and inadequate treatment of relapses. Even with good supportive care, the mortality is significant in such patients. Tuberculosis is a problem in some regions. It is a standard practice to screen the patient for the presence of tuberculosis before starting corticosteroids, and to exclude that condition during subsequent management.

The patients with nephrotic syndrome are managed according to standard recommendations. However, ciclosporin is used as a last resort, in view of its cost and difficulty of monitoring its blood levels. Most patients appear to enter permanent remission in the first half of the second decade of life, and only in occasional instances do relapses continue into the third decade.

In Asia, non-minimal renal histological lesions constitute about 5–10% of nephrotic syndrome in children. The pattern and response of such patients is not different from that reported from developed countries.

Steroid-resistant nephrotic syndrome

In India, there is an impression that the incidence of focal segmental glomerulosclerosis may be increasing.

Several centres have treated such patients with aggressive immunosuppressive regimens, with short-term benefits in a significant proportion of cases. Patients with moderate to severe mesangial proliferative lesions do not appear to respond to any form of specific therapy and a majority have a progressive course. In India, most children with membranoproliferative glomerulonephritis do not have an identified aetiology. The usual therapy consists of long-term alternate-day prednisolone and control of hypertension.

The underlying renal histological features, response to corticosteroids and the long-term outcome in African black children are, however, quite different from those in Arab children and children of Asian origin. Minimal change, steroid-responsive nephrotic syndrome is very uncommon in Nigerian children (8.9%) and South African black children (13.7%), and there is a high incidence of steroid-resistant nephrotic syndrome [10–12]. Twenty-two per cent of children with nephrotic syndrome in Nigeria had membranoproliferative glomerulonephrits (MPGN); such a high incidence of MPGN has not been found in other countries. Focal segmental glomerulosclerosis (FSGS) was identified in only 2.5% of Nigerian children but in 28% of children in South Africa, in black as well as non-black children. Such regional differences are difficult to explain. However, it is likely that seemingly similar histological lesions may involve different genetic as well as environmental aetiological factors in various population groups.

Secondary nephrotic syndrome

In Asia, secondary causes of nephrotic syndrome constitute less than 5% of all cases. Both lupus nephritis and hepatitis B-induced membranous nephropathy are more common in East Asian countries. The latter condition has a benign long-term course.

Quartan malarial nephropathy

A large proportion of children with nephrotic syndrome in Nigeria and Uganda have underlying renal histological lesions ascribed to *Plasmodium malariae* infection. The light-microscopic abnormalities consist of thickening of the glomerular capillary wall, mainly involving the subendothelial aspect of the basement membrane. Mesangial cellular proliferation is usually absent. Immunofluorescence examination shows deposits of IgG, IgM and C3 along the capillary walls. *Plasmodium malariae* antigen has been detected in these deposits in about 30% of cases. Electron microscopy shows fusion of foot processes, thickening of capillary basement membrane, and small lacunae scattered throughout the basement membrane. This form of nephrotic syndrome is resistant to corticosteroids and immunosuppressive drugs. The clinical course is characterized by progressive deterioration of renal function, with most patients developing ESRD within 5–10 years of initial presentation. The peculiar prevalence of nephrotic syndrome due to quartan malarial nephropathy apparently confined to Nigeria and Uganda is difficult to explain. It has been suggested that other infective agents may also be involved.

Hepatitis B nephropathy

Studies from South Africa report a very high incidence of hepatitis B nephropathy in black children. The underlying renal histological lesion is mostly membranous nephropathy. Patients often manifest a severe nephrotic state, since heavy proteinuria occurs against a background of malnutrition. They are not treated with corticosteroids and only supportive management is provided. The long-term prognosis of hepatitis B-associated membranous nephropathy is good, with a cumulative probability of remission of 64% at 4 years and 84% at 10 years, with very few developing chronic renal failure [11].

Congenital syphilis

Congenital syphilis as a cause of congenital nephrotic syndrome has been observed frequently in South Africa. The disorder responds to penicillin.

HIV-associated nephropathy

The incidence of HIV infection is very high in adults in many African countries. Children become infected by vertical transmission. Despite this, HIV nephropathy is mainly seen in older children: the survival of HIV-infected children in Africa is generally very poor.

Key points: Nephrotic syndrome

- The incidence of steroid-sensitive nephrotic syndrome (SSNS) is low in black Africans but similar to that seen in Western countries among Asians and Arabs.

- It is standard practice to screen the patient for the presence of tuberculosis before starting corticosteroids and to exclude that condition during subsequent management.

- The incidence of serious infections is high because of delayed and inadequate treatment of relapses.

- The incidence of focal segmental glomerulosclerosis may be increasing.

- Lupus nephritis and hepatitis B-induced membranous nephropathy are more common in East Asian countries.

- Hepatitis B nephropathy is also common in black South Africans.

- A large proportion of children with nephrotic syndrome in Nigeria and Uganda have an underlying renal histological lesion ascribed to *Plasmodium malariae* infection.

- Congenital syphilis and HIV-associated nephropathy are other important causes of nephrotic syndrome.

Post-streptococcal acute glomerulonephritis

The incidence of post-streptococcal acute glomerulonephritis (PSAGN) has been declining in many countries, although the disease is still common in China, southern India, Thailand, Mexico, Nigeria, and South Africa. In one study, it was responsible for 2.5–10.7/1000 hospital admissions [5]. It was frequently seen at referral hospitals in Delhi, India until the mid-1980s. The antecedent infections were pharyngitis and pyoderma in almost equal proportions, but in south India pyoderma was much more common. A report from South Africa showed that history of pyoderma was very prominent in black children, and a study from different parts of Nigeria showed that 45–79% of children with PSAGN had antecedent pyoderma or infected scabies [1,3,5].

The clinical features and indications for renal biopsy are similar to those in the developed world (see Chapter 20). It is usually a self-limiting disease but rarely may require dialysis, and there is 1–2% mortality in the acute stages from left ventricular failure and hypertensive encephalopathy, otherwise complete recovery is the rule. A large proportion of those requiring prolonged dialysis are those with rapidly progressive glomerulonephritis (RPGN), who will eventually develop chronic renal failure. Although there are no long-term follow-up studies from developing countries, studies from other parts of the world suggest that progressive renal damage is uncommon [17–19].

Acute nephritic syndrome

With the falling incidence of PSAGN, several uncommon conditions are detected in patients with one or more features of acute glomerulonephritis, whilst other characteristic features of the individual disorder may be initially absent or mild. Some of these include renal vasculitis, most commonly Henoch–Schönlein purpura, lupus nephritis, IgA nephropathy, infections such as bacterial endocarditis and infected shunts and prostheses. IgA nephropathy is more common in East Asian countries.

Renal vasculitis

The incidence of various renal vasculitic disorders appears to be lower in the Indian subcontinent, as indicated by experience at referral centres. However, the pattern and the clinical course is similar to that observed in developed countries. The only exception is Takayasu's disease, which is an important cause of renovascular hypertension in children in the Indian subcontinent, Thailand, and some other countries. Takayasu's disease chiefly affects the aorta and the proximal parts of its major branches. Involvement of descending aorta and renal arteries is common and responsible for hypertension. All three layers of the vessel wall initially show inflammatory lesions, which eventually result in fibrosis and narrowing or occlusion of the lumen. Involvement of the aortic arch and carotid vessels leads to absence of radial pulses.

The early phase of the disease, characterized by fever, cough, weight loss, joint pains, and anaemia, often goes unrecognized. The incidence of tuberculosis is higher in these patients and it has been suggested that an abnormal response to some tubercular antigen may be causally related. Tubercle bacilli or characteristic granuloma have not been demonstrated in the vasculitic lesions. Renal arterial narrowing has been treated with angioplasty and other surgical procedures. Occasionally, renal autotransplantation has been effective in curing the hypertension.

Lupus nephritis

Renal involvement in systemic lupus erythematosus is common and more severe in children in China and East Asian countries, including Hong Kong and Taiwan, with 40–50% having type IV diffuse proliferative lesions.

Key points: Glomerulonephritis

- The incidence of post-streptococcal acute glomerulonephritis has been declining in many countries, although it is still common in China, southern India, Thailand, Mexico, Nigeria, and South Africa.

- Pyoderma or infected scabies are common sites of antecedent infection.

- Takayasu's disease is an important cause of renovascular hypertension in children in the Indian subcontinent, Thailand, and some other countries.

- Renal involvement in systemic lupus erythematosus is common and more severe in children in China and East Asian countries.

Acute renal failure

Acute renal failure (ARF) is a common problem in hospital practice. The clinical presentation of children with ARF is often late and mortality may be up to 50% [3]. Children with ARF are offered standard treatment and some of them will have access to acute dialysis in the major hospitals. The causes of ARF differ from those in developed countries and there are additional regional variations. The pattern has changed over the past two decades. Widespread use of oral rehydration therapy for acute gastroenteritis has greatly decreased the occurrence of severe dehydration, and ARF as a complication is rare. Post-dysenteric haemolytic uraemic syndrome was the most common cause of ARF in the Indian subcontinent during the 1970s to 1980s, but its incidence has now markedly decreased. ARF associated with major surgery is encountered at the few centres where such procedures are undertaken. Similarly, tertiary care paediatric intensive care units encounter patients with ARF in association with sepsis, shock, and coagulopathy and multi-organ failure. Falciparum malaria, leptospirosis, and snake-bite are important causes of ARF in India and some other Asian countries. Hanta virus infections was frequently responsible for ARF in Korea but has now declined.

In Africa, ARF is a common cause of hospital admission for children. The more frequent causes of ARF include acute gastroenteritis with severe dehydration, cholera in some West African countries, septicaemia, and acute glomerulonephritis. Herbal toxins and diethylene glycol poisoning have also been observed in Nigeria [20,21]. The latter was a contaminant of liquid paracetamol preparations. In Durban, South Africa, herbal medicines containing extracts of the tuber *Callilepis laureola* were reported to be a common cause of ARF. Severe hepatic injury was associated and the condition was almost always fatal.

Post-dysenteric haemolytic uraemic syndrome

Haemolytic uraemic syndrome (HUS) following shigella dysentery was first reported from Bangladesh and thereafter from different centres in India. A large number of such patients were seen at referral hospitals, whereas previously HUS was rare. Most patients were infants and toddlers and had suffered from severe dysentery that responded poorly to antibiotics. HUS developed acutely, with pallor and oliguria and altered sensorium. Renal impairment was usually severe and prolonged, with most patients requiring dialysis. Coagulation studies were suggestive of disseminated coagulopathy (although confirmatory tests were not done), but severe bleeding manifestations were rare. The patients often had prolonged intestinal bleeding due to severe proctocolitis. Renal histology showed characteristic features of glomerular thrombotic microangiopathy with a larger proportion of patients showing renal cortical necrosis. The patients were treated with supportive care and no form of specific therapy was used. The mortality was high due to prolonged renal failure and difficulties in maintaining adequate nutrition. The impression gathered from experience with post-dysenteric HUS in several countries is that the renal injury may be more severe than that observed in HUS due to verotoxin-producing *Escherichia coli*. The latter form has not been encountered in Asian countries except Japan. It is of interest that the incidence of HUS in India has greatly reduced with the decline in the virulent form of shigella dysentery.

As indicated before, HUS is an important cause of acute renal failure in children in Argentina. A majority of cases are associated with a diarrhoeal illness caused by verotoxin-producing *E. coli*, usually of serotype O157:H7 and occasionally others. HUS is often severe, with 50% of patients having oliguria for more than 1 week. Neurological involvement (convulsions, focal deficits) was commonly observed in the acute stage, but usually improved with dialysis, and permanent sequelae were rare. The mortality rate was initially high but reduced subsequently with improved supportive care, chiefly nutritional and dialysis support. While children with relatively milder renal injury completely recover, a significant proportion of those with prolonged anuria develop progressive renal damage and chronic renal failure.

A large number of cases of HUS following shigella dysentery have been reported recently from South Africa and Zimbabwe. These reports describe a severe form of HUS with about 90% of patients having oliguric renal failure, and half of them needing dialysis. There was a very high incidence of a variety of complications such as encephalopathy, convulsions, protein-losing enteropathy, hepatitis, and myocarditis. In the South African report there was 17% mortality in the acute stage and 32% of patients developed chronic renal failure. The mortality rate in Zimbabwe was 40%. The experience in these countries is similar to that reported from India. HUS associated with *E. coli* producing a shigella-like toxin appears to be rare in Africa, as also in most developing countries.

Falciparum malaria

Falciparum malaria is an important cause of ARF in north-eastern parts of India, Bangladesh, Thailand, and possibly in other neighbouring countries. Although vivax malaria is widely prevalent in the Indian subcontinent, it rarely leads to ARF. In recent years falciparum malaria has shown resistance to commonly used antimalarial drugs. Heavy parasitization of red blood cells leads to impairment of renal microcirculation through several mechanisms. Damage to the red blood cell (RBC) membrane makes them rigid and less deformable. Such cells tend to adhere to platelets and leucocytes. Glycosylphosphatidylinositol moieties of the malarial parasites attach to monocytes through the CD-14 receptor, to release tumour necrosis factor, which is followed by an increase in cytokines and inflammatory mediators contributing to volume depletion. Knobs form on the surface of parasitized RBCs, which have a special affinity for adhesion molecules. Blood viscosity is also increased from a rise in fibrinogen and acute-phase reactant proteins. Histologically tubular degeneration and tubular necrosis are observed, being most prominent in the distal tubules and less severe in the proximal tubules and collecting ducts. Tubular cells may show haemosiderin pigment. Peritubular capillaries are sometimes seen to be clogged with parasitized RBCs. Glomeruli may show mild mesangial proliferation and prominence of mesangial matrix. Deposits of IgM and C3 may be observed in glomerular capillaries.

Clinical features include the usual manifestations of malaria, often complicated by severe vomiting and hypotension. ARF is indicated by increasing blood levels of urea and creatinine, since in a majority of patients ARF is of non-oliguric type. In an occasional patient with glucose-6-phosphate dehydrogenase (G-6PD) deficiency, severe intravascular haemolysis may occur and further add to the problems of management. Multi-organ involvement has rarely been reported.

Quinine and artemether are used for the treatment of falciparum malaria. ARF is managed with standard supportive care. The outcome depends chiefly upon the extent and severity of involvement of other organs.

Leptospirosis

Leptospirosis is a common cause of ARF in South India and the Philippines. *Leptospira interrogans* has over 200 serotypes. Both wild and domestic animals serve as reservoirs. The organisms invade the renal tubules and are excreted in urine. Human infection follows contact of skin with infected urine. Clinical infection varies from mild to extremely severe. The former is characterized by fever, myalgia, and conjunctival suffusion, whereas jaundice, bleeding manifestations, pneumonia, and ARF may occur in severe cases. The illness is often biphasic, with an initial 'septicaemic' phase lasting 4–7 days, after which the patient appears to improve and becomes afebrile. A few days thereafter fever, jaundice, and bleeding phenomena occur. In the early phase, urine examination may show mild proteinuria, leucocyturia, and granular casts. ARF is non-oliguric in 20–50% cases. Renal injury is thought to result from direct leptospiral invasion and non-specific factors such as hypovolaemia, hyperviscosity, coagulopathy, complement activation, and the release of inflammatory mediators. Renal histological changes consist of mesangial proliferation and neutrophilic infiltration in early stages, interstitial infiltration with mononuclear cells, and later tubular necrosis. Immunofluorescence examination shows deposits of C3, C1Q and IgM in the mesangium. Intact leptospira have been shown to be present in the glomeruli, peritubular capillaries, interstitium, and tubular lumen in early stages.

Penicillin, tetracycline, and doxycycline and some other antibiotics are effective in treatment. ARF is managed with supportive care. In hypercatabolic cases, intensive dialysis may be necessary. Exchange blood transfusion may be carried out in patients with severe hepatic dysfunction and bleeding manifestations.

Snake-bite

In rural areas and coastal regions of India and in Thailand, snake-bite is a frequent cause of ARF. Common poisonous snakes include Russell's viper, saw-scaled viper, and sea snakes. The severity of organ injury depends upon the site of bite and the amount of venom injected, the promptness and effectiveness of the antivenom administered, and other supportive measures. Renal damage results from hypotension, intravascular haemolysis, coagulopathy, and direct toxicity of the venom. Rhabdomyolysis is an important feature of sea-snake bite. Acute tubular necrosis is the usual histological finding. With early institution of adequate supportive measures, most patients recover.

Scorpion sting and other envenomations

In infants and small children, stings by poisonous scorpions (which abound in hilly terrain), wasps, and bees may occasionally cause severe toxicity with hypotension and shock. A delay in instituting appropriate management may lead to ARF.

Drugs and toxins

Outbreaks of ARF ascribed to ingestion of ethylene glycol contaminating liquid preparations of paracetamol have occasionally been reported. A large number of children with such ARF were reported from Bangladesh and there was considerable mortality. There is often prolonged oligoanuria and appropriate dialytic support may not be available. Indiscriminate use of aminoglycosides and other nephrotoxic agents are frequently suspected to have a role in children with ARF due to a variety of causes.

Key points: Acute renal failure

- Clinical presentation of children with ARF is often late and mortality may be up to 50% [3].

- Falciparum malaria, leptospirosis, and snakebite are important causes of ARF in India and some other Asian countries.

- Hantavirus infection was previously frequently responsible for ARF in Korea but has now declined.

- Herbal toxins and diethylene glycol poisoning have also been observed in Nigeria.

- ARF due to intravascular haemolysis in G-6PD deficiency is usually mild.

- HUS following shigella infection is declining in some countries.

- The aetiological infection in HUS varies from country to country.

G-6PD deficiency and intravascular haemolysis

The prevalence of glucose-6-phosphate dehydrogenase deficiency is high in some population groups in northern India and some parts of Nigeria. Exposure to oxidant drugs, chiefly antimalarials but occasionally one of a host of others, may cause severe intravascular haemolysis. The patient acutely develops pallor, weakness, mild jaundice, and haemoglobinuria. In an occasional case ARF occurs, indicated by rising levels of blood urea and creatinine. Urine output is usually maintained. With adequate supportive care, the outcome is excellent, with the exception of an occasional patient with an underlying acute or chronic hepatic disease.

Chronic renal failure and renal replacement therapy

Various forms of chronic glomerulonephritis, congenital anomalies, obstructive uropathy, urinary tract infections and reflux nephropathy, and hereditary conditions are the important causes of chronic renal failure. Renal replacement therapy is possible only in a small fraction of cases, chiefly for socio-economic reasons, although it is available to a much larger proportion of adult patients. A study from Nigeria suggested that 7.5 children/million population per year develop ESRD [1]. The true figure is likely to be more, since many patients do not get referred to major hospitals. Data from South Africa indicate that among black children, FSGS and other forms of steroid-resistant nephrotic syndrome are responsible for more than 60% of children requiring renal replacement therapy. Limited data from Nigeria indicate a similar pattern, whereas in non-black children the predominant causes include reflux nephropathy, renal dysplasia, and polycystic kidney disease. Facilities for renal replacement therapy are well established in South Africa, most of North Africa, and some parts of East Africa.

Urinary tract infections and related problems

In Africa, as in many other developing countries, the incidence of urinary tract infections (UTI) and their contribution to eventual ESRD is not well known, although recent studies from South Africa indicate that UTI may be widely prevalent. UTI often goes undetected, and even when diagnosed it is treated by general practitioners and appropriate imaging studies are not carried out. In regions where malaria is endemic, febrile illnesses are frequently treated with antimalarial drugs, and only a failure of response leads to a search for other possible causes. Vesico-ureteric reflux (VUR) and reflux nephropathy appear to be uncommon in black African children, as indicated by data from South Africa. The practice of circumcision may have a protective role against UTI [22]. However, in unskilled hands the procedure may lead to phimosis and complications from obstruction to urine flow.

Nephrolithiasis

Bladder stones are still common in young children in several countries, although the incidence has declined in some parts, such as northern India. The stones are usually single, composed of calcium oxalate and do not usually recur after removal. Malnutrition and infection are not significant aetiological factors. The stone formation is in some way related to consumption of a predominantly cereal diet with little animal protein and passage of a concentrated urine during episodes of diarrhoeal dehydration. Upper urinary tract calculi are occasionally seen in children, with an underlying metabolic abnormality, such as hypercalciuria, detectable in about half the cases.

Schistosomiasis

Schistosoma hematobium infestation is common in Egypt and East Africa. Involvement of venous plexuses around the bladder and ureter by the adult worms, where they lay eggs, causes dysuria and haematuria. Eventually fibrotic lesions of the ureter develop and lead to obstructive uropathy, usually in the third decade. Schistosomiasis probably does not play a significant role in inducing glomerular injury.

Conclusions and recommendations

Developing countries face the gigantic problem of socio-economic upliftment. Unless universal primary

> ## Key points: Urine infection and related topics
>
> - Recent studies from South Africa indicate that UTI may be widely prevalent.
>
> - Vesico-ureteric reflux (VUR) and reflux nephropathy appear to be uncommon in black African children.
>
> - Bladder stones are still common in young children in several countries, although the incidence has declined in some parts, such as northern India.
>
> - *Schistosoma hematobium* infestation is common in Egypt and East Africa and causes dysuria and haematuria and eventually obstructive uropathy.

healthcare is provided and the preventable and infectious diseases controlled, tertiary care will remain available to a very small minority of the population, with a heavy bias towards adult patients. The development of paediatric nephrology begins with a paediatric nephrologist, who has received appropriate training, usually over an extended period, and who is committed to this speciality. He must spearhead the efforts to establish a division or unit of paediatric nephrology with the aims of providing specialized services and undertake educative and investigative activities.

Paediatric nephrologists have a great responsibility for educating and training paediatricians, general physicians (who often treat children), and paramedical staff, as well as the community at large. The goals are the prevention of renal diseases in children, their recognition, appropriate initial or emergency management, and referral to a tertiary facility. Appropriate educative and instructive material should be prepared.

National and regional paediatric nephrology societies can be formed and regular meetings held to avoid academic isolation. Paediatric nephrology units should be established at medical college hospitals and standard treatment facilities developed. Peritoneal dialysis can be provided with minimal inputs but requires skill training of technical staff. These units need to co-operate closely and interact with the adult nephrology departments, pathologists, microbiologists, imaging departments, paediatric surgeons, and nutritionists.

Role of developed countries and international societies

The most serious difficulty in the development of paediatric nephrology in developing countries is the lack of proper training in various aspects of the discipline. In a number of countries in Asia and Africa there is not even a single paediatric nephrologist. Financial support is the major problem. Excellent clinical training is often available at some of the more developed developing countries (such as India, South Africa), though the training centres are usually located in large cities with a very high cost of living. Some national societies provide training fellowships. However, a complete instruction programme in paediatric nephrology, such as that established in USA, should be the ultimate aim. Collaborative arrangements between centres in advanced countries and developing countries on a long-term basis would be of great help in strengthening local academic and research efforts.

References

1. Eke F.U. and Eke N.N. Renal disorders in children: a Nigerian study. Pediatr Nephrol. 1994, 8, 1–3.
2. Hendrickse R.G. and Gilles H.M. The nephrotic syndrome and other renal diseases in children in western Nigeria. East Afr Med J. 1963, 40, 186–201.
3. Abdurrahman M.B., Babaoye F.A. and Aikionhbare H.A. Childhood renal disorders in Nigeria. Pediatr Nephrol. 1990, 4, 88–93.
4. Okoro B.A. and Okafor H.U. Pattern of renal disorders in children in Enugu. Pediatr Nephrol. 1998, 12, C182.
5. Thomson P.D. Renal problems in black South African children. Pediatr Nephrol. 1997, 11, 508–512.
6. Diniz J.S.S. Aspects of Brazilian paediatric nephrology. Pediatr Nephrol. 1988, 2, 271–276.
7. Rollins N.S., Wittenberg D.F., Coovadia H.M., Pillay D.G., Karas A.J. and Sturm A.W. Epidemic shigella dysenteriae type 1 in Natal. J Trop Pediatr. 1995, 41, 281–284.
8. Attolou V., Bigot A., Ayivi B. and Gninafon M. Renal complications associated with human acquired immunodeficiency virus infection in a population of hospital patients at the hospital and university national center in Cotonou. Sante. 1998, 8, 283–286.
9. Hendrickse R.G., Adeniyi A., Edington G.M., Glasgow E.F., White R.H.R. and Houba V. Quartan malaria nephrotic syndrome collaborative clinicopathological study in Nigerian children. Lancet. 1972, May 27, 1143–1149.
10. Abdurrahman M.B., Aikhionbare H.A., Babaoye F.A., Sathiakumar N. and Narayana P.T. Clinicopathological features of childhood nephrotic syndrome in northern Nigeria. Q J Med. 1990, 75, 563–576.
11. Bhimma R., Coovadia H.M. and Adhikari M. Nephrotic syndrome in South African children: changing perspectives over 20 years. Pediatr Nephrol. 1997, 11, 429–434.
12. Asinobi A.O., Gbadegesin R.A., Adeyemo A.A., Akang E.E., Arowolo F.A., Abiola O.A. and Osinusi K. The predominance of membranoproliferative glomerulonephritis in childhood nephrotic syndrome in Ibadan, Nigeria. West Afr J Med. 1999, 18, 203–206.
13. Elzouki A.Y., Amin F. and Jaiswal O.P. Prevalence and pattern of renal disease in eastern Libya. Arch Dis Child. 1983, 58, 106–109.
14. Abdurrahman M.B. The role of infectious agents in the aetiology and pathogenesis of childhood nephrotic syndrome in Africa. J Infections. 1984, 8, 100–109.
15. Van Buuren A.J., Bates W.D. and Muller N. Nephrotic syndrome in Namibian children. S Afr Med J. 1999, 89, 1088–1091.
16. International study of kidney disease in children. Nephrotic syndrome in children: Prediction of histopathology from clinical and laboratory characteristics at time of diagnosis. Kidney Int. 1978, 13, 159–165.
17. Baldwin D.S., Gluck M.C., Schacht R.G. and Gallo G. The long term course of poststreptococcal glomerulonephritis. Ann Intern Med. 1974, 80, 342–358.
18. Roy S., Pitcock J.A. and Etteldorf JN. Prognosis of acute post- streptococcal glomerulonephritis in childhood: prospective study and review of the literature. Adv Pediatr. 1976, 35–69.
19. Tejani A. and Ingulli E. Post streptococcal glomerulonephritis current clinical and pathologic concepts. Nephron. 1990, 55, 1–5.
20. Kadiri S., Ogunlesi A., Osinfade K. and Akinkugbe O.O. The causes and course of acute tubular necrosis in Nigerians. Afr J Med Med Sci. 1992, 21, 91–96.
21. Editorial. Acute renal failure secondary to ingestion of adulterated paracetamol syrup, Plateau and Oyo states June–September 1990. Nigerian Bulletin of Epidemiology. 1991, 1, 5–7.
22. Craig J.C., Knight J.F., Sureshkumar P., Mantz E. and Roy L.P. Effect of circumcision on incidence of urinary tract infection in preschool boys. J Pediatr 1996, 128,15–22.

28 | *Reference data for paediatric nephrology*

Richard C.L. Holt, Jane E. Connell, and G. Michael Addison

Introduction

This chapter is divided into three sections:

1. Reference values:
   - Biochemistry: blood, serum/plasma, urine, endocrine
   - Haematology
   - Immunology
   - Ultrasound measurements of renal dimensions
   - Bladder capacity

2. Renal function and useful formulae
   - Glomerular filtration rate
   - Tubular function
   - Total body water and extracellular fluid volume
   - Body surface area

3. Physiological diagrams and tables
   - Immunological mechanisms of glomerular injury
   - Laboratory characteristics of immune-mediated glomerular diseases
   - Complement cascade
   - Endocrinology and the kidney
   - Renin–angiotensin system
   - Plasma calcium and phosphate homeostasis
   - Diuretics

In sections 2 and 3, we have aimed to include useful summaries of selected areas in paediatric nephrology. These are intended to provide an overview of the more factually complex aspects, rather than a complete summary of renal physiology and pathology.

Reference values

Biochemistry

Reference ranges are for guidance only. Obtaining accurate values from healthy children is difficult, especially for the less commonly used investigations. The values given here are those used in the authors' own hospital. Some have been locally derived and others modified from the literature. It should be remembered that many of the literature-derived values have come from relatively small groups of patients and the confidence intervals of these ranges are wide. This accounts for the irregular appearance of some age-related values, when a smooth change with age would be expected. Paediatricians are encouraged to consult with the local laboratory to verify reference ranges, especially for the more methodologically dependent analytes such as enzymes and hormones.

Blood

Analyte	Age	Reference range
Acid Base (blood gases)		
pH	2–4 weeks	7.38–7.47
	>1 month	7.35–7.44
PCO$_2$	2–4 weeks	19–45 mmHg
	1–3 years	28–40 mmHg
	3–7 years	31–40 mmHg
	7–12 years	32–41 mmHg
	12–18 years	34–43 mmHg
PO$_2$ (in room air)		80–100 mmHg
Actual bicarbonate	<1 month	17–26 mmol/l
	1 month–1 year	17–28 mmol/l
	>1 year	20–29 mmol/l
Base excess	Newborn	−10 to −2 mmol/l
	Infant	−7 to −1 mmol/l
	Child	−4 to +2 mmol/l

Serum/plasma		
Alanine transferase (ALT)	<1 month	90 IU/l
	>1 month	45 IU/l
Albumin	<1 month	25–35 g/l
	1–6 months	28–44 g/l
	Child	30–45 g/l
Alkaline phosphatase (ALP)	<1 month	150–600 IU/l
	1 month to 2 years	150–1100 IU/l
	2–8 years	150–900 IU/l
	Puberty	200–1200 IU/l
	Adult	50–275 IU/l
Bicarbonate		20–26 mmol/l
Bilirubin, total	Child	<17 μmol/l
	Full term infant:levels will rise from birth to approximately 150 μmol/l at 5–6 days and then fall to normal childhood levels by day 10	
Calcium (total)	Premature	1.50–2.5 mmol/l
	Up to 2 weeks	1.90–2.8 mmol/l
	Child	2.2–2.7 mmol/l
Calcium (ionized)	All	1.0–1.5 mmol/l
Chloride	All	98–110 mmol/l
Cholesterol, total	<1 month	1.1–2.6 mmol/l
	1 month to 2 years	1.2–4.7 mmol/l
	2–16 years	<5.0 mmol/l
Creatine kinase (CK)	<2 weeks	<600 IU/l
	2–4 weeks	<400 IU/l
	1–12 months	<300 IU/l
	>1 year	<190 IU/l
Creatinine	1 week	40–125 μmol/l
	2 weeks	35–105 μmol/l
	3 weeks	25–90 μmol/l
	4 weeks	20–80 μmol/l
	6 months	20–50 μmol/l
	2 years	25–60 μmol/l
	6 years	30–70 μmol/l
	10 years	30–80 μmol/l
	>10 years (male)	65–120 μmol/l
	>10 years (female)	50–110 μmol/l
Glucose (fasting)	Up to 1 month	2.5–5.5 mmol/l
	Child	3.0–6.5 mmol/l
Magnesium	All	0.65–1.0 mmol/l
Osmolality (plasma)	All	275–295 mmol/kg
Phosphate	1 month	1.4–2.8 mmol/l
	1 year	1.2–2.2 mmol/l
	3 years	1.1–2.0 mmol/l
	12 years	1.0–1.8 mmol/l
	15 years	0.95–1.5 mmol/l
Potassium	1 month	3.5–6.0 mmol/l
	Child	3.5–5.0 mmol/l
Protein, total	1 month	45–70 g/l
	1 year	55–72 g/l
	>1 year	62–82 g/l

Analyte	Age	Reference range
Sodium	<1 month	130–145 mmol/l
	>1 month	135–145 mmol/l
Triglycerides (fasting)	<1 month	0.1–0.9 mmol/l
	1–24 months	0.4–1.4 mmol/l
	Child/teens	0.4–1.5 mmol/l
Urate	1–12 months	0.08–0.50 mmol/l
	1–10 years	0.12–0.32 mmol/l
	11–15 years (male)	0.16–0.47 mmol/l
	11–15 years (female)	0.14–0.35 mmol/l
Urea	1–12 months	2.0–5.0 mmol/l
	1–12 years	2.5–6.0 mmol/l
	12–15 years	3.0–7.5 mmol/l

Urine

Albumin : creatinine ratio (first morning urine)	All	<2.1 mg albumin/mmol creatinine
Albumin excretion rate	All	<12 µg/min
Calcium	Child	<0.1 mol/kg/24 h
	Adult	2.5–7.5 mmol/24 h
Calcium:creatinine ratio (first morning or postprandial sample)	All	<0.74
Catecholamines	See Table 28.1	

Table 28.1 Urinary catecholamine levels

Age (years)	Upper limit (97.5th centile) in mmol/mol creatinine			
	Noradrenaline	Dopamine	HMMA	HVA
0.0	0.30	2.0	18	24
0.5	0.27	1.9	17	23
1.0	0.25	1.75	15	22
1.5	0.20	1.6	12	20
2.0	0.18	1.4	11	18
3.0	0.16	1.2	9	15
4.0	0.15	1.0	8	12.5
5.0	0.14	0.95	7.5	11
6.0	0.13	0.9	7	10
7.0	0.12	0.85	6.5	9
8.0	0.12	0.8	6	8
9.0	0.11	0.75	5.7	7.5
10.0	0.11	0.7	5.5	7
12.0	0.10	0.6	5.2	6
14.0	0.08	0.55	5	5
16.0	0.07	0.5	5	4.5

These ranges are based on 24-hour urine collections. Use the age range nearest the patient's age. HMMA, hydroxy-methoxy-mandelic acid; HVA, homovanillic acid.

		Basal (mmol/kg)[a]	Maximal (mmol/kg)
Osmolality (urine)			
	1–14 days	180–400	210–650
	2–4 weeks		780–1100
	1–6 months	50–600	900–1250
	6–24 months		1000–1350
	2–15 years	50–1400	1050–1400

[a] Basal urine osmolality depends on recent intake and losses of water and solute. A normal kidney can produce urine ranging from very dilute to maximally concentrated, and therefore a measurement on a random urine is not a useful test of renal concentrating capability.

Oxalate	up to 13 years	<0.35 mmol/24 h
	13–16 years (male)	0.19–48 mmol/24 h
	13–16 years (female)	0.27–0.52 mmol/24 h
Protein : creatinine ratio (first morning urine)	All	<20 mg protein/mmol creatinine

Endocrine biochemistry

Analyte	Age	Reference range
Aldosterone	3–7 days	0.20–5.1 nmol/l
	1 week to 1 month	0.14–4.4 nmol/l
	1–12 months	0.14–2.5 nmol/l
	1–2 years	0.14–1.4 nmol/l
	2–10 years	0.10–0.9 nmol/l
	10–15 years	0.10–0.5 nmol/l

NB Aldosterone concentrations are influenced by sodium balance. These ranges are for guidance only and assume normal sodium intake.

Cortisol		200–700 nmol/l (09.00 hours)
		<150 nmol/l (24.00 hours)
Plasma renin activity (PRA)	Premature	10–170 ng/ml/h
	1–7 days	2–35 ng/ml/h
	1–12 months	2.5–37 ng/ml/h
	1–5 years	1–10 ng/ml/h
	5–15 years	0.5–3 ng/ml/h

These ranges assume normal sodium balance with the patient supine and at rest. Low sodium intake and upright posture can increase PRA by up to four times.

Parathyroid hormone (intact PTH)		12–81 pg/ml (normocalcaemic patients)

Haematology

The intervals stated are '95% limits' i.e. include 95% of the normal population. Tables 28.2 and 28.3 are based upon data for full-term, iron-sufficient children. The values in Table 28.4 are based upon infants who have received 1 mg vitamin K i.m. at birth. Adapted from [1].

The reference range for red cell folate is 100–750 μg/l for full-term infants and throughout childhood. Serum folate (range 5–30 μg/l) is regarded as a less reliable index of folate stores. The reference range for serum B_{12} is 145–700 ng/l.

Immunology

The following reference intervals are based upon the data used in the authors' institution. However, values may vary depending upon methodology. For specialized investigations (e.g. autoantibodies), it is not possible to offer meaningful values in this text. Readers are advised to consult their local laboratory for more detailed guidance.

Serum complement components (all ages)

C_3 0.83–1.46 g/l
C_4 0.20–0.52 g/l

Serum immunoglobulin levels

See Table 28.5.

Table 28.2 Blood count indices

	Hb (g/dl)	MCV (fl)	Retic (%)	WCC × 10^9/l	Neut ×10^9/l	Lymph ×10^9/l	Mono ×10^9/l	Eos ×10^9/l
Birth to 1 week	14.0–22.0	90–125	3.0–7.0 day 0; 0.1–2.0 day 7	9.0–30.0 day 0; 9.0–40.0 day 4	2.9–14.5 day 0; 1.8–5.4 day 5	2.0–11.0 day 0; 2.0–17.0 day 7	0.0–1.9	0.0–0.8
2 weeks	12.5–20.0	86–120	0.1–2.0	6.0–15.0	1.8–5.4	2.0–17.0	0.1–1.7	0.0–0.8
1 month	11.0–18.0	85–120	0.1–2.0	6.0–15.0	1.0–8.5	2.5–16.5	0.1–1.2	0.0–0.8
2 months	10.0–13.5	80–115	0.1–2.0	6.0–15.0	1.0–8.5	2.5–16.5	0.1–1.2	0.0–0.7
3–6 months	10.0–13.5	75–105	0.1–2.0	6.0–15.0	1.0–8.5	4.0–13.5 6 months	0.1–1.2	0.0–0.7
0.5–2 years	10.5–13.5	70–86	0.1–2.0	6.0–15.0	1.5–8.0	3.0–13.5	0.1–1.2	0.0–0.7
2–6 years	11.0–14.0	73–85	0.1–2.0	6.0–15.0	1.5–8.0	2.0–9.5	0.1–0.8	0.0–0.7
6–12 years	11.5–15.5	77–95	0.1–2.0	5.0–15.0	1.5–8.0	1.5–7.0	0.1–0.8	0.0–0.5
12–16 years (M)	13.0–16.0	78–98	0.1–2.0	4.0–13.0	1.8–8.0	1.2–5.2	0.1–0.8	0.0–0.5
12–16 years (F)	12.0–16.0	78–100	0.1–2.0	4.0–13.0	1.8–8.0	1.2–5.2	0.1–0.8	0.0–0.5

The reference range for platelet count is 150–400 × 10^9/l and is not age-dependent.
Hb, haemoglobin; MCV, mean corpuscular volume; Retic, reticulocytes; WCC, white cell count; Neut, neutrophils; Lymph, lymphocytes; Mono, monocytes; Eos, eosinophils.

Table 28.3 Haematinic indices

	Serum iron (μmol/l)	Iron-binding capacity (μmol/l)	Transferrin saturation (%)	Ferritin (μg/l)
2 weeks	11–36	18–50	30–39	25–200
1 month	10–31	20–52	35–94	200–600[a]
2 months	3–29	24–64	21–63	50–200
4 months	3–29	40–68	7–53	20–200
6 months	5–24	40–76	10–43	7–142
0.5–4 years	5–25	48–79	10–40	7–142
5–10 years	5–30	43–91	10–45	7–142
11–15 years	5–30	52–100	11–45	7–142

[a] Serum ferritin levels rise in the first month, as a result of neonatal haemolysis and low erythropoietin production at this age.

Table 28.4 Coagulation indices

	Prothrombin time (seconds)	APTT (seconds)	Fibrinogen (g/l)
Term newborn	10.8–13.9	31.3–54.5	1.56–4.00
3 months to adulthood	10.8–13.9	26.6–40.3	1.56–4.00

APTT,: Activated Partial Thromboplastin Time.

Tables 28.2, 28.3, and 28.4 reprinted from Diagnosis in Paediatric Haematology. Smith H. 1996 by permission of the publisher Churchill Livingstone.

Table 28.5 Serum immunoglobulin concentrations

Age	IgM (g/l)	IgG (g/l)	IgA (g/l)
Newborn	0.06–0.15	7.98–11.82	0.01–0.05
1–3 months	0.18–0.39	2.99–5.27	0.08–0.34
4–6 months	0.25–0.57	2.31–5.89	0.10–0.46
7–12 months	0.29–0.73	4.24–8.45	0.19–0.54
1–2 years	0.33–0.77	5.31–9.32	0.26–0.73
2–3 years	0.40–0.76	6.81–10.32	0.34–1.07
3–5 years	0.36–0.70	6.73–11.11	0.65–1.18
6–8 years	0.57–2.66	7.68–17.28	0.77–1.67
9–11 years	0.57–2.66	7.68–17.28	0.70–1.89
12–16 years	0.57–2.66	7.68–17.28	0.84–2.09
Adult	0.57–2.66	7.68–17.28	0.89–4.46

Ultrasound measurements of renal dimensions

Han and Babcock studied 122 children, aged from term newborn to 17 years, with no urinary tract disease [2]. Renal length was measured by ultrasound and correlated with age, height and weight. There was no difference in renal length between right and left kidneys and no difference in renal length between boys and girls of the same age/height/weight.

The data are presented in Fig. 28.1 as nomograms with predicted mean renal lengths and 95% prediction

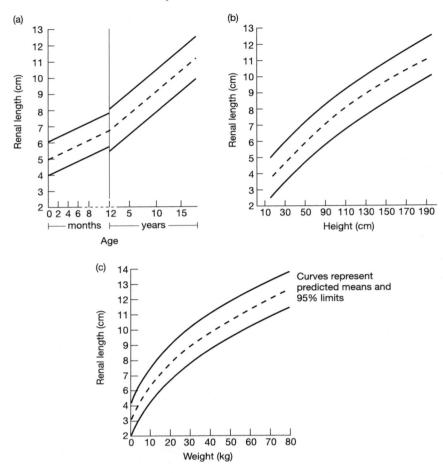

Fig. 28.1 Renal length versus (a) age; (b) height; and (c) weight [2]. Reprinted with permission from the American Journal of Roentgenology.

limits. In preparation of the nomogram of renal length versus age, a separate correlation was performed for infants less than 1 year old, as there was less variation in the data for this group: this statistical treatment accounts for the apparent discontinuity in the nomogram.

Bladder capacity

Bladder capacity has been estimated by several different methods. However, measurements may be unreliable in some studies that included anaesthetized patients.

Kaefer *et al.* reviewed the bladder capacity of children who had undergone radionuclide cystography while awake [3]. Children were excluded from analysis if they had symptoms of bladder dysfunction, urine cultures revealed intercurrent infection, or if abnormalities were detected on cystography (vesico-ureteric reflux, neurogenic bladder, infravesical obstruction). The remaining 2066 children were included in the study.

Analysis showed that there was a non-linear relationship between age and bladder capacity (Fig. 28.2). Statistical methods were used to estimate percentiles. It was observed that girls tended to have larger bladder capacities than boys, but this finding did not reach statistical significance.

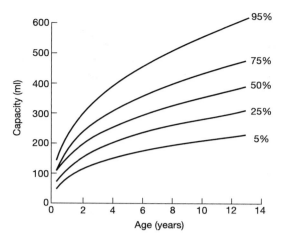

Fig. 28.2 Relationship between bladder capacity and age. From Kaefer M et al. Estimating normal bladder capacity in children. J Urol 1997; 158: 2261–2264 with permission from Lippincott Williams and Wilkins.

Renal function and useful formulae

Assessment of glomerular filtration rate

As glomerular and tubular functions are interdependent, assessment of glomerular filtration rate (GFR) provides an indication of overall level of renal function. Although GFR cannot be measured directly in clinical practice, an estimation of GFR may be made by a number of methods.

General principles

An estimate of GFR can be obtained by measuring the clearance of a solute, which is:

• exclusively excreted by the kidney;

• freely filtered at the glomerulus; and

• not subject to significant tubular secretion or reabsorption.

This can be expressed by the standard formula:

$$C_x = (U_x \times V)/P_x \qquad (28.1)$$

where:

C_x = clearance of solute x;
U_x = urine concentration of solute x;
V = volume of urine over a given time period;
P_x = plasma concentration of solute x.

Since human GFR varies diurnally and with dietary protein load, precautions should be taken to standardize these factors where possible, e.g. estimation of GFR at a fixed time of day in fasting subjects.

Inulin clearance

Inulin is a polysaccharide of plant origin. It fulfils the criteria described above and can, therefore, be used as a marker molecule to estimate GFR.

In summary, the method involves the administration of an intravenous bolus of inulin, followed by a continuous infusion of the solution to maintain the plasma inulin concentration at a constant level. After a period of equilibration, a diuresis is induced by oral or intravenous fluid administration and serial timed urine collections are commenced. Inulin concentration is measured in plasma samples obtained at approximately the midpoint of each urine collection period. The inulin excretion rate ($U_{Inulin} \times V$) and plasma inulin concentration for each time period are then used to calculate GFR from equation 28.1. A mean value is calculated from the serial GFR results.

The chief advantage of this technique is accuracy, and inulin clearance remains the 'gold standard' for comparison of other methods. Disadvantages include the need to administer an exogenous marker substance and the requirement for accurately measured, timed urine collections, which are frequently difficult to obtain in paediatric practice. Previously, there were additional problems in the preparation of the inulin solution and in the measurement of plasma inulin concentration, although developments of the technique have led to improvements in these areas.

In practice, the definitive accuracy of the inulin clearance method is rarely required to guide clinical decisions and this technique is principally a research tool.

Creatinine clearance

Creatinine is an endogenous product of muscle metabolism. As a small molecule (molecular weight 113), it is freely filtered at the glomerulus. A timed urine collection and plasma creatinine concentration may be used to derive an estimate of GFR from equation 28.1.

The attractions of this method include a relatively simple principle, wide availability in clinical practice, and the avoidance of an exogenous marker injection. Unfortunately, it relies upon a timed urine collection, with the limitations that this carries in the paediatric setting.

A further problem is inherent inaccuracy, as creatinine is excreted by tubular secretion as well as glomerular filtration, leading to overestimation of GFR. This issue may be overcome by oral administration of cimetidine prior to the creatinine clearance study. Cimetidine has been found to inhibit tubular secretion of creatinine and estimates of GFR obtained from 'cimetidine-primed' creatinine clearance have been shown to be in close agreement with formal inulin clearance [4].

Haycock–Schwartz formula

The Haycock–Schwartz formula may be used to draw an approximate estimate of GFR from the plasma creatinine concentration, without the need for a timed urine collection [5,6]. This formula is based on the argument that:

- in equation 28.1, the rate of creatinine excretion is represented by $(U_{Cr} \times V)$;

- at steady state, the rate of creatinine excretion must be equal to the body's rate of creatinine production;

- a mathematical expression representing the rate of creatinine production may, therefore, be substituted into equation 28.1 in place of the term $(U_{Cr} \times V)$;

- the body's rate of creatinine production is directly proportional to muscle mass; in turn, muscle mass is related to height in individuals of normal nutritional status;

- hence, $(k \times h)$ represents the rate of creatinine production:

$$pGFR = (k \times h)/P_{Cr} \qquad (28.2)$$

where:

$pGFR$ = predicted glomerular filtration rate (in ml/min/1.73 m^2);
k = an empirically derived value relating height to muscle mass;
h = height (in cm);
P_{Cr} = plasma concentration of creatinine (in μmol/l or mg/dl).

Values of k vary for different age groups, to reflect increasing relative muscle mass during childhood and adolescence. The same formula may be used with both European and North American units for P_{Cr}, with appropriate adjustment of k values. Commonly quoted k values are given in Table 28.6 as a guideline [7]. Since methods of creatinine measurement vary between laboratories, k values should ideally be validated for local use.

In using the Haycock–Schwartz formula, it is important to remember that:

1. The formula's validity rests upon the assumption of a biochemical 'steady state'. For practical purposes, it may be reasonable to make this assumption in monitoring a relatively stable outpatient, but the formula is rendered invalid in circumstances where there are rapid changes in level of renal function, e.g. acute renal failure.

2. At low levels of GFR (advanced chronic renal failure), tubular secretion may contribute a significant proportion of the total creatinine excretion, leading to overestimation of residual GFR.

3. k values represent body mass of individuals with normal nutritional status: in malnourished chronically ill children, lower muscle mass may lead to lower levels of P_{Cr}, causing a misleading overestimate of GFR.

4. Measurement of creatinine and prediction of GFR are subject to inherent inaccuracies. A trend in pGFR may be a clinically useful tool, but absolute values should not be relied upon in isolation. Where more accurate absolute values are

Table 28.6 Values for k for use in the Haycock–Schwartz formula (adapted from [7])

Age group	k value (P_{Cr} in μmol/l)	k value (P_{Cr} in mg/dl)
Preterm neonates	24	0.27
Term neonates	33	0.37
Normal infants 0–12 months	40	0.45
Boys and girls 2–12 years	49	0.55
Girls 13–21 years	49	0.55
Boys 13–21 years	60	0.70

required, GFR should also be estimated by an alternative method for comparison.

Note that equation 28.3 may be used to convert between European and North American units for creatinine:

$$P_{Cr} \ (\mu mol/l) = P_{Cr} \ (mg/dl) \times 88 \qquad (28.3)$$

Plasma disappearance method

This method uses an alternative approach. For a marker substance, which fulfils the general criteria required for GFR estimation, the rate of decline of plasma concentration after bolus intravenous administration will reflect the rate at which the substance is cleared from the plasma by glomerular filtration. This technique avoids the need for timed urine collections.

[51Cr]EDTA is commonly used as a marker in this type of study [8]. Chromium-51 emits β-particles, allowing quantification of the compound in plasma. After bolus injection, there is a period of equilibration, followed by an exponential decline in plasma concentration. This rate of decline may be defined by the plasma concentration measured at two time points (typically 2 and 3 hours after administration of [51Cr]EDTA). Mathematical modelling allows derivation of GFR.

The plasma disappearance method offers the advantage of greater accuracy than creatinine-based methods. However, the accuracy of this technique is dependent upon knowledge of the exact dose of marker administered. Errors are most likely to be introduced during injection. Therefore, it is important to ensure that the [51Cr]EDTA is given through a well-sited cannula (without side ports) and that the cannula is adequately flushed following the bolus injection. It should be noted that this method tends to overestimate GFR at high-normal levels of renal function. Accuracy is also unreliable in patients who are oedematous or dehydrated. Despite these caveats, GFR estimation by the plasma disappearance method is a clinically useful tool, which has found particular application in the monitoring of slowly deteriorating GFR.

The radiation dose to the patient is low. As the compound is excreted in urine, exposure risks may be minimized by diuresis and frequent micturition.

Reference values for GFR are given in Table 28.7 [9].

Tubular function

A summary of tubular function is shown in Table 28.8. As the glomerular filtrate passes along the tubules, selective reabsorption and secretion by the tubular epithelium alters its volume and constituents to produce urine and maintain fluid, electrolyte, and acid–base homeostasis.

The majority of solutes are reabsorbed in the proximal tubule with fine-tuning occurring in the distal segments. Reabsorption of metabolic end products is poor. Transport of solutes is either active (dependent on ATP hydrolysis), or passive (down concentration or electrical gradients). Water moves by osmosis.

Fractional excretion

This is most commonly used in calculation of the fractional excretion of sodium (FE_{Na}), which may be useful in assessment of volume status and acute oliguric renal impairment.

$$FE_x = (U_x/P_x) \times (P_{Cr}/U_{Cr}) \times 100 \qquad (28.4)$$

where:

FE_x = fractional excretion of solute x (expressed as %);
U_x = urine concentration of solute x;
P_x = plasma concentration of solute x;

Table 28.7 GFR in children of different ages (adapted from Chantler [9]) with permission from Blackwell Science Ltd.

Age	Mean GFR (ml/min/1.73 m²)	Range (±2SD)
Birth	20.3	–
7 days	38	26–60
1 month	48	28–68
2 months	58	30–86
6 months	77	41–103
9 months	103	49–157
12 months	115	65–160
2 years	127	89–165
4 years	127	89–165
8 years	127	89–165
12 years	127	89–165
Adult	131	88–174

Table 28.8 Tubular function indicating sites of reabsorption of major components of glomerular filtrate

Substance	Tubular handling (% transported)	Mechanism of transport
Proximal tubule (iso-osmotic filtrate)		
(i) Reabsorption		
Na^+	65%	Active via basolateral $Na^+K^+ATPase$ and apical Na^+/H^+ exchanger, Na^+ coupled co-transport and Na^+ channels
Cl^-	50%	Passive
K^+	70%	Active Na^+ co-transport and passive paracellular diffusion
Ca^{2+}	60%	Mostly passive paracellular, driven by Na^+
Mg^{2+}	30%	Passive paracellular
Inorganic phosphate	80%	Active Na^+ cotransport (inhibited by PTH)
HCO_3^-	80%	Passive, dependent on H^+ secretion and carbonic anhydrase activity (converted to CO_2 and H_2O)
Nutrients	>99%	Active Na^+ co-transport of glucose, amino acids, and vitamins
H_2O	65%	Osmosis
Proteins	Variable	Pinocytosed by tubule cells, digested to amino acids
(ii) Secretion		
H^+	Variable	Active via Na^+/H^+ exchanger
Loop of Henle (countercurrent multiplier increases osmolality at papillary tip with iso-osmotic/hypo-osmotic filtrate in the cortex)		
(i) Reabsorption		
Na^+	25%	Passive (in thin ascending limb), active co-transport via NaK2Cl transporter (thick ascending limb)
H_2O	10%	Osmosis (thin descending limb)
HCO_3^-	10–15%	Passive (thick ascending limb)
K^+	25%	Active via NaK2Cl transporter and passive diffusion
Mg^{2+}	65%	Passive paracellular and active transcellular in thick ascending limb (increased by PTH)
Ca^{2+}	20%	Passive paracellular (thick ascending limb)
Distal tubule (hypo-osmotic filtrate)		
(i) Reabsorption		
Na^+	5%	Active, NaCl co-transport
Ca^{2+}	5–10%	Active transcellular, via PTH-activated Ca^{2+} channels
Inorganic phosphate	10%	Active, Na^+ co-transport
Mg^{2+}	5%	Passive
(ii) Secretion		
K^+	Variable	Active via K^+ channel or KCl transporter

Table 28.8 Continued

Substance	Tubular handling (% transported)	Mechanism of transport
Collecting duct (hyper-osmotic filtrate)		
(i) Reabsorption		
Na^+	2–5%	Active via epithelial Na^+ channels regulated by ADH and aldosterone
K^+	Variable	Active, apical H^+/K^+ ATPase
Ca^{2+}	<2%	Active
Inorganic phosphate	2–3%	Active, Na^+ co-transport
H_2O	Variable	Osmosis, permeability dependent on ADH
HCO_3^-	5%	Passive
Urea	Variable	Passive
(ii) Secretion		
K^+	Variable	Active, basolateral Na^+/K^+ ATPases
H^+	Variable	Active, H^+/K^+ATPase or H^+ ATPases
HCO_3^-	Variable	Active

P_{Cr} = plasma concentration of creatinine;
U_{Cr} = urine concentration of creatinine.

U_x, P_x, P_{Cr}, and U_{Cr} should be in compatible units. For calculation of FE_{Na}, U_{Na}, and U_{Cr} may be measured from a 'spot' urine sample.

FE_{Na} may assist in distinguishing between renal hypoperfusion ('prerenal failure') and established acute tubular necrosis as causes of acute non-obstructive oliguric renal impairment. Blood and urine samples must be obtained prior to administration of diuretics. Data from adult studies indicate that FE_{Na} greater than 2.5% suggests established acute tubular necrosis, whereas FE_{Na} less than 1% suggests renal hypoperfusion [10] (also see Chapter 2).

Tubular reabsorption

It is seldom necessary to formally quantify tubular reabsorption in clinical practice. In its simplest terms, tubular reabsorption of any solute may be given as:

$$TR_x = 100 - FE_x \qquad (28.5)$$

where:

TR_x = tubular reabsorption of solute x (expressed as %);
FE_x = fractional excretion of solute x, as defined in equation 28.4.

Equation 28.5 may be used to assess tubular reabsorption of inorganic phosphate (TRP) from a 24-hour urine collection. TRP ranges from 80 to 95% in normal children. However, TRP is influenced by changes in GFR. Therefore, T_mP_i/GFR is often the preferred method for assessment of tubular phosphate handling, as standardization for GFR is incorporated. An additional advantage is that T_mP_i/GFR may be calculated from a preprandial early morning urine specimen, without the need for a 24-hour urine collection:

$$T_mP_i/GFR = P_{Pi} - [(U_{Pi} \times P_{Cr})/U_{Cr}] \qquad (28.6)$$

where:

T_mP_i/GFR = maximum rate of tubular phosphate reabsorption per unit GFR;
P_{Pi} = plasma concentration of inorganic phosphate;
U_{Pi} = urine concentration of inorganic phosphate;
P_{Cr} = plasma concentration of creatinine;
U_{Cr} = urine concentration of creatinine.

Normal values of T_mP_i (mean ± SD) are relatively high throughout childhood and adolescence, with a post-pubertal decline to near-adult levels by age 17 years. This pattern reflects the need for P_i to be retained during growth, to allow P_i incorporation into the skeleton [11].

Boys:	Age 6 years:	2.02 ± 0.29 mmol/l
	Age 17 years:	1.38 ± 0.21 mmol/l
Girls:	Age 6 years:	1.84 ± 0.27 mmol/l
	Age 17 years:	1.29 ± 0.16 mmol/l

Total body water and extracellular fluid volume

Data occasionally useful in biochemical assessment are shown in Table 28.9.

Table 28.9 Total body water and extracellular fluid data

Age	Total body water (% body weight)	ECF (% body weight)
0–10 days	77	42
1–120 days	73	34
0.5–2 years	62	27
2–9 years	63	25
10–15 years (male)	59	20
10–15 years (female)	56	20

Body surface area

In clinical practice, body surface area is most conveniently calculated using the Mosteller formula [12]:

$$S = \sqrt{[(h \times w)/3600]} \qquad (28.7)$$

where:

S = body surface area (in m^2);
h = height (cm);
w = weight (kg).

This formula has been shown to be faster to calculate and less prone to error than the use of a surface area nomogram [13].

Physiological diagrams and tables

Immunological mechanisms of glomerular injury (Table 28.10)

There are three main mechanisms of immune-mediated glomerular disease:

1. *Type III hypersensitivity reactions* (immune complex deposition in glomerular basement membrane (GBM) activating complement and cell-mediated attack), e.g. post-infectious glomerulonephritis, IgA nephropathy.

2. *Vasculitis* (renal blood vessels affected as part of a systemic inflammatory disorder), e.g. Henoch-Schönlein purpura (HSP), systemic lupus erythematosus (SLE), and polyarteritis nodosa (PAN).

3. *Type II hypersensitivity reactions* (autoantibodies to antigenic glycoprotein in GBM and subsequent recruitment of complement and phagocytes), e.g. Goodpasture's disease.

In these conditions, the mediators of glomerular damage include:

- complement;

- polymorphonuclear (PMN) leucocytes;

- nephritic factors (inactivate inhibitors of the complement cascade, resulting in complement activation and hypocomplementaemia);

- clotting factors.

Minimal change nephrotic syndrome (MCNS) is an exception to these general mechanisms. By definition, renal biopsy demonstrates no significant evidence of antibody deposition or immune cell infiltration in MCNS. It is likely that the proteinuria of MCNS is induced by a soluble mediator of T lymphocyte origin, via mechanisms that are not yet understood.

The complement cascade

- Complement consists of more than 40 soluble or membrane-bound inactive proteins manufactured by the liver (serum concentrations of 3–4 g/l).

- Activation by classical or alternative pathways leads to a sequential proteolytic cascade, culminating in the final membrane attack pathway (Fig. 28.3).

- Resultant release of inflammatory mediators, phagocytosis by opsonization, and cell lysis. C4a, C3a and C5a are anaphylatoxins. C3b leads to opsonization and C5a and C3a are chemotactic.

Table 28.10 Laboratory characteristics of immune-mediated glomerular disease

Disorder	Pathology	Direct immunofluorescence	C3	C4
Immune complex mediated GN				
Post-streptococcal[a]	Diffuse proliferative ± crescents	Granular deposits IgG, C3 along GBM	L	N
IgA nephropathy	Mesangial proliferation	IgA, C3, properidin ± IgG in mesangium	N	N
Membranous	Thickened GBM	Granular deposits IgG, C3 along GBM	N	N
Membranoproliferative (types I and II)	Mesangial proliferation and capillary thickening	Granular deposits IgG, C3 along GBM	L	N/L
Vasculitis				
Henoch–Schönlein nephropathy	Variable; mesangial proliferation	Mesangial IgA, C3; resembles IgA nephropathy	N	N
SLE	Variable	Granular deposits IgG, IgM, C3, C4 along GBM	L	L
Polyarteritis nodosa[b]	Vascular fibrinoid necrosis	Negative	N	N
Wegener's granulomatosis[c]	Focal proliferative + crescents	Negative	N	N
Cryoglobulinaemia	Mesangial proliferation and capillary proliferation	IgG, IgM, C3 along capillary wall	L	L
Autoantibody mediated GN				
Anti-GBM nephritis[d]	Diffuse proliferative ± crescents	Linear deposits IgG, C3 along GBM	N	N
Other				
Minimal change	Loss of epithelial foot processes on EM	Nil significant	N	N
Focal segmental glomerulosclerosis (idiopathic)	Collapse of capillaries; wrinkling of GBM; ↑ mesangial matrix	Mesangial IgM ± C3, C1q, C4, IgG, IgA, fibrin	N	N

[a] Evidence of prodromal streptococcal infection, e.g. positive antistreptolysin-O titre (ASOT), positive bacterial cultures.
[b] Positive pANCA.
[c] Positive cANCA.
[d] Positive anti-glomerular basement membrane antibody, association with HLA-DR2
L, low levels; N, normal.

Regulation is achieved by specific regulatory proteins and by the lability and dilution of activated components.

Endocrinology and the kidney

Hormones acting on, or produced by, the kidney are summarized in Table 28.11. Erythropoietin is a glycosylated protein produced mainly by the kidney (in type 1 fibroblastoid cells of the peritubular interstitium) and to a lesser extent, the liver (main site of production in the fetus and neonate). Erythropoietin physiology is outlined in Fig. 28.4. Recombinant human erythropoietin is administered subcutaneously 2–3 times weekly to treat anaemia due to CRF (main complications are polycythaemia and hypertension).

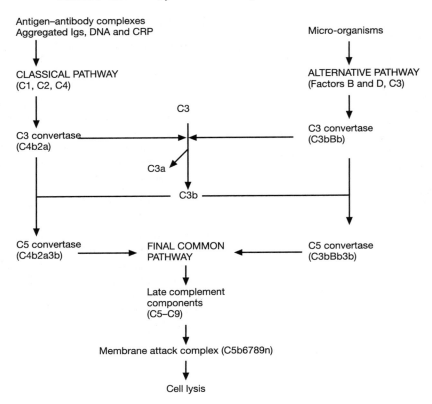

Fig. 28.3 The complement cascade.

Table 28.11 Hormones acting on and produced by the kidney

Hormone	Site of production	Site of action	Effects
Hormones acting on the kidney			
Antidiuretic hormone	Hypothalamus – secreted by posterior pituitary	DT and CD	↑H_2O absorption (via V_1 receptors), vasoconstriction (via V_2 receptors)
Aldosterone	Zona glomerulosa of adrenal cortex	DT and CD, promotes apical Na^+ channels and Na/K ATPases	↑NaCl and H_2O reabsorption; ↑K^+ and H^+ secretion
Atrial natriuretic peptide	Atrial myocytes – released on atrial distension	DT and CD inactivates apical Na^+ channels	↓NaCl absorption, ↑GFR and renal blood flow
Parathyroid hormone	Parathyroid gland	PT, DT and thick asc. limb of loop of Henle	↑Ca^{2+} absorption, ↓P_i absorption
Hormones produced by the kidney			
Renin	Juxtaglomerular apparatus	PT	↑NaCl and H_2O reabsorption, ↑H^+ secretion vasoconstriction (via angiotensin and aldosterone)
Erythropoietin	Fibroblastoid cells	Bone marrow	Erythropoiesis
Prostaglandins	Cortex and medulla	Local effects	Vasodilatation ↑Na^+ and H_2O excretion, ↑GFR
1,25-$(OH)_2$-D_3	Proximal nephron	Gut, bone, parathyroid glands	↑Ca^{2+} and P_i absorption, ↑Ca^{2+} and P_i release, ↓ PTH release

PT, proximal tubule; DT, distal tubule; CD, collecting duct; 1,25-$(OH)_2$-D_3; 1,25-dihydroxyvitamin D_3.

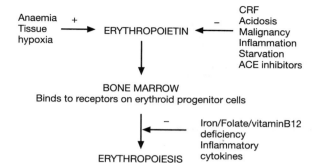

Fig. 28.4 Control of erythropoiesis, indicating the key role of erythropoietin.

Renin–angiotensin system

The renin–angiotensin system (Fig. 28.5) is primarily involved in the regulation of blood pressure, renal blood flow, and fluid/electrolyte homeostasis.

- Renin is a protease produced by the juxta-glomerular cells in the afferent arteriole in response to decreased renal perfusion (renal baroreceptor), decreased distal tubular chloride concentration (detected by the macula densa), or sympathetic stimulation.

- Angiotensin converting enzyme is membrane bound, mostly on vascular endothelium.

- Angiotensin II acts via two major receptor subtypes, AT_1 and AT_2. These differ in location and second messenger systems. AT_1 is predominant and responsible for the vasoconstrictive and growth-promoting effects of angiotensin II. AT_2 receptors are thought to have a role in apoptosis.

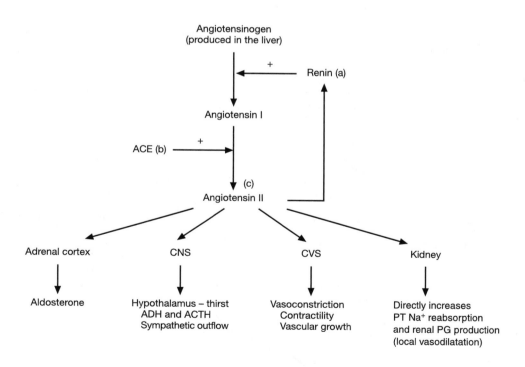

Fig. 28.5 The renin–angiotensin system. ACE, angiotensin converting enzyme; CNS, central nervous system; CVS, cardiovascular system; PT, proximal tubule; PG, prostaglandin.

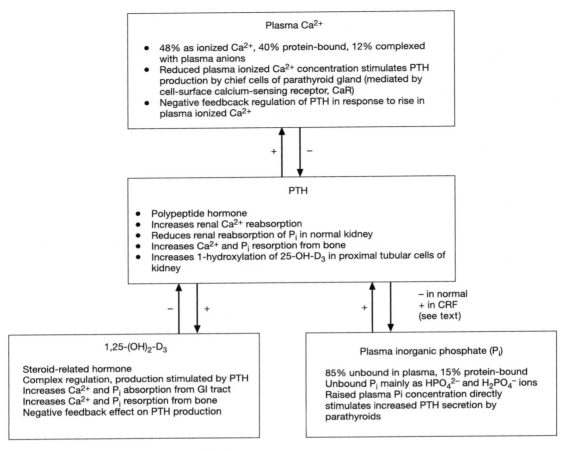

Fig. 28.6 Control of plasma calcium and phosphate. For explanation, see text.

Plasma calcium and phosphate homeostasis

Plasma calcium and phosphate homeostasis is shown in Fig. 28.6, highlighting the central role played by parathyroid hormone (PTH). Calcitonin exerts a weak effect to reduce plasma calcium concentration. This is omitted from Fig. 28.6 for clarity.

In CRF, falling production of $1,25\text{-}(OH)_2\text{-}D_3$ leads to a rise in PTH secretion. PTH stimulates Ca^{2+} and P_i resorption from bone. Under normal circumstances, P_i liberation from bone would be offset by a concomitant PTH-mediated reduction in renal P_i reabsorption. In CRF, the kidney is unable to mount the normal phosphaturic response to PTH, therefore plasma P_i concentration rises. Elevated plasma P_i leads to further stimulation of the parathyroid glands. This is recognized to be a crucial factor in the development of parathyroid hyperplasia, secondary hyperparathyroidism, and renal osteodystrophy. Hence dietary P_i restriction and P_i-binding agents form the basis for prophylaxis and therapy of renal osteodystrophy. It is generally recommended that vitamin D analogues (e.g. alfacalcidol) should not be introduced until plasma P_i concentration has been satisfactorily controlled by these measures, due to the tendency of vitamin D compounds to increase gastrointestinal absorption of P_i.

Table 28.12 Mechanisms of action of commonly used diuretics

Diuretic	Mechanism of action	Effect
Osmotic diuretics (mannitol)	Filtered and not reabsorbed; produce osmotic diuresis	$\downarrow H_2O$ reabsorption from proximal tubule $\downarrow Na^+$, Cl^-, K^+ reabsorption
Carbonic anhydrase inhibitors (acetazolamide)	Block reaction of $CO_2 + H_2O$, prevent HCO_3^- reabsorption and Na^+/K^+ exchange in proximal tubule	Potency + $\downarrow Na^+$, K^+, HCO_3^- reabsorption
Loop diuretics (furosemide)	Inhibit NaK2Cl co-transport in medullary thick ascending limb of the loop of Henle	Potency + + + $\downarrow Na^+$, K^+, Cl^- reabsorption $\downarrow$urinary concentration
Thiazides (bendroflumethiazide)	Inhibit apical NaCl co-transport in early distal tubule by binding to Cl^- binding site	Potency + + $\downarrow Na^+$, K^+, Cl^-, Mg^{2+} and $\uparrow Ca^{2+}$ reabsorption
Potassium sparing (i) spironolactone	Aldosterone antagonist	Potency + $\downarrow Na^+$ reabsorption and K^+ secretion
(ii) amiloride	Inhibits epithelial sodium channel in the collecting duct	Potency + $\downarrow Na^+$ reabsorption and K^+ secretion

Diuretics

Diuretics have effects on tubular transport, which lead to increased urinary water and electrolyte loss. The mechanisms of action of the commonly used diuretics are shown in Table 28.12.

Acknowledgements

The authors are grateful to Dr Mansel Haeney, Consultant Immunologist, Hope Hospital, Salford for assistance in preparation of the immunology section.

References

1. Smith H. *Diagnosis in Paediatric Haematology*. Edinburgh: Churchill Livingstone (1996).
2. Han BK, Babcock DS. Sonographic Measurements and Appearance of Normal Kidneys in Children. *AJR*. 1985; 145: 611–16.
3. Kaefer M, Zurakowski D, Bauer SB, Retik AB, Peters CA, Atala A, Treves ST. Estimating Normal Bladder Capacity in Children. *J Urol*. 1997; 158: 2261–2264.
4. Hellerstein S, Berenbom M, Alon US, Warady BA. Creatinine clearance following cimetidine for estimation of glomerular filtration rate. *Pediatr Nephrol*. 1998; 12: 49–54.
5. Schwartz GJ, Haycock GB, Edelmann CM Jr, Spitzer A. A Simple Estimate of Glomerular Filtration Rate in Children Derived From Body Length and Plasma Creatinine. *Pediatrics*. 1976; 58: 259–263.
6. Counahan R, Chantler C, Ghazali S, Kirkwood E, Rose F, Barratt TM. Estimation of Glomerular Filtration Rate from Plasma Creatinine in Children. *Arch Dis Child*. 1976; 51: 875–78.
7. Schwartz GJ, Brion LP, Spitzer A. The Use of Plasma Creatinine Concentration to Estimate Glomerular Filtration Rate in Infancy, Childhood and Adolescence. *Pediatr Clin North Am*. 1987; 34: 571–90.
8. Chantler C, Garnett ES, Parsons V, Veall N. Glomerular Filtration Rate Measurement In Man By The Single Injection Methods Using ^{51}Cr-EDTA. *Clin Sci*. 1969; 37: 169–80.
9. Chantler C. The Kidney. In: Godfrey S and Baum JD, eds. Clinical Paediatric Physiology. Oxford: Blackwell Scientific Publications 1979, pp. 356–98.
10. Miller TR, Anderson RJ, Linas SL *et al*. Urinary Diagnostic Indices in Acute Renal Failure: a Prospective Study. *Ann Intern Med*. 1978; 89: 47–50.
11. Kruse K, Kracht U, Gupfert G. Renal Threshold Phosphate Concentration. *Arch Dis Child*. 1982; 57: 217–23.
12. Mosteller RD. Simplified Calculation of Body Surface Area. *New Eng J Med*. 1987; 317: 1098.
13. Briars GL, Bailey BJR. Surface Area Estimation: Pocket Calculator v Nomogram. *Arch Dis Child*. 1994; 70: 246–47.

Index

Note: Entries in bold type refer to illustrations.

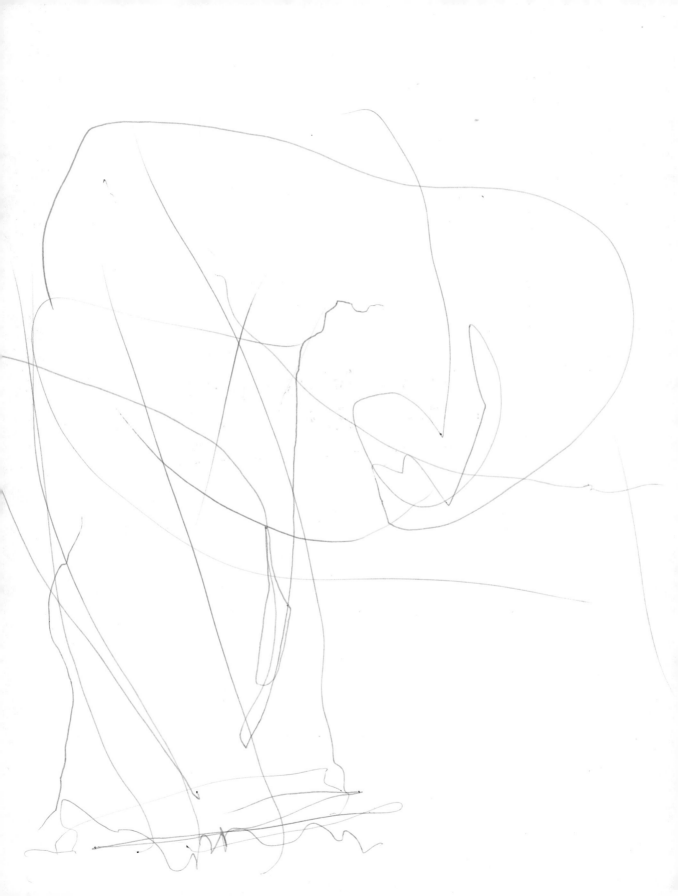